Current Insights on Lipid-Based Nanosystems

Current Insights on Lipid-Based Nanosystems

Editors

Ana Catarina Silva
João Nuno Moreira
José Manuel Sousa Lobo

MDPI • Basel • Beijing • Wuhan • Barcelona • Belgrade • Manchester • Tokyo • Cluj • Tianjin

Editors
Ana Catarina Silva
Faculty of Health Sciences
and UCIBIO/MEDTECH
Faculty of Pharmacy
University Fernando Pessoa
and University of Porto
Porto
Portugal

João Nuno Moreira
CNC—Center for
Neurosciences and
Cell Biology
Faculty of Medicine (Polo 1)
University of Coimbra
Coimbra
Portugal

José Manuel Sousa Lobo
UCIBIO/MEDTECH
Laboratory of Pharmaceutical
Technology
Faculty of Pharmacy
University of Porto
Porto
Portugal

Editorial Office
MDPI
St. Alban-Anlage 66
4052 Basel, Switzerland

This is a reprint of articles from the Special Issue published online in the open access journal *Pharmaceuticals* (ISSN 1424-8247) (available at: www.mdpi.com/journal/pharmaceuticals/special_issues/lipid_based_nanosystems).

For citation purposes, cite each article independently as indicated on the article page online and as indicated below:

LastName, A.A.; LastName, B.B.; LastName, C.C. Article Title. *Journal Name* **Year**, *Volume Number*, Page Range.

ISBN 978-3-0365-6166-0 (Hbk)
ISBN 978-3-0365-6165-3 (PDF)

Contents

Ana Catarina Silva, João Nuno Moreira and José Manuel Sousa Lobo
Editorial—Current Insights on Lipid-Based Nanosystems
Reprinted from: *Pharmaceuticals* **2022**, *15*, 1267, doi:10.3390/ph15101267 1

Cláudia Pina Costa, Sandra Barreiro, João Nuno Moreira, Renata Silva, Hugo Almeida and José Manuel Sousa Lobo et al.
In Vitro Studies on Nasal Formulations of Nanostructured Lipid Carriers (NLC) and Solid Lipid Nanoparticles (SLN)
Reprinted from: *Pharmaceuticals* **2021**, *14*, 711, doi:10.3390/ph14080711 7

Ibrahim M. Abdulbaqi, Reem Abou Assi, Anan Yaghmur, Yusrida Darwis, Noratiqah Mohtar and Thaigarajan Parumasivam et al.
Pulmonary Delivery of Anticancer Drugs via Lipid-Based Nanocarriers for the Treatment of Lung Cancer: An Update
Reprinted from: *Pharmaceuticals* **2021**, *14*, 725, doi:10.3390/ph14080725 31

Vijay Gyanani, Jeffrey C. Haley and Roshan Goswami
Challenges of Current Anticancer Treatment Approaches with Focus on Liposomal Drug Delivery Systems
Reprinted from: *Pharmaceuticals* **2021**, *14*, 835, doi:10.3390/ph14090835 71

Viliana Gugleva, Nadezhda Ivanova, Yoana Sotirova and Velichka Andonova
Dermal Drug Delivery of Phytochemicals with Phenolic Structure via Lipid-Based Nanotechnologies
Reprinted from: *Pharmaceuticals* **2021**, *14*, 837, doi:10.3390/ph14090837 99

Stefan R. Stefanov and Velichka Y. Andonova
Lipid Nanoparticulate Drug Delivery Systems: Recent Advances in the Treatment of Skin Disorders
Reprinted from: *Pharmaceuticals* **2021**, *14*, 1083, doi:10.3390/ph14111083 137

Ruvanthi N. Kularatne, Rachael M. Crist and Stephan T. Stern
The Future of Tissue-Targeted Lipid Nanoparticle-Mediated Nucleic Acid Delivery
Reprinted from: *Pharmaceuticals* **2022**, *15*, 897, doi:10.3390/ph15070897 167

Masoud Moghadaszadeh, Mehdi Khayyati, Adel Spotin, Roghayeh Norouzi, Abdol Sattar Pagheh and Sonia M. R. Oliveira et al.
Scolicidal and Apoptotic Activities of 5-hydroxy-1, 4-naphthoquinone as a Potent Agent against *Echinococcus granulosus* Protoscoleces
Reprinted from: *Pharmaceuticals* **2021**, *14*, 623, doi:10.3390/ph14070623 185

Fakhara Sabir, Gábor Katona, Ruba Ismail, Bence Sipos, Rita Ambrus and Ildikó Csóka
Development and Characterization of *n*-Propyl Gallate Encapsulated Solid Lipid Nanoparticles-Loaded Hydrogel for Intranasal Delivery
Reprinted from: *Pharmaceuticals* **2021**, *14*, 696, doi:10.3390/ph14070696 195

Sabrina Knoke and Heike Bunjes
Transfer Investigations of Lipophilic Drugs from Lipid Nanoemulsions to Lipophilic Acceptors: Contributing Effects of Cholesteryl Esters and Albumin as Acceptor Structures
Reprinted from: *Pharmaceuticals* **2021**, *14*, 865, doi:10.3390/ph14090865 217

pharmaceuticals

MDPI

Editorial

Editorial—Current Insights on Lipid-Based Nanosystems

Ana Catarina Silva [1,2,*], João Nuno Moreira [3,4] and José Manuel Sousa Lobo [1]

1 UCIBIO/REQUIMTE, MEDTECH, Laboratory of Pharmaceutical Technology, Department of Drug Sciences, Faculty of Pharmacy, University of Porto, 4050-313 Porto, Portugal
2 FP-I3ID (Instituto de Investigação, Inovação e Desenvolvimento), FP-BHS (Biomedical and Health Sciences Research Unit), Faculty of Health Sciences, University Fernando Pessoa, 4249-004 Porto, Portugal
3 CNC—Center for Neurosciences and Cell Biology, Center for Innovative Biomedicine and Biotechnology (CIBB), Faculty of Medicine (Polo 1), University of Coimbra, Rua Larga, 3004-504 Coimbra, Portugal
4 Pólo das Ciências da Saúde, Faculty of Pharmacy, CIBB, Univ. Coimbra—University of Coimbra, Azinhaga de Santa Comba, 3000-548 Coimbra, Portugal
* Correspondence: acsilva@ufp.edu.pt

Lipid-based nanosystems, including solid lipid nanoparticles (SLN) and nanostructured lipid carriers (NLC), cationic lipid nanoparticles, nanoemulsions and liposomes, have been extensively studied to improve drug delivery through different administration routes. The main advantages of these systems are the ability to protect, transport and control the release of lipophilic and hydrophilic molecules (either small-molecular-weight molecules and macromolecules), the use of generally recognized as safe (GRAS) excipients that minimize the toxicity of the formulations, and the possibility to modulate pharmacokinetics and enable the site-specific delivery of encapsulated payloads. In addition, the versatility of lipid-based nanosystems has further been demonstrated for the delivery of vaccines, protection of cosmetic actives, and improvement of moisturizing properties of cosmetic formulations.

Currently, lipid-based nanosystems are well established and there are already different commercially approved formulations in different human disorders. This success has actually paved the way to diversify the pipeline of development, to address unmet medical needs for several indications, such as cancer, neurological disorders, and autoimmune, genetic and infectious diseases.

This Special Issue aims to update readers on the latest research on lipid-based nanosystems, both at the preclinical and clinical levels. A series of 15 articles (six reviews and nine studies) is presented, with authors from 12 different countries, showing the globality of the investigations that are being carried out in this area.

Ana Catarina Silva et al. [1] revised the state of the art of in vitro cell models to perform studies with drug-loaded SLN and drug-loaded NLC nasal formulations. The authors concluded that specific in vitro cell culture models, such as the human nasal epithelial cells (HNEpC) and the human nasal septum quasidiploid tumour cells (RPMI 2650), are needed to assess the cytotoxicity of nasal formulations and to understand the mechanisms of nasal drug transport and absorption. In addition, the authors reported the great potential of using 3D nasal casts to test the effectiveness of formulations for reaching the upper part of the nasal cavity, which is critical for successful nose-to-brain delivery. These models are manufactured from computed tomography scans of the human nasal cavity and enable the analysis of the factors interfering with nasal drug deposition, including the nasal cavity area, type of administration device and angle of application, inspiratory flow rate, among others. Although 3D models are already being used to test nasal formulations, this remains an open field of research, as their validation by regulatory authorities is required.

Habibah A. Wahab et al. [2] highlighted the potential of lipid-based nanocarriers for pulmonary drug delivery for the treatment of lung cancer. The authors presented

Citation: Silva, A.C.; Moreira, J.N.; Lobo, J.M.S. Editorial—Current Insights on Lipid-Based Nanosystems. *Pharmaceuticals* **2022**, *15*, 1267. https://doi.org/10.3390/ph15101267

Received: 23 September 2022
Accepted: 8 October 2022
Published: 14 October 2022

considerations of the physiological, physicochemical and technological aspects of efficient inhalable anticancer drugs delivery systems based on lipid-based nanocarriers, and their pioneering role in the treatment of lung cancer. Lipid-based nanocarriers are able to transport drugs with different physicochemical characteristics, show enhanced permeability and retention effects for passive targeting, and can be functionalized to provide active targeting. Recent preclinical studies show that inhalable lipid-based nanocarriers can be concentrated in the lungs, from where they diffuse into the blood stream and lymphatic system, reaching cancer cells. However, the authors point out that research in this area needs to advance towards in vivo and clinical studies. In the field of anticancer therapies, Vijay Gyanani et al. [3] presented a brief review on the challenges of conventional therapies and the use of liposomes as a targeting strategy for the delivery of anticancer drugs. The authors discussed the challenges and limitations of conventional anticancer treatments (chemotherapy, radiotherapy and surgery), such as drug resistance, severity and side effects, and highlighted future research opportunities in this field. The use of active targeted liposomes remains challenging due to antigen and receptor heterogeneity, immunogenicity and low drug encapsulation efficiency, while passive targeted liposomes overcome the limitations of immunogenicity. However, there are manufacturing and clinical challenges associated with active and passive liposomes, primarily related to translating preclinical into clinical efficacy.

Viliana Gugleva et al. [4] provided a review of the therapeutic properties of different classes of phenolic compounds used for dermal application, including their effects on oxidation processes, inflammation, vascular pathology, immune response, precancerous and oncological lesions or formations, and microbial growth. The authors also presented several examples of promising results from studies with phenolic compounds encapsulated in lipid-based nanocarriers (nanoemulsions, liposomes, SLN and NLC), which aimed to improve their solubility, stability, skin permeation and therapeutic activity. On the use of lipid-based nanocarriers to improve drug delivery to the skin, Stefanov and Velichka Y. Andonova [5] presented the state of the art on recent developments in the application of these nanocarriers in topical formulations to treat skin disorders as an alternative to the conventional formulations, reducing systemic toxicity. So far, lipid-based nanocarriers have been shown to provide a flexible platform for safe, effective and biocompatible topical drug delivery, as they do not cause cytotoxicity or morphological changes through the skin.

Stephan T. Stern et al. [6] described current trends in the development of the next generation of tissue-targeted lipid nanoparticles containing nucleic acids for different therapeutic applications, including cancer, and neurological, cardiovascular and infectious diseases. The researchers underlined the interest of using lipid nanoparticles to actively target nucleic acids to the vascular endothelium through receptor-mediated transcytosis and paracellular transport, which must rely on tissue-selective receptor expression that can be identified through modern ligand–receptor identification techniques, such as phage display. Tissue targeting can be achieved by manipulating the composition of lipid nanoparticles, binding to targeting ligands or introducing cell membrane-derived components into the nanoparticles. In addition, modification in lipid components or nucleic acid cargo can be used to prepare stimuli-responsive lipid nanoparticles that react to internal or external stimuli to release their cargo.

Ehsan Ahmadpour et al. [7] evaluated in vitro the scolicidal and apoptotic activity of liposomes loaded with juglone (5-hydroxy-1,4-naphthoquinone) against protoscoleces, a larval stage of the cestode *Echinococcus granulosus* that causes helminth diseases. All tested concentrations of juglone-loaded liposomes induced scolicidal effects, although only concentrations of 800 μg/mL and 400 μg/mL induced 100% mortality. Furthermore, caspase-3 mRNA expression was higher after exposure with juglone-loaded liposomes compared to the control. From these findings, the authors concluded that optimal doses of juglone-loaded liposomes have potent scolicidal effects on the *Echinococcus granulosus* cestode, although this evidence must be confirmed in vivo.

Ildikó Csóka et al. [8] demonstrated in vitro the advantages of combining SLN and hydrogels to improve the intranasal delivery of antioxidants, increasing absorption and residence time in the nasal mucosa. The researchers used the quality-by-design (QbD) approach and the central composite design to optimize a chemically linked hyaluronic acid hydrogel containing n-propyl gallate-loaded SLN for intranasal delivery as a promising alternative for the treatment of brain tumours, such as glioblastoma multiforme, avoiding the need to cross the blood–brain barrier and improving patients' compliance. The results showed a lower burst effect and sustained release profile from the hydrogel containing n-propyl gallate-loaded SLN, when compared to the n-propyl gallate-loaded SLN alone. In addition, the cumulative permeation of n-propyl gallate from the hydrogel was 3- to 60-fold higher than that of n-propyl gallate-loaded SLN alone and native n-propyl gallate, respectively.

Sabrina Knoke and Heike Bunjes [9] investigated the release of poorly water-soluble drugs from nanoemulsions for intravenous administration in release media containing components that mimic physiological acceptors in vivo. In this study, the transfer of fenofibrate, retinyl acetate and orlistat from nanoemulsion droplets to lipid-containing hydrogel particles that mimic lipoproteins was investigated. Additionally, the transfer of the same drugs from nanoemulsion droplets to bovine serum albumin was investigated. The results showed a slower transfer rate for the lipid-containing hydrogel particles to the highest logP drugs. Thereby, the researchers suggested using lipid-containing hydrogel particles as a useful tool to compare different lipophilic acceptors to assess drug release from colloidal systems. In contrast, albumin was not relevant as a lipophilic acceptor for the drugs studied.

Xin Guo et al. [10] tested the efficacy of novel lipids to improve the activity of doxorubicin-loaded liposomes against solid tumours. In this study, three lipids containing imidazole groups were incorporated into the membrane of liposomes coated with polyethylene glycol (PEG), creating pH-sensitive convertible liposomes. The results demonstrated that imidazole lipids trigger a greater release of doxorubicin from liposomes conjugated with phosphatidylethanolamine and PEG. Thus, the researchers suggested that the use of pH-sensitive convertible liposomes that balance tissue penetration, cell binding and drug release, would induce ideal activity against solid tumours.

Aziz Unnisa et al. [11] used a three-factor, three-level Box–Behnken design to optimize dapagliflozin-loaded SLN for oral administration. The effectiveness of the optimized formulation for the management of type 2 diabetes, by reducing blood glucose levels, was tested in streptozotocin-induced diabetic rats. The results showed a two-fold increase in oral drug absorption, when compared to a commercial formulation of pure dapagliflozin.

Maria Carmo Pereira et al. [12] evaluated in vivo the toxicity of multi-dose intravenous administration of neutral liposomes and cationic liposomes for drug delivery. The results showed that the administration of 10 doses of cationic liposomes resulted in a mortality of 45%, while the administration of the same doses of neutral liposomes showed no mortality. From this study, the researchers concluded that neutral liposomes are safe carriers for the administration of repeated doses of drugs.

Rompicherla Narayana Charyulu et al. [13] used a full factorial design to optimize an oral formulation of silymarin-loaded phytosomes, aiming to improve the hepatoprotective activity of the encapsulated compound. The researchers performed in vivo studies in a tetrachloromethane-induced hepatotoxicity rat model and observed a six-fold increase in systemic bioavailability after the oral administration of the optimized silymarin phytosomal formulation, compared to pure silymarin. From these findings, the researchers concluded that phytosomes may be suitable nanocarriers to improve the oral bioavailability of phytoconstituents with poor aqueous solubility.

Shaymaa Wagdy El-Far et al. [14] used a response surface D-optimal factorial design to optimize drug-free niosome formulations, in which model drugs used for colorectal cancer treatment were encapsulated. The amphiphilic characteristics of the niosomes allowed the encapsulation of oxaliplatin (hydrophilic model drug) and placlitaxel (hydrophobic model drug). The results showed that both drugs increased the anticancer activity against HT-29 colon cancer cells, up to two- to threefold, after encapsulation in niosomes, when compared to free drugs. Thus, the researchers concluded that niosomes could be used to improve the therapeutic outcomes of oxaliplatin and paclitaxel against colorectal cancer.

Randa Mohammed Zaki et al. [15] developed a new generation of liposomes containing a high concentration of glycerol, which were called glycerosomes. In this study, the central composite rotatable design was used to optimize an oral formulation of quetiapine fumarate-loaded glycerosomes that showed highly improved brain and plasma drug bioavailability, when compared to an oral drug suspension. From these findings, the researchers proposed the use of quetiapine fumarate-loaded glycerosomes as promising alternative carriers to improve the oral delivery of quetiapine fumarate.

We would like to thank all the authors of this Special Issue for contributing with high-quality works. We also acknowledge all the reviewers, who critically evaluated the articles. In addition, we would like to thank to the Assistant Editor, Ms. Evelyn Du, for her kind help.

Funding: The Applied Molecular Biosciences Unit—UCIBIO, which is financed by national funds from Fundação para a Ciência e a Tecnologia—FCT (UIDP/04378/2020 and UIDB/04378/2020), supported this work.

Conflicts of Interest: The authors declare no conflict of interest.

References

1. Costa, C.P.; Barreiro, S.; Moreira, J.N.; Silva, R.; Almeida, H.; Sousa Lobo, J.M.; Silva, A.C. In Vitro Studies on Nasal Formulations of Nanostructured Lipid Carriers (NLC) and Solid Lipid Nanoparticles (SLN). *Pharmaceuticals* **2021**, *14*, 711. [CrossRef] [PubMed]
2. Abdulbaqi, I.M.; Assi, R.A.; Yaghmur, A.; Darwis, Y.; Mohtar, N.; Parumasivam, T.; Saqallah, F.G.; Wahab, H.A. Pulmonary Delivery of Anticancer Drugs via Lipid-Based Nanocarriers for the Treatment of Lung Cancer: An Update. *Pharmaceuticals* **2021**, *14*, 725. [CrossRef] [PubMed]
3. Gyanani, V.; Haley, J.C.; Goswami, R. Challenges of Current Anticancer Treatment Approaches with Focus on Liposomal Drug Delivery Systems. *Pharmaceuticals* **2021**, *14*, 835. [CrossRef] [PubMed]
4. Gugleva, V.; Ivanova, N.; Sotirova, Y.; Andonova, V. Dermal Drug Delivery of Phytochemicals with Phenolic Structure via Lipid-Based Nanotechnologies. *Pharmaceuticals* **2021**, *14*, 837. [CrossRef] [PubMed]
5. Stefanov, S.R.; Andonova, V.Y. Lipid Nanoparticulate Drug Delivery Systems: Recent Advances in the Treatment of Skin Disorders. *Pharmaceuticals* **2021**, *14*, 1083. [CrossRef] [PubMed]
6. Kularatne, R.N.; Crist, R.M.; Stern, S.T. The Future of Tissue-Targeted Lipid Nanoparticle-Mediated Nucleic Acid Delivery. *Pharmaceuticals* **2022**, *15*, 897. [CrossRef]
7. Moghadaszadeh, M.; Khayyati, M.; Spotin, A.; Norouzi, R.; Pagheh, A.S.; Oliveira, S.M.R.; Pereira, M.d.L.; Ahmadpour, E. Scolicidal and Apoptotic Activities of 5-hydroxy-1, 4-naphthoquinone as a Potent Agent against Echinococcus granulosus Protoscoleces. *Pharmaceuticals* **2021**, *14*, 623. [CrossRef]
8. Sabir, F.; Katona, G.; Ismail, R.; Sipos, B.; Ambrus, R.; Csóka, I. Development and Characterization of n-Propyl Gallate Encapsulated Solid Lipid Nanoparticles-Loaded Hydrogel for Intranasal Delivery. *Pharmaceuticals* **2021**, *14*, 696. [CrossRef]
9. Knoke, S.; Bunjes, H. Transfer Investigations of Lipophilic Drugs from Lipid Nanoemulsions to Lipophilic Acceptors: Contributing Effects of Cholesteryl Esters and Albumin as Acceptor Structures. *Pharmaceuticals* **2021**, *14*, 865. [CrossRef] [PubMed]
10. Huang, R.; Gyanani, V.; Zhao, S.; Lu, Y.; Guo, X. Imidazole-Based pH-Sensitive Convertible Liposomes for Anticancer Drug Delivery. *Pharmaceuticals* **2022**, *15*, 306. [CrossRef] [PubMed]
11. Unnisa, A.; Chettupalli, A.K.; Al Hagbani, T.; Khalid, M.; Jandrajupalli, S.B.; Chandolu, S.; Hussain, T. Development of Dapagliflozin Solid Lipid Nanoparticles as a Novel Carrier for Oral Delivery: Statistical Design, Optimization, In-Vitro and In-Vivo Characterization, and Evaluation. *Pharmaceuticals* **2022**, *15*, 568. [CrossRef] [PubMed]
12. Andrade, S.; Loureiro, J.A.; Ramirez, S.; Catumbela, C.S.G.; Soto, C.; Morales, R.; Pereira, M.C. Multi-Dose Intravenous Administration of Neutral and Cationic Liposomes in Mice: An Extensive Toxicity Study. *Pharmaceuticals* **2022**, *15*, 761. [CrossRef]
13. Shriram, R.G.; Moin, A.; Alotaibi, H.F.; Khafagy, E.-S.; Al Saqr, A.; Abu Lila, A.S.; Charyulu, R.N. Phytosomes as a Plausible Nano-Delivery System for Enhanced Oral Bioavailability and Improved Hepatoprotective Activity of Silymarin. *Pharmaceuticals* **2022**, *15*, 790. [CrossRef]

14. El-Far, S.W.; Abo El-Enin, H.A.; Abdou, E.M.; Nafea, O.E.; Abdelmonem, R. Targeting Colorectal Cancer Cells with Niosomes Systems Loaded with Two Anticancer Drugs Models; Comparative In Vitro and Anticancer Studies. *Pharmaceuticals* **2022**, *15*, 816. [CrossRef] [PubMed]
15. Zaki, R.M.; Alfadhel, M.M.; Alossaimi, M.A.; Elsawaf, L.A.; Devanathadesikan Seshadri, V.; Almurshedi, A.S.; Yusif, R.m.; Said, M. Central Composite Optimization of Glycerosomes for the Enhanced Oral Bioavailability and Brain Delivery of Quetiapine Fumarate. *Pharmaceuticals* **2022**, *15*, 940. [CrossRef] [PubMed]

pharmaceuticals

MDPI

Review

In Vitro Studies on Nasal Formulations of Nanostructured Lipid Carriers (NLC) and Solid Lipid Nanoparticles (SLN)

Cláudia Pina Costa [1], Sandra Barreiro [2], João Nuno Moreira [3,4], Renata Silva [2], Hugo Almeida [1], José Manuel Sousa Lobo [1] and Ana Catarina Silva [1,5,*]

1 UCIBIO/REQUIMTE, MEDTECH, Laboratory of Pharmaceutical Technology, Department of Drug Sciences, Faculty of Pharmacy, University of Porto, 4050-313 Porto, Portugal; claudiaspinacosta@gmail.com (C.P.C.); hperas5@hotmail.com (H.A.); slobo@ff.up.pt (J.M.S.L.)

2 UCIBIO/REQUIMTE, Laboratory of Toxicology, Department of Biological Sciences, Faculty of Pharmacy, University of Porto, 4050-313 Porto, Portugal; sandrafcbarreiro@gmail.com (S.B.); rsilva@ff.up.pt (R.S.)

3 CNC—Center for Neuroscience and Cell Biology, Center for Innovative Biomedicine and Biotechnology (CIBB), Faculty of Medicine (Pólo I), University of Coimbra, 3004-504 Coimbra, Portugal; jmoreira@ff.uc.pt

4 UC—University of Coimbra, CIBB, Faculty of Pharmacy, Pólo das Ciências da Saúde, Azinhaga de Santa Comba, 3000-548 Coimbra, Portugal

5 FP-ENAS (UFP Energy, Environment and Health Research Unit), CEBIMED (Biomedical Research Centre), Faculty of Health Sciences, University Fernando Pessoa, 4249-004 Porto, Portugal

* Correspondence: ana.silva@ff.up.pt or acsilva@ufp.edu.pt

Abstract: The nasal route has been used for many years for the local treatment of nasal diseases. More recently, this route has been gaining momentum, due to the possibility of targeting the central nervous system (CNS) from the nasal cavity, avoiding the blood−brain barrier (BBB). In this area, the use of lipid nanoparticles, such as nanostructured lipid carriers (NLC) and solid lipid nanoparticles (SLN), in nasal formulations has shown promising outcomes on a wide array of indications such as brain diseases, including epilepsy, multiple sclerosis, Alzheimer's disease, Parkinson's disease and gliomas. Herein, the state of the art of the most recent literature available on in vitro studies with nasal formulations of lipid nanoparticles is discussed. Specific in vitro cell culture models are needed to assess the cytotoxicity of nasal formulations and to explore the underlying mechanism(s) of drug transport and absorption across the nasal mucosa. In addition, different studies with 3D nasal casts are reported, showing their ability to predict the drug deposition in the nasal cavity and evaluating the factors that interfere in this process, such as nasal cavity area, type of administration device and angle of application, inspiratory flow, presence of mucoadhesive agents, among others. Notwithstanding, they do not preclude the use of confirmatory in vivo studies, a significant impact on the 3R (replacement, reduction and refinement) principle within the scope of animal experiments is expected. The use of 3D nasal casts to test nasal formulations of lipid nanoparticles is still totally unexplored, to the authors best knowledge, thus constituting a wide open field of research.

Keywords: nasal administration; nanostructured lipid carriers; solid lipid nanoparticles; in vitro cell cultures; 3D nasal casts

Citation: Costa, C.P.; Barreiro, S.; Moreira, J.N.; Silva, R.; Almeida, H.; Sousa Lobo, J.M.; Silva, A.C. In Vitro Studies on Nasal Formulations of Nanostructured Lipid Carriers (NLC) and Solid Lipid Nanoparticles (SLN). *Pharmaceuticals* **2021**, *14*, 711. https://doi.org/10.3390/ph14080711

Academic Editor: Dimitris Tsiourvas

Received: 20 June 2021
Accepted: 21 July 2021
Published: 23 July 2021

1. Introduction

The nasal route had been widely used for several years for the local treatment of nasal diseases, through the administration of corticosteroids, decongestants, and antihistamines [1]. More recently, the possibility of reaching the brain through the nose without the need to cross the blood−brain barrier (BBB) has gained attention, especially to improve the treatment of central nervous system (CNS) disorders, including epilepsy, Alzheimer's disease, Parkinson's disease, multiple sclerosis, gliomas, among others [2,3]. As the BBB is vital to protect the brain from exogenous substances, it acts as an obstacle to the passage of most drugs. This barrier is a semipermeable membrane that maintains the CNS homeostasis, providing nutrient exchange between the brain and the blood. The presence of tight junctions of endothelial capillary cells restricts the passage of drugs, with smaller molecules weighing less than 400 Da and lipophilic molecules being the only ones that can easily cross this barrier [4–8].

Different strategies have been investigated to increase the drug passage through the BBB, such as electromagnetic force-field techniques and mini-pump-assisted intracranial delivery. However, these methods are invasive and can lead to the passage of toxins to the brain, being nonselective and neurotoxic [9–11]. Thus, it is essential to find new ways to avoid the need to bypass the BBB to target drugs to the brain. In this area, intranasal administration has emerged as the only direct drug delivery route to the brain via the olfactory and trigeminal nerves, without the need to pass into the systemic circulation and cross the BBB. Nonetheless, it is important to keep in mind that after intranasal administration, part of the drug is absorbed into the systemic circulation and reaches the brain through the BBB [3]. In addition, the use of lipid nanoparticles, such as solid lipid nanoparticles (SLN) and nanostructured lipid carriers (NLC), to promote the targeting of drugs to the brain after intranasal administration, has been suggested as a promising alternative to the conventional treatments of brain disorders [1,3,12,13].

This review provides the state of the art of the in vitro studies with nasal formulations containing lipid nanoparticles, reported in the past two years. The manuscript starts with anatomical and physiological considerations of the nasal route, followed by the requisites of nasal formulations. Subsequently, the most used in vitro cell models for performing studies with nasal formulations, and relevant outcomes observed with liquid and semisolid nasal formulations of SLN and NLC are described. Finally, the use of in vitro nasal cavity and computational models to predict the in vivo performance of nasal formulations is reported.

2. Nasal Route

2.1. Anatomical and Physiological Considerations

The anatomical and physiological characteristics of the different regions of the nasal cavity are summarized in Table 1 and the location of each region is shown in Figure 1 [12–14].

Table 1. Characteristics of the different regions of the nasal cavity (data from [3,9,13,15–17]).

Region	Surface Area	Location	Characteristics	Vascularization	Epithelium
Vestibule	0.6 cm^2	Anterior part	• Poor permeability and small surface area that limits drug absorption. • Presence of mucus and hairs or vibrissae, which constitute an important defense mechanism, preventing the entrance of toxic particles, pathogens and allergens from the external environment into the body.	Low	Squamous epithelium
Respiratory region	130 cm^2	Middle part and lateral walls	• High permeability and large surface area, being the region where the greatest absorption of drugs occurs. • Divided into three turbinates: inferior, middle and superior. • Provides drug absorption to the systemic circulation. • Direct pathway of drug transport to the brain via the trigeminal nerve. • Presents cilia, microvilli and mucus. • Occurrence of mucociliary clearance mechanism.	High	Respiratory epithelium: ciliated pseudostratified and columnar epithelium

Table 1. *Cont.*

Region	Surface Area	Location	Characteristics	Vascularization	Epithelium
Olfactory region	10 cm^2	Upper part	• Located above the respiratory region and below the cribriform plate. • Includes superior turbinate, and a small upper portion of the middle turbinate. • Enables drug access from the nose to the brain via the olfactory bulb, bypassing the blood–brain barrier (BBB). • Responsible for detecting odors.	High	Olfactory epithelium

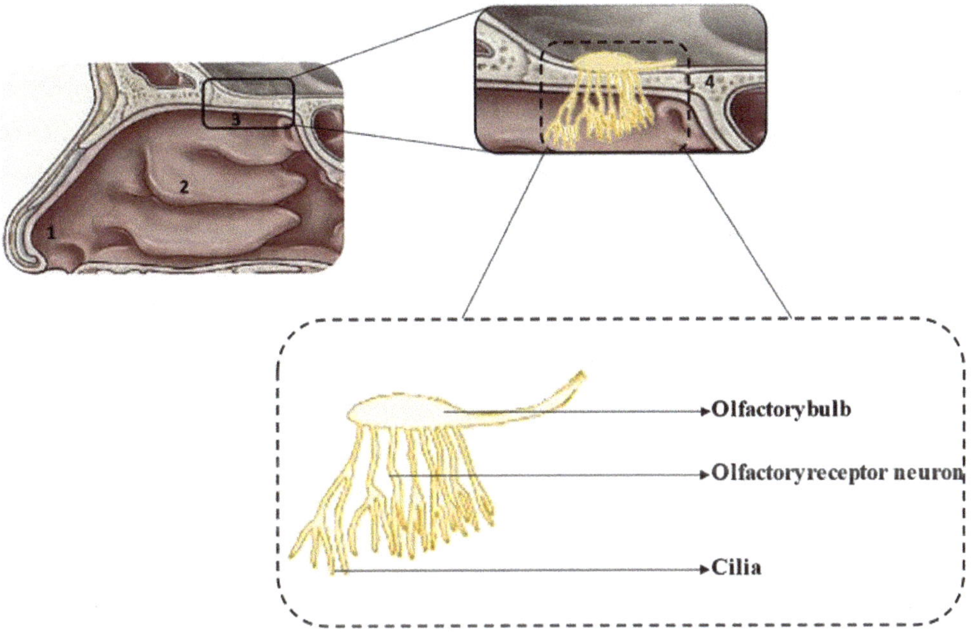

Figure 1. Schematic representation of the nasal cavity (**top**) and olfactory region (**bottom**): 1—vestibule, 2—respiratory region, 3—olfactory region, 4—cribriform plate.

2.2. Nose-to-Brain Delivery

After nasal administration, different pathways of drug transport from the nose to the brain can occur, which have been divided into direct transport, indirect transport and a combination of both. Besides, some drug can be eliminated by the mucociliary clearance mechanism before reaching the olfactory or/and respiratory regions. To our knowledge, there is no confirmation of the exact transport mechanism followed by intranasal drugs, which seems to be influenced by the drug's molecular characteristics, formulation consistency (liquid or semi-solid) and type of application device. Thus, it is impossible to assess the exact amount of drug reaching the brain after intranasal administration via a specific transport mechanism, although good approaches have been reported in in vivo studies that compared the results of the amount of drug reaching the brain after intranasal and intravenous administrations. In addition, toxicological concerns were raised related to the possibility of an accumulation of excipients in the brain and the risk of impairment of the mucociliary clearance mechanism. Figure 2 summarizes the different drug pathways after nasal administration [2,3,6,18].

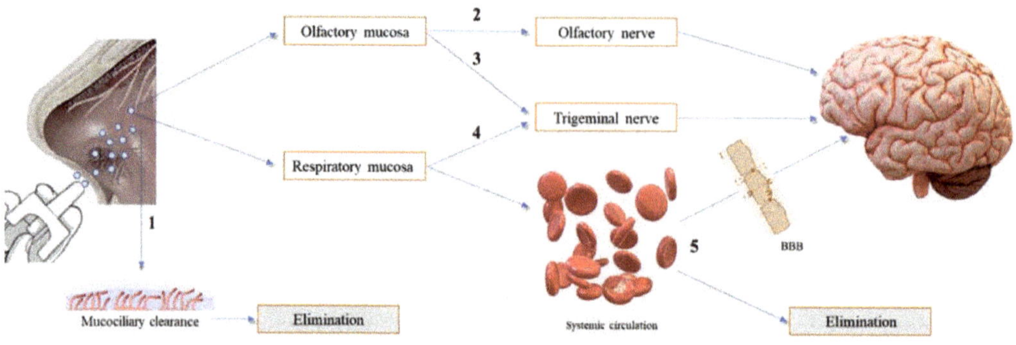

Figure 2. Overview of the different drug pathways after nasal administration. (1) The drug is eliminated by the mucociliary clearance mechanism. (2) The drug reaches the olfactory mucosa, passes through the olfactory nerve, via intraneuronal and/or extraneuronal transport, and reaches the brain. (3) The drug reaches the olfactory mucosa, passes through the trigeminal nerve and reaches the brain via the cribriform plate. (4) The drug reaches the respiratory mucosa, passes through the trigeminal nerve and reaches the brainstem. (5) The drug reaches the respiratory mucosa, is absorbed into the systemic circulation, and diverges between passage to the brain, upon crossing the blood–brain barrier (BBB), and elimination, before reaching the brain.

2.3. Requisites of Nasal Formulations

Some factors of the nasal formulations can interfere with drug absorption and should be considered. For instance, these formulations should be isotonic (i.e., osmolality between 280 mOsm/Kg and 310 mOsm/Kg) and have a pH close to that of the nasal cavity (5.0–6.8), to avoid discomfort, mucosal irritation and/or damage to the cilia, after administration [13,19]. In addition, the drug excipients used should be compatible with the nasal mucosa to avoid irritation and toxicity [20,21].

One of the main disadvantages of intranasal administration is the rapid elimination of the drug through mucociliary clearance (a physiological defense mechanism that eliminates foreign substances every 15–30 min). To avoid this, substances that interact with the mucus can be added to the formulations. The mucus is composed of water, mucin and other proteins, electrolytes, enzymes and lipids [15]. Mucin is a negatively charged glycoprotein and, therefore, positively charged formulations can easily bind it through electrostatic interactions, which facilitates mucoadhesion. In contrast, negatively charged formulations can penetrate mucin chains and hydrogen bonds can be formed, which improves mucoadhesion [13,22].

New strategies to overcome the drawbacks of the nasal formulations have been investigated. For example, the use of nanocarriers, such as lipid nanoparticles, to achieve prolonged release, protection against enzymatic degradation and improve targeting to the brain [23]. The use of permeation enhancers, including mucoadhesive polymers and in situ hydrogels to improve drug retention time in the nasal mucosa and, consequently, drug absorption is also a commonly used strategy [23]. There are already marketed nasal formulations (e.g., Nasonex and Rhinocort) that increase viscosity after administration, improving the retention time of the drug in the nasal cavity [13].

3. In Vitro Cell Models to Evaluate the Effectiveness of Nasal Formulations

There are different models available to assess the nose-to-brain drug delivery that can be used to determine the drug absorption and permeability through the nasal cavity, to evaluate its pharmacokinetic, toxicity and possible drug transport interactions [24]. Indeed, different in vitro, in vivo and ex vivo models are widely used to assess nose to brain drug transport [24]. While in vivo models allow nasal absorption and pharmacokinetic studies and ex vivo models allow the performance of nasal perfusion studies, in vitro models are useful to predict drug permeability, allowing exploration of the underlying mechanism(s) of drug absorption and transport through the nasal route [24,25].

Regardless of the remarkable information that can be achieved from in vivo studies, the extrapolation of the results to humans is still challenging given the significant differences between species in what concerns the structure of the upper airway and the epithelial cell populations of the mucosal surface tissue covering the nasal routes. Additionally, in vivo studies often require a large number of animals and higher drug amounts [26].

Recently, many distinct nasal in vitro models have been developed. Accordingly, cell culture models and excised nasal mucosae are important and useful in in vitro models to study the characteristics underlying the metabolic barrier capacity of the nasal epithelium, and for drug permeability studies [27,28]. Moreover, by using cultured human nasal epithelial cells (both primary cells and/or immortalized cell lines) an accurate prediction of the drug metabolism, toxicity and transport across the nasal tissue in humans may be successfully accomplished and may even provide results with a more direct clinical relevance [26,29]. In fact, the use of standardized in vitro nasal epithelial cell cultures in pharmacological and toxicological studies offers diverse advantages, including the possibility of controlling/monitoring experimental conditions, the potential exclusion of pre- and post-mucosal issues, the execution of a quicker and more efficient evaluation of permeability, metabolism and toxicity and their underlying mechanisms, and the limited needs of animal studies, therefore reducing costs [26,27]. However, in vitro models for nasal drug delivery studies remain often imperfect, as they still lack a cell line that adequately mimics the nasal epithelium [29,30].

In vitro cell culture models are an ideal alternative for permeability screening studies. They present several advantages when compared with other models, namely in situ or in vivo models, as they allow the rapid evaluation of the permeability profiles of a given drug, and the possibility to test molecules that could be harmful if tested directly in vivo [25]. Additionally, the use of in vitro models with human cells does not involve the same ethical problems and regulatory impediments as the studies performed with in vivo models [25,30].

The efficacy of a drug administered in the nasal cavity will depend on the anatomic region where its absorption takes place, between the nasal epithelium and the lungs [26]. Nasal cells or tissue excised from the nasal cavity may be originated from different nasal domains, including the vestibular area, the atrium, the turbinates (superior, medium and inferior) and the olfactory epithelium [27]. To perform transport and metabolic studies, the respiratory epithelium, a pseudostratified ciliated columnar epithelium in the region of the medium and inferior turbinates, is the most relevant [27]. This region has a particular architecture that highly influences the absorption of a given drug, as it holds ciliated columnar cells with many mitochondria in the apical side, basal cells, nonciliated columnar cells with microvilli, goblet cells with mucous granules and a fully developed Golgi apparatus [27].

At the nasal mucosa, the absorption of intranasally administered drugs is highly influenced by both passive diffusion and carrier-mediated transport processes. The transporters here implicated belong to the two most important families of transporter proteins: the ATP binding cassette (ABC) and the solute carrier (SLC) superfamilies. ABC transporters, efflux pumps including P-glycoprotein (P-gp, encoded by the *ABCB1* gene) and multidrug resistance-associated proteins (MRPs), represent a family of transporters that uses the energy resulting from ATP hydrolysis to carry their substrates across biological membranes and against their concentration gradients [31,32]. Additionally, the SLC gene family translates a wide group of protein membrane carriers that are present in many organelle or cellular membranes. This transporter superfamily includes several passive transporters, ion-coupled transporters and exchangers. Nevertheless, the information available on the expression and functionality of the SLC transporters in the human nasal mucosa, as well as in the existing nasal in vitro models, remains fairly scarce when compared with data reported in other epithelial barriers and tissues, such as in the liver, intestine or lungs [31].

In order to study the permeability of drugs through the respiratory epithelium, and its underlying mechanisms, several in vitro models are used, including excised tissue (human, bovine, porcine, and others), primary human nasal epithelial cell cultures and immortalized cell lines [28,30,33,34]. Excised tissues represent the closest physiological approach in terms of histology, transporter expression and cell type distribution [35,36]. In fact, both excised tissue (organotypic explants) and primary cell cultures are morphologically closer to the airway mucosa, presenting proper tissue architecture and differentiation, but the poor accessibility, the lack of standardization and the existing interspecies differences (nonhuman alternatives) limits their applicability in drug transport and permeability studies [30,33,34,37,38]. In addition, the reproducibility of organotypic explants and primary cell cultures is often challenging due to the genetic variability, inter- and intraindividual differences between the donors, and the uncontrollable environmental variables preceding tissue harvest. They have complex isolation procedures and limited lifespan, are difficult to maintain in culture, time-consuming, less reproducible, and more expensive [28,30,33]. On the other hand, immortalized cell lines are easily maintained in culture and offer higher reproducibility and genetic homogeneity, being the most convenient in vitro models of the nasal epithelial barrier, even though lacking the real organ complexity originated by the presence of cilia, mucus and blood vessels [35]. However, although epithelial cell lines are the most used for drug transport studies, there still is a lack of cell lines that completely mimic the nasal epithelium [28,30,33]. Currently, the available immortalized nasal cell lines include the NAS 2BL, a rat nasal epithelial tumor cell line, BT cell line, bovine turbinate obtained from new-born bovine turbinate tissue, and RPMI 2650 cells, this last one being the only human nasal cell line that could be properly used for drug transport studies [26,35,39]. Because of this deficiency, and despite the known differences in the morphologies of different cell lines, many research groups have been using bronchial epithelial cells as a surrogate for nasal epithelial cells, such as the human bronchial epithelial cell line Calu-3 [26,29].

The choice of a proper cell culture model is influenced by different factors, including the level of cell differentiation required. In addition, the selected cell culture techniques (air−liquid interface or immersion cultures) and cell growth conditions (seeding density, cell confluency, media supplements, culture periods, cell culture on a collagen coating) certainly may influence the cells' phenotype differentiation, and their morphological and functional features. As a result, the expression of drug transporters or drug metabolizing enzymes may be different from the human respiratory epithelium, altering the permeability profile of a drug [25,27,40].

As mentioned, the cell culture conditions will highly influence the results of permeability and transport, metabolism, or toxicity studies. For instance, the cell-support membranes (uncoated or coated extracellular matrix) selected for permeability studies, the cells' electrical properties, the cellular confluency and tight junction generation, the differentiation pattern of the cell monolayer (morphologically well differentiated with ciliated, nonciliated and secretory cells), and the developed ciliary activity, mucus secretion, and metabolic activity, [26,40]. The nasal epithelium morphologically and functionally resembles the respiratory epithelium of the lower airways, which can be useful to culture differentiated nasal, tracheal or bronchial epithelium cells [26].

The cell culture models can be compared, and their integrity assessed through the evaluation of the permeation coefficients of different marker compounds and the transepithelial electrical resistance (TEER) determination, which indicates tight junction development [26,28]. For instance, the human nasal mucosa obtained from the inferior turbinates demonstrated TEER values of ranging from 40 up to 120 Ω cm^2, thus being moderately different from excised animal tissues (from 90 up to 180 Ω cm^2) [30,34]. In addition, and when compared with human nasal excised tissues, primary cell lines often yield more tight junctions with significantly higher TEER values (600–3100 Ω cm^2) [34,36]. This difference in the TEER values could lead to an underestimation of the permeability, particularly of more hydrophilic compounds, typically transported by paracellular pathways [26].

The common pathways for drug transport across the nasal epithelium are similar to other epithelia in the body, being the two main routes involved in transepithelial drug permeability across the nasal epithelium, the transcellular and the paracellular transport pathways [26]. Thereby, in vitro cell culture models are a useful tool to discriminate passive and active transepithelial drug transport [26].

3.1. Human Nasal Epithelial Cells (HNEpC)

Human nasal epithelial cells (HNEpC) can be obtained from the nasal tissues of patients submitted to endonasal surgery of polyps, septum deviation, hyperplastic conchae or even nasal reconstruction [26]. Primary cell cultures of HNEpC present some disadvantages related to the shortage of human nasal tissue available from one donor, the short-term cultures, the heterogeneity within cultures and between cell cultures, significant variability between donors and cell culture difficulties [26,31,37,40]. Nevertheless, and although respiratory epithelial cells can only be passed two or three successive times, these cells can be subcultured into confluent monolayers, while retaining the capacity to differentiate into ciliated and secretory cells [26,37,40].

Primary cell cultures are the most reliable in resembling the native airway epithelium and, therefore, are suitable for drug transport studies [40]. HNEpC retain morphological and functional characteristics similar to the native human nasal epithelium, showing mucin secretion, expression of mucins (MUC5AC, MUC5B and MUC8), microvilli and cilia, aminopeptidase, and tight junction proteins [40]. However, the use of different media, culture interfaces, and time in culture have substantial consequences on the human nasal cell ultrastructure, barrier formation, and transporter expression [40]. For example, the use of liquid cell cultures of primary HNEpC allows the formation of monolayers of simple cuboidal cells, while when cultured at an air–liquid interface, the same HNEpC cells can differentiate into multilayers similar to the original nasal tissues as far as structure, mRNA and immune responses are concerned [37].

3.2. Human Nasal Septum Quasidiploid Tumour Cells (RPMI 2650)

The human nasal septum quasidiploid tumor cells (RPMI 2650) were initially obtained, in 1962, from an anaplastic squamous cell carcinoma of the human nasal septum [26,35,41]. RPMI 2650 cells are often used to study drug metabolism and toxicity as they produce different cytokeratins, retain the ability for mucus secretion and exhibit identical metabolic activity to the human nasal mucosa. Furthermore, these cells are quite stable throughout continued passaging, maintaining their quasidiploid karyotype in culture [24,27,29,35].

Depending on the selected cell support or extracellular matrix, RPMI 2650 cells in culture may form clusters of round and slightly flattened cells, or may tend to spread [28]. When compared to excised human nasal tissue, these cells present similar aminopeptidase activity, expressing lysosomal aminopeptidase, leucine aminopeptidase and aminopeptidases N, A and B, enzymes that often influence the nasal permeability of peptides and proteins [26].

The RPMI 2650 cells were initially shown to be poorly differentiated into goblet or ciliated cells, did not express tight junctions and lacked the cell polarization that is essential for nasal drug transport studies [28,29]. However, over the last years, the RPMI 2650 cell model has been also used for drug permeability studies, through the application of specific air–liquid interface and liquid-covered culture conditions that lead to the formation of a tight barrier and confluent monolayers [12,24,28,30,35]. The apical and basolateral sides of the liquid-covered cell culture model are filled with culture medium, showing the presence of flattened ciliated cells and mucin expression [12,24]. In addition, in the air–liquid interface cell model, initially the apical and basolateral sides are filled with culture medium, and the apical side is aerated later. Moreover, the culture medium of the basolateral side is changed on alternate days, which creates a high similarity with living nasal tissue. This model contains ciliated cells, a high expression of mucin genes, expresses tight junction proteins and develops sufficient transepithelial electrical resistance, providing an adequate environment for cytotoxicity and permeability screening studies [12,24,28,30].

Overall, the RPMI 2650 cell model has similar physiologic barrier properties particularly for passive transport, and it has been the only human cell line used for nasal drug transport studies [28,30]. Upon specific culture conditions, the RPMI 2650 cell model has previously shown the ability of forming a permeable organotypic barrier with a tight uniform cell multilayer, exhibiting TEER values similar to the physiological, and permeation coefficients in the same range of those found in the human nasal mucosa [12,30].

The RPMI 2650 cell line expresses a variety of cell junction proteins, including ZO-1, occludin, claudin-1, E-cadherin, and β-catenin [36]. It was shown to moderately express genes encoding the multidrug resistant proteins (ABCB), being the most abundant ABCB6. Additionally, ABCC1 expression was the greatest amongst the multidrug resistance associated proteins (MRP/ABCC) [30]. In the human nasal respiratory mucosa, ABCC1 was present in ciliated epithelial cells with higher expression levels in serous glandular cells [30,31]. The RPMI 2650 cell line also expresses ABCB1 (P-gp), which is found in the normal mucosa of human nasal turbinates [30]. Concerning SLC transporters, the SLC19A2, SLC25A1, and SLC38A2 were the most abundant, and members of the SLC3 and SLC7 families, amino acid transporters, were found to be highly expressed (SLC3A1, SLC3A2, SLC7A6, SLC7A8, and SLC7A11), the SLC15A2 being well expressed in these cells [30].

Although more complex and difficult to handle and grow, co-cultures containing a collagen matrix of human nasal fibroblasts covered by a monolayer of RPMI 2650 cells have been developed to conduct transport and permeability studies. These co-cultures mimic the permeation barrier properties of nasal mucosa and simulate a non-pseudostratified and non-ciliated human nasal epithelium [28].

3.3. *Human Lung Cancer Cells (Calu-3)*

The human bronchial epithelial cell line Calu-3 represents a promising in vitro model of the upper airway epithelial barrier [36]. This submucosal adenocarcinoma cell line was obtained from the bronchial airways of a 25-year-old white Caucasian male. The Calu-3 cells are capable of forming differentiated, tight and polarized layers of a combined phenotype, including ciliated and secretory cells, have microvilli, express several cell junction proteins (tight junctions, desmosomes and zonulae adherens) and contain mucin granules [26,36]. Despite its origin, the Calu-3 cell line has characteristics similar to serous nasal cells, being useful for nasal permeability studies [42].

Regarding the culture conditions, studies have shown that the air—liquid culturing interface shows a closer resemblance of these cells to the in vivo airway epithelia, when compared to liquid—liquid culturing conditions, in terms of morphology, mucus production and barrier integrity, with TEER values close to the observed in primary human tracheo-bronchiolar cells [36]. At an air–liquid interface, Calu-3 cells form a confluent polarized cell monolayer with tight junctions and a uniform mucus layer [26].

The Calu-3 cell line provides an alternative in vitro model of the airway epithelia for drug permeability assessments, being easily maintained in culture, reproducible, with a wide passage range and ethical acceptability [36].

Calu-3 cell cultures may provide a valuable model for studying mucin gene expression and synthesis, electrolyte transport, epithelial barrier properties and their regulation mechanisms, as they highly express MUC1 and MUC5/5AC mRNA, and MUC5/5AC mucins, as well as functional cytochrome P450 isozymes (CYP1A1, CYP2B6 and CYP2E1) [26,42]. They can also be useful in permeability screening studies for the nasal and lung permeability potential of drugs [26,42].

3.4. *Human Epithelial Colorectal Adenocarcinoma Cells (Caco-2)*

The Caco-2 cell line was originally obtained from a human colon adenocarcinoma. Under normal culture conditions on semiporous filter membranes, these cells can differentiate into enterocytes. It is the most suitable model to study the absorption and permeability of drugs and drug formulations though the intestinal epithelium but is often used as a screening model to evaluate the nasal absorption of formulations after its differentiation [12,24,42].

Caco-2 cells can create polarized monolayers of columnar epithelial cells with brush border and tight junctions, improving TEER values. Among the advantages of these cells is the occurrence of both passive and active transports, including the expression of important uptake (SLC15A1, SLC22A1, SLC22A2, SLC22A3, SLCO2B1) and efflux transporters (P-gp/MDR1/ABCB1, BCRP/ABCG2, MRP2/ABCC2, MRP4/ABCC4) [43].

The Caco-2 cell model is widely used to assess the paracellular transport through the nasal epithelia. However, this model is unable to explain the effect of nasal mucus, mucins and clearance and physiological factors that interfere with drug permeability [24]. The same as other immortalized cell culture models, Caco-2 cells display heterogeneous populations that can lead to different permeabilities as a consequence of the cell source, number of cell passages, initial seeding density, transport experiment conditions, cell culture media, filter size and composition, and the transport buffer composition and pH. However, this variability can be reduced by standardization of the culture conditions and permeability assay [43].

3.5. *Others*

The Madin–Darby canine kidney (MDCK) cells, isolated from canine distal renal tissue (distal tubule epithelium), similarly to Caco-2 cells, differentiate into columnar epithelial cells and form tight junctions, when cultured on semiporous membranes. They have lower TEER and shorter culture times than Caco-2 cells [42,43]. MDCK cells express canine efflux transporters, namely Mdr1 (P-gp), Mrp1, Mrp2, Mrp5, and also functionally express uptake transporters, such as Oct2 (as expected in cells from renal origin), and transporters for monocarboxylic acids and peptides [43]. MDCK cells are a potential alternative to mimic the transport across the BBB because of the expression of P-gp and tight junction proteins, such as claudin-1, claudin-4 and occludin, which are important to form a restrictive paracellular barrier with tight junctions. Although useful, MDCK cells present several differences from the nasal mucosa, not being an ideal alternative for nasal permeability studies [42].

Concerning human bronchial epithelial cell lines, and similarly to the Calu-3 cell line, 16HBE14o- (16HBE) cell monolayers have been used as models of the airway epithelium due to their morphological characteristics, barrier properties and expression of drug transporters that are present in vivo [44,45]. The 16HBE cells are human bronchial epithelial cells firstly isolated from a 1-year-old male and then immortalized with the SV40 plasmid. Although it is being used as an in vitro model of several respiratory diseases, the potential for the application of the 16HBE cells in nasal permeability studies remains unclear [46]. In culture, and when reaching confluency, 16HBE cells form tight junctional seals, become polar and show apical microvilli, and present the cAMP-regulated CFTR (cystic fibrosis transmembrane conductance regulator, a chloride channel), they are able to develop TEER values similar to the ones seen in the Calu-3 airway epithelial cell line model and normal bronchial epithelia in primary culture [45,46].

4. Solid Lipid Nanoparticles (SLN) and Nanostructured Lipid Carriers (NLC) for Nasal Delivery

The inclusion of lipid nanoparticles, such as SLN and NLC, in nasal formulations can improve the effectiveness of drugs. Regarding their advantages over other colloidal carriers, lipid nanoparticles have been described as superior carriers for nasal drug delivery. For instance, they enable the direct transport of drugs from the nose to the brain, via olfactory and trigeminal nerves, and adhere to the olfactory epithelium, increasing contact time with the nasal mucosa. In addition, they provide prolonged drug release, drug protection from nasal enzymatic degradation and have low or no toxicity due to the use of generally recognized as safe (GRAS) excipients [1–3,47,48].

To understand the specific features of lipid nanoparticles for nasal delivery, it is important to first clarify their specific characteristics. Briefly, SLN were first created and consist of aqueous dispersions of nanoparticles made by one solid lipid and stabilized by one or two emulsifiers. Their solid matrix enables prolonged release, while protecting the encapsulated molecules. Although SLN appear to be effective drug carriers, some drawbacks have been observed, in particular, poor storage stability related to the occurrence of lipid polymorphic transitions that originate molecule release and nanoparticle aggregation. To circumvent these problems, NLCs were developed, which also consist of aqueous dispersions of nanoparticles with a solid lipid matrix composed of one solid lipid and one liquid lipid and stabilized by one or two emulsifiers. The presence of oil within the lipid matrix causes a more disordered internal structure that leads to fewer lipid polymorphic transitions during storage, producing higher stability.

Thereby, the use of SLN and NLC has been extensively investigated to improve drug delivery through different administration routes, as they show advantages over other nanosystems, including the use of GRAS excipients, easy industrial manufacture, high encapsulation efficiency, protection and prolonged release of lipophilic molecules, and good storage stability. In this field, very complete review articles are available [49–63].

4.1. In Vitro Studies with Nasal Formulations of NLC and SLN

The use of aqueous dispersions of SLN and NLC show limitations in some administration routes, including cutaneous, ocular and nasal. For instance, the low viscosity of these dispersions decreases the contact time with the locale of application, reducing the therapeutic effectiveness of the drug. To avoid this, different strategies have been used, including the incorporation of SLN and NLC in conventional semisolid formulations, such as hydrogels, creams and ointments, or the addition of viscosifying agents, mucoadhesive polymers or in situ gelling polymers, directly to the aqueous phase of the SLN and NLC dispersions [53,64–67]. Examples of viscosifying agents used in nasal formulations containing lipid nanoparticles include gellan gum, poloxamers, and carbomers [12,68,69], while commonly used mucoadhesive polymers are hypromellose, carbomers, alginate, hyaluronic acid, chitosan, polyethylene glycol, cyclodextrins, polyacrylic acid and cellulose derivatives, such as carboxymethylcellulose, hydroxypropyl methylcellulose and methylcellulose. Examples of in situ gelling polymers include poloxamers, such as poloxamer 407 and 188, gellan gum, pectin, sodium alginate, carrageenan and xyloglucan [12,13,18,20,69,70].

Regarding nasal administration, the use of liquid and semisolid formulations has been investigated and it seems that both formulations promote the efficacy of drugs for different therapeutic applications. In the following sections, examples of the most relevant studies are reported. The main outcomes of these studies are summarized in Table 2. Over the past two years, about ten studies have been published investigating the use of SLN or NLC for intranasal delivery, mainly for the treatment of neurological disorders.

Table 2. Relevant outcomes from in vitro studies with nasal formulations of solid lipid nanoparticles (SLN) and nanostructured lipid carriers (NLC).

Type of Lipid Nanoparticle Formulation	Drug	Targeted Disease	Cell Line	Relevant Results	Reference
SLN-liquid	Curcumin	CNS disorders	Mouse fetal fibroblasts	• High cell viability (80%) for curcumin-loaded NLC and curcumin-loaded SLN, in a concentration range of 1–10 μg/mL. • No significant difference in cell viability was observed between the drug-loaded lipid nanoparticles, blank nanoparticles and free curcumin. • At a concentration of 20 μg/mL, a slight reduction in cell viability was observed.	[76]
SLN-liquid	Dopamine and grape seed extract	Parkinson's disease	SH-SY5Y neuroblastoma and Olfactory ensheathing	• None of the three formulations (grape seed-derived extract dopamine-loaded SLN, dopamine-loaded SLN and grape seed-derived extract-loaded SLN) presented cytotoxicity to olfactory ensheathing cells and SH-SY5Y neuroblastoma cells, in a concentration range of 18–75 μM and 4–34.5 μM for dopamine and grape seed-derived extract, respectively.	[74]
NLC-liquid	Ketoconazole	Meningoencephalitis	Fungal cells	• In the yeast-extract peptone dextrose medium, the fungal growth inhibition effect of ketoconazole-loaded NLC was significant at concentrations above 0.5 μg/mL, having shown a growth inhibition of 92%, compared to a 50% inhibition shown by the ketoconazole solution. • In the RPMI 1640 medium, the cell inhibition rate was 4-fold higher for the ketoconazole-loaded NLC formulation than for the ketoconazole solution.	[71]
SLN-liquid	Nalbuphine	Pain management	Human embryonic kidney (HEK-293)	• A concentration up to 750 μM was shown to be nontoxic to HEK-293 cells. • Percent cell survival was 100% for nalbuphine concentrations of 100, 250 and 500 μM, 80% for a concentration of 750 μM and almost 75% for a concentration of 1000 μM.	[77]

Table 2. *Cont.*

Type of Lipid Nanoparticle Formulation	Drug	Targeted Disease	Cell Line	Relevant Results	Reference
SLN-semisolid	Paeonol	CNS disorders	RPMI 2650	• Cell viability of the in situ gel containing paeonol-loaded SLN, paeonol-loaded SLN, blank SLN, and blank in situ gel over a concentration range of 0.001–10 μg/mL was greater than 90%, indicating good biocompatibility. • The fluorescence intensity of dead cells was similar for the four formulations tested, indicating good cell viability.	[80]
NLC-liquid	Pioglitazone	Alzheimer's disease	SH-SY5Y	• The LC50 was 16.626 μg/mL for pure pioglitazone and 17.387 μg/mL for NLC loaded with pioglitazone. • Cell viability was similar for both formulations, being 69.15% for NLC loaded with pioglitazone and 66.89% for pure pioglitazone at a concentration of 10 μg/mL.	[72]
SLN-liquid	*Pueraria* flavone	CNS disorders	Caco-2	• Greater cellular uptake was observed for *Pueraria* flavone-loaded SLN modified with borneol and stearic acid, followed by *Pueraria* flavone-loaded SLN modified with borneol, *Pueraria* flavone-loaded SLN and *Pueraria* flavone free, at 37 °C and 4 °C, at concentrations 100, 200 and 400 mg/mL of *Pueraria* flavone. • Cellular uptake of all formulations was achieved at the highest temperatures and concentrations.	[75]
NLC-liquid	Tacrine	Alzheimer's disease	SH-SY5Y	• Blank NLC and tacrine-loaded NLC, at the same concentration, showed similar cell viability. • The cell viability of tacrine-loaded NLC conjugated to an amphipathic peptide drastically decreased compared to tacrine-loaded NLC at the same concentration. • The use of a concentration up to 10 μM of tacrine was considered safe.	[73]

Table 2. *Cont.*

Type of Lipid Nanoparticle Formulation	Drug	Targeted Disease	Cell Line	Relevant Results	Reference
NLC-liquid	Tenofovir disoproxil fumarate	Acquired Immune Deficiency Syndrome (AIDS)	bEnd.3 cerebral cortex	• The two different tenofovir disoproxil fumarate-loaded NLC showed cell viability similar to blank NLC at a concentration of 5, 10 and 50 µg/mL. • Cell viability decreased in a concentration of 100 µg/mL of tenofovir disoproxil fumarate after 72 h in both formulations. • The use of emulsifiers did not cause any cytotoxicity below 100 µg/mL of tenofovir disoproxil fumarate-loaded NLC.	[78]
NLC-semisolid	Teriflunomide	Glioma	Human U-87	• Based on the percentage of viable cells, pure teriflunomide and the in situ gel containing teriflunomide-loaded NLC showed greater cytotoxicity compared to teriflunomide-loaded NLC. • After 48 h, cell viability was 4% for pure teriflunomide, 6% for in situ gel, and 48.2% for NLC, for a concentration of 100 µg/mL. • The IC50 concentration was 78.5 µg/mL for NLC, followed by the in situ gel at 7 µg/mL and by teriflunomide at 4.8 µg/mL.	[79]

4.1.1. Liquid Formulations

Du et al. [71] developed ketoconazole-loaded NLC for nose-to-brain delivery in the treatment of cryptococcus neoformans-mediated meningoencephalitis, which is a critical infectious disorder of the CNS. These authors investigated this strategy because the therapeutic effectiveness of conventional treatments is limited due to the poor penetration across the BBB. The developed ketoconazole-loaded NLC presented appropriate particle size, good stability and the fluorescence images demonstrated that the optimized formulations were able to penetrate the C. neoformans capsules. The in vitro antifungal activity against the cryptococcus neoformans was evaluated in the ketoconazole-loaded NLC and ketoconazole solution in fungal cells, using the yeast-extract peptone dextrose and RPMI 1640 medium. The results showed that the fungal growth inhibition was significant at concentrations above 0.5 µg/mL, for the yeast-extract peptone dextrose medium, with a growth inhibition of 92% for ketoconazole-loaded NLC and 50% for ketoconazole solution. In the RPMI 1640 medium, the cell inhibition rate was four-fold higher for the NLC formulation than the ketoconazole solution. Furthermore, the ketoconazole-loaded NLC exhibited greater inhibition rates even at low concentrations, indicating a higher cell uptake.

Jojo et al. [72] evaluated the nasal cytotoxicity of optimized pioglitazone-loaded NLC formulation for the treatment and management of Alzheimer's disease. This antidiabetic drug has been extensively investigated because the most common cause of dementia in the elderly is a metabolic disorder associated to an impaired brain insulin signalling. SH-SY5Y neuroblastoma cells were used to conduct in vitro studies, evaluating the nasal cytotoxicity of pioglitazone-loaded NLC and pure pioglitazone, through cell viability and the lethal concertation 50 (LC50). Based on the results, the LC50 was 16.626 μg/mL for pure pioglitazone and 17.3874 μg/mL for pioglitazone-loaded NLC. In addition, the cell viability was similar for both formulations, being 69.15% for pioglitazone-loaded NLC and 66.89% for pure pioglitazone at a concentration of 10 μg/mL. The results showed that there was no significant change between the NLC formulation and the pure drug, indicating that pioglitazone-loaded NLC is safe for neuronal cells. In another study, Silva et al. [73] evaluated the in vitro cytotoxicity of tacrine-loaded NLC and tacrine-loaded NLC conjugated to an amphipathic peptide in SH-SY5Y neuroblastoma cell lines. The formulation cytotoxicity was evaluated through the MTT assay and SBR assay. From the results, when comparing the same concentration of empty NLC and tacrine-loaded NLC, the cell viability was similar. However, the cell viability of tacrine-loaded NLC conjugated to an amphipathic peptide at the same concentration decreased dramatically. Therefore, a concentration up to 10 μM of tacrine was considered safe. These results showed that tacrine-loaded NLC is safe for neuronal cells, being a promising formulation for the management of Alzheimer's disease. Trapani et al. [74] compared the in vitro cytotoxicity of grape seed-derived extract dopamine-loaded SLN, dopamine-loaded SLN and grape seed-derived extract-loaded SLN. The conjugation of dopamine with an antioxidant grape seed-derived proanthocyanidin reduces the oxidative stress observed in Parkinson's disease. The in vitro studies were carried out in SH-SY5Y neuroblastoma cells and olfactory ensheathing cells. One day after the beginning of the tests, it was observed that none of the formulations presented cytotoxicity to the olfactory ensheathing cells and to the SH-SY5Y neuroblastoma cells, in a concentration range of 18–75 μM and 4–34.5 μM of dopamine and grape seed-derived extract, respectively. Therefore, the authors concluded that the tested formulations can be used to improve Parkinson's disease therapy.

Wang et al. [75] studied the in vitro efficacy of intranasal *Pueraria* flavone solution, *Pueraria* flavone-loaded SLN, *Pueraria* flavone-loaded SLN modified with borneol and *Pueraria* flavone-loaded SLN modified with borneol and stearic acid. Pueraria flavone is extracted from the *Pueraria thoom sonii* and *Pueraria lobata* and is used for the management of CNS diseases, such as Parkinson's disease and Alzheimer's disease. In this study, the cellular uptake of the different formulations was tested in Caco-2 cells. The results showed a higher cellular uptake for *Pueraria* flavone-loaded SLN modified with borneol and stearic acid and *Pueraria* flavone-loaded SLN modified with borneol, when compared to *Pueraria* flavone-loaded SLN and pure *Pueraria* flavone at a concentration of 100 mg/mL, 200 mg/mL and 400 mg/mL of *Pueraria* flavone. In addition, a higher cellular uptake was observed for higher temperatures and higher concentrations. From the results of their study, the authors concluded that the modified SLN containing *Pueraria* flavone could be used to improve the management of neurodegenerative diseases.

Malvajerd et al. [76] developed curcumin-loaded SLN and curcumin-loaded NLC to study their potential for brain delivery in the treatment of CNS disorders. Before performing in vivo experiments, the researchers evaluated the in vitro cytotoxicity of the formulations in mouse fetal fibroblast cells using the MTT assay. The results showed a high cell viability (abound 80%) for curcumin-loaded SLN and for curcumin-loaded NLC at concentrations of 1–10 μg/mL, while a slight decrease in cell viability was observed at higher concentrations (20 μg/mL). Thus, the authors concluded that no remarkable cytotoxicity was observed in any of the tested formulations of lipid nanoparticles containing curcumin.

Khanna et al. [77] evaluated the safety of exposing nalbuphine-loaded SLN to human embryonic kidney cells (HEK-293). In this study, the in vitro cytotoxicity of nalbuphine-loaded SLN was tested in a drug concentration range of 100–1000 μM. The results showed a cell viability of 100% for concentrations of 100, 250 and 500 μM, a viability of 80% for a concentration of 750 μM and a viability of almost 75% for a concentration of 1000 μM. These results suggested that nalbuphine-loaded SLN containing drug concentrations up to 750 μM is safe for use in the management of pain.

Sarma et al. [78] investigated the in vitro cytotoxicity of two different tenofovir disoproxil fumarate-loaded NLC, one with Tween 80 and the other with Tween 80 and Pluronic

F68, in bEnd.3 cells of the cerebral cortex, after 24 h and 72 h of exposure. Similar cell viability was observed for both formulations, and at both times, at concentrations of 5, 10 and 50 μg/mL. After 72 h, cell viability decreased at concentrations of 100 μg/mL for both formulations. From these results, the authors concluded that the use of emulsifiers did not cause differences in cytotoxicity. In addition, at concentrations up to 100 μg/mL, tenofovir disoproxil fumarate-loaded NLCs are safe for intranasal administration. Based on these findings, the use of the tenofovir disoproxil fumarate-loaded NLCs for the treatment of Acquired Immune Deficiency Syndrome (AIDS) was proposed.

4.1.2. Semisolid Formulations

Gadhave et al. [79] developed a carbopol-gellan gum in situ gel containing teriflunomide-loaded NLC for the treatment of gliomas. Gellan gum is a natural anionic polysaccharide capable of forming a hydrogel in the presence of cations in the nasal cavity. In this sense, the objective of using gellan gum, as a gelling agent, and carbopol 974P, as a mucoadhesive polymer, was to increase the contact time of the formulation in the nasal cavity, promoting drug absorption. The antitumor activity of the in situ gel containing teriflunomide-loaded NLC, teriflunomide-loaded NLC and pure teriflunomide was evaluated in human U-87 glioma cells. The results showed that pure teriflunomide and the in situ gel containing teriflunomide-loaded NLC had higher cytotoxicity compared to teriflunomide-loaded NLC. After 48 h, cell viability was 4% for pure teriflunomide, 6% for in situ gel containing teriflunomide-loaded NLC and 48.2% for teriflunomide-loaded NLC, at a concentration of 100 μg/mL. The IC_{50} was 78.5 μg/mL for the teriflunomide-loaded NLC, followed by 7 μg/mL for the in situ gel teriflunomide-loaded NLC and 4.8 μg/mL for the pure teriflunomide. Therefore, it was concluded that the in situ gel containing teriflunomide-loaded NLC and pure teriflunomide were more cytotoxic than teriflunomide-loaded NLC.

Sun et al. [80] evaluated the in vitro cytotoxicity in RPMI 2650 cells of an in situ gel containing paeonol-loaded SLN, paeonol-loaded SLN, blank SLN and a blank in situ gel, using the MTT method. The cell viability of all tested formulations, in the concentration range of 0.001–10 μg/mL, was higher than 90%, indicating biocompatibility. Additionally, the cell viability of blank SLN and paeonol-loaded SLN, without removing the free emulsifiers used to prepare these formulations, decreased with increasing concentration, with strong cytotoxicity being observed at 1000 μg/mL, presenting cell viability of 24.20% and 25.90%, respectively. Furthermore, the live/dead double staining method showed similar dead cell fluorescence intensity in all tested formulations, which was in agreement with the MTT results and indicated good cell viability.

5. Nasal Cavity Models

The deposition of drugs in the nasal cavity upon administration remains challenging. Ensuring drug release to the target area of the nasal cavity is essential to obtain the therapeutic effect. Factors that interfere with the pattern of nasal deposition of drugs include [68,81–83]: differences in nasal geometries between individuals, age being fundamental, since adults and children have different lengths and areas of the nasal cavity; nasal application device and the respective flow used; complexity of the structure of the nasal cavity; how the patients administer (e.g., whether or not they are breathing); formulation characteristics (e.g., particle size and viscosity). To overcome these drawbacks, the use of nasal cavity models (or nasal casts) and computational models to predict the deposition of drugs in the nasal cavity have been investigated.

Extensive progress in imaging technology and reconstruction software has enabled the 3D reproduction of the human nasal cavity with the correct geometry and dimensions to visualize drug deposition patterns in specific regions [82,84]. To produce a 3D nasal cast it is necessary to have an image of the human nasal cavity, which can be obtained by computed tomography (CT)-scan or magnetic resonance imaging (MRI) [85–87].

Most 3D models are transparent to allow visualization of the formulation path within the nasal cast (Figure 3). However, it is possible to use a color change method to quantify drug deposition by photometric or colorimetric analysis. Silicone is one of the most used materials to manufacture nasal casts, being described as the most realistic. However, as all nasal casts, silicone casts do not replicate the entire complexity of the nasal cavity, such as nasal valve dynamics or mucociliary clearance. Notwithstanding, the 3D nasal casts allow the visualization of the influence of breathing patterns (with and without airflow), consistency of formulations (liquid, powder or gels), variables of the nasal device (e.g., spray angle and plume characteristics) and the formulation deposition location [68,82,84,87–89].

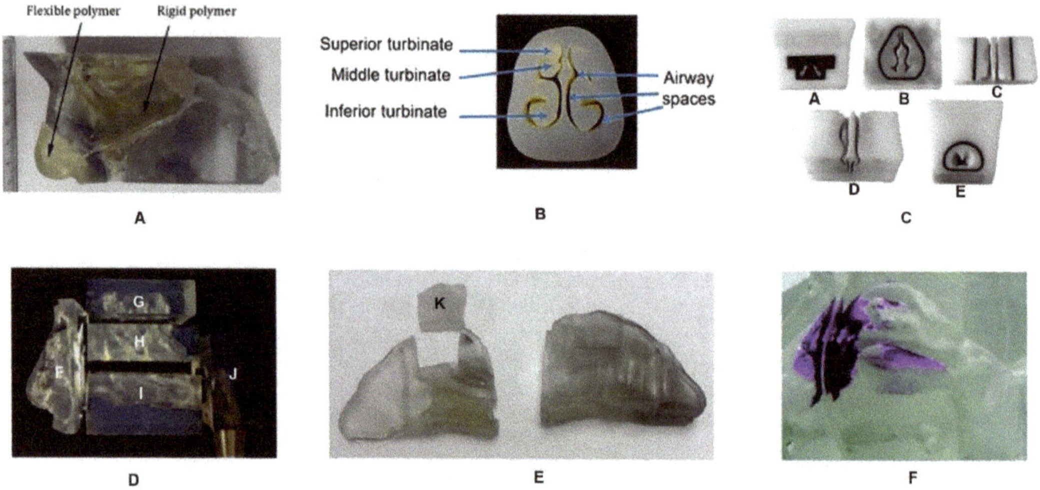

Figure 3. Examples of different nasal casts: (**A**) 7-year-old child; (**B**) MRI image of a 12-year-old child; (**C**) made from CT-scan of an adult; (CA) nostrils, (CB) nasal vestibule, (CC) lower turbinates, (CD) middle and upper turbinates, (CE) nasopharynx; (**D**) CT-scan of a patient, (DF) anterior region, (DG) upper turbinates, (DH) middle turbinates, (DI) lower turbinates, (DJ) nasopharynx; (**E**) MRI image of a 53-year-old man, K—olfactory region; (**F**) silicone transparent commercial cast with Sar-gel (adapted from [90], with permission from Elsevier).

Nizic et al. [68] used a commercial silicone cast to study the deposition profile of melatonin-loaded pectin/hypromellose microspheres. A respiratory pump was connected to the nasal cast to simulate air inspiration and to observe the differences between inspiratory airflow of 0 L/min and 20 L/min. A nasal insufflator was used to pump the formulation into the nasal cavity cast in one nostril, while the other nostril was closed. Lactose monohydrate was added to increase the fraction of microspheres deposited within the nasal cavity. The results showed a higher drug deposition with an inspiratory flow of 0 L/min than 20 L/min, in all regions of the nasal cavity. It was also observed that the incorporation of lactose monohydrate increased the deposition efficiency in the upper part and in the turbinates of the nasal cavity by 40%, being $8.3 \pm 0.2\%$ for the olfactory region and $30.9 \pm 4.5\%$ for the turbinates. The same authors [70] evaluated the nasal deposition of in situ gels of fluticasone containing different polymers (sodium hyaluronate, pectin and gellan gum), in the same nasal cast, using different inspiration flow rates (0, 30 and 60 L/min) and different angles of administration (30°, 52.5° and 75°). In addition, Sar-gel, which is an indicator paste that runs purple when it contacts with water, was used to cover the nasal cast and allow visualization of the drug deposition. The results showed that a decrease in the angle of administration from 75° to 30° significantly increased drug deposition in the turbinates, while an increase in the inspiratory flow resulted in drug deposition close to the nasal valve. The use of sodium hyaluronate produced a greater influence on the turbinates deposition pattern, compared to gellan gum. Furthermore, the results of the nasal deposition of in situ gels containing 0.058% of fluticasone and 0.31% of surfactant are shown in Figure 4. Different gelling polymers, angles of administration and inspiratory flow rates were tested.

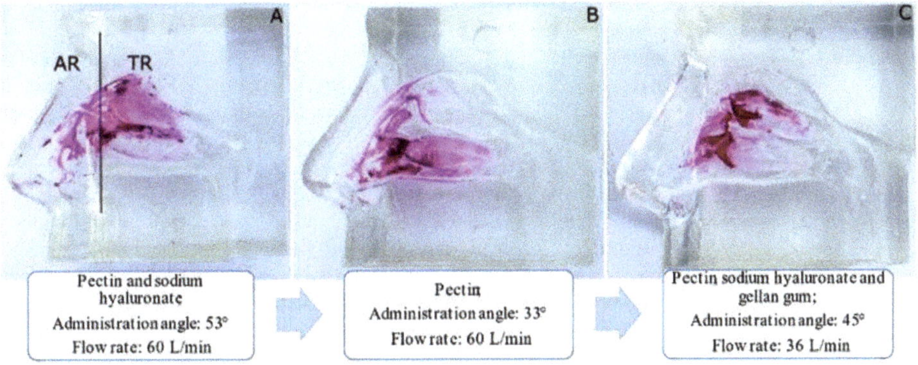

Figure 4. Evaluation of the deposition of fluticasone in situ gels in a 3D nasal cast covered with Sar-gel. (**A**) in situ gels of pectin and sodium hyaluronate, with an administration angle of 53° and a flow rate of 60 L/min; (**B**) in situ gel of pectin, with an administration angle of 33° and a flow rate of 60 L/min, (**C**) in situ gel of pectin, sodium hyaluronate and gellan gum, with an administration angle of 45° and a flow rate of 36 L/min (adapted from [70], with permission from Elsevier).

From Figure 4, it can be observed that the use of a 3D model of transparent silicone coated with Sar-gel facilitated the visualization of the behavior of the drug in the nasal cast. Furthermore, it was observed that the angle of administration strongly influenced drug deposition between the upper and lower part of the turbinates region, and the combination of three in situ gelling polymers with a low inspiratory flow rate reduced drug deposition in the region of the turbinates.

Recently, the same researchers [85] developed a 3D nasal cast from a CT-scan of a 62-year-old healthy patient, produced by stereolithography using a 3D system and printed on transparent rigid plastic. A respiratory pump was connected to the nasal cast, simulating inspiration, and the differences between an inspiratory airflow of 0 L/min and 20 L/min were analyzed. The Miat spray device was used to administer a dexamethasone sodium phosphate powder formulation to the nasal cavity, with angles of 0°, 60° and 75°. The amount of drug deposited in the olfactory region ranged from 5.1 ± 0.9% to 17.0 ± 1.6%. In addition, it was observed the highest drug deposition with an administration angle of 75° and an inspiratory flow rate of 0 L/min. Gholizadeh et al. [91] compared the drug deposition of a thermosensitive in situ gel of tranexamic acid with a tranexamic acid solution, in the same nasal cast covered with Sar-gel. The results showed that the amount of drug deposited with the thermosensitive in situ gel was 68.52 ± 2.60%, while with the drug solution was 62.79 ± 2.92%. In addition, the deposition pattern remained unchanged from the 20 min for the in situ gel, while for the drug solution it was unstable, showing leakage and runoff. Based on the results, it was concluded that the viscosity of the formulations influenced drug deposition and the use of a mucoadhesive agent increased the residence time in the nasal cavity.

Xi et al. [82] compared the differences in deposition patterns of four commercially available spray pumps (Apotex, Astelin, Miaoling and Nasonex) and four nebulizers (Drive Voyager Pro, Respironics Ultrasonic, Pari Sinus and Philips Respironics) in a nasal cast reconstructed from an MRI scan of an adult male, 3D printed, made of polypropylene and covered with Sar-gel. Higher deposition was observed in the olfactory region with Miaoling, followed by Astelin, Apotex and Nasonex, although most of the deposition occurred in the vestibule and only a small portion reached the upper part of the nasal cavity. Regarding nebulizers, deposition was lower than that of nasal sprays, with Drive Voyager Pro being the one with a higher deposition in the upper part of the nasal cavity.

From these results, the authors concluded that the standard nasal delivery systems tested are inadequate to significantly reach the olfactory region of the nasal cavity. In this regard, the same researchers compared the deposition with normal and bidirectional nasal delivery techniques, and the results showed that the latter increased the efficiency of delivery in the olfactory region [92].

Warnken et al. [88] developed ten 3D nasal casts produced from the nasal CT scan of five adults and five children to assess deposition variations related to the nasal geometries and dimensions. The influence of the plume angle (patient-specific angle, 30°, 40°, 60° and 75°) of the nasal sprays on the deposition efficiency in the turbinates was studied. The minimum coronal cross-section areas of the tested nasal casts (corresponding to the nasal valve area in each individual) ranged from 114.0 mm^2 to 299.2 mm^2 and the length ranged from 59.2 mm to 88.0 mm. Cromolyn sodium deposition was evaluated in the anterior region, turbinates, upper region and nasopharynx. The results showed a higher deposition of cromolyn sodium in the turbinates, in adults and in children, compared to the deposition in the upper region of the nasal cavity. Furthermore, it was observed that turbinate deposition decreased with increasing the administration angle. In contrast, in the upper region of the nasal cavity, no significant differences were observed with increasing the administration angle, and no deposition was detected in the upper region of some of the nasal casts tested. In addition, a higher deposition of cromolyn sodium in the turbinates was observed in the assessment of patient-specific angle in comparison with the other angles tested, with no significant differences between adults and children. From these results, the authors concluded that nasal sprays are inadequate devices for the efficient administration of drugs in the upper region of the nasal cavity, as the drug was only detected in six of the ten nasal casts tested. Hosseini and Golshahi [93], who also used 3D nasal casts to test drug deposition, obtained different results. These researchers observed the occurrence of higher drug deposition in the olfactory region of adults ($3.55 \pm 1.29\%$), followed by children ($3.15 \pm 0.57\%$) and toddlers ($2.21 \pm 0.95\%$). In addition, higher deposition was also observed in the superior turbinates of adults ($2.53 \pm 0.88\%$), followed by children ($2.46 \pm 0.47\%$) and toddlers ($2.10 \pm 0.41\%$). In this study, researchers also concluded that the use of different nasal delivery devices interferes with drug deposition. They tested two nasal spray pumps (Flonase and Flonase SensimistTM) and one atomization device (MAD nasalTM) and observed the occurrence of olfactory deposition in adults with Flonase and Flonase SensimistTM, being higher with the former. However, the occurrence of olfactory deposition in children and toddlers was not observed with any of the nasal delivery devices tested [94].

Computational Models

Computational and mathematical approaches to predict the drug deposition in different regions of the nasal cavity are also used to analyze the path followed by nasal formulations upon administration. For instance, Setty [86] developed the eBrain by translating the MRI data into an interactive 3D model that uses graphics and integrates medical images and physiological data. The eBrain allows intranasal drug delivery to be studied under various conditions, predicting the experimental results based on algorithms, design and other set up requirements. In another study, Tian et al. [95] evaluated nasal deposition of inhaled nanoparticles from low to moderate breathing using 3D computer models obtained from the CT scans of a 48-year-old man and a Sprague Dawley rat. This study aimed to visualize the olfactory deposition in nasal cavities with different geometries. For example, in humans the olfactory region comprises about 10% of the nasal cavity, while in rats it occupies about 50% of the nasal cavity. Empirical equations were developed to quantitatively predict the deposition of different nanoparticle sizes under different breathing conditions.

6. Conclusions

The research of novel formulations for nasal drug administration, namely incorporating lipid nanoparticles, such as SLN and NLC, has been attracting the interest of the scientific community. In this respect, the possibility of targeting drugs from the nose to the brain, avoiding the need to cross the BBB, and thus possibly tackling unmet medical needs associated with several CNS disorders, has been a major driver.

Among the different studies required while engineering novel nasal formulations of lipid nanoparticles, the ones performed with in vitro cell cultures mimicking the nasal epithelium have enabled mechanistic insights into cell uptake, as well as into their cytotoxicity, essential for estimating the safe concentration to be used in the following studies.

To further test the effectiveness of nasal formulations in reaching the upper part of the nasal cavity, critical for successful nose-to-brain delivery, the use of nasal cavity models encompasses a great potential. Their manufacture, relying on 3D CT scans of the human nasal cavity or computational models of this cavity, has brought about major improvements in the recapitulation of some features of the nasal cavity. They enable analysis of the factors interfering with nasal drug deposition, such as nasal cavity area, type of administration device and angle of application, inspiratory flow rate, presence of mucoadhesive agents, among others. Notwithstanding, they do not preclude the use of confirmatory in vivo studies, a significant impact on the 3R (replacement, reduction and refinement) principle within the scope of animal experiments is expected. The use of 3D nasal casts to test nasal formulations of lipid nanoparticles is still totally unexplored, to the authors' best knowledge, thus constituting a wide open field of research.

Author Contributions: Conceptualization, C.P.C., A.C.S. and J.N.M.; investigation, C.P.C.; writing—original draft preparation, C.P.C., A.C.S., R.S., S.B. and H.A.; writing—review and editing, A.C.S., R.S., J.N.M. and J.M.S.L.; All authors have read and agreed to the published version of the manuscript.

Funding: This work was supported by Fundação para a Ciência e a Tecnologia (FCT) (SFRH/136177/2018, Portugal), by the Applied Molecular Biosciences Unit-UCIBIO, which is financed by national funds from FCT (UIDP/04378/2020 and UIDB/04378/2020), and CIBB (FCT reference: UIDB/04539/2020).

Institutional Review Board Statement: Not applicable.

Informed Consent Statement: Not applicable.

Data Availability Statement: Data sharing not applicable.

Conflicts of Interest: The authors declare no conflict of interest.

References

1. Cunha, S.; Amaral, M.H.; Lobo, J.M.S.; Silva, A.C. Lipid Nanoparticles for Nasal/Intranasal Drug Delivery. *Crit. Rev. Ther. Drug. Carrier. Syst.* **2017**, *34*, 257–282. [CrossRef]
2. Costa, C.P.; Moreira, J.N.; Sousa Lobo, J.M.; Silva, A.C. Intranasal delivery of nanostructured lipid carriers, solid lipid nanoparticles and nanoemulsions: A current overview of in vivo studies. *Acta Pharm. Sin. B* **2021**, *11*, 925–940. [CrossRef]
3. Costa, C.; Moreira, J.N.; Amaral, M.H.; Sousa Lobo, J.M.; Silva, A.C. Nose-to-brain delivery of lipid-based nanosystems for epileptic seizures and anxiety crisis. *J. Control. Release* **2019**, *295*, 187–200. [CrossRef] [PubMed]
4. Xie, J.; Shen, Z.; Anraku, Y.; Kataoka, K.; Chen, X. Nanomaterial-based blood-brain-barrier (BBB) crossing strategies. *Biomaterials* **2019**, *224*, 119491. [CrossRef] [PubMed]
5. Veronesi, M.C.; Alhamami, M.; Miedema, S.B.; Yun, Y.; Ruiz-Cardozo, M.; Vannier, M.W. Imaging of intranasal drug delivery to the brain. *Am. J. Nucl. Med. Mol. Imaging* **2020**, *10*, 1–31. [PubMed]
6. Islam, S.U.; Shehzad, A.; Ahmed, M.B.; Lee, Y.S. Intranasal Delivery of Nanoformulations: A Potential Way of Treatment for Neurological Disorders. *Molecules* **2020**, *25*, 1929. [CrossRef]
7. Binda, A.; Murano, C.; Rivolta, I. Innovative Therapies and Nanomedicine Applications for the Treatment of Alzheimer's Disease: A State-of-the-Art (2017-2020). *Int. J. Nanomed.* **2020**, *15*, 6113–6135. [CrossRef]
8. Wang, Z.; Xiong, G.; Tsang, W.C.; Schätzlein, A.G.; Uchegbu, I.F. Nose-to-Brain Delivery. *J. Pharmacol. Exp. Ther.* **2019**, *370*, 593–601. [CrossRef]
9. Bahadur, S.; Pardhi, D.M.; Rautio, J.; Rosenholm, J.M.; Pathak, K. Intranasal Nanoemulsions for Direct Nose-to-Brain Delivery of Actives for CNS Disorders. *Pharmaceutics* **2020**, *12*, 1230. [CrossRef]

10. Küçüktürkmen, B.; Bozkır, A. A New Approach for Drug Targeting to the Central Nervous System: Lipid Nanoparticles. In *Nanoarchitectonics in Biomedicine*; Grumezescu, A.M., Ed.; William Andrew Publishing: Norwich, NY, USA, 2019; Chapter 10; pp. 335–369.
11. Akhtar, A.; Andleeb, A.; Waris, T.S.; Bazzar, M.; Moradi, A.-R.; Awan, N.R.; Yar, M. Neurodegenerative diseases and effective drug delivery: A review of challenges and novel therapeutics. *J. Control. Release* **2021**, *330*, 1152–1167. [CrossRef]
12. Erdő, F.; Bors, L.A.; Farkas, D.; Bajza, Á.; Gizurarson, S. Evaluation of intranasal delivery route of drug administration for brain targeting. *Brain Res. Bull.* **2018**, *143*, 155–170. [CrossRef]
13. Tan, M.S.A.; Parekh, H.S.; Pandey, P.; Siskind, D.J.; Falconer, J.R. Nose-to-brain delivery of antipsychotics using nanotechnology: A review. *Expert. Opin. Drug. Deliv.* **2020**, *17*, 839–853. [CrossRef]
14. Agrawal, M.; Saraf, S.; Saraf, S.; Dubey, S.K.; Puri, A.; Patel, R.J.; Ajazuddin, V.R.; Murty, U.S.; Alexander, A. Recent strategies and advances in the fabrication of nano lipid carriers and their application towards brain targeting. *J. Control. Release* **2020**, *321*, 372–415. [CrossRef]
15. Pires, A.; Fortuna, A.; Alves, G.; Falcão, A. Intranasal drug delivery: How, why and what for? *J. Pharm. Pharm. Sci.* **2009**, *12*, 288–311. [CrossRef]
16. Hussein, N.R.; Omer, H.; Elhissi, A.; Ahmed, W. Advances in Nasal Drug Delivery Systems. In *Advances in Medical and Surgical Engineering*; Academic Press: Cambridge, MA, USA, 2020; Chapter 15; pp. 279–311.
17. Djupesland, P.G.; JMessina, J.C.; Mahmoud, R.A. The nasal approach to delivering treatment for brain diseases: An anatomic, physiologic, and delivery technology overview. *Ther. Deliv.* **2014**, *5*, 709–733. [CrossRef] [PubMed]
18. Gänger, S.; Schindowski, K. Tailoring Formulations for Intranasal Nose-to-Brain Delivery: A Review on Architecture, Physico-Chemical Characteristics and Mucociliary Clearance of the Nasal Olfactory Mucosa. *Pharmaceutics* **2018**, *10*, 116. [CrossRef]
19. Xu, J.; Tao, J.; Wang, J. Design and Application in Delivery System of Intranasal Antidepressants. *Front. Bioeng Biotechnol* **2020**, *8*, 626882. [CrossRef]
20. Javia, A.; Kore, G.; Misra, A. Polymers in Nasal Drug Delivery: An. Overview. In *Applications of Polymers in Drug Delivery*, 2nd ed.; Misra, A., Shahiwala, A., Eds.; Elsevier: Amsterdam, The Netherlands, 2021; Chapter 11; pp. 305–332.
21. Dhas, N.L.; Kudarha, R.R.; Mehta, T.A. Intranasal Delivery of Nanotherapeutics/Nanobiotherapeutics for the Treatment of Alzheimer's Disease: A Proficient Approach. *Crit Rev. Ther Drug Carrier Syst* **2019**, *36*, 373–447. [CrossRef] [PubMed]
22. Pangua, C.; Reboredo, C.; Camión, R.; Gracia, J.M.; Martínez-López, A.L.; Agüeros, M. Mucus-Penetrating Nanocarriers. In *Theory and Applications of Nonparenteral Nanomedicines*; Kesharwani, P., Taurin, S., Greish, K., Eds.; Academic Press: Cambridge, MA, USA, 2021; Chapter 7; pp. 137–152.
23. Agrawal, M.; Saraf, S.; Saraf, S.; Dubey, S.K.; Puri, A.; Gupta, U.; Kesharwani, P.; Ravichandiran, V.; Kumar, P.; Naidu, V.G.M.; et al. Stimuli-responsive In situ gelling system for nose-to-brain drug delivery. *J. Control. Release* **2020**, *327*, 235–265. [CrossRef]
24. Sarma, A.; Das, M.K. Nose to brain delivery of antiretroviral drugs in the treatment of neuroAIDS. *Mol. Biomed.* **2020**, *1*, 15. [CrossRef]
25. Hoang, V.D.; Uchenna, A.R.; Mark, J.; Renaat, K.; Norbert, V. Characterization of human nasal primary culture systems to investigate peptide metabolism. *Int. J. Pharm.* **2002**, *238*, 247–256. [CrossRef]
26. Dimova, S.; Brewster, M.E.; Noppe, M.; Jorissen, M.; Augustijns, P. The use of human nasal in vitro cell systems during drug discovery and development. *Toxicol. Vitr.* **2005**, *19*, 107–122. [CrossRef]
27. Merkle, H.P.; Ditzinger, G.; Lang, S.R.; Peter, H.; Schmidt, M.C. In vitro cell models to study nasal mucosal permeability and metabolism. *Adv. Drug Deliv. Rev.* **1998**, *29*, 51–79. [PubMed]
28. Wengst, A.; Reichl, S. RPMI 2650 epithelial model and three-dimensional reconstructed human nasal mucosa as in vitro models for nasal permeation studies. *Eur. J. Pharm. Biopharm.* **2010**, *74*, 290–297. [CrossRef] [PubMed]
29. Bai, S.; Yang, T.; Abbruscato, T.J.; Ahsan, F. Evaluation of human nasal RPMI 2650 cells grown at an air-liquid interface as a model for nasal drug transport studies. *J. Pharm. Sci.* **2008**, *97*, 1165–1178. [CrossRef] [PubMed]
30. Kreft, M.E.; Jerman, U.D.; Lasič, E.; Rižner, T.L.; Hevir-Kene, N.; Peternel, L.; Kristan, K. The Characterization of the Human Nasal Epithelial Cell Line RPMI 2650 Under Different Culture Conditions and Their Optimization for an Appropriate in vitro Nasal Model. *Pharm. Res.* **2015**, *32*, 665–679. [CrossRef]
31. Dolberg, A.M.; Reichl, S. Expression of P-glycoprotein in excised human nasal mucosa and optimized models of RPMI 2650 cells. *Int. J. Pharm.* **2016**, *508*, 22–33. [CrossRef]
32. Gil-Martins, E.; Barbosa, D.J.; Silva, V.; Remião, F.; Silva, R. Dysfunction of ABC transporters at the blood-brain barrier: Role in neurological disorders. *Pharmacol. Ther.* **2020**, *213*, 107554. [CrossRef]
33. Sibinovska, N.; Žakelj, S.; Roškar, R.; Kristan, K. Suitability and functional characterization of two Calu-3 cell models for prediction of drug permeability across the airway epithelial barrier. *Int. J. Pharm.* **2020**, *585*, 119484. [CrossRef]
34. Gonçalves, V.S.S.; Matias, A.A.; Poejo, J.; Serra, A.T.; Duarte, C.M.M. Application of RPMI 2650 as a cell model to evaluate solid formulations for intranasal delivery of drugs. *Int. J. Pharm.* **2016**, *515*, 1–10. [CrossRef]
35. Mercier, C.; Perek, N.; Delavenne, X. Is RPMI 2650 a Suitable In Vitro Nasal Model. for Drug Transport. Studies? *Eur. J. Drug Metab. Pharm.* **2018**, *43*, 13–24. [CrossRef] [PubMed]
36. Sibinovska, N.; Žakelj, S.; Kristan, K. Suitability of RPMI 2650 cell models for nasal drug permeability prediction. *Eur. J. Pharm. Biopharm.* **2019**, *145*, 85–95. [CrossRef]

37. Charles, D.D.; Fisher, J.R.; Hoskinson, S.M.; Medina-Colorado, A.A.; Shen, Y.C.; Chaaban, M.R.; Widen, S.G.; Eaves-Pyles, T.D.; Maxwell, C.A.; Miller, A.L.; et al. Development of a Novel ex vivo Nasal Epithelial Cell Model. *Supporting Colonization With Human Nasal Microbiota. Front. Cell. Infect. Microbiol.* **2019**, *9*, 165. [CrossRef]
38. Keller, L.-A.; Merkel, O.; Popp, A. Intranasal drug delivery: Opportunities and toxicologic challenges during drug development. *Drug Deliv. Transl. Res.* **2021**, 1–23.
39. Hood, A.T.; Currie, D.; Garte, S.J. Establishment of a rat nasal epithelial tumor cell line. *In Vitro Cell Dev. Biol.* **1987**, *23*, 274–278. [CrossRef]
40. Kreft, M.E.; Tratnjek, L.; Lasič, E.; Hevir, N.; Rižner, T.L.; Kristan, K. Different Culture Conditions Affect. *Drug Transporter Gene Expression, Ultrastructure, and Permeability of Primary Human Nasal Epithelial Cells. Pharm. Res.* **2020**, *37*, 170.
41. Moore, G.E.; Sandberg, A.A. Studies of a human tumor cell line with a diploid karyotype. *Cancer* **1964**, *17*, 170–175. [CrossRef]
42. Furubayashi, T.; Inoue, D.; Nishiyama, N.; Tanaka, A.; Yutani, R.; Kimura, S.; Katsumi, H.; Yamamoto, A.; Sakane, T. Comparison of Various Cell Lines and Three-Dimensional Mucociliary Tissue Model. *Systems to Estimate Drug Permeability Using an In Vitro Transport. Study to Predict Nasal Drug Absorption in Rats. Pharmaceutics* **2020**, *12*, 79.
43. Volpe, D.A. Drug-permeability and transporter assays in Caco-2 and MDCK cell lines. *Future Med. Chem.* **2011**, *3*, 2063–2077. [CrossRef]
44. Sarmento, B.; Andrade, F.; Baptista da Silva, S.; Rodrigues, F.; Neves, J.; Ferreira, D. Cell-based in vitro models for predicting drug permeability. *Expert Opin. Drug Metab. Toxicol.* **2012**, *8*, 607–621. [CrossRef]
45. Forbes, B.; Shah, A.; Martin, G.P.; Lansley, A.B. The human bronchial epithelial cell line 16HBE14o- as a model system of the airways for studying drug transport. *Int. J. Pharm.* **2003**, *257*, 161–167. [CrossRef]
46. Callaghan, P.J.; Ferrick, B.; Rybakovsky, E.; Thomas, S.; Mullin, J.M. Epithelial barrier function properties of the 16HBE14o- human bronchial epithelial cell culture model. *Biosci. Rep.* **2020**, *40*, BSR20201532. [CrossRef]
47. Ghasemiyeh, P.; Mohammadi-Samani, S. Solid lipid nanoparticles and nanostructured lipid carriers as novel drug delivery systems: Applications, advantages and disadvantages. *Res. Pharm. Sci.* **2018**, *13*, 288–303.
48. Cunha, S.; Almeida, H.; Amaral, M.H.; Sousa Lobo, J.M.; Silva, A.C. Intranasal lipid nanoparticles for the treatment of neurodegenerative diseases. *Curr. Pharm. Des.* **2017**, *23*, 6553–6562. [CrossRef]
49. Silva, A.C.; Santos, D.; Ferreira, D.; Lopes, C.M. Lipid-based Nanocarriers As An. *Alternative for Oral Delivery of Poorly Water-Soluble Drugs: Peroral and Mucosal Routes. Curr. Med. Chem.* **2012**, *19*, 4495–4510.
50. Silva, A.C.; González-Mira, E.; Sousa Lobo, J.M.; Amaral, M.H. Current progresses on nanodelivery systems for the treatment of neuropsychiatric diseases: Alzheimer's and schizophrenia. *Curr. Pharm. Des.* **2013**, *19*, 7185–7195. [CrossRef]
51. Almeida, H.; Amaral, M.H.; Lobão, P.; Silva, A.C.; Sousa Lobo, J.M. Applications of polymeric and lipid nanoparticles in ophthalmic pharmaceutical formulations: Present and future considerations. *J. Pharm. Pharm. Sci.* **2014**, *17*, 278–293. [CrossRef]
52. Silva, A.C.; Amaral, M.H.; Sousa Lobo, J.M.; Lopes, C.M. Lipid nanoparticles for the delivery of biopharmaceuticals. *Curr. Pharm. Biotechnol.* **2015**, *16*, 291–302. [CrossRef]
53. Garcês, A.; Amaral, M.H.; Sousa Lobo, J.M.; Silva, A.C. Formulations based on solid lipid nanoparticles (SLN) and nanostructured lipid carriers (NLC) for cutaneous use: A review. *Eur. J. Pharm. Sci.* **2018**, *112*, 159–167. [CrossRef]
54. Silva, A.C.; Amaral, M.H.; Sousa Lobo, J.M.; Almeida, H. Editorial: Applications of Solid Lipid Nanoparticles (SLN) and Nanostructured Lipid Carriers (NLC): State of the Art. *Curr. Pharm. Des.* **2017**, *23*, 6551–6552. [CrossRef]
55. Mehnert, W.; Mäder, K. Solid lipid nanoparticles: Production, characterization and applications. *Adv. Drug Deliv. Rev.* **2012**, *64*, 83–101. [CrossRef]
56. Müller, R.H.; Mäder, K.; Gohla, S. Solid lipid nanoparticles (SLN) for controlled drug delivery–a review of the state of the art. *Eur. J. Pharm. Biopharm.* **2000**, *50*, 161–177. [CrossRef]
57. Müller, R.H.; Radtke, M.; Wissing, S.A. Solid lipid nanoparticles (SLN) and nanostructured lipid carriers (NLC) in cosmetic and dermatological preparations. *Adv. Drug Deliv. Rev.* **2002**, *54*, S131–S155. [CrossRef]
58. Pardeike, J.; Hommoss, A.; Müller, R.H. Lipid nanoparticles (SLN, NLC) in cosmetic and pharmaceutical dermal products. *Int. J. Pharm.* **2009**, *366*, 170–184. [CrossRef]
59. Muller, R.H.; Shegokar, R.; Keck, C.M. 20 years of lipid nanoparticles (SLN & NLC): Present state of development & industrial applications. *Curr. Drug Discov. Technol.* **2011**, *8*, 207–227.
60. Müller, R.H.; Petersen, R.D.; Hommoss, A.; Pardeike, J. Nanostructured lipid carriers (NLC) in cosmetic dermal products. *Adv. Drug Deliv. Rev.* **2007**, *59*, 522–530. [CrossRef]
61. Weber, S.; Zimmer, A.; Pardeike, J. Solid Lipid Nanoparticles (SLN) and Nanostructured Lipid Carriers (NLC) for pulmonary application: A review of the state of the art. *Eur. J. Pharm. Biopharm.* **2014**, *86*, 7–22. [CrossRef]
62. Üner, M. Preparation, characterization and physico-chemical properties of Solid Lipid Nanoparticles (SLN) and Nanostructured Lipid Carriers (NLC): Their benefits as colloidal drug carrier systems. *Die Pharm. Int. J. Pharm. Sci.* **2006**, *61*, 375–386.
63. Wissing, S.A.; Kayser, O.; Müller, R.H. Solid lipid nanoparticles for parenteral drug delivery. *Adv. Drug Deliv. Rev.* **2004**, *56*, 1257–1272. [CrossRef]
64. Almeida, H.; Amaral, M.H.; Lobão, P.; Sousa Lobo, J.M. In situ gelling systems: A strategy to improve the bioavailability of ophthalmic pharmaceutical formulations. *Drug Discov. Today* **2014**, *19*, 400–412. [CrossRef]
65. Almeida, H.; Amaral, M.H.; Lobão, P.; Sousa Lobo, J.M. Applications of poloxamers in ophthalmic pharmaceutical formulations: An overview. *Expert Opin. Drug Deliv.* **2013**, *10*, 1223–1237. [CrossRef]

66. Wang, Q.; Zuo, Z.; Cheung, C.K.C.; Leung, S.S.Y. Updates on thermosensitive hydrogel for nasal, ocular and cutaneous delivery. *Int. J. Pharm.* **2019**, *559*, 86–101. [CrossRef]
67. Karavasili, C.; Fatouros, D.G. Smart materials: In situ gel-forming systems for nasal delivery. *Drug Discov. Today* **2016**, *21*, 157–166. [CrossRef] [PubMed]
68. Nižić, L.; Potás, J.; Winnicka, K.; Szekalska, M.; Erak, I.; Gretić, M.; Jug, M.; Hafner, A. Development, characterisation and nasal deposition of melatonin-loaded pectin/hypromellose microspheres. *Eur. J. Pharm. Sci.* **2020**, *141*, 105115. [CrossRef] [PubMed]
69. Chonkar, A.; Nayak, U.; Udupa, N. Smart Polymers in Nasal Drug Delivery. *Indian J. Pharm. Sci.* **2015**, *77*, 367–375.
70. Nižić, L.; Ugrina, I.; Špoljarić, D.; Saršon, V.; Kučuk, M.S.; Pepić, I.; Hafner, A. Innovative sprayable in situ gelling fluticasone suspension: Development and optimization of nasal deposition. *Int. J. Pharm.* **2019**, *563*, 445–456. [CrossRef] [PubMed]
71. Du, W.; Li, H.; Tian, B.; Sai, S.; Gao, Y.; Lan, T.; Meng, Y.; Ding, C. Development of nose-to-brain delivery of ketoconazole by nanostructured lipid carriers against cryptococcal meningoencephalitis in mice. *Colloids Surf. B Biointerfaces* **2019**, *183*, 110446. [CrossRef]
72. Jojo, G.M.; Kuppusamy, G.; De, A.; Karri, V.V.S.N.R. Formulation and optimization of intranasal nanolipid carriers of pioglitazone for the repurposing in Alzheimer's disease using Box-Behnken design. *Drug Dev. Ind. Pharm.* **2019**, *45*, 1061–1072. [CrossRef] [PubMed]
73. Silva, S.; Marto, J.; Gonçalves, L.; Almeida, A.J.; Vale, N. Formulation, Characterization and Evaluation against SH-SY5Y Cells of New Tacrine and Tacrine-MAP Loaded with Lipid Nanoparticles. *Nanomaterials* **2020**, *10*, 2089. [CrossRef]
74. Trapani, A.; Guerra, L.; Corbo, F.; Castellani, S.; Sanna, E.; Capobianco, L.; Monteduro, A.G.; Manno, D.E.; Mandracchia, D.; Di Giola, S.; et al. Cyto/Biocompatibility of Dopamine Combined with the Antioxidant Grape Seed-Derived Polyphenol Compounds in Solid Lipid Nanoparticles. *Molecules* **2021**, *26*, 916. [CrossRef]
75. Wang, L.; Zhao, X.; Du, J.; Liu, M.; Feng, J.; Hu, K. Improved brain delivery of pueraria flavones via intranasal administration of borneol-modified solid lipid nanoparticles. *Nanomedicine* **2019**, *14*, 2105–2119. [CrossRef]
76. Sadegh Malvajerd, S.; Azadi, A.; Izadi, Z.; Kurd, M.; Dara, T.; Dibaei, M.; Zadeh, M.S.; Javar, H.A.; Hamidi, M. Brain Delivery of Curcumin Using Solid Lipid Nanoparticles and Nanostructured Lipid Carriers: Preparation, Optimization, and Pharmacokinetic Evaluation. *ACS Chem. Neurosci.* **2019**, *10*, 728–739. [CrossRef] [PubMed]
77. Khanna, K.; Sharma, N.; Rawat, S.; Khan, N.; Karwasra, R.; Hasan, N.; Kumar, A.; Jain, G.K.; Nishad, D.K.; Khanna, S.; et al. Intranasal solid lipid nanoparticles for management of pain: A full factorial design approach, characterization & Gamma Scintigraphy. *Chem. Phys. Lipids* **2021**, *236*, 105060.
78. Sarma, A.; Das, M.K.; Chakraborty, T.; Das, S. Nanostructured lipid carriers (NLCs)-based intranasal Drug Delivery System of Tenofovir disoproxil fumerate (TDF) for brain targeting. *Res. J. Pharm. Technol.* **2020**, *13*, 5411–5424.
79. Gadhave, D.; Rasal, N.; Sonawane, R.; Sekar, M.; Kokare, C. Nose-to-brain delivery of teriflunomide-loaded lipid-based carbopol-gellan gum nanogel for glioma: Pharmacological and in vitro cytotoxicity studies. *Int. J. Biol. Macromol.* **2021**, *167*, 906–920. [CrossRef]
80. Sun, Y.; Li, L.; Xie, H.; Wang, Y.; Gao, S.; Zhang, L.; Bo, F.; Yang, S.; Feng, A. Primary Studies on Construction and Evaluation of Ion.-Sensitive in situ Gel Loaded with Paeonol-Solid Lipid Nanoparticles for Intranasal Drug Delivery. *Int. J. Nanomed.* **2020**, *15*, 3137–3160. [CrossRef]
81. Schroeter, J.D.; Tewksbury, E.W.; Wong, B.A.; Kimbell, J.S. Experimental measurements and computational predictions of regional particle deposition in a sectional nasal model. *J. Aerosol. Med. Pulm. Drug Deliv.* **2015**, *28*, 20–29. [CrossRef] [PubMed]
82. Xi, J.; Yuan, J.E.; Zhang, Y.; Nevorski, D.; Wang, Z.; Zhou, Y. Visualization and Quantification of Nasal and Olfactory Deposition in a Sectional Adult Nasal Airway Cast. *Pharm. Res.* **2016**, *33*, 1527–1541. [CrossRef] [PubMed]
83. Sosnowski, T.R.; Rapiejko, P.; Sova, J.; Dobrowolska, K. Impact of physicochemical properties of nasal spray products on drug deposition and transport in the pediatric nasal cavity model. *Int. J. Pharm.* **2020**, *574*, 118911. [CrossRef] [PubMed]
84. Djupesland, P.G. Nasal drug delivery devices: Characteristics and performance in a clinical perspective-a review. *Drug Deliv. Transl. Res.* **2013**, *3*, 42–62. [CrossRef]
85. Nižić Nodilo, L.; Ugrina, I.; Špoljarić, D.; Amidžić Klarić, D.; Jakobušić Brala, C.; Perkušić, M.; Pepić, I.; Lovrić, J.; Saršon, V.; Safundžić Kučuk, M.; et al. A Dry Powder Platform for Nose-to-Brain Delivery of Dexamethasone: Formulation Development and Nasal Deposition Studies. *Pharmaceutics* **2021**, *13*, 795. [CrossRef] [PubMed]
86. Setty, Y. EBrain: A Three Dimensional Simulation Tool to Study Drug Delivery in the Brain. *Sci. Rep.* **2019**, *9*, 6162. [CrossRef] [PubMed]
87. Sawant, N.; Donovan, M.D. In Vitro Assessment of Spray Deposition Patterns in a Pediatric (12 Year-Old) Nasal Cavity Model. *Pharm. Res.* **2018**, *35*, 108. [CrossRef]
88. Warnken, Z.N.; Smyth, H.D.C.; Davis, D.A.; Weitman, S.; Kuhn, J.G.; Williams 3rd, R.O. Personalized Medicine in Nasal Delivery: The Use of Patient-Specific Administration Parameters To Improve Nasal Drug Targeting Using 3D-Printed Nasal Replica Casts. *Mol. Pharm.* **2018**, *15*, 1392–1402. [CrossRef]
89. Pu, Y.; Goodey, A.P.; Fang, X.; Jacob, K. A Comparison of the Deposition Patterns of Different Nasal Spray Formulations Using a Nasal Cast. *Aerosol. Sci. Technol.* **2014**, *48*, 930–938. [CrossRef]
90. Deruyver, L.; Rigaut, C.; Lambert, P.; Haut, B.; Goole, J. The importance of pre-formulation studies and of 3D-printed nasal casts in the success of a pharmaceutical product intended for nose-to-brain delivery. *Adv. Drug Deliv. Rev.* **2021**, *175*, 113826. [CrossRef]

91. Gholizadeh, H.; Messerotti, E.; Pozzoli, M.; Cheng, S.; Traini, D.; Young, P.; Kourmatzis, A.; Caramella, C.; Ong, H.X. Application of a Thermosensitive In Situ Gel of Chitosan-Based Nasal Spray Loaded with Tranexamic Acid for Localised Treatment of Nasal Wounds. *AAPS PharmSciTech* **2019**, *20*, 299. [CrossRef]
92. Xi, J.; Wang, J.; Si, X.A.; Zhou, Y. Nasal dilation effects on olfactory deposition in unilateral and bi-directional deliveries: In vitro tests and numerical modeling. *Eur. J. Pharm. Sci.* **2018**, *118*, 113–123. [CrossRef] [PubMed]
93. Hosseini, S.; Golshahi, L. An in vitro evaluation of importance of airway anatomy in sub-regional nasal and paranasal drug delivery with nebulizers using three different anatomical nasal airway replicas of 2-, 5- and 50-Year old human subjects. *Int. J. Pharm.* **2019**, *563*, 426–436. [CrossRef]
94. Hosseini, S.; Wei, X.; Wilkins, J.V., Jr.; Fergusson, C.P.; Mohammadi, R.; Vorona, G.; Golshahi, L. In Vitro Measurement of Regional Nasal Drug Delivery with Flonase,(®) Flonase(®) Sensimist™ and MAD Nasal™ in Anatomically Correct Nasal Airway Replicas of Pediatric and Adult Human Subjects. *J. Aerosol. Med. Pulm. Drug Deliv.* **2019**, *32*, 374–385. [CrossRef]
95. Tian, L.; Shang, Y.; Chen, R.; Bai, R.; Chen, C.; Inthavong, K.; Tu, J. Correlation of regional deposition dosage for inhaled nanoparticles in human and rat olfactory. *Part. Fibre Toxicol.* **2019**, *16*, 6. [CrossRef] [PubMed]

pharmaceuticals

MDPI

Review

Pulmonary Delivery of Anticancer Drugs via Lipid-Based Nanocarriers for the Treatment of Lung Cancer: An Update

Ibrahim M. Abdulbaqi [1,2], Reem Abou Assi [1,2], Anan Yaghmur [3], Yusrida Darwis [1,*], Noratiqah Mohtar [1], Thaigarajan Parumasivam [1], Fadi G. Saqallah [1] and Habibah A. Wahab [1,*]

1 School of Pharmaceutical Sciences, Universiti Sains Malaysia, Minden, Penang 11800, Malaysia; ibrahimm.abdulbaqi@student.usm.my (I.M.A.); reemabouassi@student.usm.my (R.A.A.); noratiqah@usm.my (N.M.); thaigarp@usm.my (T.P.); fadi_saqallah@student.usm.my (F.G.S.)
2 College of Pharmacy, Al-Kitab University, Altun kupri, Kirkuk 36001, Iraq
3 Department of Pharmacy, Faculty of Health and Medical Sciences, University of Copenhagen, Universitetsparken 2, DK-2100 Copenhagen Ø, Denmark; anan.yaghmur@sund.ku.dk
* Correspondence: yusrida@usm.my (Y.D.); habibahw@usm.my (H.A.W.); Tel.: +604-6534588 (Y.D.); +604-6532211 (H.A.W.)

Abstract: Lung cancer (LC) is the leading cause of cancer-related deaths, responsible for approximately 18.4% of all cancer mortalities in both sexes combined. The use of systemic therapeutics remains one of the primary treatments for LC. However, the therapeutic efficacy of these agents is limited due to their associated severe adverse effects, systemic toxicity and poor selectivity. In contrast, pulmonary delivery of anticancer drugs can provide many advantages over conventional routes. The inhalation route allows the direct delivery of chemotherapeutic agents to the target LC cells with high local concertation that may enhance the antitumor activity and lead to lower dosing and fewer systemic toxicities. Nevertheless, this route faces by many physiological barriers and technological challenges that may significantly affect the lung deposition, retention, and efficacy of anticancer drugs. The use of lipid-based nanocarriers could potentially overcome these problems owing to their unique characteristics, such as the ability to entrap drugs with various physicochemical properties, and their enhanced permeability and retention (EPR) effect for passive targeting. Besides, they can be functionalized with different targeting moieties for active targeting. This article highlights the physiological, physicochemical, and technological considerations for efficient inhalable anticancer delivery using lipid-based nanocarriers and their cutting-edge role in LC treatment.

Keywords: lung cancer; targeted drug delivery; lipid-based nanocarriers; pulmonary delivery; dry powder inhalers; aerosols; liposomes; nanoemulsions; nanotechnology

Citation: Abdulbaqi, I.M.; Assi, R.A.; Yaghmur, A.; Darwis, Y.; Mohtar, N.; Parumasivam, T.; Saqallah, F.G.; Wahab, H.A. Pulmonary Delivery of Anticancer Drugs via Lipid-Based Nanocarriers for the Treatment of Lung Cancer: An Update. *Pharmaceuticals* **2021**, *14*, 725. https://doi.org/10.3390/ph14080725

Academic Editors: Ana Catarina Silva, João Nuno Moreira and José Manuel Sousa Lobo

Received: 1 June 2021
Accepted: 20 July 2021
Published: 27 July 2021

1. Introduction

Lung cancer (LC) is one of the major medical challenges worldwide. It is globally ranked as one of the most commonly diagnosed cancers, representing about 11.4% of all the reported cases and it is the leading cause for cancer-related deaths, responsible for approximately 18% of all cancer mortalities in both sexes combined [1,2]. In the United States alone, the American Cancer Society predicted that there will be around 235,760 new cases of LC (accounting for 12.4% of all the new diagnosed cancers) and around 131,880 deaths (accounting for 21.7% of all cancer deaths) in 2021. More persons die from LC annually than from cancer of the prostate, breast and colon combined [3,4]. Furthermore, the World Health Organization (WHO) estimates through the Global Cancer Observatory that from 2020 to 2040 the LC incidence and mortality rates for both men and women and all ages will increase by 64.4% and 67.5%, respectively [5,6].

LC may develop as a result of different environmental and genetic factors and their interactions. Tobacco smoking remains the primary cause; smokers are found to have 10- to 30-fold increased risk of developing LC in comparison to non-smokers. Other important factors include second-hand smoke, exposure to industrial and environmental hazards such as radon, asbestos, metals including chromium, cadmium and arsenic, exposure to different organic chemicals, ionizing radiation and a positive history of respiratory illnesses (e.g., bronchitis, emphysema, and tuberculosis). In families, first-degree relatives of LC probands have a 2- to 3-fold increased risk of LC and other malignancies, many of which are not smoking-related [7].

LC is classified into two main types, small cell lung cancer (SCLC) and non-small cell lung cancer (NSCLC). The latter is subdivided depending on the tumor tissue histology into three main histologic categories, including adenocarcinoma, squamous cell carcinoma, and large-cell carcinoma. NSCLC represents approximately 85% of all lung cancers, while SCLC is responsible for the remaining percentage [7,8]. The detection of LC at its early stages is crucial for best therapy outcomes, but unfortunately, the symptoms typically start to appear only at the advanced stages of the disease and sometimes they are masked by other concurrent respiratory conditions. Accordingly, the majority of patients are diagnosed with LC while the disease is at its advanced stages and turned out to be incurable with currently available treatments [9] with very poor prognosis and a 5-year survival rates of only 21% [4].

The treatment strategy depends on the type, stage of LC and the physical state of the patient. The currently available conventional treatment methods may include surgery, high doses of intravenous chemotherapeutic agents, radiation therapy, targeted therapies, immunotherapy, and photodynamic or laser therapy [7,10]. Generally, surgery is confined to the early stages of LC and is typically combined with chemotherapy and/or radiation therapy to eradicate the cancerous tissue [9,11]. The use of single chemotherapeutic agents (such as cisplatin, paclitaxel, and etoposide) or their combinations remain the main treatment method for LC. However, the therapeutic efficacies of these cytotoxic drugs are limited due to their poor selectivity, the development of multidrug resistance, and besides, their use is associated with severe adverse effects and systemic toxicity symptoms including anemia, nausea, vomiting, nephrotoxicity and neurotoxicity which in turn limit their use [12,13]. Therefore, and for a complete cure and eradication of LC, there is an immediate need to use and investigate the possible potential roles of different routes of drug administration such as the pulmonary route and novel drug delivery systems such as nanoscale materials that are highly effective with excellent targeting abilities against the LC cells and display improved toxicity profiles.

Nanotechnology represents a powerful tool in the hands of researchers today for enhancing the currently available classical therapies and developing new therapeutic strategies and diagnostic tools to combat LC. The extensive research in this field has yielded a wide range of nanosystems (including the lipid-based nanocarriers) that have the potential to dramatically change how LC is treated nowadays [13–15]. This is attributed to their ability to entrap drugs with different physicochemical properties, suitability for combination therapy, and enhanced permeability and retention (EPR) effect which makes them highly effective in passive targeting, besides; their surface could be functionalized with different targeting moieties for active targeting, so they can selectively target cancerous cells and neoplasms.

In this contribution, the potential role, advantages, and challenges associated with using the pulmonary route to deliver anticancer drugs via lipid-based nanocarriers are presented. The physicochemical aspects that should be considered for efficient delivery, the recent technologies, materials, and lung delivery devices used to formulate and deliver different anticancer drug-loaded lipid-based nanocarriers are discussed. Furthermore, the advances in using the inhalable lipid-based nanocarriers for combating LC and their evaluation on the in vitro, in vivo, and clinical studies are presented.

2. Methodology

The literature selection in this review was performed by manually searching the PubMed, Google Scholar, ScienceDirect, and Wiley Library databases for published literature on inhalable chemotherapy via lipid-based nanocarriers using various keywords such as (Inhaled/aerosolized/nebulized/dry powder inhalers/inhalable chemotherapy for LC, inhaled liposomes for LC, aerosolized solid lipid nanoparticles (SLNs) for LC, DPIs of nanostructured lipid carriers (NLCs) for LC, inhalable nanoemulsions (NEs) for LC, lipid-based nanoparticles for LC, etc.). For liposomes, examples of the most recent (2010–2021) studies about inhalable anticancer drug-loaded liposomal formulations that involved in vivo studies were included in this study. All the published research work for the other types of lipid-based nanocarriers (i.e., NEs, SLNs, NLCs, niosomes, and others) designed as inhalable anticancer drug-loaded formulations for the treatment and/or diagnosis of LC were reviewed in this study.

3. Inhalable Anticancer Therapy via Lipid-Based Nanocarriers: Main Advantages and Critical Challenges

Drug delivery for the treatment of LC using lipid-based nanocarriers is achieved mainly via the intravenous and pulmonary routes of administration. Regional drug delivery methods at the tumor site are also considered for certain cases.

Pulmonary delivery of anticancer drugs via lipid-based nanoparticles for LC treatment is a growing and expanding area of research. This route of drug administration is non-invasive (needle free), provides better patient compliance, and can be self-administered. It can be used to overcome the drawbacks associated with the oral or intravenous routes that may include high levels of systemic toxicity, poor aqueous solubility of the anticancer agents, low drug accumulation within the tumor, and high rates of tumor relapse [16].

The use of inhalable lipid-based nanocarriers could provide many advantages over the conventional routes for LC treatment, especially for patients with surgically unresectable LC. Pharmacokinetically, inhalation allows the delivery of chemotherapeutic agents to the target cancer cells and avoids the hepatic metabolism; thus, rapid onset of action, lower dosing and fewer systemic distribution and toxicities are expected [17]. Moreover, the alveolar region in the lungs has a large surface area of ~100 m^2, extensive vasculature, and limited drug-metabolizing enzymatic activity compared to other organs such as the liver and the gastrointestinal tract. In addition, the alveolar epithelium is extremely thin (0.1–0.2 μm), which is much thinner than that in the upper bronchial tree (50–60 μm). Thus, drug absorption and bioavailability in the targeted region may be further improved [18,19]. Additionally, phospholipids, which are major constituents of many lipid-based nanoparticles, especially liposomes, are present in the lungs and constitute almost 90% of lung surfactants [20]. This favors the design of more biocompatible lipid-based formulation and enhances lung tolerability to the delivered anticancer agent. All these factors may significantly decrease treatment failures, development of drug resistance, and chemotherapy interruptions that are responsible for the repopulation of cancerous cells. Subsequently, tumors refractory to traditional systemic chemotherapy could also potentially respond to inhalational therapy.

Pulmonary drug delivery via lipid-based carriers allows anticancer drugs to target and reach various lung tumors via different pathways. After deposition in the respiratory tract, the inhaled drug can target lung tumors by directly penetrating the tumor via the achievement of elevated local concentrations and significantly high concentration gradients of therapeutic agents at the lung tumor site. Certain types of lung tumors such as squamous cell carcinomas or bronchioloalveolar cell carcinomas that are found next to or within the airways might take up the deposited drug by direct penetration. Furthermore, drugs delivered to the lung by inhalable lipid carriers can be absorbed into the local blood circulations. Due to the communication between the bronchial and pulmonary circulations, sufficient drug concentration could reach lung tumors that lack a direct connection with the main airways depending on the tumor site. The bronchial vasculature nourishes lung tumors if they are located in the conducting region, while the pulmonary circulation feeds them if they are sited at the respiratory region [21–23]. However, the absorption, lung clearance mechanisms, biodistribution, and tumor penetration of inhaled drug-loaded particles are subject to many factors such as the physicochemical properties of the drug/particles, the characteristics and composition of the used formulation, the site of dug deposition, the histological features of the respiratory system, the associated pathological condition. In this regard, Haque et al. evaluated how inhaled liposomal formulation affects existing lung disease by comparing the pulmonary pharmacokinetic behavior of drug-loaded ^{3}H-labelled PEGylated liposomes after intratracheal administration to healthy rats and rats with bleomycin-induced lung inflammation by following both ^{3}H label and drug. The results showed that liposomes were initially cleared more rapidly from inflamed lungs than from the healthy ones but exhibited similar rates of lung clearance after three days. This was interesting given that mucociliary clearance was more efficient from healthy lungs, despite evidence of higher mucus retention in inflamed lungs and reduced association of the liposomes with lung tissue. The plasma pharmacokinetics of ^{3}H-phosphatidylcholine revealed higher liposomal bioavailability and more prolonged absorption from inflamed lungs. Concentrations of the pro-inflammatory cytokine IL-1β were increased in bronchoalveolar lavage fluid after a single pulmonary dose of liposomes to rats with inflamed lungs, but no other significant changes in inflammatory lung markers were identified in healthy or bleomycin-challenged rats [24]. Moreover, inhaled drugs are also drained by the lymphatic system; they were commonly detected in the lungs' lymph nodes (Figure 1). Consequently, these nodes are considered as potential targets for the inhaled drug to suppress cancer metastasis to and from the lungs [25–27]. Videira et al. described the biodistribution of radiolabeled (^{99m}Tc) solid lipid nanoparticles (SLNs) following their pulmonary delivery to male Wistar rats. A 60 min dynamic image acquisition was performed in a gamma-camera, followed by static image collection at 30 min intervals up to 4 h post inhalation. Radiation counting was performed in organ samples collected after the animals were sacrificed. The results revealed a significant uptake of the radiolabeled SLNs into the lymphatics after inhalation and a high distribution rate in periaortic, axillar, and inguinal lymph nodes [28]. Due to all these remarkable advantages inhalation therapy is having the potential to become an effective and safe delivery method for the treatment of LC.

Despite the aforementioned advantages, we should bear in mind that the pulmonary drug delivery of anticancer drugs via lipid-based nanocarriers for LC treatment is confronted by some challenges and limitations. One of the major concerns is the lung tolerance and the potential risk of local pulmonary toxicity and adverse effects because of the cytotoxic activity of anticancer drugs themselves. Besides, the lungs' health of LC patients is often impaired either due to LC complications or because of the presence of other concomitant lung diseases such as asthma or chronic obstructive pulmonary diseases that can significantly affect patients' ability to tolerate the inhalable anticancer therapy.

Results from the so far conducted and published clinical trials (see Section 7) of nebulized liposomal chemotherapeutics such as 9-nitrocamptothecin (9NC) (phase I) [29], cisplatin (CIS) (phase I and Ib/IIa), (NCT00102531) [30–32] for the treatment of LC revealed that they have relatively safe profiles. The most reported side effects or dose-limiting toxicities (DLT) were mainly related to the respiratory tract, where grade 3 chemical pharyngitis and grade 3 bronchitis are reported as the most severe side effects [29,30]. To reduce these adverse effects, prophylactic doses of bronchodilators and/or corticosteroids before starting the anticancer inhalation therapy were used and/or recommended in clinical trials; they were found to help controlling these effects [29,33–35].

Furthermore, the inhaled drug-loaded particles are faced by various lung clearance mechanisms depending on various factors (Figure 1). These mechanisms can clear these particles from the lungs before reaching their targeted sites or reduce their residence time before exerting their desired therapeutic effects. The mucociliary clearance is the predominant mechanism in the conducting zone; the inhaled particles will be carried from the bronchial region to the larynx and then transferred to the gastrointestinal tract by swallowing. Almost 80 to 90 percent of the inhaled particulates can be excreted from the central and upper airways by this mechanism within 24 h. The lining mucus blanket (with thickness up to 30 μm) secreted by the goblet cells in this region represents another barrier. Additionally, particles on the alveolar epithelium (respiratory zone) may be phagocytosed by alveolar macrophages leading to lysosomal degradation, or they are taken to the upper respiratory tract by mucociliary escalator. The macrophages tend to engulf particles with geometric size of 0.5 to 5 μm. The alveolar epithelium, on the other hand, is covered by lung surfactants which can aid in drug dissolution and diffusion. If drugs are dissolved, they are either absorbed by the blood or lymphatic circulations or subjected to enzymatic degradation [36–40]. Lipid-based nanocarriers were employed efficiently to overcome these challenges and obtain improved therapeutic outcomes by ensuring longer drug-residence time and sustained release of therapeutic agents in the targeted sites of the lungs. Xu et al. developed a spray-dried liposomal formulation of vincristine and tested the absorption and tissue distribution of the drug after the intratracheal administration of the formulation in male SD rats. The liposomal formulation was able to enhance the pharmacokinetic behavior of the drug by decreasing drug clearance and elimination half-life by 83.2% and 81.1%, respectively, compared to the free drug solution [41]. After pulmonary delivery of paclitaxel-loaded, surface-modified solid lipid nanoparticles (SLNs) with a folate-grafted copolymer of polyethylene glycol (PEG) and chitosan, the formulation was found to significantly prolong the pulmonary exposure to the drug to up to 6 h in vivo (in female CD-1 and BALB/c mice) and limit the systemic distribution of the drug compared to inhaled Taxol-like formulation [42].

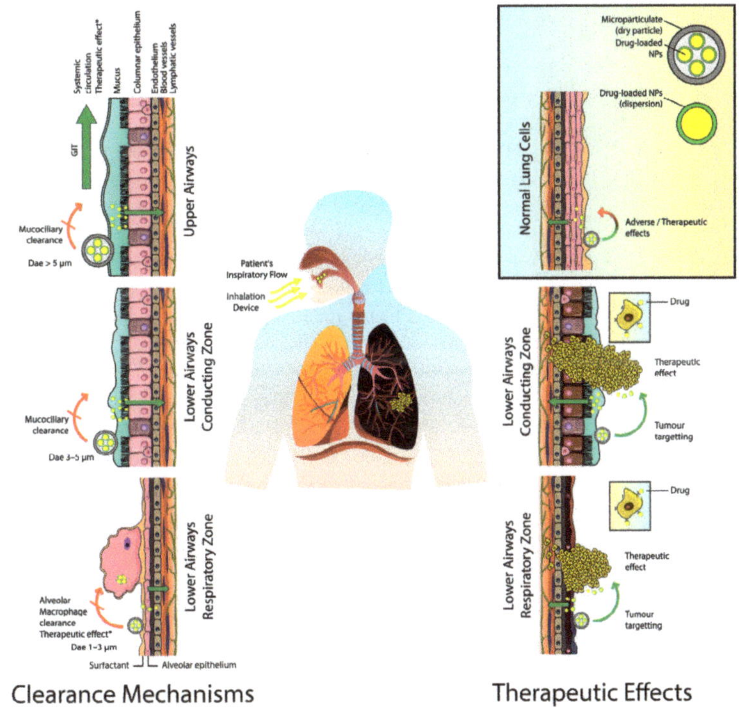

Figure 1. The involved clearance mechanisms and therapeutic effects of the inhaled anticancer agents-loaded nanocarriers. D_{ae}, aerodynamic diameter; GIT, gastrointestinal tract; NPs, nanoparticles. * Therapeutic effects are obtained via expression/secretion of anticancer proteins or induction of anticancer immune responses.

4. Physicochemical Considerations, Passive, and Active Targeting For Efficient Pulmonary Delivery of Anticancer Drugs via Lipid-Based Nanocarriers

The physicochemical properties of the anticancer drugs, nano or microcarriers, should be well considered while designing inhalation formulations because they will affect the drug residence time within the lungs and, consequently, the therapeutic efficacy. In order to achieve the required pharmacodynamic effects, anticancer agents must be available to cancerous cells within a minimum period of time. Drugs that are readily absorbed by the lungs may then be ineffective in treating the disease. Generally, lipophilic drugs with (log P > 0) are absorbed rapidly from the lungs because of their higher ability to diffuse in the lipid membranes. In contrast, hydrophilic drugs (log P < 0) tend to have longer lung residence times [43]. As a result, formulation techniques to increase lung residence of the lipophilic drugs and prolong their exposure time to cancer must be adopted.

Aerosols of drug-loaded lipid-based nanoparticles (either as liquid dispersions or dry powders) can be deposited via various mechanisms such as inertial impaction, sedimentation, and Brownian diffusion on the respiratory epithelium. These mechanisms are governed primarily by the aerodynamic diameter (D_{ae}) of the generated aerosol particles. The D_{ae} is the most precise parameter for measuring the aerosol particle size. It can correlate the particles' dynamic behavior as it is calculated based on their geometric size, density, and dynamic shape. There is a consensus in the literature that for efficient pulmonary delivery, the inhaled particles should be with D_{ae} of (1–5 μm) to reach the lower respiratory tract and in the range of (1–3 μm) for the respiratory zone. Particles with ($D_{ae} > 5$) μm will be deposited in the upper respiratory tract, while smaller particles those with ($D_{ae} < 0.5$) μm are expected to be emitted out of the body via the expiratory airflow [44–47]. The lipid-based nanocarriers, can be aerosolized and delivered to the lungs as dispersions by nebulization. At the same time, due to their extremely small geometric size, they must be incorporated in secondary carriers (microparticles) to be delivered as dry powders. Various particle engineering techniques were applied for their preparation and are discussed in Section 5.

Particle shape can also substantially contribute to the developed inhaled anticancer formulation's therapeutic efficiency because it can determine the extent of alveolar macrophage clearance. The relationship between different particles' shapes (i.e., elliptical disks, spherical, oblate ellipsoids, rectangular disks, and worm-like shape) and the time that was taken for their clearance by phagocytosis was previously investigated [48,49]. It was found that the shape and orientation of these particles significantly affect their phagocytosis clearance time. Phagocytosis was initiated for all shapes in at least one orientation. Due to macrophages' attachment to their principal axes, elliptical discs were engulfed in less than 6 min. Regardless of the macrophage attachment point, the spherical particles were also cleared immediately. Interestingly, macrophage attachment to the flat surfaces or minor axes of the rectangular, elliptical disks, and oblate ellipsoids failed to clear these particles even after two h [48]. Furthermore, because of their low curvature region, worm-like shaped particles resulted in significantly less phagocytosis clearance than the spherical particles [49]. By the use of particle-engineering technologies, lipid based nanocarriers could be embedded in microparticles of different morphologies for possibly enhancing their delivery.

The surface charges of the inhaled particles could also influence their cellular uptake in addition to their clearance and retention in the lungs. The positively charged particles were reported to have better penetration into tumor cells because of their higher binding tendency with tumor cells [36]. Furthermore, cationic nanoparticles were shown to be taken up quickly by the lung epithelial cells and or macrophages shortly after their administration, unlike neutral and anionic nanoparticles of the same hydrodynamic diameters. Therefore, cationic nanoparticles are retained for a longer time within lung cells, limiting their translocation to lymph nodes and bloodstream [50].

Targeting cancerous cells via drug-loaded lipid-based nanoparticles could be done by the passive and active methods. Generally, via passive targeting, nanoparticles tend to leak preferentially into cancer tissue via permeable tumor vessels and are then retained in the tumor bed due to reduced lymphatic drainage. This phenomenon is known as the enhanced permeability and retention (EPR) effect [51]. However, the EPR effect is suggested to offer less than a twofold increment in drug delivered by a nanocarrier to tumors in comparison to critical healthy organs, resulting in subtherapeutic concentrations that are not sufficient to cure most cancers [52]. On the other hand, the active targeting can enhance the therapeutic efficacy and increase the selectivity of drug delivery by attaching targeting ligands (which bind to specific receptors on the tumor cells and endothelium) to the surfaces of nanocarriers [53]. The surfaces of the lipid-based nanocarriers are highly tunable and could be functionalized using with more than one type of functional groups and surface modification techniques to provide stealth characteristics (PEGylation), and active targeting towards the cancerous cells [54,55]. The main targeting sites in LC may include the overexpressed receptors on the surfaces of the cancer cells (e.g., epidermal growth factor receptor (EGFR), folate receptors (FRs), transferrin receptors (TfRs)), cellular organelles (e.g., mitochondria, lysosomes) and the LC microenvironment (e.g., vascular cell-adhesion molecules, cluster-of-differentiation 44, matrix-metalloproteases) [56]. The strategies of developing positively charged or surface modified uni, di, or multifunctional lipid-based nanocarriers using different ligands and targeting moieties for active targeting of LC are adopted by many researchers. The results of these studies in enhancing the pulmonary delivery and therapeutic efficiency of anticancer drugs on the in vitro and in vivo levels are discussed and summarized in Section 6 of this article. Another active targeting method of malignant cells can be achieved by the development of "stimuli-responsive" nanocarriers by taking advantage of the natural physiological conditions within the target tissue, such as elevated temperature or alteration in pH, or through the application of external stimuli such as a magnetic field or ultrasonic waves [54]. However, the potential role of different types of inhaled stimuli-responsive lipid-based nanoparticles, such as the thermo-sensitive, pH-sensitive, magnetic-field, and ultrasound responsive nanocarriers in the treatments of LC, is rarely investigated. In one study, inhaled magnetic and thermo-responsive lipid vehicles were incorporated with superparamagnetic iron-oxide nanoparticles and budesonide for controlled and targeted pulmonary delivery. The formulated dry powders had a fine particle fraction (FPF) of 30%. The formulations were shown to have an accelerated drug release rate at hyperthermic temperatures (45 °C). The authors concluded that the developed lipid matrix is a good and effective drug vehicle in targeted and controlled inhalation therapy [57].

In addition to the discussed physicochemical aspects, the pathophysiological aspects of the lungs should also be considered while developing an inhalable formulation for the treatment of LC. These might include LC type and stage, concomitant diseases such as asthma, chronic obstructive pulmonary diseases, and their associated changes to normal lung physiology should also be considered while developing an inhaled formulation for the treatment of LC. These considerations are well-reviewed and discussed elsewhere [36,58].

5. Devices for the Pulmonary Drug Delivery of Anticancer Drug-Loaded Lipid-Based Nanocarriers

Drug-loaded lipid-based nanoformulations are delivered to lungs as liquid-based (i.e., solutions, dipersions) or solid-based (i.e., dry powders) aerosol systems. Nebulizers, dry powder inhalers (DPIs), pressurized metered-dose inhalers (pMDIs), and soft-mist inhalers are the main types of devices to deliver therapeutic agents into the lungs.

For effective therapeutic outcomes, higher doses (ranging from one to tens of mg) of inhaled anticancer drugs must be deposited in the lungs. The pMDIs and soft-mist inhalers can only deliver smaller drug doses of less than 1 mg; therefore, they are rarely used to deliver anticancer drugs [59,60]. On the other side, nebulizers and DPIs are suitable for delivering higher drug doses necessary for the inhaled chemotherapeutic agents to act on the cancerous cells and tumors. Therefore, these devices have the potential to be used effectively for inhalable-based anticancer therapy.

Nebulizers are liquid-based aerosol delivery devices. Different types of these devices are available, including jet, vibrating mesh, and ultrasonic nebulizers; they deliver aerosols to the lungs as finely atomized droplets with high FPF over certain periods of time using compressed gas flow, oscillating perforated membrane, or piezoelectric crystals vibrating at high frequency, respectively [61]. They are the most used delivery systems of anticancer drugs-loaded lipid-based nanoparticles in preclinical studies and the only used ones in pilot studies and clinical trials (see Section 7). Nebulizers have many potential benefits. They generate large amounts of aerosolized droplets with an aerodynamic size of <5 μm from solutions or nanoparticles dispersions to be deposited in the lungs. Also, they need minor patient collaboration and are suitable for patients with chronic pulmonary illnesses such as LC who cannot perform active inhalation or receiving mechanical ventilation [62]. However, for the delivery of therapeutic doses, the nebulization process may need to continue over a long period and for multiple cycles. Furthermore, during nebulization, large amounts of the produced aerosols are not inhaled but instead, they are lost in the nebulizer or released into the air leading to air contamination. Therefore, the nebulization of anticancer drugs needs to be performed under hospital settings only, as specific protective and safety measures should be taken to protect healthcare givers and neighbors and prevent their exposure to chemotherapeutic agents. On the other hand, factors such as pH, osmolality, and viscosity of the developed inhaled nanoformulations dispersions should be well characterized and optimized for efficient delivery and prevent coughing, lung mucosa irritation, and bronchoconstriction [27,63,64]. Furthermore, the nebulization process of lipid-based nanoparticles using the different types of nebulizers could significantly affect the size, drug loading, and the in vitro release rate of these carriers. It was reported that during nebulization by jet nebulizer, the multilamellar liposomes (with particle size (PS) of up to several microns) exhibited a decrease in PS, while unilamellar liposomes (with PS from 30 to 150 nm) have shown an increase in PS [65]. By testing the nebulization of paclitaxel-loaded lipid nanocapsules using jet, ultrasonic, and mesh nebulizers of different brands, it was revealed that vibrating mesh nebulizers were able to generate aerosols of lipid nanocapsules with good performance and stability [66]. The excipients of nanoparticles could also contribute to the stabilization of nanoparticles structure during the nebulization process. It was reported that the incorporation of cholesterol and PEGylated phospholipids in the liposomal formulations could result in an increase in liposome membrane stability in the broncho-alveolar lavage or during nebulization [67,68]. Therefore, the proper selection of nebulization technique and formulation excipients should be very well considered while developing lipid-based nanocarriers for the LC via nebulization. They could significantly contribute to the nanoparticle stability and consequently the therapeutic outcome of the developed formulation.

On the other hand, the solid-based delivery aerosol systems (i.e., DPIs) can overcome the previously mentioned drawbacks of nebulizers as they have many advantages and unique features [69]. They are easy to use, can be self-administered, portable, do not need hospitalization, cost-effective, and can efficiently deliver high doses of anticancer drugs or drug-loaded nanocarriers as dry powder to the lungs [70]. DPIs are breath-actuated using the patient's inspiration for a short time with negligible drug exhalation, causing no air contamination during use. Furthermore, the dry powders have higher long-term stability, suitable for the formulation of lipophilic drugs [71]. Besides, DPIs can be produced as disposable devices, consequently limiting the contamination of the device and the environment [72]. Recently, many preclinical studies were published, including the development of inhaled anticancer drugs using DPIs for the treatment of LC, which reflects the growing interest in this approach [73–75]. However, the development of dry powders for such drugs for DPIs necessitates the need for taking extra protective and safety measures by the researchers and personnel in the industrial facilities if the formulation is to be commercialized.

Nowadays, there is a wide range of the available classical DPIs in the markets, and the number will keep increasing. The main differences among these DPIs lie in their design, airflow resistances, formulations' type and excipients, and dry powder production techniques and dispersion methods [76,77]. These mentioned device and formulations related-variables, in addition to the patient-related variations such as the patient's respiratory health and performance, may significantly affect the performance of these devices and lead to some variations in their drug deposition efficiencies into the lungs [78].

To ensure efficient powder aerosolization and delivery of drugs, the production of classical DPIs needs many optimization steps where the milled and micronized drug particles are usually formulated as three main particle types, namely: carrier-based, agglomerate-based (spheronized), and engineered particles. In the carrier-based type, the drug particles are attached physically to large inactive carrier particles such as lactose (if lactose was the used carrier they are called as lactose blends), while the agglomerates are composed of aggregates of the micronized drug. The engineered particles are usually composed of spray-dried particles of drug solubilized in an inert hydrophobic carrier [79].

On the other hand, nanocarriers-based DPIs also require many steps to create the inhalable drug-loaded nanocarriers dry powder beside the initial preparation and optimization of the drug-loaded nanocarriers processes. As discussed previously, the inhaled particles' D_{ae} must be in the range of (1–5 μm). Since the lipid-based nanoparticles possess too small D_{ae} (due to their small particle size and or density) so they are not suitable by themselves for efficient deposition in the respiratory tract, where they may be exhaled out of the respiratory system. Besides, lipid-based nanoparticles' high surface free energy due to their small size and enormous surface area can lead to particle aggregation, making their handling as a dry powder very difficult because of the poor flowability [44,80]. Overcoming these limitations of these nanoparticles can be done by particle engineering. One of the available potential solutions is to embed nanocarriers into microstructures (microparticles) with the required aerodynamic properties [81–84]. These nano in microparticles are also known as nanoaggregates or Trojan particles [85,86]. They must be engineered to have good dispersion properties to quickly dissolve and redisperse to release the initial nanocarriers in lung fluids upon delivery. The lipid-based nanocarriers, could be encapsulated into these microscale structures.

The excipients used in the formulation of dry powders of the nano in microparticles are typically hydrophilic excipients such as lactose, trehalose, dextran, and mannitol [87,88]. However, other additional materials were investigated such as L-leucine [89,90], hydroxypropyl β -cyclodextrin, polyvinyl alcohol, whey protein, maltodextrin, and gum Arabic [91].

Different techniques were used to produce dried lipid-based nanoparticles with or without excipients to generate stable, well-characterized, and inhalable particulates. These include spray-drying, freeze-drying (lyophilization), spray freeze-drying, milling, supercritical fluid drying, and electrohydrodynamic (electrospraying and electrospinning) methods. The pros and cons of these techniques, the critical variables that should be considered during formulation, and the properties of dry powders produced are well discussed and reviewed elsewhere [92,93].

Effervescent technology was also used to overcome the lipid-based nanoparticles' size-related limitations and enhance their lungs' release. It is done by embedding and co-drying of nanoparticles with an effervescent matrix, the typical excipients used in effervescent-based dry powders may include sodium carbonate, citric acid, and ammonium hydroxide.

The concept was first introduced by Ely et al. 2007 for polymer-based nanoparticles using ciprofloxacin as a drug model [94]. The technology was applied later to develop inhalational dry powders of cytotoxic drug-loaded lipid [95] or polymer-based nanoparticles [96,97] to treat LC. In one study, a comparison between inhalable effervescent-based and non-effervescent nanostructured lipid particles of 9-Bromo-noscapine was performed. The results showed that both formulations had good mean particle and aerodynamic size of 19.4 ± 6.1 nm and 3.1 ± 1.8 μm and 13.4 ± 3.2 nm and 2.3 ± 1.5 μm respectively. The cellular studies in A549 LC cells revealed that the effervescent-based formulation had enhanced cytotoxicity, apoptosis, and cellular uptake compared to the non-effervescent one. The in vivo studies were performed on Swiss albino male mice. The analysis of drug pharmacokinetics and distribution following inhalation demonstrated the superiority of effervescent-based formulation that exhibited 1.12 and 1.75-fold enhancement in drug half-life compared to non-effervescent formulation or drug powder [95].

6. Inhalable, Anticancer Drug-Loaded Lipid-Based Nanocarriers

The lipid-based nanocarriers are gaining significant interest by researchers working on the development of novel formulations for the pulmonary delivery of anticancer drugs owing to their biocompatible, biodegradable, non-toxic, and non-irritant nature, the ability to entrap and deliver diverse molecules in a controlled manner with enhanced bioavailability, ability to transport across blood vessels and different membranes and barriers in addition to the ease of preparation and scale-up [98–102]. Furthermore, their surfaces are highly tunable and can be functionalized by different ligands to target the cancerous cells in the lungs. Taking into consideration that the majority of the newly discovered anticancer drugs belong to class II drugs according to the biopharmaceutical classification system (i.e., have poor water solubility and poor oral bioavailability) is turning lipid-based nanoparticles to be an excellent choice for researchers in this field. Lipid-based nanoparticles are the first type of drug delivery systems translated from principle to clinical application and now represent a well-developed, established, and evolving technology platform with significant clinical acceptability [103]. Each type of lipid-based carrier has a unique structure, as shown in Figure 2. In this review, the most recent studies about the inhalable anticancer drug-loaded liposomal formulation that include in vivo studies are discussed in the following section and summarized in Table 1. While all the published research work for the other types of lipid-based nanocarriers (i.e., nanoemulsions NEs, solid lipid nanoparticles SLNs, nanostructured lipid carriers NLCs, niosomes, and the others) are discussed in the following sections and summarized in Table 2.

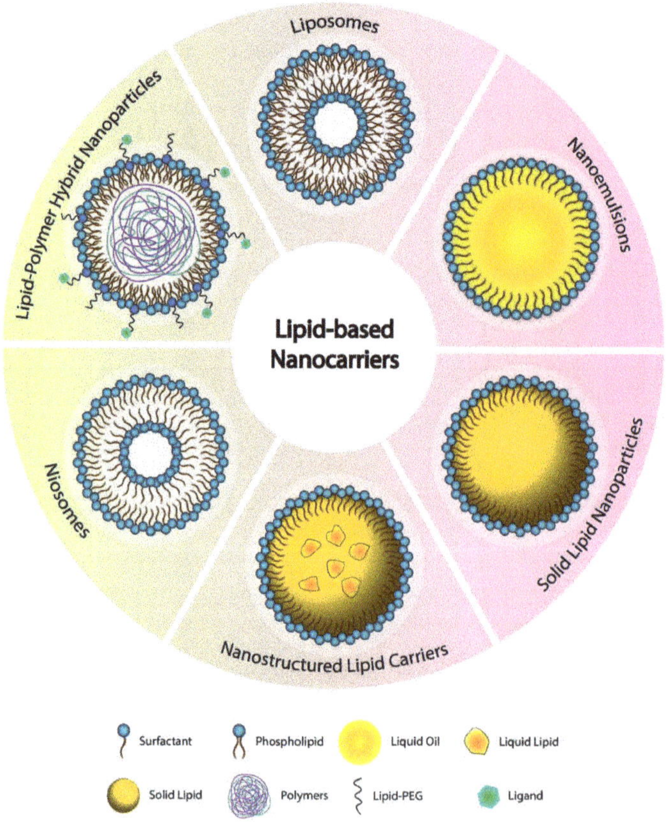

Figure 2. The various types of the lipid-based nanocarriers.

Table 1. Summary of the recently published in vivo studies about the inhalable anticancer drugs-loaded liposomal formulations for the treatment of LC.

Drug/Agent	Composition	Aim	Targeting Moiety/Strategy	Form	Delivery Method/Device	Cell line/Species	Main Outcomes	Ref.
HC & 5-Aminolevulinic acid	SPC, cholesterol, & octadecylamine	Chemo-sonodynamic therapy for metastatic LC	Cationic liposomes	Liquid	Intratracheal/Insufflator (IA-EC, Penn-Century, Inc., USA)	Formulation evaluation on metastatic LC-bearing mice: Female Balb/c mice (19–21g).	Synergistic effect of the inhaled chemotherapy and sonodynamic therapy led to improved apoptosis of cancer cells	[104]
CpG & Poly I:C	DOTAP & DPPC	To locally deliver immunotherapy against LC	N/A	Liquid	Intratracheal instillation	Tumor growth evaluation using murine B16F10 model of metastatic LC, Specific-pathogen-free female C57BL/6 Nrj mice (age, 6–8 weeks).	Delayed tumor growth caused via both agents. Inhalation of the CpG was superior to its intraperitoneal injection in slowing the growth of lung metastases with enhanced antitumor activities.	[105]
Paclitaxel	Soybean lecithin & cholesterol.	The investigation of delivering locally live carriers (paclitaxel-in-liposomes-in-bacteria) to combat LC.	Dry liposomes internalized into bacteria (*E. coli* or *L. casei*)	Liquid	Intratracheal instillation	Anti-cancer effects evaluation using male SD rats (180–220 g)	Liposomes in E-coli: highest anticancer effect, with the downregulation of VEGF and HIF-1α and the improvement of cancer cell apoptosis	[106]
Curcumin	Lecithin, cholesterol, stearylamine, poloxamer 188, 2-hydroxypropyl-β-cyclodextrin	To overcome the curcumin poor aqueous solubility and oral bioavailability	N/A	DP	Intratracheal instillation	MTT assay on A549 Cell line. Pharmacokinetic studies using Albino rats (220–260 g)	The liposomes formulation surpassed curcumin powder in the rate and extent of lung tissue absorption and mean residence time within the lung tissues.	[107]
Curcumin	Soybean lecithin & cholesterol	To evaluate the efficacy of curcumin-loaded liposomes	N/A	DP	Insufflator (DP4M, Penn-Century Inc., USA).	MTT assay On BEAS-2B, A549 cells line. Anti-cancer activity evaluation using male SD rats (190–200g).	Liposomes curcumin dry powder showed higher anticancer effects and selectivity than free form.	[108]
Lenvatinib-bound to magnetic iron oxide NP	N/A	To investigate the use of inhaled liposomes encapsulating targeted NP contrast agent (TNCA) for diagnosing purposes	Lenvatinib	Liquid	Atomizer	Tomography studies using C57BL/6 mice both sexes (age, 6–8 weeks).	The sensitivity and accuracy of computerized tomography imaging for the diagnosis of early-stage NSCLC was improved.	[109]

Table 1. *Cont.*

Drug/Agent	Composition	Aim	Targeting Moiety/ Strategy	Form	Delivery Method/ Device	Cell line/Species	Main Outcomes	Ref.
Doxorubicin	DPPC, Poloxamer 188	To formulate thermosensitive doxorubicin-loaded liposomes	Hybrid liposomes	Liquid	Intratracheal administration	WST assay on A549 and Raw 264.7 cells lines. The evaluation of lactate dehydrogenase activity and tumor necrosis factor alpha secretion in cell-free bronchoalveolar lavage fluid using Wistar rats (male, age, 13 weeks).	The formulated liposomes administered via the pulmonary route maybe useful for treating LC.	[110]
Doxorubicin & ASO, or siRNA	DOTAP & cholesterol.	To evaluate the use of a nose-only exposure chamber for inhalation and delivery of doxorubicin or nucleic acids	ASO, or siRNA	Liquid	One-jet Collison nebulizer (BGI Inc., Waltham, MA, USA)	Evolution of formulation's distribution and tumor growth size reduction using Nude nu/nu mice (age, 6–8 weeks).	The developed formulation inhalation resulted in tumor volume reduction of more than 90%, whereas only about 40% reduction was achieved after intravenous injection of the free drug.	[111]
Doxorubicin	DSPC, DSPE-PEG2000, DSPE-PEG-COOH, & cholesterol	To investigate the efficacy of active drug targeting via TF receptor-mediated uptake.	TF- PEG liposomes	Liquid	An AeroProbe intracorporeal nebulizing catheter connected to a catheter control unit	Tumor induction evaluation using female athymic Rowett nude (rnu) rats (age, 8–10 weeks).	More animals survived in the TF–liposomes groups than in the other treatment regimes, and their lung tissue generally had fewer and smaller tumors.	[112]
Quercetin	SPC, DSPE-PEG2000, cholesterol & DSPE-PEG2000-MAL-T7 conjugate	To augment therapeutic efficacy of quercetin-targeting TF receptors.	T7 (HAIYPRH) peptide	Liquid	Microsprayer® Aerosolizer Pulmonary Aerosol-Kit for Mouse (Penn-Century Inc., PA, USA)	MTT assay on A549 and MRC-5 cells lines. Apoptosis, cell-cycle analysis, cellular uptake, and tumor-spheroid penetration and inhibition studies on A549 cell line. Biodistribution study and therapeutic efficacy using male BALB/c nude mice (age, 7–8 weeks).	The developed formulation significantly enhanced the anticancer activity of the drug and lifespan of mice.	[113]

Table 1. *Cont.*

Drug/Agent	Composition	Aim	Targeting Moiety/ Strategy	Form	Delivery Method/ Device	Cell line/Species	Main Outcomes	Ref.
Triptolide	SPC, DSPE-PEG2000, DSPE-PEG2000-MALCPP33	To explore the pulmonary delivery of dual-ligand modified and triptolide-loaded liposomes modified triptolide-loaded liposomes	Anti-CA IX antibody & CPP33 dual ligands	Liquid	Microsprayer Aerosolizer Pulmonary Aerosol Kit for Mouse Model PAK-MSA	Wound healing, apoptosis, penetration, and cytotoxic damage in 3 D tumor spheroids on A549 cell line. Pharmacokinetic study using male SD rats (250 ± 20 g)	The formulation significantly enhanced the anticancer efficacy of the drug without apparent systemic toxicity.	[114]
Docetaxel	PC, cholesterol, DSPE-PEG-FA/DSEP-PEG-COOH/Co-spray	To compare the physicochemical properties, and antitumor activities of different targeted liposomal formulations	Folic acid conjugate	Liquid	Intratracheal administration	MTT assay, cellular uptake, endocytic routes study and metabolism assay on A549 and SPCA1 cells lines. bio-distribution studies using SD rats (180–220 g).	The co-spray drying did change the properties, while tracheal administration of the dry powder provided higher drug exposure at the tumor site without increasing the exposure of other organs	[75]
Temozolomide	PC, cholesterol & auric tetrachloride	To investigate the possible therapeutic effects of intratracheal inhalation of the developed liposomes-gold NP	N/A	Liquid	Intratracheal administration using Microsprayer IA-1C system (Penn-Century, Philadelphia, PA, USA)	Study the developed formulation's effects on lung homogenate MDA, GSH and inflammatory cytokines as well as on serum CYFRA 21-1 and IGF-1 level using male BALB/c mice (22–30 g).	The developed liposomes formulations succeed to improve all biochemical data and histological patterns.	[115]
Gemcitabine-HCl	HSPC, DSPG, mPEG2000-DSPE.	To formulate and evaluate gemcitabine-HCl -loaded liposomes	PEG- liposomes	DP	Intratracheal administration	MTT assay and cellular uptake on A549 cell line. Maximum tolerated dose, oedema index, acute toxicity study, and pharmacokinetic studies using Wistar rats (200–220 g).	Better pulmonary pharmacokinetic profile of the loaded formulation with lower toxicity to lung tissues than that of drug solution	[116]
Vincristine	SPC, & cholesterol.	To improve efficacy, lung exposure and decrease the clearance of the drug	N/A	DP	Intratracheal administration	MTT assay on MCF-7 and A549 cells lines. Absorption and tissue distribution study male SD rats (250 g).	The developed formulation had improved pharmacokinetic behavior of increased maximum concentration and systemic exposure and decreased elimination half-life in comparison to the free drug.	[41]

Table 1. *Cont.*

Drug/Agent	Composition	Aim	Targeting Moiety/ Strategy	Form	Delivery Method/ Device	Cell line/Species	Main Outcomes	Ref.
Gefitinib	SPC & cholesterol.	Comparative study of intratracheally administered of gefitinib- liposomes via intratracheally and orally administered free drug	N/A	DP	Intratracheal administration	Pharmacokinetic and biodistribution study using male SD rats (180–200 g).	Intratracheally administered liposomal powder showed higher in vivo therapeutic effect with reduction of inflammation, weak lung injury, and high apoptosis than intratracheally or administered free drug.	[117]
Sorafenib tosylate	Phospholipon 90H® & cholesterol	To enhance the physicochemical properties of sorafenib tosylate	N/A	DP	Revolizer device (Cipla Inc.)	NA	The loaded formulation offered biphasic release pattern, burst release in the first 6 h followed by sustained release up to 72 h	[73]

Anti-CA IX: Anti-carbonic anhydrase IX; ASO: Antisense oligonucleotides; CpG: Unmethylated oligodeoxynucleotides containing CpG motifs; DOTAP: Dioleoyltrimethylammoniumpropane; DP: Dry powder; DPPC: Dipalmitoylphosphatidylcholine; DSPC: Distearoyl-sn-glycero-3-phosphocholine; DSPE-PEG2000: Glycero-3-phospho-ethanolamine-N-[methoxy(polyethylene glycol)-2000]; DSPE-PEG-COOH: Glycero-3-phosphoethanolamine-N-[carboxy(polyethylene glycol)-2000]; FA: Fatty acids; HC: Hydroxycamptothecin; HSPC: Hydrogenated soy phosphatidylcholine; NP: Nanoparticles; PC: Phosphatidylcholine; Poly I:C: polyinosinic-polycytidylic acid double-stranded RNA; SD: Sprague–Dawley; siRNA: Small interfering RNA; SPC: Soy-phosphatidylcholine; TF: Transferrin.

Table 2. Summary of all the published preclinical studies on the developed anticancer drugs-loaded lipid-based nanocarriers for the treatment of LC.

Drug/Agent	Composition	Aim	Targeting Moiety/ Strategy	Form	Delivery Method/ Device	Cell line/Species/Subjects	Main Outcomes	Ref.
				NEs				
Docetaxel	PKOE, lauric FA, myristic FA, lecithin, Tween 85®, Span 85®, & glycerol	To select biocompatible excipients and perform aerodynamic characterization of nebulized NEs.	N/A	Liquid	OMRON MicroAIR nebulizer	MTT assay on A549 and MRC-5 cell lines	The NEs characteristics nominated it as potential inhalable carriers for docetaxel.	[118]
Docetaxel & Curcumin	PKOE, lauric FA, myristic FA, lecithin, Tween 85®, Span 85®, & glycerol	To formulate and optimize aerosolized NEs encapsulating docetaxel and curcumin	N/A	Liquid	OMRON MicroAIR nebulizer	N/A	The optimized NE offered desirable physicochemical and aerodynamic properties for inhalation therapy.	[119]
Curcuminoids	Limonene or oleic acid with Tween 80® & ethanol	To prepare nebulized curcuminoid-loaded NEs	N/A	Liquid	Sidestream jet nebulizer	Comet assay on human lymphocytes cells	Both NEs characteristics surpassed the saline-based suspensions of curcuminoid, with no genotoxicity.	[120]

Table 2. *Cont.*

Drug/Agent	Composition	Aim	Targeting Moiety/ Strategy	Form	Delivery Method/ Device	Cell line/Species/Subjects	Main Outcomes	Ref.
Quercetin	PBE, Tween 80®, lecithin & glycerol	To enhance quercetin solubility and cytotoxic selectivity	N/A	Liquid	OMRON MicroAIR nebulizer	MTT assay on A549 and MRC-5 cell lines	Loaded NEs characteristics and release profile were within the pulmonary delivery selection criteria requirements with stable and selective cytotoxic manners.	[121,122]
				SLNs				
Blank formulation	Lipid mixture (Softisan® & Phospholipon® 90G) & Solutol® HS15 as surfactant.	To evaluate the short-term toxicity of inhaled blank SLNs	N/A	Liquid	A jet-driven aerosol generator system (nebulizer)	MTT assay, neutral red uptake assay on A549 cell line and WST-1 assay using organotypic lung tissue cultures. Short term safety study on female BALB/c mice (age, 8–12 weeks).	This blank SLNs is suitable for pulmonary drug delivery via inhalation. No in vivo record of upregulation in lactate dehydrogenase and inflammation indicators levels	[123]
Erlotinib	Compritol 888 ATO®, Tween 80®, poloxamer 407®.	To get rapid drug deposition in lungs, with improved drug therapeutic efficiency and less systemic side effects	N/A	Liquid & DP	N/A	MTT assay on A549 cell line	The developed loaded SLNs surpassed the free drug with a cumulative drug release profile and significant higher anticancer activity.	[124]
Epirubicin	Compritol 888 ATO®, lecithin, poloxamer 188®.	To overcome major side effects including hematological and cardiac toxicity.	N/A	Liquid	Pari inhalier boy nebulizer	Crystal violet cytotoxicity assay on A549 cell line. Pharmacokinetic study using male SD rats, (250 ± 20 g)	The suitable SLNs characteristics offered a decrease in drug loss, with possible ability to deliver the drug into the deep lung, enhanced cytotoxicity and pharmacokinetics (~ 2 folds)	[125]
Afatinib & paclitaxel	Stearic acid & poloxamer 188®.	To explorer the co-delivery outcome of those drugs.	N/A	Liquid & DP	In vitro: Turbospin, a single dose powder inhaler device. In vivo: a dry powder insufflator	Growth-inhibitory curves study on H1975 and PC9/G cell lines. Short-term safety evaluation, pharmacokinetic and tissue distribution using male SD rats, (180–220 g)	The SLNs characteristics offered extremely high retention in the induction port for both drugs and with no interaction between them or the excipients. Pharmacokinetically, SLNs offered 96 h of a two-stage release and high lung concentration, with no signs of other critical organs distribution	[126]

Table 2. *Cont.*

Drug/Agent	Composition	Aim	Targeting Moiety/ Strategy	Form	Delivery Method/ Device	Cell line/Species/Subjects	Main Outcomes	Ref.
Paclitaxel	Glyceryl-stearate, cholesterol, vitamin E TPGS & sodium taurocholate.	To targeted deliver poor soluble drug	Folate-PEG/chitosan	Liquid	MicroSprayer Aerosolizer IA-1C (endotracheal route)	Cellular uptake on HeLa (CCL-2), M109-HiFR cell lines. Pharmacokinetic study using female (CD-1 and BALB/c mice.	The coated SLNs entered folate receptor (FR)-expressing HeLa and M109-HiFR cells in vitro, and M109 tumors in vivo after pulmonary delivery. The formulation prolonged the pulmonary exposure to paclitaxel up to 6 h and limited systemic distribution.	[42]
Myricetin	Gelucires (G 39/01, 50/13, 44/14) & compritol®	To enhance the nutraceutical solubility, stability, and delivery	NA	DP	N/A	MTT assay, and cellular uptake on A549 cell line.	Gelucire-based SLNs were proved to improve the physiochemical properties, release, and anticancer effects of the drug.	[127]
Gefitinib	Lecithin, cholesterol, stearic acid, & PEG2000	To glucosamine targeted	Glucosamine	DP	N/A	MTT assay, and cellular uptake on A549 cell line.	The satisfactory aerosol formulation cellular uptake study clearly demonstrated that functionalization of SLNs with glucosamine promote the accumulation of SLNs within GLUT1 overexpressing cells	[74]
NLCs								
Celecoxib	Compritol®, miglyol®, & sodium taurocholate	Evaluation of anticancer synergetic activity of aerosolized celecoxib-NLCs in combination with IV docetaxel.	N/A	Liquid	Inexpose™ nebulizer	MTT assay on A549 cell line. Tumor size reduction evaluation using nu/nu mice (age, 4–6 weeks).	In vivo study proved the synergetic effects of celecoxib-NLCs inhalation and docetaxel IV.	[128]
Paclitaxel	Stearic acid (or glyceryl monostearate) oleic acid, Tween 80®, Tween 20®, or Tween 40®.	To compare the oral paclitaxel solution with the paclitaxel-NLCs inhaled delivery	N/A	DP	DP insufflator	Intracellular uptake assay in Caco-2 cell line. Organ distribution of loaded NLCs using male Wistar rats, 180–200 g.	Inhaled paclitaxel-NLCs showed excellent local delivery and organ selectivity when accumulated mainly in lung and in compared to pure drug solution oral intake	[129]
Doxorubicin or paclitaxel	Precirol ATO 5®, squalene, Tween 80®	To provide selective local and targeted inhalation lung delivery.	Synthetic analog LHRH/DSPE-PEG2000 and siRNA	DP	Collision nebulizer connected to nose-only exposure chamber for inhalation	Cellular uptake and the intracellular localization on A549 cell line. Tumor size reduction evaluation using athymic nu/nu mice	The developed inhaled NLCs showed high efficiency and selectivity for tumor-targeted local delivery.	[130]

Table 2. *Cont.*

Drug/Agent	Composition	Aim	Targeting Moiety/ Strategy	Form	Delivery Method/ Device	Cell line/Species/Subjects	Main Outcomes	Ref.
Paclitaxel	Precirol ATO 5®, squalene, Tween 80®	To compare the NLC cytotoxicity and selectivity via I.V. and inhalation routes.	LHRH-PEG2000-siRNA	Liquid	Collison nebulizer	MTT assay on A549, H1781, and H3255 cell lines. NLCs organ distribution and tumor size evaluation using nude mice.	Efficient accumulation and retention of the inhaled NLCs in the mice lungs, with no signs of systematic cytotoxicity compared to I.V. route.	[131]
				LPHNs				
siRNA	PLCGA & DPPC	To downregulate the genes involved in the pathogenesis of LC through the local siRNA delivery	N/A	Liquid	Vibrating mesh nebulizer	MTT assay on A549 and 16HBE14o cell lines	The developed NLCs offered a peculiar triphasic siRNA release lasting for 5 days, with a prolonged inhibition of ENaC protein expression.	[132]
				Niosomes				
Gemcitabine & cisplatin	Tween 65®, Span 60®, cholesterol, sodium dodecyl sulfate, glycerol	To develop dual drug inhalable niosomes with efficacy but lower dose, and side effects.	N/A	Liquid	OMRON MicroAIR nebulizer	MTT assay on A549 and MRC5 cell lines	Developed NLCs cytotoxicity reduced against the tested cell lines when compared with free drug.	[133]
Curcumin	Span 80®, diethyl ether, with or without cholesterol	To formulate C.-niosomes for effective lung delivery	Cationic niosomes	DP	Nebulizer	MTT assay and cellular uptake on A549 cell line	The cholesterol-containing carriers surpassed the cholesterol-free carriers in terms of antiproliferative effects and a higher endocytosis.	[134]
				Sterosomes				
Metformin	Cholesterol, stearylamine or myristic acid	To evaluate the safety, tolerability, & pharmacokinetics of inhaled metformin sterosomes	N/A	Liquid	Jet nebulizer	MTT assay on A549 cell line. Clinical study ($n = 6$, 3 males and 3 females age > 18)	The formulated carriers significantly increased the biological half-life area under the curve, and mean residence time of metformin in all healthy volunteers after inhalation.	[135]
				Lipid Nanocapsules				
Paclitaxel	Captex 8000®, Lipoid S75-3®, & Solutol® HS 15.	To encapsulate paclitaxel in lipid nanocapsules	N/A	Liquid	Jet, ultrasonic and mesh nebulizers of different brands.	Growth inhibition assay on NCI-H460 human lung cancer cells	LNC dispersions could be made into aerosols by using mesh nebulizers without altering the LNC structure.	[66]

DP: Dry powder; DPPC: Dipalmitoylphosphatidylcholine; DSPE-PEG2000: Glycero-3-phospho-ethanolamine-N-[methoxy(polyethylene glycol)-2000]; FA: Fatty acids; LHRH: Luteinizing hormone-releasing hormone; PBE: Palm-based ester; PKOE: Palm kernel oil esters; PLCGA: Poly(lactic-co-glycolic) acid; SD: Sprague–Dawley; siRNA: Small interfering RNA.

6.1. Liposomes

Liposomes are the primary and the most widely studied systems of the lipid-based nanocarriers for the delivery of anticancer agents using different targeting strategies for the treatment of various tumors, including LC. They are first reported and described by Bangham and his colleagues in 1960 [136]. In the subsequent years, several phospholipid bilayer structures were defined, originally called bangosomes and then liposomes, as a result of combining two Greek words, "lipos" meaning fat, and "soma" signifying "body" [137]. Liposomes are self-assembled unilamellar or multilamellar spherical vesicular systems typically composed of one or more phospholipids bilayers surrounding an aqueous core (Figure 2). Liposomal properties vary considerably depending on their lipid composition, preparation method, size, surface charge and functionalization moiety. Liposomes are typically prepared using phospholipids of various origins (natural sources such as egg yolk and soybean oil, or synthetic), cholesterol and surfactants. Generally, liposomal constituents are mimicking the biological membranes and naturally present in the pulmonary surfactants that make them non-immunogenic, biodegradable and biocompatible. The size range of liposomal systems varies between 30 nm up to several micrometers [138,139]. The surface of the liposomes is highly tunable and could be functionalized using various formulation and targeting moieties. Furthermore, because of their unique structure and composition, liposomes are able to incorporate and deliver anticancer agents (such as chemotherapeutics, genes, and peptides) of highly diverse physicochemical properties and lipophilicities, where they can enhance the therapeutic efficacy by passive or active lung targeting, reduce toxicity and improve the pharmacokinetic profile of the incorporated drugs/agents [140]. All these properties turned liposomes to be excellent candidates and active area of research for pulmonary delivery and LC therapy.

Recently, inhaled hydroxycamptothecin-loaded cationic liposomes were used with concomitant intratracheally delivered sonosensitizer (5-aminolevulinic acid) for the combined chemo-sonodynamic (Chemo-STD) therapy for metastatic LC. Liposomes were prepared using the thin film method and composed of soybean phosphatidylcholine, cholesterol, and octadecylamine. The in vivo cytotoxicity studies showed that the combined Chemo-STD therapy had better cytotoxicity effects than using the hydroxycamptothecin-loaded cationic liposomes or the SDT only. The in vivo studies on metastatic LC-bearing mice showed that the highest anticancer activity was obtained using the inhaled combined Chemo-SDT than the single therapy via either inhaled or intravenously administered hydroxycamptothecin-loaded cationic liposomes or the SDT alone. The authors suggested that the synergistic effect of the inhaled chemotherapy and STD led to improved apoptosis of cancer cells and the enhanced production of reactive oxygen species [104].

Inhalable cationic liposomal formulations loaded with unmethylated oligodeoxynucleotides containing CpG motifs (CpG) and polyinosinic-polycytidylic acid (poly I:C) double-stranded RNA were also prepared recently as locally delivered immunotherapy against LC where liposomes could increase the uptake of the loaded nucleic acids by the lung phagocytes thereby the activation of toll-like receptors within endosomes. Dioleoyltrimethylammoniumpropane (DOTAP) and dipalmitoylphosphatidylcholine (DPPC) were used in the preparation of liposomes. The formulations were tested in vivo using murine B16F10 model of metastatic LC. Delayed tumor growth was observed via both agents (i.e., poly I:C and CpG). However, increased pulmonary levels of interferon-γ were observed with CpG only. Inhalation of the CpG was superior to its intraperitoneal injection to slow the growth of lung metastases and to induce the production of granzyme B, a pro-apoptotic protein, and interferon-γ, monokine induced by the gamma interferon (MIG) and the (regulated upon activation, normal T cell expressed and presumably secreted) (RANTES), T helper type 1 cytokines and chemokines, in the lungs. These antitumor activities of CpG were efficiently enhanced by CpG loading in liposomal formulations [105].

Functionalized inhalable dry powder of folic acid-conjugated liposomal formulation of docetaxel was developed for the treatment of LC [75]. The folic acid-conjugated liposomes were prepared by the thin-film hydration method and were composed of phosphatidylcholine, cholesterol, DSPE-PEG$_{2000}$-FA, and DESP-PEG$_{2000}$-COOH. The prepared liposomal dispersions were then co-spray dried with mannitol and leucine at different concentrations. The particle size (PS), dispersity (Đ), zeta potential (ZP), and entrapment efficiency (EE%) of the re-dispersed liposomes were 346.8 ± 4.7 nm, 0.401, −29.3 ± 1.8 mV, and 99.5 ± 0.3%, respectively. While the liposomal dry powder had D_{ae}, FPF, spray drying production yield (PY), angle of repose (θ), Carr's index and Hausner ratio of 3.10 ± 0.005 μm, 10.0 ± 0.1%, 61.9% ± 0.5%, 36.8 ± 0.4 °, 32.1 ± 1.86 and 1.47 ± 0.04, respectively. The morphological studies of re-dispersed liposomes showed that they were spherical as before; instead, they had irregular shapes attributed to the effects of the spray drying process. The results of in vivo studies on Sprague Dawley rats showed a 45-fold higher concentration of docetaxel in the lungs of the studied rats at 30 min after the tracheal administration compared with the intravenously administered formulation. Higher drug exposure at the tumor site was obtained by the tracheal administration of the dry powder without exposure increment to other organs. The authors concluded that the inhaled dry powders might be clinically effective for the treatment of LC [75].

Liposomal dry powder formulation of curcumin was developed as an inhalable treatment for primary LC to overcome the drug-associated drawbacks such as low water solubility, poor bioavailability, and rapid metabolism that significantly limits clinical applications. The liposomes were initially prepared using the thin film method and were composed of soybean lecithin and cholesterol. The resulted liposomes were then lyophilized in the presence of mannitol as a cryoprotectant to obtain the final liposomal curcumin dry powder. The rehydrated curcumin-loaded liposomes had PS and Đ of (94.65 ± 22.01 nm) and (0.26 ± 0.01), respectively. While the liposomal power had D_{ae} of 5.81 μm with FPF of 46.71%, rendering the powder suitable for pulmonary delivery. The in vitro cell culture studies showed significantly greater and faster cellular uptake of curcumin-loaded liposomes by human LC A549 cells than free curcumin. Furthermore, the high cytotoxicity of curcumin-loaded liposomes on A549 cells and their low cytotoxic activity against normal human bronchial BEAS-2B epithelial cells produced a high selection index partly due to increased cell apoptosis. The in vivo studies were performed by directly spraying curcumin liposomal powder, curcumin powder, and gemcitabine into the lungs of male Sprague–Dawley (SD)rats with LC through the trachea. Higher anticancer effects were obtained by developed liposomal curcumin powder than the other two tested medications in terms of pathology and the expression of various cancer-related markers such as VEGF, malondialdehyde, TNF-α, caspase-3, and BCL-2. Accordingly, the developed curcumin liposomal dry powder formulation has the potential to be used as inhalation therapy for LC [108].

The use of bacterial therapy is an emerging treatment technique for various cancers and may represent a promising strategy to combat LC when locally delivered by inhalation. Recently, inhaled live carriers (paclitaxel-in-liposomes-in-bacteria) were prepared and evaluated for the treatment of primary LC. The paclitaxel-load liposomes were prepared using the thin film method and composed of soy phosphatidylcholine and cholesterol. The drug-loaded liposomes were then internalized by electroporation into bacteria (*Escherichia coli* or *Lactobacillus casei*) to get LP-in-*E. Coli* (LPE) or LP-in-*L. Casei* (LPL). The PS, Đ, ZP and EE% of the developed paclitaxel-load liposomes were 64.3 ± 2.4 nm, 0.35 ± 0.08, −9.96 ± 0.48 mV and 97.2 ± 0.5% respectively. In vitro cytotoxicity studies on the A549 cell line revealed that LPE caused the highest inhibition of cellular proliferation compared to LPL, paclitaxel-loaded liposomes, a mixture of paclitaxel-load liposomes and bacteria. Paclitaxel-in-liposomes-in-bacteria delivered the cargos into the cells quicker than the other tested samples. The results of the in vivo studies on primary LC animal model using male Sprague–Dawley (SD) showed that among all the studied formulations, LPE had the highest anticancer effect with the downregulation of vascular endothelial growth factor (VEGF) and hypoxia-inducible factor 1-alpha (HIF-1α) and the enhancement of malignant cell apoptosis following the intratracheal administration. Furthermore, the live bacterial carriers significantly improved the expressions of (tumor necrosis factor- α, interleukin 4, and interferon-γ) immune markers and (leukocytes and neutrophils) immune cells [106].

6.2. Nanoemulsions

The first record in the history of nanoemulsions (NEs) began in 1943 with Hoar and Schulman [141]. However, it was not until 1993 that the term "nanoemulsions" or "ultrafine emulsion" was first reported, reflecting a formulation with a nanoscale droplet size (PS) of 20 nm to 200 nm, a transparent and semi-translucent appearance, and long-term thermodynamic stability against sedimentation by preventing flocculation, aggregation, coalescence, and Ostwald ripening [142,143]. Generally, the International Union of Pure and Applied Chemistry (IUPAC) does not yet have a fixed PS range for NEs [144], while the US FDA is considering NEs PS in the nanoscale range (approximately 1–100 nm) [145]. However, NEs prepared for pulmonary delivery must comply with the PS parameter set for this route.

NEs have gained popularity from the fact that they can be formulated from natural or synthetic excipients that are generally recognized as safe (GRAS) or approved by the US FDA [143,146,147]. Their structure is illustrated in Figure 2. In chemotherapy delivery, NEs superiority over conventional delivery systems originates from their ability to achieve the required therapeutic effect by enhancing the solubility and bioavailability of poorly soluble drugs, which may significantly contribute to decreasing drugs' dosing and frequency as the drug is released in a sustained release manner over longer times [148,149]. Since vascularized tissues surround the cancer cells, NEs can easily accumulate in these tissues because of the small PS that gives them the advantage to pass through such barriers [150] via direct transcellular or paracellular transport. By proper selection of formulation excipients, they could have the ability to inhibit the P-gp efflux, thus enhancing cellular and mucosal permeability of the incorporated anticancer drug [118]. Besides, NEs lipophilic core is augmenting the nanosystem's stability by protecting the drug/compound against the enzymatic hydrolysis allowing better drug delivery [151].

NEs can be categorized as simple or multiple emulsions depending on whether the core is either water or oil and the complexity of the carrier [147]. As far as pulmonary drug delivery is concerned, NEs can be classified into three generations; first-generation are prepared by spontaneous emulsification and composed of oil, surfactants, co-solvents, and a selected aqueous phase such as deionized water or saline solution [151,152]. The second-generation NEs contain the same materials as the first, but their droplets are additionally decorated with specific polymers (chitosan, hyaluronan, hydroxypropyl methylcellulose (HPMC)) to enhance mucoadhesive properties, while the third generation droplets are decorated with ligands and/or polymers for targeted drug delivery [59]. As a nonequilibrium system and a spontaneous formation is unfeasible, high energy input is applied to form NEs. This can be achieved by homogenizing the aqueous phase with an immiscible oil phase using low-and/or high-energy emulsification techniques. The size of the droplets will depend heavily on the hydrophilic-lipophilic balance (HLB) values of the NEs' excipients [153], the type of instruments used, and their process parameters, such as time, stirring speed, temperature, and sample composition [147].

Although NEs may be constructed using long, medium, short-chain fatty acids or any mixture of them, however, it is noted that the inhaled NEs prepared for the delivery of conventional (non-cytotoxic) drugs were mostly composed of either medium [154–156] or long-chain fatty acids separately [152,157]. In contrast, inhaled NEs for anticancer delivery are usually prepared using a mixture of both (i.e., the long and medium-chain fatty acids), as illustrated in the following sections. Future studies could focus on comparing the impact of the fatty acid chain lengths on the suitability, efficiency, and biocompatibility of the inhaled anticancer NEs for lung delivery [158,159].

In addition to the oil phase, selecting a proper surfactant system is essential for the proper development of NEs for pulmonary delivery. The use of non-ionic surfactants is more prevalent than ionic surfactants in the formulation of NEs, due to the suggested deterioration of the biological membrane by their use. The superiority of non-ionic surfactants also comes from their ability to enhance poorly soluble drug dissolution, particle size, shape, and stability [160]. NEs safety is another concern that is primarily associated with the use of synthetic emulsifiers and is a key issue that needs to be addressed in particular to the adverse negative interactions between lipids and surfactants of the lung alveoli [161]. Most synthetic emulsifiers may trigger toxic symptoms with prolonged administration, including the potential binding of anionic emulsifiers to proteins, enzymes, and phospholipid membranes in the human body, resulting in various adverse reactions, such as enzyme dysfunction, protein structure modification, and membrane cell phospholipid [162]. Consequently, replacing synthetic emulsifiers and excipients with natural substitutes is one of the novelties on-demand in the construction of the NEs. Co-solvents may also be included in the formulation of NEs. Glycerol is used as the preferred co-solvent in almost every inhaled NEs for the lung delivery of anticancer drugs. This could be due to its ability to modify the aerodynamic distribution of the PS of the emitted aerosol droplets and to produce a slower dissolution rate, with the potential to modify the cell permeability of the loaded drugs, which can significantly impact their lung absorption and distribution [163,164].

Since NEs behave similarly to solutions, these formulations tend to exhibit significant improvements in their in vitro aerosolization performance when nebulized compared to other suspended nanoformulations' types [165,166]. Although there are various solidification techniques for the production of NEs as dry powders, no dry powder of anticancer drug-loaded NEs were produced. All the developed NEs were aerosolized using nebulizers only.

NEs of docetaxel were recently formulated using biocompatible excipients for the drug pulmonary delivery to overcome the drug's low solubility and improve its bioavailability and efficacy. A mixture of medium (lauric fatty acids and palm kernel oil esters) and long-chain fatty acid (myristic fatty acids) were used as the oil phase in these NEs. The surfactants system was composed of non-ionic (Tween 80® and Span 80®) and amphipathic (lecithin) surfactants as they are known to be non-toxic, biocompatible, and unaffected by pH. The optimized docetaxel-loaded NEs formulation had a spherical shape with PS, ZP, and entrapment efficacy (EE%) of 94.35 ± 0.77 nm, −38.64 ± 1.43 mV, and 100%, respectively. Besides, the optimized NEs were also shown to have neutral pH, with an osmolality of (301 ± 1.00 mOsm/kg) and viscosity of (1.92 ± 0.08 cP) that are suitable for the pulmonary delivery. The optimized NEs were aerosolized using OMRON MicroAIR nebulizer and were evaluated using the Andersen cascade impactor method. The nebulized NEs showed desirable aerosolization properties for pulmonary delivery where the D_{ae} and the FPF were 3.02 ± 0.26 and 92.76 ± 0.63, respectively. The in vitro cell culture studies found that the final formulation is more selective on human lung carcinoma cells (A549) than the normal cell (MRC-5). It was concluded that the developed NEs are potential carriers for docetaxel in targeting LC via the inhalation route [118].

Aerosolization of NEs for pulmonary delivery for LC using docetaxel and curcumin were also reported by the same group. The NEs for both drugs (separately) were designed with a mixture of medium (palm kernel oil ester) and long (safflower seed oil) chain fatty acids and a set of non-ionic (Tween 85® and Span 85®) and amphipathic (lecithin) surfactants, as well as glycerol as a co-solvent. Both formulations were characterized and found to have the required physicochemical and aerosolization properties suitable for inhalation [119].

The in-vitro aerosolization and toxicity of curcuminoids NEs for LC were investigated by Al Ayoub et al.; the formulated NEs were composed of medium (limonene) and long (oleic acid) fatty acids as oil phases, Tween 80® as the surfactant, and ethanol as the co-surfactant. Based on the loaded amount of curcumin (100–500 µg/mL), the developed NEs had the PS of (13–39 nm) and Đ of (0.1–0.2) as well as osmolality, pH, and viscosity in the range of (336 to 600 mOsm/kg), (6–7), and (1.1–1.7 mPas) respectively. The nebulized NEs prepared with limonene oil had FPF and D_{ae} ranged from 50% and 4.6 µm to 45% and 5.6 µm, respectively; whereas the FPF and D_{ae} of the nebulized NEs prepared with oleic acid oil ranged from 46% and 4.9 µm to 44% and 5.6 µm, respectively. Genotoxicity using Comet assay showed that the developed NEs are nontoxic at the tested curcuminoid doses suggesting the safety and suitability of the developed NEs. The authors recommend further pre-clinical and clinical studies [120]. However, additional cytotoxicity evaluation and in vitro release study are also essential in such formulations.

Quercetin is a flavonoid phytochemical that is suggested to treat LC via its antiproliferative and antimetastatic effect on A549 cells through the impact on the cytoskeleton and repressing the metastatic capacity of LC via suppressing, as well as promoting apoptosis in LC [167]. NEs of quercetin were employed to enhance the lung delivery of this poorly soluble flavonoid for the treatment of LC. The in vitro cytotoxicity studies showed some selectivity of the quercetin-loaded NEs towards the A549 cells line without affecting the normal cells [121,122].

Although the used excipients in all these studies are considered safe, but the long-term safety studies due to possible adverse interactions with lung surfactants and efficacy of developed formulations against LC are strongly encouraged at the in vitro and preclinical level before reaching to clinical trials.

Like other lipid-based formulations, NEs that are working through passive targeting, are facing limitations in recognizing cancer or normal cells. Active targeting of the nanoemulsions could be approached by modifying the surface of these carriers, where the attached ligand (monoclonal antibodies, transferrin, folic acid, hyaluronic acid, aptamer, or antibody fragments) aids in recognition of the target tumor cells [146]. The development of anticancer-loaded NEs for active targeting decorated with ligands such as the folate-targeted NEs loaded with docetaxel [168] and transferrin-targeted docetaxel NEs [169] for ovarian cancer are already developed but currently limited for intravenous delivery. Inhaled NEs with active targeting moieties for the treatment of LC as far as we are aware, are not explored yet.

6.3. Solid-Lipid Nanoparticles (SLNs)

Solid lipid nanocarriers (SLNs) were introduced in 1991 as an upgrade to the traditional colloidal drug delivery systems. They are best represented as a mixture of liposomes and niosomes containing phospholipids and surfactant molecules, with a submicron PS ranging from 40 to 1000 nm [170,171]; they are derived from oil-in-water (O/W) emulsions by replacing liquid lipids with a lipid matrix that is solid at room and body temperatures [172], as illustrated in Figure 2. The use of solid lipids instead of liquid oils can result in controlled release of drugs as the mobility of the drug in a solid lipid matrix is significantly lower than that of liquid oil [173]. SLNs are composed of physiologically tolerated and safe lipids such as fatty acids (e.g., stearic acid), monoglycerides (e.g., glycerol monostearate), diglycerides (e.g., glycerol behenate), triglycerides (e.g., tripalmitin, tristearin, trilaurin), waxes (e.g., cetyl palmitate), or steroids (e.g., cholesterol) that are dispersed with an appropriate surfactant phase [174]. Next to the design of the inhalation devices, drug carrier's selection is equally important in assuring the sufficient stability and appropriate size delivery of the loaded drug, thus, lipids and surfactants selection is an essential factor for SLNs characteristics [175]. Generally, high-pressure homogenization and microemulsion methods are being the most commonly used for the preparation of SLNs.

Pharmacokinetically, SLNs, and liposomes have been reported to be eliminated from the lungs at comparable rates, even though SLNs are deposited after intratracheal instillation in the upper respiratory tract and, in particular, through the mucociliary escalator and do not stimulate significant inflammatory reactions [176]. The inhaled radiolabelled SLNs biodistribution showed significant uptake in lymphatics, with a high rate of distribution in periaortic, axillary, and inguinal lymph nodes and these findings indicate that SLNs may have the potential to be efficient carriers for lymphoscintigraphy or pulmonary therapy [28]. Besides, some SLNs may remain mostly intact in the pulmonary area, which may lead to longer lung retention times [177].

As safety and lung tolerability are of the essential parameters to be considered while developing formulations for pulmonary delivery, some studies preferred to assess the toxicity of the inhaled blank SLNs before deciding to load them with active materials. For instance, a blank SLNs formulation was designed using a lipid matrices mixture of triglycerides (Softisan®) and phosphatidylcholine (Phospholipon® 90G), Solutol®HS15 as a surfactant, and double-distilled water. The high-pressure homogenization method was used for the preparation. The produced SLNs had PS, Đ, and ZP of 98.4 nm, 0.148, and −14.6 mV, respectively. The MTT assay and neutral red uptake assay (NRU) on the A549 cell line for 24 h showed the blank SLNs ability to reduce this cell line viability with calculated half-maximal effective concentration (EC_{50}) of 3090 μg/mL and 2090 μg/mL, respectively. The organotypic cultures of lung tissue showed that the SLNs reduced the metabolic activity of the used murine precision-cut lung slices after incubating it with SLNs for 24 h and using WST-1 assay at EC_{50} of 575 μg/mL. The SLNs were nebulized by a jet-driven aerosol generator system. The in vivo cytotoxicity study on female BALB/c mice for 16 days showed no significant changes or upregulation in lactate dehydrogenase levels as an exponent of low levels of damage to the cell membrane, as well as bronchoalveolar lavage fluid protein as an indicator of cytotoxicity in lung tissues, and different inflammation indicators (TNF-a, IL-8 (A549), IL-6, and chemokine KC) [123]. Interestingly, this system was reported without loading it with an active ingredient; moreover, such evaluation should be conducted using both LC and normal cell lines to get a complete understanding of the developed SLNs' cytotoxicity and selectivity.

Inhaled SLNs were also used to get rapid drug deposition in lungs, less systemic side effects, and improved drug therapeutic efficiency of erlotinib (a quinazoline derivative with antineoplastic properties). The SLNs were synthesized from Compritol 888 ATO® (solid lipid), Tween 80® (surfactant), and Poloxamer 407® (an aqueous phase surfactant) using the hot homogenization method [124]. The erlotinib-loaded SLNs owned a PS (< 100 nm), Đ (0.367), DL% (4.17%), and EE% of (78.21%). For aerosolization of the developed NLCs, they were further spray dried in the absence and presence of mannitol (as an inert bulking agent). The dry powder of aerosolized erlotinib-loaded SLNs in the presence of mannitol had D_{ae} (3.93), emitted dose (ED)% (94.91), FPF% (30.98), and geometric standard deviation (GSD) of (4.339). The TEM and scanning electron microscopy (SEM) micrographs of both liquid and powder SLNs indicated a regular and spheroidal shape with smooth surfaces. The in vitro release studies using the dialysis membrane method showed that here was no burst release from the formulated SLNs and cumulative drug release occurred with a steady rate to reach approximately 12% at 8 h, as compared to ~18% with free drug. Besides, the MTT assay revealed significantly higher anticancer activity of the erlotinib-loaded SLNs against A549 cells in comparison to the free drug and after 18 h of incubation. However, no in vivo studies were performed for the elevation of organs distribution and anticancer activity were performed in this study.

Epirubicin which is an anthracycline and a stereoisomer of doxorubicin that has shown activity against various types of tumors including LC, but its use is associated with major side effects including hematological and cardiac toxicity, thus specific targeting through simple, safe and stable formulations is highly recommended. Accordingly, Epirubicin-loaded SLNs were prepared. The SLNs were composed of soy lecithin, compritol 888 ATO®, and poloxamer 188®. The produced SLNs had the characterization of PS, ZP and EE% of 223.7 nm, −30.6mV, 78.9% respectively. The formulation was nebulized using (Pari Inhalierboy, Starnberg, Germany). No significant changes in PS ZP or EE% were observed after nebulization [125]. The nebulized formulations were evaluated for their in vitro deposition by a Twin Stage Impinges (TSI). The blank SLNs, epirubicin-loaded SLNs and pure epirubicin solution showed respirable fractions (RF) of 77.03%, 78.46%, and 59.51%, respectively indicating the decrease in drug loss, besides the SLN possible ability to deliver the drug into the deep lung. The cytotoxicity on A549 cells using 0.1% crystal violet after incubation for 24 h revealed the improved cytotoxic effects of the developed SLNs in comparison to the free drug. Pharmacokinetically, and upon analyzing plasma and lung samples via HPLC, aerosolized epirubicin-loaded SLNs showed excellent lung deposition characteristics compared to epirubicin solution in male Sprague–Dawley rats, while the plasma area under the curve values for epirubicin-loaded SLNs was 2.07-fold higher than that after epirubicin solution suggesting the potential suitability of the developed inhaled SLNs for pulmonary delivery to treat LC.

SLNs were employed also for the co-delivery of afatinib and paclitaxel for the treatment of epidermal growth factor receptor tyrosine kinase resistant NSCLC. In this study, afatinib was first loaded in SLNs composed of stearic acid and poloxamer 188 and had PS, Đ, and EE% of 358.3 nm, 0.167, and 87.9% respectively. Furthermore, these SLNs were lyophilized using trehalose (as a cryoprotectant) and loaded with paclitaxel into poly-lactide-co-glycolide-based porous microspheres. These inhaled microspheres systems are characterized with D_{ae}, FPF, fine particle dose (FPD), and GSD of 3.26 and 3.25 μm, 23.04 and 24.07%, 41.01 and 59.66 μg, 2.26 and 2.32, as well as EE% 53–70.85% of afatinib and paclitaxel, respectively. These final formulations showed an initial in vitro drug release for paclitaxel (20%) and afatinib (30%), with extremely high retention (more than 65%) in the induction port (17.21 ± 0.22% for afatinib and 16.00 ± 1.52% for paclitaxel), and no interaction between drugs and carriers when characterized by FTIR and NMR spectroscopy [126]. On the cellular level, there was a significant synergistic effect between afatinib and paclitaxel and superior treatment capability of the final loaded microspheres for drug-resistant NSCLC on H1975 and PC9/G cells. The pharmacokinetics and tissue distribution results demonstrated that afatinib and paclitaxel in the microspheres exhibited 96 h of a two-stage release and high lung concentration. The final loaded microspheres did not distribute to other critical organs. These results revealed that the drug combination therapy using these nanocarriers is highly promising for treating drug-resistant LC.

6.4. Nanostructured Lipid Carriers (NLCs)

The nanostructured lipid carriers (NLCs) represent an advanced type of the SLNs. These carriers can overcome the SLNs-related disadvantages, such as the drug loading capacity and formulation stability challenges by creating a less structured solid lipid matrix via mixing fluid lipid with solid lipid (as shown in Figure 2), resulting in less drug expulsion during storage [173,178,179]. NLCs are the products of o/w emulsion process, hence the available surfactants typically have a high HLB range, and ideally dissolved in the external aqueous phase of the emulsion [160]. Besides, these nanocarriers can be used to circumvent the limitations associated with conventional cancer chemotherapy such as poor drug solubility, and multiple drug-resistance by enhancing chemotherapy's targeting and selectivity index [180,181]. Additionally, NLCs are suitable to carry drugs with different physicochemical properties, natural compounds and small interfering RNA (e.g., siRNA), where the latter is currently trending as an NLCs conjugate due to its proved ability in recognizing a homologous mRNA sequence in the cancer cell and induce its degradation [182]. In this regard, and chemistry wise, a smooth conjugation between thiol-modified DNA or RNA molecules (e.g., siRNA) and the NLCs surface occurs by biodegradable disulfide (S–S) bonds. Further conjugations with NLC include polymers conjugation (e.g., PEG) with targeting fractions (e.g., luteinizing-hormone releasing hormone (LHRH) peptide) [183,184]. However, the key drawback of NLCs is the need to use organic solvents to initially solubilize the hydrophobic drugs before loading [185], as well as the short-term stability of the liquid NLCs compared to the solid ones [186,187]. Like the previously discussed lipid-based nanocarriers, the use of NLCs as localized inhaled dosage forms is still under investigation mainly as active carriers for anti-tuberculosis [188], genetic disorders such as lung cystic fibrosis [189], antibiotics lung delivery [190,191], in addition to LC therapies. In LC, NLCs are often used to resolve p-glycoprotein (P-gp) efflux, and drug resistance which is generally associated with over-expression of MRP1 protein (responsible for cancer cell drug efflux) and BCL2 protein (responsible for anti-apoptotic cellular defense) [192–195].

Inhaled NLCs were used for the pulmonary delivery of various drugs and approaches for LC treatment. The cyclooxygenase-2 enzyme, which is responsible for the progression and growth of NSCLC and found to be up-regulated among different cancers [196,197].

Thus, the efficacy of inhaled celecoxib-loaded NLCs in NSCLC in combination with IV administered docetaxel was evaluated using a metastatic A549 tumor model in Nu/Nu mice. The NLCs were initially prepared using a hot melt homogenization technique via mixing compritol (solid lipid), miglyol (liquid lipid), and sodium taurocholate (surfactant). The PS, Đ, ZP, drug content, DL, EE% of the NLC produced were 211 nm, 0.22, 25.30 mV, 1.8 mg/mL, 4 *w/w*%, and 95.6%, respectively. The celecoxib-loaded NLCs were nebulized using Inexpose™ (SCIREQ Scientific Respiratory Equipment Inc, Montreal, QC, Canada). The aerosolized NLCs had D_{ae} and FPF were 1.58 μm and 76.2%, respectively. The isobologram of the interaction between docetaxel and celecoxib-NLC in the A549 NSCLC cell line suggests moderate synergistic activity. While the analysis of the 28-days in vivo studies showed that treatment with inhaled celecoxib-NLC, IV docetaxel, and the combination of both treatments decreased tumor volume by 25%, 37%, and 67%, respectively, without a substantial decrease in mice weight compared to control group. Besides, the inhaled celecoxib-NLCs, IV docetaxel, and combined therapy have also decreased vascular endothelial growth factor expressions in regressive tumors by 0.27, 0.44, and 0.65 times, respectively, compared to control. The quantitative proteomic analysis shows a significant reduction in the regulation of multiple proteins demonstrating enhanced anticancer activity in combination therapy compared to docetaxel treatment alone [128].

A comparison in lung deposition was evaluated in vivo using Wistar rats between pulmonary delivered paclitaxel loaded-NLCs (as a dry powder delivered using insufflators (Penny Century, PA, USA)) and orally administered methanolic PBS suspension of the drug [129]. The NLCs were prepared by the emulsification and ultrasonication method using various surfactants. The solid and liquid lipids phase consisted of stearic acid (or glyceryl monostearate) and oleic acid at different concentrations, while the aqueous phase was composed of different amounts of Tween 80®, Tween 20®, or Tween 40®. The statistical analysis showed that the low lipid ratio, the high levels of surfactant concentration and, the medium homogenization speed provided favorable ranges of PS, Đ, and ZP values for Tween 20® (178.7 nm, 0.158, −15.22 mV), Tween 80® (243.1 nm, 0.225, −16.12 mV), and Tween 60® (298.2 nm, 0.281, −22.23 mV). The NLCs formulated with Tween 20® showed the highest uptake of Caco-2 cells, which could be attributed to Tween 20® ability to inhibit P-gp efflux [198]. As a result, the Tween 20®-based NLCs were further spray-dried using leucine as anti-adherent to produce NLCs powder with PS, Đ, ZP, and an in vitro release of 283.4 nm, 0.226, −25.12 mV, 64.9%, respectively. The dried NLCs had good powder and flow properties with a D_{ae} of 3.53 μm. Lungs' uptake of the drug from the powdered NLCs was higher than the plain drug suspension. This could be attributed to the less clearance of the drug from the lungs due to the slow release of the drug from the NLCs and the retention of the drug in lipid nanoparticles. This indicates the superiority of local delivery via the pulmonary route [129].

The concept of multifunctional NLCs-based delivery systems substantially enhanced the efficiency of NSCLC therapy with suggested abilities to limit the adverse side effects of the treatments, primarily when targeting strategies are used and administered via inhalation. In this regard, multifunctional anticancer (doxorubicin or paclitaxel) and siRNA-loaded NLCs for pulmonary delivery via nebulization were developed for the treatment of LC. The NLCs were functionalized with a modified synthetic analog of luteinizing hormone-releasing hormone (LHRH) as a targeting moiety. In addition, they were conjugated with (1,2-Distearoyl-sn-glycero-3-phosphoethanolamine-poly(ethylene glycol) (DSPE- PEG). The developed doxorubicin-NLCs were primarily used to evaluate cellular uptake and the intracellular localization due to the intrinsic fluorescence of doxorubicin, while the paclitaxel-NLCs were used to assess the anticancer efficacy of the formulation. After the preparation process, the final NLC was purified via dialysis (MWC 10,000) and lyophilized with mannitol (5%) as a cryoprotectant. In vivo orthotopic model of human LC in nu/nu mice was used to evaluate the anticancer activity and tissue distribution. After inhalation, the developed NLCs efficiently delivered their payload into LC cells, leaving healthy lung tissues unaffected compared with IV injection. The tumor size decreased from 117 mm^3

to 20.8 mm^3 and 2.6 mm^3 upon treatment with LHRH-NLC- paclitaxel, and LHRH-NLC-paclitaxel -siRNAs, respectively. The obtained results showed the high efficiency of the inhaled NLCs for tumor-targeted local delivery, specifically LC cells. As a result, effective suppression of tumor growth and prevention of adverse side effects on healthy organs [130].

The same concept in the latter study was used recently to developed paclitaxel tumor-targeted NLCs using the melted ultrasonic method after successfully mixing Precirol ATO 5® (solid lipid), squalene (liquid lipid), and soybean phosphatidylcholine (emulsifier) with the aqueous phase, which was composed of Tween 80® (surfactant) and (N-[1-(2,3-dioleoyloxy)propyl]-N,N,N-trimethylammonium) "DOTAP" (a cationic lipid which grants positive charge to NLC) in deionized distilled water, while paclitaxel was dissolved in dimethyl sulfoxide (DMSO). PEG2000 was the most suitable choice for the linkage of LHRH peptide with the NLCs, and later it was further conjugated with siRNA. The LHRH-NLC-siRNAs-paclitaxel-loaded nanoparticles had distinct spherical shape with PS, ZP, and loading efficiency of 113 nm, +45 mV, and 98%, respectively. On the cellular level, the toxicity of the developed formulation was superior to the traditionally available epidermal growth factor inhibitor, gefitinib, in three types of cells, including H1781, H3255, and A549 cells lines, as such sensitivity was linked to the presence of LHRH. The in vivo study was performed using an orthotopic NSCLC mouse model. The NLCs formulations were administered via IV and inhalation (using a Collison nebulizer (BGI, Inc., Waltham, MA, USA) methods. The results showed that developed multifunctional NLCs had a suggested efficient accumulation and retention in the lungs when inhaled compared to the IV route. The immunoperoxidase assay indicated that the formulation did not induce an immune response in human peripheral blood lymphocytes. Besides, no signs of toxicity were observed (in vivo) in the (liver, kidney, spleen, heart, lung, brain) of nude mice following inhalation or IV administration [131].

In summary, NLCs are potential carriers for the pulmonary delivery of anticancer drugs, they were successfully developed for this purpose using GRAS materials. They have the advantage to be efficiently functionalized using different ligands for active targeting. Besides, they can be aerosolized using nebulization or converted to dry powders to be used in DPIs. The results from the in vitro and in vivo studies are highly promising in the treatment of LC. However, these lipid-based nanocarriers were not tested in any clinical trial yet.

6.5. Miscellaneous Inhaled Lipid-Based Nanocarriers

A number of certain types of lipid-based nanocarriers were addressed for the delivery of anticancer for the treatment of LC via inhalation is available but at a very limited scale. Among these are the lipid-polymer hybrid nanoparticles (LPHNs), these nanocarriers incorporate the advantages of both liposomes and polymeric nanoparticles into one novel drug delivery platform [199]. LPHNs are typically consist of a biodegradable polymeric hydrophobic core and an outer shell made of lipid or lipid-ligand [200] (Figure 2). LPHNs may offer some benefits, such as physical stability and biocompatibility; their surfaces are highly tunable so they are suitable for the passive and active drug targeting, they also provide controlled release of drugs [201]; reduced systemic toxicity; and therefor they can potentially enhance efficacy of anticancer drugs [202]. However, despite all these potential advantages, these nanocarriers are not well explored for the pulmonary delivery.

In one study, LPHNs were used in the downregulation of genes involved in the pathogenesis of severe lung diseases such as LC through the local siRNA delivery. The developed LPHNs were composed of poly(lactic-co-glycolic) acid and dipalmitoylphosphatidylcholine as siRNA inhalation formulation and prepared using the emulsion/solvent diffusion method. The optimized formulation was found to have PS and ZP in the range of (135 to 169 nm) and (−16 to −30 mV), respectively, with $Đ < 0.130$ and EE% of 75%. The formulation possessed a peculiar triphasic release profile, characterized by an initial burst, with more than 50% of siRNA released in the first hours, followed by a slow-release phase lasting a couple of days and a final fast release time period after 4–5 days. The nebulized formulation was having D_{ae} < 5.39 µm. Before each experiment, freeze-dried HLPNs were dispersed in 0.5 mM sodium chloride. The stability of the developed siRNA-loaded LPHNs was confirmed by TEM analysis of freeze-dried formulation in the presence of mannitol before and after nebulization in the Vitrocell Cloud system (Vitrocell Systems GmbH, Waldkirch, Germany). On the cellular level, these LPHNs were able to penetrate into cells effectively and are localized intracellularly on the TCCC cell line leading to an effective in vitro gene silencing (on A549 cells line) in the form of knocking down both aENaC and bENaC subunit proteins up to 72 h. The developed nanosystem was muco-inert and stable inside artificial mucus with no cytotoxic or acute proinflammatory effect toward any of the cell components of the co-culture model. The results demonstrated the high potential of using HLPNs as carriers for pulmonary delivery of siRNA [132].

These hybrid nanocarriers are having excellent potential for the pulmonary delivery of drugs, and their possible role in delivering inhaled anticancer drugs is not well investigated and could be considered for future studies in this field.

Niosomes are also among the systems that are rarely investigated for inhaled anticancer therapy to treat LC. Niosomes are also known as non-ionic surfactant-based vesicles (Figure 2). These carriers gained much interest in the pharmaceutical field due to their excellent abilities to encapsulate and efficiently deliver drugs/agents of different physicochemical properties via different routes of drug administration. Furthermore, their production is easy to scale up at low costs. Besides, these nanoparticles demonstrated to be more stable than liposomes during the formulation phase or upon storage. The required pharmacokinetic properties can be achieved by optimizing the components or modifying the surface of niosomes [203]. Particle size and zeta potential are essential to the pharmacokinetics, bio-distribution, toxicity, and stability of niosomes and should be well considered [204,205].

Inhalable cationic niosomes of curcumin were developed for effective and local delivery to LC cells [134], to circumvent the poor physicochemical and biopharmaceutical limitations of curcumin associated with its oral and parenteral administration, such as the poor and unpredictable bioavailability at the site of action and the extensive first-pass metabolism and irregular bio-distribution [206,207]. The developed niosomes were prepared using the reverse-phase evaporation method and composed of span 80®, diethyl ether, and chloroform with or without cholesterol. The prepared formulations were further freeze-dried using mannitol as a cryoprotectant. The resulted curcumin-loaded niosomes (containing cholesterol) (Cur-C-SUNS) were cationic and unilamellar with PS (97.4 nm), ZP (+28.5 mV), and %EE of (83.3%). While the freeze-dried niosomes prepared without cholesterol (Cur-SUNS) had a smaller PS (83.8 nm), and ZP value of (−3.02 mV), and EE% of (78.8%). The in vitro release of the powdered niosomes using dialysis membrane technique was enhanced by (30.1%), which could be due to the amorphization of nanovesicles that ultimately enhanced the solubility and release rate of the drug [208]. The optimized formulation (Cur-C-SUNS) was able to inhibit the A549 cells proliferation at the IC50 of 3.1 µM, which is significantly lower than 7.5 µM for Cur-SUNS and curcumin dispersion (< 32 µM). The in vitro cellular uptake results illustrated higher endocytosis of Cur-C-SUNS as compared to Cur-SUNS due to electrostatic interaction between cationic nanovesicles and negatively charged plasma membrane of A549 cells [134]. Although the obtained in vitro results were promising, no further in vivo studies were performed to investigate the potential roles of inhaled niosomes for the delivery of anticancer drugs for LC treatment.

Sterosomes, are new and promising non-phospholipid type of liposomes drug delivery nanoparticles, typically they composed of stearylamine and cholesterol. They are named as 'sterosomes' owing to their high sterol content. These carriers are highly tunable and suggested to have better stability and longer circulation and residence time than the classical liposomes [209,210].

Sterosomes were recently reported to deliver the widely used antidiabetic drug (metformin) as an inhalation dosage form because it was shown to have anticancer activities via inhibition of cellular proliferation of many cancers, including LC. The safety, tolerability and pharmacokinetics of inhaled metformin sterosomal formulation or solution. In this study, cholesterol was mixed with stearylamine or myristic acid followed by dissolving accurately weighed quantities of the solid chemicals in a mixture of benzene/methanol. The PS, %EE and ZP of the developed formulation have ranged approximately from 288.7 to 578 nm, 71% to 89% and + 16.2 to + 63.2 mV, respectively. The Đ values were generally <0.4. The measured D_{ae}, GSD and FPF values for aerosolized metformin-loaded sterosomes by jet nebulizer were 3.3 μm, 2.114, 62.36 respectively. The MTT assay on A549 cell lines (for 48 h) showed that survival rate after exposure to metformin-containing sterosomes was very low <50%. The clinical study in this work (3 females: 3 males) at average age of 32 years old showed that the volunteers noted the greasy and ammonia-like smell of metformin sterosomal preparation. The entire process of aerosol administration of the prepared metformin-loaded sterosomes and metformin solution was generally feasible and well tolerated. The metformin-loaded sterosomes enhanced the half-life, area under the curve, and mean residence time of metformin in all healthy volunteers after inhalation of a single dose of 750 mg of metformin sterosomal formulation [135]. Authors have addressed some limitations of this study such as the relatively small number of subjects which could lead to improper variability in the results, and the lack of comparison between multiple and different doses. More extensive clinical trials with long-term follow-up are needed to confirm the safety and efficacy of the developed formulation.

7. Inhalable Anticancer Drug-Loaded Lipid-Based Nanocarriers in Clinical Trials

Despite the proven advantages offered by inhalable anticancer therapy via lipid-based nanocarriers in preclinical studies, the number of conducted clinical trials is still limited (Table 3). In addition, the most advanced development of inhaled anticancer therapy was performed up to phase II only; consequently, no inhaled lipid-based nanocarrier product reached the market yet. This could be attributed to the associated challenges of using this route of administration, as discussed in Section 3 of this review.

Table 3. Summary of clinical trials that have been conducted on the inhalable anticancer drug-loaded lipid-based nanocarriers for the treatment of LC.

Drug	Cisplatin	Cisplatin	9-nitrocamptothecin
NCT Number	N/A *	NCT00102531	N/A **
Phase	Phase I	Phase Ib/IIa	Phase I
Nanocarrier Type	Liposomes	Liposomes	Liposomes
Nanocarrier composition	Dipalmitoyl phosphatidylcholine (DPPC) and Cholesterol	Dipalmitoyl phosphatidylcholine (DPPC) and Cholesterol	Dilauroyl phosphatidylcholine (DLPC)
Drug dose	1.5–60 mg/m^2	24 and 36 mg/m^2	6.7–26.6 μg/kg/day
Study duration	1 to 4 consecutive days in 3-weeks cycles.	The given dose was administered on a 2-weeks cycles.	The given dose was administered for 1 to 8 weeks followed by a 2-weeks rest cycles.
Delivering device	Nebulizer	Nebulizer	Nebulizer
Droplet size	3.7 ± 1.9 μm	3.7 ± 1.9 μm	1–3 μm
No. of Subjects	17	19	25
Type of carcinoma	NSCLC (16) SCLC (1)	High-grade, progressive, or recurrent osteosarcoma in the lungs (secondary LC).	Primary or metastatic LC.
Subjects' gender	F + M	F + M	F + M
Age, mean (years)	41.8–70.7, 56.6	13–27, 18 ± 3	33–84, 58.5
Main adverse events	Dyspnea, vomiting, nausea, cough, hoarseness, and eosinophilia.	Dyspnea, nausea, cough, and wheezing.	Pharyngitis, fatigue, nausea, vomiting, cough, anemia, neutropenia, anorexia, and skin rash

Table 3. *Cont.*

Main findings	A significant reversible (in 94% of the subjects) decrease in forced expiratory volume in 1 s (FEV_1) was observed after one cycle.	Most of the adverse events occurred at the higher given dose (36 mg/m^2).	A decrease in pulmonary function tests during treatment was noticed.
	No significant change in the diffusing lung capacity for carbon monoxide.	No significant or long-lasting systematic adverse events were noticed.	No hematological toxicities were noticed.
	No dose-limiting toxicity was observed at the maximum delivered dose.	No significant change in the pulmonary function testing parameters.	Inhaled 9NC plasma levels were like those observed after oral ingestion.
	No systematic adverse effects of cisplatin were noticed.	Serum concentrations of inhaled cisplatin were lower than those of intravenous cisplatin.	A dose-dependent increment in both C max and AUC values at the two lower doses; 6.7 and 13.3 µg/kg/day, but not at the highest dose.
	Only 10–15% of the dose reached the site of action.	Systemic cisplatin exposure was minimal.	Partial remissions were observed in 2 patients with uterine cancer, and stabilization occurred in 3 patients with primary lung cancer.
	Very low plasma platinum levels only with the longest repeated inhalations.	No significant difference in cisplatin deposition within the tumors and the surrounding lung tissue.	Higher levels of 9NC were found in the lungs compared to those in the plasma by the end of treatment.
	70% of the subjects showed a stable disease, while 23% of them had a progressive disease.	Two patients had stable disease after 2 cycles, underwent metastasectomy, and remained free from pulmonary recurrence 1 year after initiation of therapy.	The recommended dose for Phase II studies was 13.3 µg/kg/day on a daily 60-min exposure, 5 consecutive days/week for 8 weeks, with a concentration of 9NC of 0.4 mg/mL in the nebulizer.
Reference	[30]	[31,32]	[29]

* Phase II clinical trial involving inhaled liposomal cisplatin formulation for the treatment of pulmonary recurrent osteosarcoma (NCT01650090) was completed in 2018 but no data were published yet. ** Totally six clinical trials were conducted furtherly; NCT00492141, NCT00250016, NCT00249990, NCT00250068, NCT00277082 and NCT00250120, where the latter was withdrawn and no published results of the first five trials have been published up to date.

Among the various types of inhalable lipid-based nanocarriers, only liposomes were evaluated in clinical trials. The safety and pharmacokinetics of aerosolized sustained-release lipid inhalation targeting (SLIT) of cisplatin in patients with lung carcinoma were investigated. Seventeen patients and one tracheostomy patient on compassionate use received treatment. The results showed that the aerosolized liposomal cisplatin was well tolerated. In addition, no DLT was observed at the maximum delivered dose. Safety data showed that no hematologic toxicity, nephrotoxicity, ototoxicity, or neurotoxicity was observed. Pharmacokinetically, very low plasma platinum levels were obtained only with the longest repeated inhalations. The aerosolized cisplatin-loaded liposomal formulation was found to be feasible and safe [30].

To evaluate the safety and efficacy of inhaled lipid cisplatin (ILC) in patients with recurrent osteosarcoma who only had pulmonary metastases, an open-label, phase Ib/IIa study was performed (NCT00102531). The study involved nineteen patients. The results showed that no patients experienced hematologic toxicity, nephrotoxicity, or ototoxicity. The inhaled liposomal cisplatin was well tolerated in heavily treated osteosarcoma patients. In addition, the typical toxicities associated with intravenous cisplatin did not appear with the inhaled therapy [31,32]. A phase II clinical trial to establish whether treatment with inhaled liposomal cisplatin (ILC) formulation is effective in delaying/preventing pulmonary relapse in osteosarcoma patients in complete surgical remission following one or two prior pulmonary relapses was completed in 2018 (NCT01650090). However, no data have been published yet [211].

Aerosolized 9-nitro-20(*S*)-camptothecin (9NC)-loaded liposomal formulation was evaluated clinically for safety and feasibility in a group of 25 patients with primary or metastatic LC. The patients received the aerosolized liposomal formulation for five consecutive days/week for 1, 2, 4, or 6 weeks followed by two weeks of rest to determine feasibility. As mentioned previously, chemical pharyngitis was the DLT at 26 mg/kg/day. After inhalation, 9NC was absorbed in a rapid and sustained manner through the lung parenchyma to the bloodstream circulation. Stabilization occurred in 3 patients with primary LC, and partial remissions were observed in 2 patients with uterine cancer. The results revealed that the pulmonary administration of 13.3 mg/kg/day of the 9NC-loaded liposomal formulation was feasible and safe. Furthermore, the researchers recommended a dose of 13.3 mg/kg/day of the liposomal formulation for phase II of the study [29].

There is other six clinical trials of aerosolized 9NC-loaded liposomes have been completed but no results were released or published to the author's best knowledge, and they are namely: (NCT00492141) for determining the effectiveness of L9NC given by aerosol in combination with temozolomide in patients with solid tumors involving the lungs (Phase II, completed in September 2009) [212], (NCT00249990) for determining efficacy and toxicity profile in metastatic or recurrent endometrial cancer (Phase II, completed in September 2007) [213], (NCT00250016) to determine the amount of aerosolized drug in patients' blood and tumor (completed in August 2007) [214], (NCT00250068) to determine the overall response rate to 9NC administered by aerosolization in patients with NSCLC any stage (Phase II, completed in December 2007) [215], (NCT00277082) to determine the concentration of the drug in the alveolar fluid over time (completed in June 2005) [216], (NCT00250120) to determine the overall response rate to the inhaled liposomal drug in patients with NSCLC at any stage (withdrawn, Phase II, completed in August 2007) [217].

With the new advancements in the fields of lipid-based nanocarriers, drug targeting, and pulmonary delivery devices, clinical studies are currently needed to reveal the promising potentials of inhalation chemotherapy.

8. Conclusions

Inhalable anticancer therapy via lipid-based nanocarriers is an exciting and growing research area. It is a promising treatment strategy to combat LC and lung metastases. Due to the unique properties of the lipid-based nanocarriers of great biocompatibility, high drug loading, and tunable surfaces for active targeting and controlled drug-release behavior, they are gaining much interest. Results from the recent studies on preclinical levels revealed that the drugs loaded in these inhalable nanocarriers will be concentrated in the lungs and then diffuse gradually into the blood circulation and the lymphatic system to target the cancerous cells. Among the currently available pulmonary devices, only nebulizers and DPIs are potentially suitable for the efficient delivery of these nanoparticles. The use of DPIs as devices for inhaled anticancer drugs loaded in lipid-based nanoparticles is quite promising as they have many advantages and could overcome the challenges associated with this route. Combining the use of lipid-based nanocarriers, DPIs devices, particle engineering, and formulation sciences opens the door for new advancements and possibilities. However, the research in this field is still in its infancy, particularly at the in vivo and clinical studies levels. The general formulation strategy should concentrate on developing uni- or multifunctional lipid-based nanocarriers for active targeting, with good drug loading and sustained release properties, embedded in well-engineered microparticles composed of safe and well-tolerated excipients of high FPF for efficient lung deposition, drug delivery, and antitumor activity.

Author Contributions: Conceptualization, I.M.A., H.A.W., Y.D.; writing—original draft preparation, I.M.A., R.A.A.; writing—review and editing, I.M.A., R.A.A., H.A.W., A.Y., Y.D.; visualization, F.G.S. and I.M.A.; supervision, H.A.W., A.Y, Y.D and T.P.; project administration, H.A.W., N.M., T.P.; funding acquisition, H.A.W., N.M., T.P., I.M.A. All authors have read and agreed to the published version of the manuscript.

Funding: This research was funded by Malaysian ministry of higher education, fundamental research grant scheme (FRGS) grant number FRGS/1/2020/SKK0/USM/01/4 (account no: 203.PFARMASI.6711891).

Institutional Review Board Statement: Not applicable.

Informed Consent Statement: Not applicable.

Data Availability Statement: Data sharing not applicable.

Acknowledgments: Ibrahim M. Abdulbaqi and Reem Abou Assi gratefully acknowledge Universiti Sains Malaysia (USM), the Institute of Postgraduate Studies (IPS), Penang, Malaysia for awarding of USM Fellowship.

Conflicts of Interest: The authors declare no conflict of interest. The funders had no role in the design of the study; in the collection, analyses, or interpretation of data; in the writing of the manuscript, or in the decision to publish the results.

References

1. Bray, F.; Ferlay, J.; Soerjomataram, I.; Siegel, R.L.; Torre, L.A.; Jemal, A. Global cancer statistics 2018: GLOBOCAN estimates of incidence and mortality worldwide for 36 cancers in 185 countries. *CA Cancer J. Clin.* **2018**, *68*, 394–424. [CrossRef]
2. World Health Organization. The Global Cancer Observatory. Cancer Fact Sheets. Available online: http://gco.iarc.fr/today/data/factsheets/cancers/15-Lung-fact-sheet.pdf (accessed on 23 April 2021).
3. American Cancer Society. Key Statistics for Lung Cancer. Available online: https://www.cancer.org/content/cancer/en/cancer/lung-cancer/about/key-statistics.html (accessed on 23 April 2021).
4. National Cancer Institute. The Surveillance, Epidemiology, and End Results (SEER) Program. Cancer Stat Facts: Lung and Bronchus Cancer. Available online: https://seer.cancer.gov/statfacts/html/lungb.html (accessed on 23 April 2021).
5. World Health Organization. International Agency for Research on Cancer. The Global Cancer Observatory (GCO). Cancer Tomorrow (Incidence). Available online: http://gco.iarc.fr/tomorrow/graphic-line?type=0&population=900&mode=population&sex=0&cancer=39&age_group=value&apc_male=0&apc_female=0#collapse-group-1-1 (accessed on 23 April 2021).
6. World Health Organization. International Agency for Research on Cancer. The Global Cancer Observatory (GCO). Cancer Tomorrow (Mortality). Available online: http://gco.iarc.fr/tomorrow/graphic-line?type=1&population=900&mode=population&sex=0&cancer=39&age_group=value&apc_male=0&apc_female=0#collapse-group-1-1 (accessed on 23 April 2021).
7. Lovly, L.H.C.M. Neoplasms of the lung. In *Harrison's Principles of Internal Medicine*, 20th ed.; Jameson, J.L., Dennis, A.S.F., Kasper, L., Hauser, S.L., Longo, D.L., Loscalzo, J., Eds.; McGraw-Hill Education: New York, NY, USA, 2018.
8. Butler, S.K. Lung cancer. In *Applied Therapeutics: The Clinical Use of Drugs*, 11th ed.; Zeind, C.S., Carvalho, M.G., Eds.; Wolters Kluwer: Philadelphia, PA, USA, 2018.
9. Postmus, P.E.; Kerr, K.M.; Oudkerk, M.; Senan, S.; Waller, D.A.; Vansteenkiste, J.; Escriu, C.; Peters, S.; on behalf of the ESMO Guidelines Committee. Early and locally advanced non-small-cell lung cancer (NSCLC): ESMO Clinical Practice Guidelines for diagnosis, treatment and follow-up. *Ann. Oncol.* **2017**, *28*, iv1–iv21. [CrossRef]
10. American Cancer Society. Treating Non-Small Cell Lung Cancer. Available online: https://www.cancer.org/cancer/lung-cancer/treating-non-small-cell.html (accessed on 23 April 2021).
11. American Cancer Society. Surgery for Small Cell Lung Cancer. Available online: https://www.cancer.org/cancer/lung-cancer/treating-small-cell/surgery.html (accessed on 23 April 2021).
12. Nurgali, K.; Jagoe, R.T.; Abalo, R. Editorial: Adverse effects of cancer chemotherapy: Anything new to improve tolerance and reduce sequelae? *Front. Pharm.* **2018**, *9*, 245. [CrossRef] [PubMed]
13. Zhao, C.Y.; Cheng, R.; Yang, Z.; Tian, Z.M. Nanotechnology for cancer therapy based on chemotherapy. *Molecules* **2018**, *23*, 826. [CrossRef] [PubMed]
14. Gonciar, D.; Mocan, T.; Matea, C.T.; Zdrehus, C.; Mosteanu, O.; Mocan, L.; Pop, T. Nanotechnology in metastatic cancer treatment: Current achievements and future research trends. *J. Cancer* **2019**, *10*, 1358–1369. [CrossRef] [PubMed]
15. National Cancer Institute. Cancer and Nanotechnology: Treatment and Therapy. Available online: https://www.cancer.gov/nano/cancer-nanotechnology/treatment (accessed on 22 December 2019).
16. Amararathna, M.; Goralski, K.; Hoskin, D.W.; Rupasinghe, H.P.V. Pulmonary nano-drug delivery systems for lung cancer: Current knowledge and prospects. *J. Lung Health Dis.* **2019**, *3*, 11–28. [CrossRef]
17. Dolovich, M.B.; Dhand, R. Aerosol drug delivery: Developments in device design and clinical use. *Lancet* **2011**, *377*, 1032–1045. [CrossRef]
18. Patton, J.S.; Byron, P.R. Inhaling medicines: Delivering drugs to the body through the lungs. *Nat. Rev. Drug Discov.* **2007**, *6*, 67–74. [CrossRef] [PubMed]
19. Lee, W.-H.; Loo, C.-Y.; Traini, D.; Young, P.M. Nano- and micro-based inhaled drug delivery systems for targeting alveolar macrophages. *Expert Opin. Drug Deliv.* **2015**, *12*, 1009–1026. [CrossRef]
20. Garmany, T.H.; Moxley, M.A.; White, F.V.; Dean, M.; Hull, W.M.; Whitsett, J.A.; Nogee, L.M.; Hamvas, A. Surfactant Composition and Function in Patients with ABCA3 Mutations. *Pediatric Res.* **2006**, *59*, 801–805. [CrossRef]
21. Kwok, P.C.L.; Chan, H.-K. *Advances in Pulmonary Drug Delivery*, 1st ed.; CRC Press: Boca Raton, FL, USA, 2016. [CrossRef]
22. Williams, R.O.; Taft, D.R.; McConville, J.T. *Advanced Drug Formulation Design to Optimize Therapeutic Outcomes*, 1st ed.; CRC Press: Boca Raton, FL, USA, 2007. [CrossRef]
23. Mangal, S.; Gao, W.; Li, T.; Zhou, Q. Pulmonary delivery of nanoparticle chemotherapy for the treatment of lung cancers: Challenges and opportunities. *Acta Pharmacol. Sin.* **2017**, *38*, 782. [CrossRef]

24. Haque, S.; Feeney, O.; Meeusen, E.; Boyd, B.J.; McIntosh, M.P.; Pouton, C.W.; Whittaker, M.; Kaminskas, L.M. Local inflammation alters the lung disposition of a drug loaded pegylated liposome after pulmonary dosing to rats. *J. Control. Release* **2019**, *307*, 32–43. [CrossRef] [PubMed]
25. Sharma, S.; White, D.; Imondi, A.R.; Placke, M.E.; Vail, D.M.; Kris, M.G. Development of inhalational agents for oncologic use. *J. Clin. Oncol.* **2001**, *19*, 1839–1847. [CrossRef]
26. Tatsumura, T.; Koyama, S.; Tsujimoto, M.; Kitagawa, M.; Kagamimori, S. Further study of nebulisation chemotherapy, a new chemotherapeutic method in the treatment of lung carcinomas: Fundamental and clinical. *Br. J. Cancer* **1993**, *68*, 1146–1149. [CrossRef] [PubMed]
27. Zarogoulidis, P.; Chatzaki, E.; Porpodis, K.; Domvri, K.; Hohenforst-Schmidt, W.; Goldberg, E.P.; Karamanos, N.; Zarogoulidis, K. Inhaled chemotherapy in lung cancer: Future concept of nanomedicine. *Int J. Nanomed.* **2012**, *7*, 1551–1572. [CrossRef]
28. Videira, M.A.; Botelho, M.F.; Santos, A.C.; Gouveia, L.F.; Pedroso de Lima, J.J.; Almeida, A.J. lymphatic uptake of pulmonary delivered radiolabelled solid lipid nanoparticles. *J. Drug Target.* **2002**, *10*, 607–613. [CrossRef]
29. Verschraegen, C.F.; Gilbert, B.E.; Loyer, E.; Huaringa, A.; Walsh, G.; Newman, R.A.; Knight, V. Clinical evaluation of the delivery and safety of aerosolized liposomal 9-nitro-20(s)-camptothecin in patients with advanced pulmonary malignancies. *Clin. Cancer Res.* **2004**, *10*, 2319–2326. [CrossRef]
30. Wittgen, B.P.; Kunst, P.W.; van der Born, K.; van Wijk, A.W.; Perkins, W.; Pilkiewicz, F.G.; Perez-Soler, R.; Nicholson, S.; Peters, G.J.; Postmus, P.E. Phase I study of aerosolized SLIT cisplatin in the treatment of patients with carcinoma of the lung. *Clin. Cancer Res.* **2007**, *13*, 2414–2421. [CrossRef] [PubMed]
31. Chou, A.J.; Gupta, R.; Bell, M.D.; Riewe, K.O.; Meyers, P.A.; Gorlick, R. Inhaled lipid cisplatin (ILC) in the treatment of patients with relapsed/progressive osteosarcoma metastatic to the lung. *Pediatr. Blood Cancer* **2013**, *60*, 580–586. [CrossRef]
32. ClinicalTrials.gov. Inhalation SLIT Cisplatin (Liposomal) for the Treatment of Osteosarcoma Metastatic to the Lung. Available online: https://clinicaltrials.gov/ct2/show/NCT00102531 (accessed on 25 June 2021).
33. Lemarie, E.; Vecellio, L.; Hureaux, J.; Prunier, C.; Valat, C.; Grimbert, D.; Boidron-Celle, M.; Giraudeau, B.; le Pape, A.; Pichon, E.; et al. Aerosolized gemcitabine in patients with carcinoma of the lung: Feasibility and safety study. *J. Aerosol Med. Pulm. Drug Deliv.* **2011**, *24*, 261–270. [CrossRef]
34. Zarogoulidis, P.; Eleftheriadou, E.; Sapardanis, I.; Zarogoulidou, V.; Lithoxopoulou, H.; Kontakiotis, T.; Karamanos, N.; Zachariadis, G.; Mabroudi, M.; Zisimopoulos, A.; et al. Feasibility and effectiveness of inhaled carboplatin in NSCLC patients. *Investig. New Drugs* **2012**, *30*, 1628–1640. [CrossRef] [PubMed]
35. Kosmidis, C.; Sapalidis, K.; Zarogoulidis, P.; Sardeli, C.; Koulouris, C.; Giannakidis, D.; Pavlidis, E.; Katsaounis, A.; Michalopoulos, N.; Mantalobas, S.; et al. Inhaled cisplatin for NSCLC: Facts and results. *Int. J. Mol. Sci.* **2019**, *20*, 2005. [CrossRef]
36. Dabbagh, A.; Abu Kasim, N.H.; Yeong, C.H.; Wong, T.W.; Abdul Rahman, N. Critical parameters for particle-based pulmonary delivery of chemotherapeutics. *J. Aerosol Med. Pulm. Drug Deliv.* **2018**, *31*, 139–154. [CrossRef] [PubMed]
37. Ruge, C.A.; Kirch, J.; Lehr, C.-M. Pulmonary drug delivery: From generating aerosols to overcoming biological barriers—Therapeutic possibilities and technological challenges. *Lancet Respir. Med.* **2013**, *1*, 402–413. [CrossRef]
38. Olsson, B.; Bondesson, E.; Borgström, L.; Edsbäcker, S.; Eirefelt, S.; Ekelund, K.; Gustavsson, L.; Hegelund-Myrbäck, T. Pulmonary drug metabolism, clearance, and absorption. In *Controlled Pulmonary Drug Delivery*; Smyth, H.D.C., Hickey, A.J., Eds.; Springer: New York, NY, USA, 2011; pp. 21–50. [CrossRef]
39. Hidalgo, A.; Cruz, A.; Pérez-Gil, J. Barrier or carrier? Pulmonary surfactant and drug delivery. *Eur. J. Pharm. Biopharm.* **2015**, *95*, 117–127. [CrossRef]
40. Lee, W.-H.; Loo, C.-Y.; Traini, D.; Young, P.M. Inhalation of nanoparticle-based drug for lung cancer treatment: Advantages and challenges. *Asian J. Pharm. Sci.* **2015**, *10*, 481–489. [CrossRef]
41. Xu, J.; Lu, X.; Zhu, X.; Yang, Y.; Liu, Q.; Zhao, D.; Lu, Y.; Wen, J.; Chen, X.; Li, N. Formulation and characterization of spray-dried powders containing vincristine-liposomes for pulmonary delivery and its pharmacokinetic evaluation from in vitro and in vivo. *J. Pharm. Sci.* **2019**, *108*, 3348–3358. [CrossRef]
42. Rosière, R.; Van Woensel, M.; Gelbcke, M.; Mathieu, V.; Hecq, J.; Mathivet, T.; Vermeersch, M.; Van Antwerpen, P.; Amighi, K.; Wauthoz, N. New folate-grafted chitosan derivative to improve delivery of paclitaxel-loaded solid lipid nanoparticles for lung tumor therapy by inhalation. *Mol. Pharm.* **2018**, *15*, 899–910. [CrossRef]
43. Carvalho, T.C.; Carvalho, S.R.; McConville, J.T. Formulations for pulmonary administration of anticancer agents to treat lung malignancies. *J. Aerosol Med. Pulm. Drug Deliv.* **2011**, *24*, 61–80. [CrossRef]
44. Yang, W.; Peters, J.I.; Williams, R.O. Inhaled nanoparticles—A current review. *Int. J. Pharm.* **2008**, *356*, 239–247. [CrossRef] [PubMed]
45. Smola, M.; Vandamme, T.; Sokolowski, A. Nanocarriers as pulmonary drug delivery systems to treat and to diagnose respiratory and non respiratory diseases. *Int J. Nanomed.* **2008**, *3*, 1–19.
46. El-Sherbiny, I.M.; Villanueva, D.G.; Herrera, D.; Smyth, H.D.C. Overcoming lung clearance mechanisms for controlled release drug delivery. In *Controlled Pulmonary Drug Delivery*; Smyth, H.D.C., Hickey, A.J., Eds.; Springer: New York, NY, USA, 2011; pp. 101–126. [CrossRef]
47. Carvalho, T.C.; Peters, J.I.; Williams, R.O., 3rd. Influence of particle size on regional lung deposition—What evidence is there? *Int. J. Pharm.* **2011**, *406*, 1–10. [CrossRef]
48. Champion, J.A.; Mitragotri, S. Role of target geometry in phagocytosis. *Proc. Natl. Acad. Sci. USA* **2006**, *103*, 4930–4934. [CrossRef]

49. Champion, J.A.; Mitragotri, S. Shape induced inhibition of phagocytosis of polymer particles. *Pharm. Res.* **2009**, *26*, 244–249. [CrossRef]
50. Choi, H.S.; Ashitate, Y.; Lee, J.H.; Kim, S.H.; Matsui, A.; Insin, N.; Bawendi, M.G.; Semmler-Behnke, M.; Frangioni, J.V.; Tsuda, A. Rapid translocation of nanoparticles from the lung airspaces to the body. *Nat. Biotechnol.* **2010**, *28*, 1300–1303. [CrossRef] [PubMed]
51. Matsumura, Y.; Maeda, H. A new concept for macromolecular therapeutics in cancer chemotherapy: Mechanism of tumoritropic accumulation of proteins and the antitumor agent smancs. *Cancer Res.* **1986**, *46*, 6387–6392. [PubMed]
52. Nakamura, Y.; Mochida, A.; Choyke, P.L.; Kobayashi, H. Nanodrug delivery: Is the enhanced permeability and retention effect sufficient for curing cancer? *Bioconjug. Chem.* **2016**, *27*, 2225–2238. [CrossRef] [PubMed]
53. Hirsjärvi, S.; Passirani, C.; Benoit, J.P. Passive and active tumour targeting with nanocarriers. *Curr. Drug Discov. Technol.* **2011**, *8*, 188–196. [CrossRef] [PubMed]
54. Kim, C.H.; Lee, S.G.; Kang, M.J.; Lee, S.; Choi, Y.W. Surface modification of lipid-based nanocarriers for cancer cell-specific drug targeting. *J. Pharm. Investig.* **2017**, *47*, 203–227. [CrossRef]
55. Yan, W.; Leung, S.S.; To, K.K. Updates on the use of liposomes for active tumor targeting in cancer therapy. *Nanomedicine* **2020**, *15*, 303–318. [CrossRef]
56. Riaz, M.K.; Riaz, M.A.; Zhang, X.; Lin, C.; Wong, K.H.; Chen, X.; Zhang, G.; Lu, A.; Yang, Z. Surface functionalization and targeting strategies of liposomes in solid tumor therapy: A review. *Int. J. Mol. Sci.* **2018**, *19*, 195. [CrossRef] [PubMed]
57. Upadhyay, D.; Scalia, S.; Vogel, R.; Wheate, N.; Salama, R.O.; Young, P.M.; Traini, D.; Chrzanowski, W. Magnetised thermo responsive lipid vehicles for targeted and controlled lung drug delivery. *Pharm. Res.* **2012**, *29*, 2456–2467. [CrossRef] [PubMed]
58. Wauthoz, N.; Rosière, R.; Amighi, K. Inhaled cytotoxic chemotherapy: Clinical challenges, recent developments, and future prospects. *Expert Opin. Drug Deliv.* **2020**, 1–22. [CrossRef]
59. Rosière, R.; Amighi, K.; Wauthoz, N. Nanomedicine-based inhalation treatments for lung cancer. In *Nanotechnology-Based Targeted Drug Delivery Systems for Lung Cancer*; Academic Press: Cambridge, MA, USA, 2019; pp. 249–268. [CrossRef]
60. Zhou, Q.T.; Tang, P.; Leung, S.S.; Chan, J.G.; Chan, H.K. Emerging inhalation aerosol devices and strategies: Where are we headed? *Adv. Drug Deliv. Rev.* **2014**, *75*, 3–17. [CrossRef] [PubMed]
61. Garrastazu Pereira, G.; Lawson, A.J.; Buttini, F.; Sonvico, F. Loco-regional administration of nanomedicines for the treatment of lung cancer. *Drug Deliv.* **2016**, *23*, 2881–2896. [CrossRef] [PubMed]
62. Longest, W.; Spence, B.; Hindle, M. Devices for improved delivery of nebulized pharmaceutical aerosols to the lungs. *J. Aerosol Med. Pulm. Drug Deliv.* **2019**, *32*, 317–339. [CrossRef] [PubMed]
63. Labiris, N.R.; Dolovich, M.B. Pulmonary drug delivery. Part II: The role of inhalant delivery devices and drug formulations in therapeutic effectiveness of aerosolized medications. *Br. J. Clin. Pharmacol.* **2003**, *56*, 600–612. [CrossRef]
64. Labiris, N.R.; Dolovich, M.B. Pulmonary drug delivery. Part I: Physiological factors affecting therapeutic effectiveness of aerosolized medications. *Br. J. Clin. Pharmacol.* **2003**, *56*, 588–599. [CrossRef]
65. Cipolla, D.; Gonda, I.; Chan, H.K. Liposomal formulations for inhalation. *Ther. Deliv.* **2013**, *4*, 1047–1072. [CrossRef]
66. Hureaux, J.; Lagarce, F.; Gagnadoux, F.; Vecellio, L.; Clavreul, A.; Roger, E.; Kempf, M.; Racineux, J.L.; Diot, P.; Benoit, J.P.; et al. Lipid nanocapsules: Ready-to-use nanovectors for the aerosol delivery of paclitaxel. *Eur. J. Pharm. Biopharm.* **2009**, *73*, 239–246. [CrossRef]
67. Anabousi, S.; Kleemann, E.; Bakowsky, U.; Kissel, T.; Schmehl, T.; Gessler, T.; Seeger, W.; Lehr, C.M.; Ehrhardt, C. Effect of PEGylation on the stability of liposomes during nebulisation and in lung surfactant. *J. Nanosci. Nanotechnol.* **2006**, *6*, 3010–3016. [CrossRef]
68. Wauthoz, N.; Amighi, K. Phospholipids in pulmonary drug delivery. *Eur. J. Lipid Sci. Technol.* **2014**, *116*, 1114–1128. [CrossRef]
69. ElKasabgy, N.A.; Adel, I.M.; Elmeligy, M.F. Respiratory tract: Structure and attractions for drug delivery using dry powder inhalers. *AAPS PharmSciTech* **2020**, *21*, 238. [CrossRef] [PubMed]
70. Gamal, A.; Saeed, H.; Sayed, O.M.; Kharshoum, R.M.; Salem, H.F. Proniosomal microcarriers: Impact of constituents on the physicochemical properties of proniosomes as a new approach to enhance inhalation efficiency of dry powder inhalers. *AAPS PharmSciTech* **2020**, *21*, 156. [CrossRef] [PubMed]
71. Lee, W.-H.; Loo, C.-Y.; Traini, D.; Young, P.M. Development and evaluation of paclitaxel and curcumin dry powder for inhalation lung cancer treatment. *Pharmaceutics* **2021**, *13*, 9. [CrossRef] [PubMed]
72. Party, P.; Bartos, C.; Farkas, Á.; Szabó-Révész, P.; Ambrus, R. Formulation and in vitro and in silico characterization of "nano-in-micro" dry powder inhalers containing meloxicam. *Pharmaceutics* **2021**, *13*, 211. [CrossRef] [PubMed]
73. Patel, K.; Bothiraja, C.; Mali, A.; Kamble, R. Investigation of sorafenib tosylate loaded liposomal dry powder inhaler for the treatment of non-small cell lung cancer. *Part. Sci. Technol.* **2021**, 1–10. [CrossRef]
74. Satari, N.; Taymouri, S.; Varshosaz, J.; Rostami, M.; Mirian, M. Preparation and evaluation of inhalable dry powder containing glucosamine-conjugated gefitinib SLNs for lung cancer therapy. *Drug Dev. Ind. Pharm.* **2020**, *46*, 1265–1277. [CrossRef]
75. Zhu, X.; Kong, Y.; Liu, Q.; Lu, Y.; Xing, H.; Lu, X.; Yang, Y.; Xu, J.; Li, N.; Zhao, D.; et al. Inhalable dry powder prepared from folic acid-conjugated docetaxel liposomes alters pharmacodynamic and pharmacokinetic properties relevant to lung cancer chemotherapy. *Pulm. Pharm. Ther.* **2019**, *55*, 50–61. [CrossRef]
76. Malamatari, M.; Charisi, A.; Malamataris, S.; Kachrimanis, K.; Nikolakakis, I. Spray drying for the preparation of nanoparticle-based drug formulations as dry powders for inhalation. *Processes* **2020**, *8*, 788. [CrossRef]

77. Yang, M.Y.; Chan, J.G.Y.; Chan, H.-K. Pulmonary drug delivery by powder aerosols. *J. Control. Release* **2014**, *193*, 228–240. [CrossRef]
78. Weers, J.; Clark, A. The impact of inspiratory flow rate on drug delivery to the lungs with dry powder inhalers. *Pharm. Res.* **2017**, *34*, 507–528. [CrossRef] [PubMed]
79. Clark, A.R.; Weers, J.G.; Dhand, R. The confusing world of dry powder inhalers: It is all about inspiratory pressures, not inspiratory flow rates. *J. Aerosol Med. Pulm. Drug Deliv.* **2019**, *33*, 1–11. [CrossRef] [PubMed]
80. Zhang, J.; Wu, L.; Chan, H.-K.; Watanabe, W. Formation, characterization, and fate of inhaled drug nanoparticles. *Adv. Drug Deliv. Rev.* **2011**, *63*, 441–455. [CrossRef] [PubMed]
81. Huang, Z.; Kłodzińska, S.N.; Wan, F.; Nielsen, H.M. Nanoparticle-mediated pulmonary drug delivery: State of the art towards efficient treatment of recalcitrant respiratory tract bacterial infections. *Drug Deliv. Transl. Res.* **2021**, 1–21. [CrossRef]
82. Bohr, A.; Water, J.; Beck-Broichsitter, M.; Yang, M. Nanoembedded microparticles for stabilization and delivery of drug-loaded nanoparticles. *Curr. Pharm. Des.* **2015**, *21*, 5829–5844. [CrossRef] [PubMed]
83. Umerska, A.; Mugheirbi, N.A.; Kasprzak, A.; Saulnier, P.; Tajber, L. Carbohydrate-based Trojan microparticles as carriers for pulmonary delivery of lipid nanocapsules using dry powder inhalation. *Powder Technol.* **2020**, *364*, 507–521. [CrossRef]
84. Assadpour, E.; Jafari, S.M. Advances in spray-drying encapsulation of food bioactive ingredients: From microcapsules to nanocapsules. *Annu. Rev. Food Sci. Technol.* **2019**, *10*, 103–131. [CrossRef]
85. Kaur, P.; Mishra, V.; Shunmugaperumal, T.; Goyal, A.K.; Ghosh, G.; Rath, G. Inhalable spray dried lipidnanoparticles for the co-delivery of paclitaxel and doxorubicin in lung cancer. *J. Drug Deliv. Sci. Technol.* **2020**, *56*, 101502. [CrossRef]
86. Anton, N.; Jakhmola, A.; Vandamme, T.F. Trojan microparticles for drug delivery. *Pharmaceutics* **2012**, *4*, 1–25. [CrossRef]
87. Abdelaziz, H.M.; Freag, M.S.; Elzoghby, A.O. Solid lipid nanoparticle-based drug delivery for lung cancer. In *Nanotechnology-Based Targeted Drug Delivery Systems for Lung Cancer*; Academic Press: Cambridge, MA, USA, 2019; pp. 95–121. [CrossRef]
88. Lechanteur, A.; Evrard, B. Influence of composition and spray-drying process parameters on carrier-free dpi properties and behaviors in the lung: A review. *Pharmaceutics* **2020**, *12*, 55. [CrossRef]
89. El-Gendy, N.; Berkland, C. Combination chemotherapeutic dry powder aerosols via controlled nanoparticle agglomeration. *Pharm. Res.* **2009**, *26*, 1752–1763. [CrossRef]
90. Varshosaz, J.; Hassanzadeh, F.; Mardani, A.; Rostami, M. Feasibility of haloperidol-anchored albumin nanoparticles loaded with doxorubicin as dry powder inhaler for pulmonary delivery. *Pharm. Dev. Technol.* **2015**, *20*, 183–196. [CrossRef]
91. Li, X.; Anton, N.; Ta, T.M.C.; Zhao, M.; Messaddeq, N.; Vandamme, T.F. Microencapsulation of nanoemulsions: Novel Trojan particles for bioactive lipid molecule delivery. *Int. J. Nanomed.* **2011**, *6*, 1313–1325. [CrossRef]
92. Chaurasiya, B.; Zhao, Y.Y. Dry powder for pulmonary delivery: A comprehensive review. *Pharmaceutics* **2020**, *13*, 31. [CrossRef] [PubMed]
93. Nikolaou, M.; Krasia-Christoforou, T. Electrohydrodynamic methods for the development of pulmonary drug delivery systems. *Eur. J. Pharm. Sci.* **2018**, *113*, 29–40. [CrossRef]
94. Ely, L.; Roa, W.; Finlay, W.H.; Löbenberg, R. Effervescent dry powder for respiratory drug delivery. *Eur. J. Pharm. Biopharm.* **2007**, *65*, 346–353. [CrossRef] [PubMed]
95. Jyoti, K.; Kaur, K.; Pandey, R.S.; Jain, U.K.; Chandra, R.; Madan, J. Inhalable nanostructured lipid particles of 9-bromo-noscapine, a tubulin-binding cytotoxic agent: In vitro and in vivo studies. *J. Colloid Interface Sci.* **2015**, *445*, 219–230. [CrossRef]
96. Roa, W.H.; Azarmi, S.; Al-Hallak, M.H.; Finlay, W.H.; Magliocco, A.M.; Löbenberg, R. Inhalable nanoparticles, a non-invasive approach to treat lung cancer in a mouse model. *J. Control. Release* **2011**, *150*, 49–55. [CrossRef] [PubMed]
97. Al-Hallak, M.H.; Sarfraz, M.K.; Azarmi, S.; Roa, W.H.; Finlay, W.H.; Rouleau, C.; Löbenberg, R. Distribution of effervescent inhalable nanoparticles after pulmonary delivery: An in vivo study. *Ther. Deliv.* **2012**, *3*, 725–734. [CrossRef]
98. Kumar, R. Lipid-based nanoparticles for drug-delivery systems. In *Nanocarriers for Drug Delivery*; Elsevier: Amsterdam, The Netherlands, 2019; pp. 249–284. [CrossRef]
99. Muller, R.H.; Keck, C.M. Challenges and solutions for the delivery of biotech drugs–a review of drug nanocrystal technology and lipid nanoparticles. *J. Biotechnol.* **2004**, *113*, 151–170. [CrossRef] [PubMed]
100. Narvekar, M.; Xue, H.Y.; Eoh, J.Y.; Wong, H.L. Nanocarrier for poorly water-soluble anticancer drugs—Barriers of translation and solutions. *AAPS PharmSciTech* **2014**, *15*, 822–833. [CrossRef] [PubMed]
101. Mohanta, B.C.; Palei, N.N.; Surendran, V.; Dinda, S.C.; Rajangam, J.; Deb, J.; Sahoo, B.M. Lipid based nanoparticles: Current strategies for brain tumor targeting. *Curr. Nanomater.* **2019**, *4*, 84–100. [CrossRef]
102. Talluri, S.V.; Kuppusamy, G.; Karri, V.V.; Tummala, S.; Madhunapantula, S.V. Lipid-based nanocarriers for breast cancer treatment—Comprehensive review. *Drug Deliv.* **2016**, *23*, 1291–1305. [CrossRef]
103. Allen, T.M.; Cullis, P.R. Liposomal drug delivery systems: From concept to clinical applications. *Adv. Drug Deliv. Rev.* **2013**, *65*, 36–48. [CrossRef]
104. Xiao, Z.; Zhuang, B.; Zhang, G.; Li, M.; Jin, Y. Pulmonary delivery of cationic liposomal hydroxycamptothecin and 5-aminolevulinic acid for chemo-sonodynamic therapy of metastatic lung cancer. *Int. J. Pharm.* **2021**, *601*, 120572. [CrossRef] [PubMed]
105. Loira-Pastoriza, C.; Vanvarenberg, K.; Ucakar, B.; Machado Franco, M.; Staub, A.; Lemaire, M.; Renauld, J.-C.; Vanbever, R. Encapsulation of a CpG oligonucleotide in cationic liposomes enhances its local antitumor activity following pulmonary delivery in a murine model of metastatic lung cancer. *Int. J. Pharm.* **2021**, *600*, 120504. [CrossRef]

106. Zhang, M.; Li, M.; Du, L.; Zeng, J.; Yao, T.; Jin, Y. Paclitaxel-in-liposome-in-bacteria for inhalation treatment of primary lung cancer. *Int. J. Pharm.* **2020**, *578*, 119177. [CrossRef]
107. Adel, I.M.; ElMeligy, M.F.; Abdelrahim, M.E.A.; Maged, A.; Abdelkhalek, A.A.; Abdelmoteleb, A.M.M.; Elkasabgy, N.A. Design and characterization of spray-dried proliposomes for the pulmonary delivery of curcumin. *Int. J. Nanomed.* **2021**, *16*, 2667–2687. [CrossRef]
108. Zhang, T.; Chen, Y.; Ge, Y.; Hu, Y.; Li, M.; Jin, Y. Inhalation treatment of primary lung cancer using liposomal curcumin dry powder inhalers. *Acta Pharm. Sin. B* **2018**, *8*, 440–448. [CrossRef]
109. Yuan, N.; Zhang, X.; Cao, Y.; Jiang, X.; Zhao, S.; Feng, Y.; Fan, Y.; Lu, Z.; Gao, H. Contrast-enhanced computerized tomography combined with a targeted nanoparticle contrast agent for screening for early-phase non-small cell lung cancer. *Exp. Ther. Med.* **2017**, *14*, 5063–5068. [CrossRef]
110. Tagami, T.; Kubota, M.; Ozeki, T. Effective remote loading of doxorubicin into DPPC/poloxamer 188 hybrid liposome to retain thermosensitive property and the assessment of carrier-based acute cytotoxicity for pulmonary administration. *J. Pharm. Sci.* **2015**, *104*, 3824–3832. [CrossRef]
111. Mainelis, G.; Seshadri, S.; Garbuzenko, O.B.; Han, T.; Wang, Z.; Minko, T. Characterization and application of a nose-only exposure chamber for inhalation delivery of liposomal drugs and nucleic acids to mice. *J. Aerosol Med. Pulm. Drug Deliv.* **2013**, *26*, 345–354. [CrossRef]
112. Gaspar, M.M.; Radomska, A.; Gobbo, O.L.; Bakowsky, U.; Radomski, M.W.; Ehrhardt, C. Targeted delivery of transferrin-conjugated liposomes to an orthotopic model of lung cancer in nude rats. *J. Aerosol Med. Pulm. Drug Deliv.* **2012**, *25*, 310–318. [CrossRef] [PubMed]
113. Riaz, M.K.; Zhang, X.; Wong, K.H.; Chen, H.; Liu, Q.; Chen, X.; Zhang, G.; Lu, A.; Yang, Z. Pulmonary delivery of transferrin receptors targeting peptide surface-functionalized liposomes augments the chemotherapeutic effect of quercetin in lung cancer therapy. *Int. J. Nanomed.* **2019**, *14*, 2879–2902. [CrossRef] [PubMed]
114. Lin, C.; Zhang, X.; Chen, H.; Bian, Z.; Zhang, G.; Riaz, M.K.; Tyagi, D.; Lin, G.; Zhang, Y.; Wang, J.; et al. Dual-ligand modified liposomes provide effective local targeted delivery of lung-cancer drug by antibody and tumor lineage-homing cell-penetrating peptide. *Drug Deliv.* **2018**, *25*, 256–266. [CrossRef] [PubMed]
115. Hamzawy, M.A.; Abo-Youssef, A.M.; Salem, H.F.; Mohammed, S.A. Antitumor activity of intratracheal inhalation of temozolomide (TMZ) loaded into gold nanoparticles and/or liposomes against urethane-induced lung cancer in BALB/c mice. *Drug Deliv.* **2017**, *24*, 599–607. [CrossRef]
116. Gandhi, M.; Pandya, T.; Gandhi, R.; Patel, S.; Mashru, R.; Misra, A.; Tandel, H. Inhalable liposomal dry powder of gemcitabine-HCl: Formulation, in vitro characterization and in vivo studies. *Int. J. Pharm.* **2015**, *496*, 886–895. [CrossRef] [PubMed]
117. Zhang, T.; Wang, R.; Li, M.; Bao, J.; Chen, Y.; Ge, Y.; Jin, Y. Comparative study of intratracheal and oral gefitinib for the treatment of primary lung cancer. *Eur. J. Pharm. Sci.* **2020**, *149*, 105352. [CrossRef] [PubMed]
118. Asmawi, A.A.; Salim, N.; Ngan, C.L.; Ahmad, H.; Abdulmalek, E.; Masarudin, M.J.; Abdul Rahman, M.B. Excipient selection and aerodynamic characterization of nebulized lipid-based nanoemulsion loaded with docetaxel for lung cancer treatment. *Drug Deliv. Transl. Res.* **2019**, *9*, 543–554. [CrossRef] [PubMed]
119. Asmawi, A.A.; Salim, N.; Abdulmalek, E.; Abdul Rahman, M.B. Modeling the effect of composition on formation of aerosolized nanoemulsion system encapsulating docetaxel and curcumin using D-optimal mixture experimental design. *Int. J. Mol. Sci.* **2020**, *21*, 4357. [CrossRef] [PubMed]
120. Al Ayoub, Y.; Gopalan, R.C.; Najafzadeh, M.; Mohammad, M.A.; Anderson, D.; Paradkar, A.; Assi, K.H. Development and evaluation of nanoemulsion and microsuspension formulations of curcuminoids for lung delivery with a novel approach to understanding the aerosol performance of nanoparticles. *Int. J. Pharm.* **2019**, *557*, 254–263. [CrossRef] [PubMed]
121. Arbain, N.H.; Basri, M.; Salim, N.; Wui, W.T.; Abdul Rahman, M.B. Development and characterization of aerosol nanoemulsion system encapsulating low water soluble quercetin for lung cancer treatment. *Mater. Today Proc.* **2018**, *5*, S137–S142. [CrossRef]
122. Arbain, N.H.; Salim, N.; Masoumi, H.R.F.; Wong, T.W.; Basri, M.; Abdul Rahman, M.B. In vitro evaluation of the inhalable quercetin loaded nanoemulsion for pulmonary delivery. *Drug Deliv. Transl. Res.* **2019**, *9*, 497–507. [CrossRef]
123. Nassimi, M.; Schleh, C.; Lauenstein, H.; Hussein, R.; Hoymann, H.; Koch, W.; Pohlmann, G.A.; Krug, N.; Sewald, K.; Rittinghausen, S. A toxicological evaluation of inhaled solid lipid nanoparticles used as a potential drug delivery system for the lung. *Eur. J. Pharm. Biopharm.* **2010**, *75*, 107–116. [CrossRef]
124. Bakhtiary, Z.; Barar, J.; Aghanejad, A.; Saei, A.A.; Nemati, E.; Ezzati Nazhad Dolatabadi, J.; Omidi, Y. Microparticles containing erlotinib-loaded solid lipid nanoparticles for treatment of non-small cell lung cancer. *Drug Dev. Ind. Pharm.* **2017**, *43*, 1244–1253. [CrossRef]
125. Hu, L.; Jia, Y.; Ding, W. Preparation and characterization of solid lipid nanoparticles loaded with epirubicin for pulmonary delivery. *Pharmazie* **2010**, *65*, 585–587. [PubMed]
126. Yang, Y.; Huang, Z.; Li, J.; Mo, Z.; Huang, Y.; Ma, C.; Wang, W.; Pan, X.; Wu, C. PLGA Porous microspheres dry powders for codelivery of afatinib-loaded solid lipid nanoparticles and paclitaxel: Novel therapy for EGFR tyrosine kinase inhibitors resistant nonsmall cell lung cancer. *Adv. Healthc. Mater.* **2019**, *8*, 1900965. [CrossRef] [PubMed]
127. Nafee, N.; Gaber, D.M.; Elzoghby, A.O.; Helmy, M.W.; Abdallah, O.Y. Promoted antitumor activity of myricetin against lung carcinoma via nanoencapsulated phospholipid complex in respirable microparticles. *Pharm. Res.* **2020**, *37*, 82. [CrossRef] [PubMed]

128. Patel, A.R.; Chougule, M.B.; Patlolla, R.; Wang, G.; Singh, M. Efficacy of aerosolized celecoxib encapsulated nanostructured lipid carrier in non-small cell lung cancer in combination with docetaxel. *Pharm. Res.* **2013**, *30*, 1435–1446. [CrossRef] [PubMed]
129. Kaur, P.; Garg, T.; Rath, G.; Murthy, R.R.; Goyal, A.K. Development, optimization and evaluation of surfactant-based pulmonary nanolipid carrier system of paclitaxel for the management of drug resistance lung cancer using Box-Behnken design. *Drug Deliv.* **2016**, *23*, 1912–1925. [CrossRef] [PubMed]
130. Taratula, O.; Kuzmov, A.; Shah, M.; Garbuzenko, O.B.; Minko, T. Nanostructured lipid carriers as multifunctional nanomedicine platform for pulmonary co-delivery of anticancer drugs and siRNA. *J. Control. Release* **2013**, *171*, 349–357. [CrossRef]
131. Garbuzenko, O.B.; Kuzmov, A.; Taratula, O.; Pine, S.R.; Minko, T. Strategy to enhance lung cancer treatment by five essential elements: Inhalation delivery, nanotechnology, tumor-receptor targeting, chemo- and gene therapy. *Theranostics* **2019**, *9*, 8362–8376. [CrossRef] [PubMed]
132. D'Angelo, I.; Costabile, G.; Durantie, E.; Brocca, P.; Rondelli, V.; Russo, A.; Russo, G.; Miro, A.; Quaglia, F.; Petri-Fink, A.; et al. Hybrid lipid/polymer nanoparticles for pulmonary delivery of siRNA: Development and fate upon in vitro deposition on the human epithelial airway barrier. *J. Aerosol Med. Pulm. Drug Deliv.* **2018**, *31*, 170–181. [CrossRef] [PubMed]
133. Saimi, M.N.I.; Salim, N.; Ahmad, N.; Abdulmalek, E.; Abdul Rahman, M.B. Aerosolized niosome formulation containing gemcitabine and cisplatin for lung cancer treatment: Optimization, characterization and in vitro evaluation. *Pharmaceutics* **2021**, *13*, 59. [CrossRef] [PubMed]
134. Jyoti, K.; Pandey, R.S.; Madan, J.; Jain, U.K. Inhalable cationic niosomes of curcumin enhanced drug delivery and apoptosis in lung cancer cells. *Indian J. Pharm. Educ. Res.* **2016**, *50*. [CrossRef]
135. Osama, H.; Sayed, O.M.; Hussein, R.R.S.; Abdelrahim, M.; Elberry, A. Design, optimization, characterization, and in vivo evaluation of sterosomes as a carrier of metformin for treatment of lung cancer. *J. Liposome Res.* **2020**, *30*, 150–162. [CrossRef] [PubMed]
136. Bangham, A.D.; Standish, M.M.; Watkins, J.C. Diffusion of univalent ions across the lamellae of swollen phospholipids. *J. Mol. Biol.* **1965**, *13*, IN26–IN27. [CrossRef]
137. Çağdaş, M.; Sezer, A.D.; Bucak, S. Liposomes as potential drug carrier systems for drug delivery. In *Application of Nanotechnology in Drug Delivery*; IntechOpen: London, UK, 2014. [CrossRef]
138. Paranjpe, M.; Muller-Goymann, C.C. Nanoparticle-mediated pulmonary drug delivery: A review. *Int. J. Mol. Sci.* **2014**, *15*, 5852–5873. [CrossRef]
139. Akbarzadeh, A.; Rezaei-Sadabady, R.; Davaran, S.; Joo, S.W.; Zarghami, N.; Hanifehpour, Y.; Samiei, M.; Kouhi, M.; Nejati-Koshki, K. Liposome: Classification, preparation, and applications. *Nanoscale Res. Lett.* **2013**, *8*, 102. [CrossRef]
140. Noble, G.T.; Stefanick, J.F.; Ashley, J.D.; Kiziltepe, T.; Bilgicer, B. Ligand-targeted liposome design: Challenges and fundamental considerations. *Trends Biotechnol.* **2014**, *32*, 32–45. [CrossRef]
141. Choudhury, H.; Gorain, B.; Chatterjee, B.; Mandal, U.K.; Sengupta, P.; Tekade, R.K. Pharmacokinetic and pharmacodynamic features of nanoemulsion following oral, intravenous, topical and nasal route. *Curr. Pharm. Des.* **2017**, *23*, 2504–2531. [CrossRef] [PubMed]
142. Jideani, Y.M.a.V.A. *Factors Affecting the Stability of Emulsions Stabilised by Biopolymers, Science and Technology Behind Nanoemulsions*; IntechOpen: London, UK, 2018.
143. Nguyen, T.T.L.; Anton, N.; Vandamme, T.F. Oral pellets loaded with nanoemulsions. In *Nanostructures for Oral Medicine*; Andronescu, E., Grumezescu, A.M., Eds.; Elsevier: Amsterdam, The Netherlands, 2017; pp. 203–230. [CrossRef]
144. Kale, S.N.; Deore, S.L. Emulsion micro emulsion and nano emulsion: A review. *Syst. Rev. Pharm.* **2017**, *8*, 39. [CrossRef]
145. Gutiérrez, J.; González, C.; Maestro, A.; Solè, I.; Pey, C.; Nolla, J. Nano-emulsions: New applications and optimization of their preparation. *Curr. Opin. Colloid Interface Sci.* **2008**, *13*, 245–251. [CrossRef]
146. Choudhury, H.; Pandey, M.; Gorain, B.; Chatterjee, B.; Madheswaran, T.; Md, S.; Mak, K.K.; Tambuwala, M.; Chourasia, M.K.; Kesharwani, P. Nanoemulsions as effective carriers for the treatment of lung cancer. In *Nanotechnology-Based Targeted Drug Delivery Systems for Lung Cancer*; Elsevier: Amsterdam, The Netherlands, 2019; pp. 217–247. [CrossRef]
147. Ngan, C.L.; Asmawi, A.A. Lipid-based pulmonary delivery system: A review and future considerations of formulation strategies and limitations. *Drug Deliv. Transl. Res.* **2018**, *8*, 1527–1544. [CrossRef] [PubMed]
148. Ganta, S.; Amiji, M. Coadministration of Paclitaxel and curcumin in nanoemulsion formulations to overcome multidrug resistance in tumor cells. *Mol. Pharm.* **2009**, *6*, 928–939. [CrossRef]
149. Agrawal, N.; Maddikeri, G.L.; Pandit, A.B. Sustained release formulations of citronella oil nanoemulsion using cavitational techniques. *Ultrason. Sonochem.* **2017**, *36*, 367–374. [CrossRef]
150. Tiwari, S.; Tan, Y.-M.; Amiji, M. Preparation and in vitro characterization of multifunctional nanoemulsions for simultaneous MR imaging and targeted drug delivery. *J. Biomed. Nanotechnol.* **2006**, *2*, 217–224. [CrossRef]
151. Gupta, S.; Kesarla, R.; Omri, A. Formulation strategies to improve the bioavailability of poorly absorbed drugs with special emphasis on self-emulsifying systems. *ISRN Pharm.* **2013**, *2013*, 848043. [CrossRef] [PubMed]
152. Shah, K.; Chan, L.W.; Wong, T.W. Critical physicochemical and biological attributes of nanoemulsions for pulmonary delivery of rifampicin by nebulization technique in tuberculosis treatment. *Drug Deliv.* **2017**, *24*, 1631–1647. [CrossRef] [PubMed]
153. Lovelyn, C.; Attama, A.A. Current state of nanoemulsions in drug delivery. *J. Biomater. Nanobiotechnol.* **2011**, *02*, 626–639. [CrossRef]

154. Nesamony, J.; Shah, I.S.; Kalra, A.; Jung, R. Nebulized oil-in-water nanoemulsion mists for pulmonary delivery: Development, physico-chemical characterization and in vitro evaluation. *Drug Dev. Ind. Pharm.* **2014**, *40*, 1253–1263. [CrossRef] [PubMed]
155. Krahn, C.L.; Raffin, R.P.; Santos, G.S.; Queiroga, L.B.; Cavalcanti, R.L.; Serpa, P.; Dallegrave, E.; Mayorga, P.E.; Pohlmann, A.R.; Natalini, C.C.; et al. Isoflurane-loaded nanoemulsion prepared by high-pressure homogenization: Investigation of stability and dose reduction in general anesthesia. *J. Biomed. Nanotechnol.* **2012**, *8*, 849–858. [CrossRef] [PubMed]
156. Amani, A.; York, P.; Chrystyn, H.; Clark, B.J. Evaluation of a nanoemulsion-based formulation for respiratory delivery of budesonide by nebulizers. *AAPS PharmSciTech* **2010**, *11*, 1147–1151. [CrossRef]
157. Li, M.; Zhu, L.; Liu, B.; Du, L.; Jia, X.; Han, L.; Jin, Y. Tea tree oil nanoemulsions for inhalation therapies of bacterial and fungal pneumonia. *Colloids Surf. B Biointerfaces* **2016**, *141*, 408–416. [CrossRef]
158. Mason, T.G.; Wilking, J.N.; Meleson, K.; Chang, C.B.; Graves, S.M. Nanoemulsions: Formation, structure, and physical properties. *J. Phys. Condens. Matter* **2006**, *18*, R635–R666. [CrossRef]
159. Qi, K.; Al-Haideri, M.; Seo, T.; Carpentier, Y.A.; Deckelbaum, R.J. Effects of particle size on blood clearance and tissue uptake of lipid emulsions with different triglyceride compositions. *JPEN J. Parenter. Enter. Nutr.* **2003**, *27*, 58–64. [CrossRef]
160. Kaur, P.; Garg, T.; Rath, G.; Murthy, R.S.R.; Goyal, A.K. Surfactant-based drug delivery systems for treating drug-resistant lung cancer. *Drug Deliv.* **2016**, *23*, 717–728. [CrossRef]
161. Mansour, H.M.; Rhee, Y.S.; Wu, X. Nanomedicine in pulmonary delivery. *Int. J. Nanomed.* **2009**, *4*, 299–319. [CrossRef]
162. Dammak, I.; Sobral, P.J.d.A.; Aquino, A.; Neves, M.A.d.; Conte-Junior, C.A. Nanoemulsions: Using emulsifiers from natural sources replacing synthetic ones—A review. *Compr. Rev. Food Sci. Food Saf.* **2020**, *19*, 2721–2746. [CrossRef]
163. Renne, R.A.; Wehner, A.P.; Greenspan, B.; Deford, H.; Ragan, H.A.; Westerberg, R.; Buschbom, R.; Burger, G.; Hayes, A.W.; Suber, R.; et al. 2-week and 13-week inhalation studies of aerosolized glycerol in rats. *Inhal. Toxicol.* **2008**, *4*, 95–111. [CrossRef]
164. Terakosolphan, W. Pharmacokinetic-Modifying Effects of Glycerol in Inhaled Medicines. Ph.D. Thesis, King's College, London, UK, 2019.
165. Darquenne, C. Aerosol deposition in the human lung in reduced gravity. *J. Aerosol Med. Pulm. Drug Deliv.* **2014**, *27*, 170–177. [CrossRef] [PubMed]
166. Kamali, H.; Abbasi, S.; Amini, M.A.; Amani, A. Investigation of factors affecting aerodynamic performance of nebulized nanoemulsion. *Iran. J. Pharm Res.* **2016**, *15*, 687–693. [PubMed]
167. Vafadar, A.; Shabaninejad, Z.; Movahedpour, A.; Fallahi, F.; Taghavipour, M.; Ghasemi, Y.; Akbari, M.; Shafiee, A.; Hajighadimi, S.; Moradizarmehri, S.; et al. Quercetin and cancer: New insights into its therapeutic effects on ovarian cancer cells. *Cell Biosci.* **2020**, *10*, 32. [CrossRef]
168. Ganta, S.; Singh, A.; Rawal, Y.; Cacaccio, J.; Patel, N.R.; Kulkarni, P.; Ferris, C.F.; Amiji, M.M.; Coleman, T.P. Formulation development of a novel targeted theranostic nanoemulsion of docetaxel to overcome multidrug resistance in ovarian cancer. *Drug Deliv.* **2016**, *23*, 968–980. [CrossRef]
169. Afzal, S.M.; Shareef, M.Z.; Kishan, V. Transferrin tagged lipid nanoemulsion of docetaxel for enhanced tumor targeting. *J. Drug Deliv. Sci. Technol.* **2016**, *36*, 175–182. [CrossRef]
170. Sajid, M.; Cameotra, S.S.; Khan, M.S.A.; Ahmad, I. Chapter 23—Nanoparticle-based delivery of phytomedicines: Challenges and opportunities. In *New Look to Phytomedicine*; Khan, M.S.A., Ahmad, I., Chattopadhyay, D., Eds.; Academic Press: Cambridge, MA, USA, 2019; pp. 597–623. [CrossRef]
171. Borges, A.; de Freitas, V.; Mateus, N.; Fernandes, I.; Oliveira, J. Solid lipid nanoparticles as carriers of natural phenolic compounds. *Antioxidants* **2020**, *9*, 998. [CrossRef] [PubMed]
172. Shah, R.; Eldridge, D.; Palombo, E.; Harding, I. *Lipid Nanoparticles: Production, Characterization and Stability*; Springer: Berlin/Heidelberg, Germany, 2015.
173. Mehnert, W.; Mäder, K. Solid lipid nanoparticles: Production, characterization and applications. *Adv. Drug Deliv. Rev.* **2001**, *47*, 165–196. [CrossRef]
174. Shah, R.; Eldridge, D.; Palombo, E.; Harding, I. Composition and structure. In *Lipid Nanoparticles: Production, Characterization and Stability*; Springer: Berlin/Heidelberg, Germany, 2015; pp. 11–22.
175. Müller, R.H.; Rühl, D.; Runge, S.A. Biodegradation of solid lipid nanoparticles as a function of lipase incubation time. *Int. J. Pharm.* **1996**, *144*, 115–121. [CrossRef]
176. Haque, S.; Whittaker, M.; McIntosh, M.P.; Pouton, C.W.; Phipps, S.; Kaminskas, L.M. A comparison of the lung clearance kinetics of solid lipid nanoparticles and liposomes by following the 3H-labelled structural lipids after pulmonary delivery in rats. *Eur. J. Pharm. Biopharm.* **2018**, *125*, 1–12. [CrossRef]
177. Huang, Z.; Huang, Y.; Wang, W.; Fu, F.; Wang, W.; Dang, S.; Li, C.; Ma, C.; Zhang, X.; Zhao, Z.; et al. Relationship between particle size and lung retention time of intact solid lipid nanoparticle suspensions after pulmonary delivery. *J. Control. Release* **2020**, *325*, 206–222. [CrossRef] [PubMed]
178. Müller, R.H.; Radtke, M.; Wissing, S.A. Solid lipid nanoparticles (SLN) and nanostructured lipid carriers (NLC) in cosmetic and dermatological preparations. *Adv. Drug Deliv. Rev.* **2002**, *54* (Suppl. S1), S131–S155. [CrossRef]
179. Müller, R.H.; Radtke, M.; Wissing, S.A. Nanostructured lipid matrices for improved microencapsulation of drugs. *Int. J. Pharm.* **2002**, *242*, 121–128. [CrossRef]
180. Ahmad, J.; Akhter, S.; Rizwanullah, M.; Amin, S.; Rahman, M.; Ahmad, M.Z.; Rizvi, M.A.; Kamal, M.A.; Ahmad, F.J. Nanotechnology-based inhalation treatments for lung cancer: State of the art. *Nanotechnol. Sci. Appl.* **2015**, *8*, 55–66. [CrossRef]

181. Wang, Y.; Zhang, H.; Hao, J.; Li, B.; Li, M.; Xiuwen, W. Lung cancer combination therapy: Co-delivery of paclitaxel and doxorubicin by nanostructured lipid carriers for synergistic effect. *Drug Deliv.* **2016**, *23*, 1398–1403. [CrossRef] [PubMed]
182. Chernikov, I.V.; Vlassov, V.V.; Chernolovskaya, E.L. Current development of siRNA bioconjugates: From research to the clinic. *Front. Pharmacol.* **2019**, *10*. [CrossRef] [PubMed]
183. Kuzmov, A.; Minko, T. Nanotechnology approaches for inhalation treatment of lung diseases. *J. Control. Release* **2015**, *219*, 500–518. [CrossRef]
184. Anderson, C.F.; Grimmett, M.E.; Domalewski, C.J.; Cui, H. Inhalable nanotherapeutics to improve treatment efficacy for common lung diseases. *WIREs Nanomed. Nanobiotechnol.* **2020**, *12*, e1586. [CrossRef]
185. Jaiswal, P.; Gidwani, B.; Vyas, A. Nanostructured lipid carriers and their current application in targeted drug delivery. *Artif. Cells Nanomed. Biotechnol.* **2016**, *44*, 27–40. [CrossRef]
186. Gerhardt, A.; Voigt, E.; Archer, M.; Reed, S.; Larson, E.; Van Hoeven, N.; Kramer, R.; Fox, C.; Casper, C. A Thermostable, flexible RNA vaccine delivery platform for pandemic response. *bioRxiv* **2021**, 1–26. [CrossRef]
187. Emami, J.; Rezazadeh, M.; Varshosaz, J.; Tabbakhian, M.; Aslani, A. Formulation of LDL targeted nanostructured lipid carriers loaded with paclitaxel: A detailed study of preparation, freeze drying condition, and in vitro cytotoxicity. *J. Nanomater.* **2012**, *2012*, 358782. [CrossRef]
188. Magalhães, J.; Pinheiro, M.; Drasler, B.; Septiadi, D.; Petri-Fink, A.; Santos, S.G.; Rothen-Rutishauser, B.; Reis, S. Lipid nanoparticles biocompatibility and cellular uptake in a 3D human lung model. *Nanomedicine* **2020**, *15*, 259–271. [CrossRef] [PubMed]
189. Garbuzenko, O.B.; Kbah, N.; Kuzmov, A.; Pogrebnyak, N.; Pozharov, V.; Minko, T. Inhalation treatment of cystic fibrosis with lumacaftor and ivacaftor co-delivered by nanostructured lipid carriers. *J. Control. Release* **2019**, *296*, 225–231. [CrossRef] [PubMed]
190. Moreno-Sastre, M.; Pastor, M.; Esquisabel, A.; Sans, E.; Vinas, M.; Fleischer, A.; Palomino Lago, E.; Bachiller, D.; Pedraz, J. Pulmonary delivery of tobramycin-loaded nanostructured lipid carriers for Pseudomonas aeruginosa infections associated with cystic fibrosis. *Int. J. Pharm.* **2016**, *498*, 263–273. [CrossRef]
191. Sans-Serramitjana, E.; Jorba, M.; Fusté, E.; Pedraz, J.L.; Vinuesa, T.; Viñas, M. Free and nanoencapsulated tobramycin: Effects on planktonic and biofilm forms of pseudomonas. *Microorganisms* **2017**, *5*, 35. [CrossRef] [PubMed]
192. Pakunlu, R.I.; Wang, Y.; Tsao, W.; Pozharov, V.; Cook, T.J.; Minko, T. Enhancement of the Efficacy of chemotherapy for lung cancer by simultaneous suppression of multidrug resistance and antiapoptotic cellular defense. *Nov. Multicompon. Deliv. Syst.* **2004**, *64*, 6214–6224. [CrossRef] [PubMed]
193. Saad, M.; Garbuzenko, O.B.; Minko, T. Co-delivery of siRNA and an anticancer drug for treatment of multidrug-resistant cancer. *Nanomedicine* **2008**, *3*, 761–776. [CrossRef]
194. Taratula, O.; Garbuzenko, O.B.; Chen, A.M.; Minko, T. Innovative strategy for treatment of lung cancer: Targeted nanotechnology-based inhalation co-delivery of anticancer drugs and siRNA. *J. Drug Target.* **2011**, *19*, 900–914. [CrossRef]
195. Garbuzenko, O.B.; Saad, M.; Pozharov, V.P.; Reuhl, K.R.; Mainelis, G.; Minko, T. Inhibition of lung tumor growth by complex pulmonary delivery of drugs with oligonucleotides as suppressors of cellular resistance. *Proc. Natl. Acad. Sci. USA* **2010**, *107*, 10737–10742. [CrossRef] [PubMed]
196. Hida, T.; Kozaki, K.-i.; Muramatsu, H.; Masuda, A.; Shimizu, S.; Mitsudomi, T.; Sugiura, T.; Ogawa, M.; Takahashi, T. Cyclooxygenase-2 inhibitor induces apoptosis and enhances cytotoxicity of various anticancer agents in non-small cell lung cancer cell lines. *Clin. Cancer Res.* **2000**, *6*, 2006–2011.
197. Shaik, M.S.; Chatterjee, A.; Jackson, T.; Singh, M. Enhancement of antitumor activity of docetaxel by celecoxib in lung tumors. *Int. J. Cancer* **2006**, *118*, 396–404. [CrossRef]
198. Abou Assi, R.; Abdulbaqi, I.M.; Seok Ming, T.; Siok Yee, C.; Wahab, H.A.; Asif, S.M.; Darwis, Y. Liquid and solid self-emulsifying drug delivery systems (SEDDs) as carriers for the oral delivery of azithromycin: Optimization, in vitro characterization and stability assessment. *Pharmaceutics* **2020**, *12*, 1052. [CrossRef]
199. Liu, J.; Cheng, H.; Le Han, Z.Q.; Zhang, X.; Gao, W.; Zhao, K.; Song, Y. Synergistic combination therapy of lung cancer using paclitaxel-and triptolide-coloaded lipid–polymer hybrid nanoparticles. *Drug Des. Dev. Ther.* **2018**, *12*, 3199. [CrossRef]
200. Yugui, F.; Wang, H.; Sun, D.; Zhang, X. Nasopharyngeal cancer combination chemoradiation therapy based on folic acid modified, gefitinib and yttrium 90 co-loaded, core-shell structured lipid-polymer hybrid nanoparticles. *Biomed. Pharmacother.* **2019**, *114*, 108820. [CrossRef]
201. Mukherjee, A.; Waters, A.K.; Kalyan, P.; Achrol, A.S.; Kesari, S.; Yenugonda, V.M. Lipid-polymer hybrid nanoparticles as a next-generation drug delivery platform: State of the art, emerging technologies, and perspectives. *Int. J. Nanomed.* **2019**, *14*, 1937–1952. [CrossRef]
202. Wang, G.; Wang, Z.; Li, C.; Duan, G.; Wang, K.; Li, Q.; Tao, T. RGD peptide-modified, paclitaxel prodrug-based, dual-drugs loaded, and redox-sensitive lipid-polymer nanoparticles for the enhanced lung cancer therapy. *Biomed. Pharmacother.* **2018**, *106*, 275–284. [CrossRef] [PubMed]
203. Ge, X.; Wei, M.; He, S.; Yuan, W.-E. Advances of non-ionic surfactant vesicles (niosomes) and their application in drug delivery. *Pharmaceutics* **2019**, *11*, 55. [CrossRef] [PubMed]
204. Shi, B.; Fang, C.; Pei, Y. Stealth PEG-PHDCA niosomes: Effects of chain length of PEG and particle size on niosomes surface properties, in vitro drug release, phagocytic uptake, in vivo pharmacokinetics and antitumor activity. *J. Pharm. Sci.* **2006**, *95*, 1873–1887. [CrossRef]
205. Tangri, P.; Khurana, S. Niosomes: Formulation and evaluation. *Int. J. Biopharm.* **2011**, *2229*, 7499.

206. Heger, M.; van Golen, R.F.; Broekgaarden, M.; Michel, M.C. The molecular basis for the pharmacokinetics and pharmacodynamics of curcumin and its metabolites in relation to cancer. *Pharm. Rev.* **2014**, *66*, 222–307. [CrossRef]
207. Merisko-Liversidge, E.; Liversidge, G.G. Nanosizing for oral and parenteral drug delivery: A perspective on formulating poorly-water soluble compounds using wet media milling technology. *Adv. Drug Deliv. Rev.* **2011**, *63*, 427–440. [CrossRef]
208. Gajra, B.; Dalwadi, C.; Patel, R. Formulation and optimization of itraconazole polymeric lipid hybrid nanoparticles (Lipomer) using Box Behnken design. *DARU J. Pharm. Sci.* **2015**, *23*, 3. [CrossRef] [PubMed]
209. Cui, Z.K.; Fan, J.; Kim, S.; Bezouglaia, O.; Fartash, A.; Wu, B.M.; Aghaloo, T.; Lee, M. Delivery of siRNA via cationic Sterosomes to enhance osteogenic differentiation of mesenchymal stem cells. *J. Control. Release* **2015**, *217*, 42–52. [CrossRef] [PubMed]
210. Cui, Z.K.; Kim, S.; Baljon, J.J.; Doroudgar, M.; Lafleur, M.; Wu, B.M.; Aghaloo, T.; Lee, M. Design and characterization of a therapeutic non-phospholipid liposomal nanocarrier with osteoinductive characteristics to promote bone formation. *ACS Nano* **2017**, *11*, 8055–8063. [CrossRef] [PubMed]
211. ClinicaTtrials.gov. Phase 2 Study of Inhaled Lipid Cisplatin in Pulmonary Recurrent Osteosarcoma. Available online: https://clinicaltrials.gov/ct2/show/NCT01650090 (accessed on 26 June 2021).
212. ClinicalTrials.gov. Aerosol L9-NC and Temozolomide in Ewing's Sarcoma. Available online: https://clinicaltrials.gov/ct2/show/NCT00492141 (accessed on 26 June 2021).
213. ClinicalTrials.gov. Phase II Study of Aerosolized Liposomal 9-Nitro-20 (S)- Camptothecin (L9NC). Available online: https://clinicaltrials.gov/ct2/show/record/NCT00249990 (accessed on 26 June 2021).
214. ClinicalTrials.gov. Pharmacology Study of Aerosolized Liposomal 9-Nitro-20 (S)-Camptothecin (L9NC). Available online: https://clinicaltrials.gov/ct2/show/NCT00250016 (accessed on 25 June 2021).
215. ClinicalTrials.gov. Study of Aerosolized Liposomal 9-Nitro-20 (S)- Camptothecin (L9NC). Available online: https://clinicaltrials.gov/ct2/show/NCT00250068 (accessed on 26 June 2021).
216. ClinicalTrials.gov. Aerosolized Liposomal Camptothecin in Patients with Metastatic or Recurrent Cancer of the Endometrium or the Lung. Available online: https://clinicaltrials.gov/ct2/show/record/NCT00277082 (accessed on 26 June 2021).
217. ClinicalTrials.gov. Pharmacology Study of Aerosolized Liposomal. Available online: https://clinicaltrials.gov/ct2/show/NCT00250120 (accessed on 26 June 2021).

pharmaceuticals

Review

Challenges of Current Anticancer Treatment Approaches with Focus on Liposomal Drug Delivery Systems

Vijay Gyanani [1,*], Jeffrey C. Haley [1] and Roshan Goswami [2]

1 Long Acting Drug Delivery, Celanese Corporation, Irving, TX 75039, USA; jeff.haley@celanese.com
2 Formulation, R&D, mAbxience, 24009 Leon, Spain; roshan.goswami30@gmail.com
* Correspondence: vijay.gyanani@celanese.com

Abstract: According to a 2020 World Health Organization report (Globocan 2020), cancer was a leading cause of death worldwide, accounting for nearly 10 million deaths in 2020. The aim of anticancer therapy is to specifically inhibit the growth of cancer cells while sparing normal dividing cells. Conventional chemotherapy, radiotherapy and surgical treatments have often been plagued by the frequency and severity of side effects as well as severe patient discomfort. Cancer targeting by drug delivery systems, owing to their selective targeting, efficacy, biocompatibility and high drug payload, provides an attractive alternative treatment; however, there are technical, therapeutic, manufacturing and clinical barriers that limit their use. This article provides a brief review of the challenges of conventional anticancer therapies and anticancer drug targeting with a special focus on liposomal drug delivery systems.

Keywords: chemotherapy; radiotherapy; active targeting; passive targeting; tumor; immunoconjugate; traditional liposome; stealth liposome; triggered release; limitations of liposomes

Citation: Gyanani, V.; Haley, J.C.; Goswami, R. Challenges of Current Anticancer Treatment Approaches with Focus on Liposomal Drug Delivery Systems. *Pharmaceuticals* **2021**, *14*, 835. https://doi.org/10.3390/ph14090835

Academic Editors: Ana Catarina Silva, João Nuno Moreira and José Manuel Sousa Lobo

Received: 29 July 2021
Accepted: 20 August 2021
Published: 24 August 2021

1. Introduction

Cancer Statistics: Need for Better Therapeutics

Cancer is a group of diseases characterized by uncontrolled growth of abnormal cells that have the latent potential to penetrate other tissues. It is the leading cause of death worldwide, amounting to nearly 7.6 million deaths globally i.e., nearly 13% of total deaths in 2008 [1] and more recently 10 million deaths in 2020 [2]. As per current estimates, the number of cancer cases may reach an unprecedented 22.2 million in 2030 [1]. Statistics in the United States are no different where cancer is the second most prevalent cause of death, next to only heart related diseases [3]. As per the American Cancer Society, about 608,570 Americans are expected to die of cancer in 2021, which accounts for approximately 1670 deaths per day and nearly a quarter of total deaths in the US [3]. These data highlight the significance of anticancer research and the necessity to discover innovative ways to treat cancer.

The main goal of anticancer therapy is to specifically inhibit the malignant activity of cancer cells, while leaving healthy cells unaffected. Conventional anticancer treatments, including chemotherapy, radiotherapy and surgery, are challenged by drug resistance, severity and side effects. Some of the challenges and limitations of these therapies are discussed.

2. Limitations and Challenges Associated with Traditional Anticancer Therapies

2.1. Cancer Surgery

Cancer surgery is perceived to be an effective tool for eliminating early-stage cancer i.e., at the tumor level. However, it is worth acknowledging that not all early-stage cancerous tissues can be surgically removed. The limitation of surgery lies in how deep seated a tumor tissue is as well as its size. If the tumor size is perilously big, it can seriously impair the regular functioning of a surrounding tissue or organ. A relevant example, post brain surgery, is negative impact on normal functioning of brain i.e., thinking, speaking, etc. In this situation, surgery may not be a first preference for treatment [4]. Another pertinent example is breast cancer where accurate determination of tumor size and position remains a challenge and, therefore, limits the success of a surgical procedure [4].

Other notable examples where surgery impacts normal functioning include permanent impairment of fertility that may be caused by prostrate, ovarian and uterine surgery [4]. Similarly, impact on vocal cords caused by lung surgery performed especially in the upper trachea and shortness of breath developed after lower lung procedures are other known examples [4].

Furthermore, while there are other glaring instances, such as Laryngectomy which eliminates the natural ability to speak, procedures such as a Glossectomy do not eliminate natural speaking but lead to slurred speech with difficulty in swallowing [4].

Irrespective of the complications associated with cancer surgery at various sites, surgery inherently carry risks such as infections, bleeding and pain associated with local nerve injury.

2.2. *Chemotherapy*

Chemotherapy is a treatment regime where a combination of drugs is administered to the body. Notably, chemotherapy remains one of only a few treatment choices for advanced-stage cancer (metastasized cancer); however, a serious deficiency of chemotherapy is the lack of its target selectivity. As the cancer cells arise from normal functioning cells that exhibit uncontrolled growth, anticancer drugs indiscriminately impact the growth of normal non-proliferative cells along with inhibiting cancer cell growth. This poor selectivity of common chemotherapeutic drugs imparts serious side effects on normal tissues such as bone marrow, hair follicles and the gastrointestinal tract [5]. To quote some examples: Carboplatin or carboplatin in conjunction with other chemotherapeutic agents have been known to induce dose-dependent hematotoxicity such as neutropenia and thrombocytopenia. Dermatological effects, specifically keratitis, are common skin reactions arising from chlorambucil administration. Also, dose-limiting glomerular and tubular dysfunction, nuclear pallor in distal nephron and mitochondrial swelling may be caused by renal accumulation of cisplatin by a membrane transport assisted process after continuous and long-term exposure [6]. Acute cardiotoxicity that may include arrhythmias, acute heart failure, inflammatory responses such as pericarditis and myocarditis and other related symptoms including apoptosis due to formation of free radicals, and cardiomyocyte dysfunction are known to be caused by accumulation of Anthracyclines, specifically doxorubicin [7]. In addition to acute toxicity, chronic cardiotoxicity such as left ventricular dysfunction is also related to anthracyclines [7]. For breast cancer treatments, emesis, neutropenia and alopecia are common symptoms of 5-fluorouracil (CMF) cyclophosphamide and methotrexate regimen [8].

Besides the above-mentioned significant examples of severe side effects of chemotherapeutic agents, there are other side effects that are not as potent but do severely limit quality of life and may lead to premature discontinuation of chemotherapy. Dermatologic reactions are most prevalent between them [9]. Common skin related adverse effects include hyperpigmentation, dryness and rash. Other common skin reactions such as erythema and swelling are generally associated with antimetabolite drugs such as CMF and capecitabine [9]. Relatively new anticancer drugs e.g., epidermal growth factor receptor (EGFR) inhibitors noticeably cause follicular rash (e.g., papulopustular rash) and dryness that can then lead to infections such as pruritis [9]. Besides skin, other common side effects are observed on mucosal membranes where conditions such as toxic epidermic necrolysis and Steven Johnson Syndrome (SJS) are caused by other drugs e.g., busulfan, chlorambucil, cyclophosphamide and procarbazine [9].

In furtherance to the adverse effects mentioned above, owing to poor selectivity/non-specificity of chemotherapeutic agents against cancer cells, the other significant limitation is the advancement of 'multi-drug resistance' (MDR) after prolonged exposure of drugs (Figure 1). Cancerous cells may grow resistance against a single chemotherapeutic agent or a combination of agents with an analogous mechanism of action but may develop into cross-resistance against other agents with differing mechanism of actions and/or targets. This transformation to cross-resistance against other therapeutic agents is called 'multi-drug resistance' (MDR). It is due to the development of MDR that heterogeneous cancer cells grow even in the presence of chemotherapeutic drugs. The development of this drug tolerance is manifested in cancer cells either as modification in a potential drug target or as augmentation of cell survival mechanisms such as DNA repair, changes in apoptotic cycles due to changes in ceramide levels, ineffective tumor suppressor protein (p53) or activation of cytochrome oxidases which is critical for cellular respiration [10].

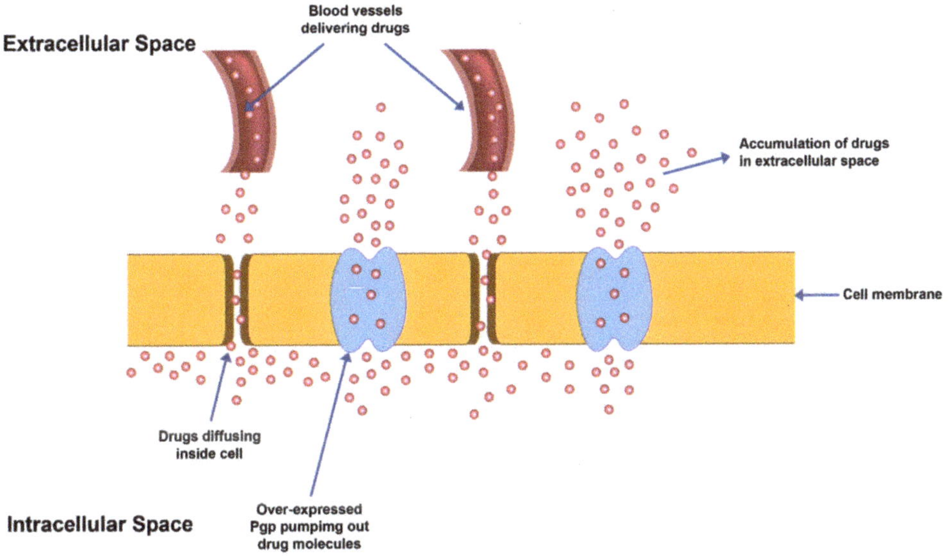

Figure 1. MDR exhibited by overexpression of Pgp transporter proteins leading to efflux of drug from cancer cells.

MDR also leads to over-expression of ATP binding cassette-based efflux transporters which in turn reduce the drug levels in the intracellular space to suboptimal levels in the cells (Figure 1).

The severity of side effects caused by chemotherapy, as well as the MDR phenomenon combined with the narrow therapeutic index of anticancer drugs, severely limits the therapeutic efficacy of chemotherapy. Furthermore, severity of side effects necessitates dose reductions of the anticancer agent which eventually leads to inefficient therapeutic outcomes and potential metastasis.

2.3. Radiotherapy

Radiotherapy is another prominent anticancer therapy and is characterized by the use of high-energy radiation for the treatment of cancer. The wide application of radiotherapy varies from eliminating tumor to reducing tumor size. One way in which radiotherapy differs from chemotherapy is that the adverse effects of radiotherapy are localized in nature (in proximity to the radiated area) as opposed to systemic adverse effects manifested by chemotherapy. The side effects of radiation therapy can be classified either as early or late effects. While early effects are reversible, late effects have propensity to be irreversible and aggravate with time. The more involved late effects are facilitated by stromal, parenchymal, inflammatory and endothelial cells.

Early adverse effects are largely skin reactions such as desquamation and erythema. On the other hand, late effects consist of conditions for example radiation-induced neuron and blood vessel injury, atrophy and fibrosis. Fibrosis is a condition defined by buildup of excessive collagen and extracellular matrix in and around radiated tissues. The early phase of fibrosis is characterized by activation of cytokine cascades which yields tumor-necrosis factor-α (TNFα), interleukins 1 and 6 and other growth factors in much similarity to the wound healing process [11]. In contrast to a regular wound healing process, however, which is a short-term process, fibrotic factor TNF β is downregulated by TNFα and connective tissue growth factor (CTGF); the fibrogenesis in tissues continues for years, resulting in fibrosis of tissues [11].

3. Targeted Drug Delivery Systems and Their Limitations

As mentioned earlier, chemotherapy finds its limitation in being indiscriminate, non-specific in its mechanism of action and development of MDR. The sum of these effects renders chemotherapy damaging to normal dividing cells and thus, causes multiple side effects and, over prolonged exposure, becomes less effective to the tumor due to the development of MDR. Notably, less than 10% of an anticancer drug reaches its target tumor tissue [12]. In addition, radiotherapy primarily is localized in its effect and may lead to fibrosis in some cases. Targeted drug delivery systems, on the other hand, specifically target cancer cells while sparing normal cells. Most of the targeted nano drug delivery systems developed in the last few decades include liposomes, antibodies, Immunoconjugates, Immunotoxins, and polymer conjugates among others. Some of these delivery systems are discussed in this review with greater emphasis on liposomal drug delivery systems. It is important to note that these delivery systems have different mechanical and physico-chemical properties than individual constituents' lipids, allowing these microstructures to incorporate highly insoluble and/or unstable drugs that can be delivered in designated dosages to the target site.

Drug delivery approaches designed for targeting tumors can be largely classified into two main types: Active and Passive targeting approaches.

Some recent examples of anticancer liposomal drug delivery systems and their targeting mechanisms is provided in Table 1.

Table 1. Some recent examples of anticancer liposomal drug delivery systems and their targeting mechanisms.

Active Ingredient/s	Trade/Brand Name	Liposome Composition	Active/Passive Targeting	Route of Administration	Indication	Ref.
Hwtp53 DNA	SGT-53	DOTAP/DOPE	Active (Anti-Transferrin scFv)	IV, in vivo, clinical	Solid tumors	[13–15]
Docetaxel prodrug	MM-310	Egg derived sphingomyelin/CH	Active (Anti-Ephrin receptor A2)	IV, in vivo, clinical	Solid tumors	[16–19]
DOX	C225-ILs-dox	DSPC/CH/mPEG-DSPE	Active (Anti-EGFR Fab fragment from mAb C225 (cetuximab))	IV, in vivo, clinical	Glioblastoma	[15,19–21]
DOX	MM-302	HSPC/CH/DSPE-PEG	Active (Anti-HER2 antibody)	IV, in vivo, clinical	Breast cancer	[22,23]
Melanoma antigens + interferon-gamma	Lipovaxin-MM	POPC/Ni-3NTA-DTDA	Active (Single domain antibody (dAb) fragment (VH))	IV, in vivo, clinical	Malignant melanoma	[15,24]
RB94 plasmid DNA	SGT-94	DOTAP/DOPE	Active (Anti-Transferrin Antibody fragment (scFv))	IV, in vivo, clinical	Solid tumor	[15,25–27]
DOX	2B3-101	HSPC/CH/DSPE-PEG	Active (Glutathione ligand)	IV, in vivo, clinical	Active brain metastasis, meningeal carcinomatosis	[18,28,29]
Tetrandrine + vincristine	-	EPC/CH/DSPE-PEG 2000	Active (Transferrin ligand)	IV, in vivo in mice	Brain glioma	[19,30]
Bleomycin	-	DOPE/CH	Active (Folic acid ligand)	In vitro	Cervical and breast cancer cell lines	[19,31]

Table 1. *Cont.*

Active Ingredient/s	Trade/Brand Name	Liposome Composition	Active/Passive Targeting	Route of Administration	Indication	Ref.
DOX	-	DOPE/DOPC/Lecithin	Active (Glycoprotein ligand)	IV, in vivo in mice	Mouse melanoma cells	[32]
ATRA	-	DPPC/CH/DSPE-mPEG2000	Passive	In vitro	Human thyroid carcinoma cell lines	[33]
ATRA	-	DOTAP/CH	Passive	In vivo in mice, IV	Lung cancer	[34]
Daunorubicin + Cytarabine	VYXEOS	DSPG/DSPC/CH	Passive	IV, in vivo, FDA approved	Secondary acute myeloid leukemia (sAML)	[15,35–37]
Paclitaxel	LEP-ETU	DOPC/CH/cardiolipin	Passive	IV, in vivo, FDA approved	Ovarian cancer	[38,39]
Vincristine	-	Sphingomyelin/CH	Passive	IV, in vivo, clinical	Philadelphia chromosome-negative (Ph-) acute lymphoblastic leukemia (ALL)	[40–42]
Verteporfin	Visudyne	DMPC/EPG	Passive	IV, in vivo, clinical	EGFR-mutated glioblastoma	[43–45]
DOX	ThermoDox	DPPC/MSPC/PEG 2000-DSPE	Passive	IV, in vivo, clinical	Hepatocellular carcinoma (HCC)	[46,47]
Paclitaxel	EndoTAG-1	DOTAP/DOPC	Passive	IV, in vivo, clinical	Pancreatic cancer	[38,48]
miR-34a	-	DOTAP/CH	Passive	IV, in vivo, clinical	Advanced solid tumors	[40,49–51]
Irinotecan	ONIVYDE	DSPC/DSPE/CH/mPEG-2000	Passive	IV, in vivo, FDA approved	Metastatic adenocarcinoma of the pancreas	[52,53]
Mitomycin-C prodrug	Promitil	HSPC/CH/DSPE-PEG	Passive	IV, in vivo, clinical	Solid tumors	[54–56]
TUSC2/FUS1	REQORSA	DOTAP/CH	Passive	IV, in vivo, clinical	Non-Small cell lung cancer	[57,58]
Eribulin mesylate	E7389-LF	HSPC/CH/PEG 2000-DSPE	Passive	IV, in vivo, clinical	Solid tumors	[15,59,60]
Navelbine	-	DSPC/CH/PEG -DSPE	Passive	In vivo in mice	Colorectal cancer cells	[61]
Curcumin	Lipocurc	DMPG/DMPC	Passive	IV, in vivo, clinical	Metastatic tumors	[62–64]
Paclitaxel	PTX-LDE	Cholesteryl oleate/Egg-PC/Miglyol 812/CH	Passive	IV, in vivo, clinical	Ovarian carcinoma	[65–67]
PKN3 siRNA	Atu027	AtuFECT01/DPhyPE/DSPE-PEG-2000	Passive	IV, in vivo, clinical	Pancreatic cancer	[25]

Abbreviation: Hwtp53, human wild type p53; DNA, Deoxyribonucleic acid; DOTAP, 1,2-Dioleoyl-3-trimethylammonium-propane; DOPE, Dioleoyl phosphatidylethanolamine; scFv, single chain variable fragment; IV, Intravenous; CH, Cholesterol; DOX, Doxorubicin; DSPC, Distearoyl phosphatidylcholine; DSPE, Distearoyl phosphoethanolamine; mPEG, methoxy Polyethylene Glycol; EGFR, Epidermal growth factor receptor; mAb, Monoclonal antibody; HSPC, Hydrogenated soybean phosphatidylcholine; PEG, Polyethylene Glycol; HER 2, Human epidermal growth factor receptor 2; POPC, palmitoyloleoyl phosphocholine; Ni-3NTA-DTDA, nitrilotriacetic acid ditetradecylamine, nickel salt; dAb, Single domain antibody; VH, variable heavy chain; DOPC, Dioleoyl phosphocholine; ATRA, all-trans-retinoic acid; DPPC, Dipalmitoyl phosphatidylcholine; DSPG, Distearoyl phosphoglycerol; DMPC, Dimyristoyl phosphocholine; EPC, egg phosphatidylglycerol; MSPC, Myristoyl-palmitoyl phosphatidylcholine; DMPG, Dimyristoyl phosphorylglycerol; Egg-PC, Egg phosphatidylcholine; PKN3, Protein Kinase N3; AtuFECT01, β-L-arginyl-2,3-L-diaminopropionic acid-N-palmityl-N-oleyl-amide trihydrochloride; DPhyPE, Diphytanoyl phosphoethanolamine.

3.1. *Active Tumor Targeting Approach*

Active targeting at the molecular level discriminates between normal and cancerous cells by acting upon their morphological, phenotypic, and biochemical differences. A common active targeting approach involves ligand–receptor or antigen–antibody binding interactions to locally deliver cytotoxic drugs to tumor cells. The precise drug delivery mechanism in most instances is via receptor-mediated endocytosis after interaction of a drug or a drug carrier molecule with a specific antigen/receptor. The cytotoxic agents are associated with tumor specific ligands either directly via a carrier molecule.

A major limitation to active targeting, however, is antigen heterogeneity. As stated earlier, different kinds of cancers or even same kind of cancer expresses different biochemical and morphological characteristics at different stages of their development which creates heterogeneity in the antigen expression (Figure 2). Receptor density is another important criterion to consider in active targeting. For a discriminatory effect, it is critical that the number of receptors are over-expressed in the cancer cells as compared to normal healthy cells (Figure 2). To illustrate this point, for enhanced breast cancer efficacy a receptor concentration of 10^5 per cell of the tyrosine-protein kinase receptor (CD340) was deemed essential [5]. Likewise, a concentration of up to 10^5 per cell of CD19 antigens was required for effective targeting of B cells by anti-CD19 antibody conjugated to liposomes [68]. Besides receptor density, during the development of cancer, shedding of antigens or their down-regulation may severely alter receptor concentration on the cell surface. Moreover, shed antigens may compete for interaction with an administered ligand, which is directed towards antigens attached to the cancer cell surface. Depending on the level of shedding, this phenomenon might impact the level of cytotoxic agent internalization to the cancer cells (Figure 2) [5]. Moreover, if the ligand–receptor binding avidity is very strong then it will impede the penetration depth of the anticancer agent in the tumor tissue due to 'binding-site barrier' where conjugated drugs are strongly bound by the first few receptor targets in the tumor tissue (Figure 2) [5]. As an example, it is reported that SK-OV-3 ovarian cancer targeting by single-chain fragment variable (SCFv) was dictated by the binding avidity of the SCFv antibody against the human epidermal growth factor 2 (HER2) receptors [69]. Binding affinity of a mutant-type Fv molecule over and above 10^{-9} M leveled off the distribution of Fv in the targeted tissue [69].

3.1.1. Antibody and Antibody Fragments

Cancer cell targeting strategies involving antibodies have employed either whole antibodies or their fragments. While whole (intact) antibodies are generally considered more stable, they possess multiple binding sites. The presence of these sites makes them vulnerable to recognition by white blood cells in the body. A common interaction and, therefore, their clearance mechanism is the binding of their Fc domain with macrophages. (Figure 2) [5]. This binding triggers a cascade of immunogenic reactions which leads to rapid clearance of antibodies from the blood circulation. Mechanisms have been developed to modify the antibodies to yield more humanized or chimeric antibodies that invoke a less intense immune reaction; however, the development and manufacturing of such systems have proven to be challenging. In addition, when whole antibodies are conjugated to nano-carriers (liposomes, nanoparticles etc.) the ability to impart multivalent decoration is severely restricted due to the steric hindrance (Figure 2).

As a potential solution, antibody fragments were introduced that have specific binding sites such as Fab, Fv or ScFv but are relatively less stable as compared to parent antibodies. Also, these fragments carry less binding avidity due to their monovalent binding sites. Furthermore, attempts to use non-antibody peptides/proteins such as RGD (Arg-Gly-Asp), folate and transferrin have yielded non-specific results due to lack of disparity or receptor density in expression of their targets among tumor and normal tissues (Figure 2) [5].

Another alternate domain that is fast catching up is targeting using nanobodies. Nanobodies are naturally found in camel, llama or whales and are more comparatively stable than whole antibodies but they still have to find their clinical relevance.

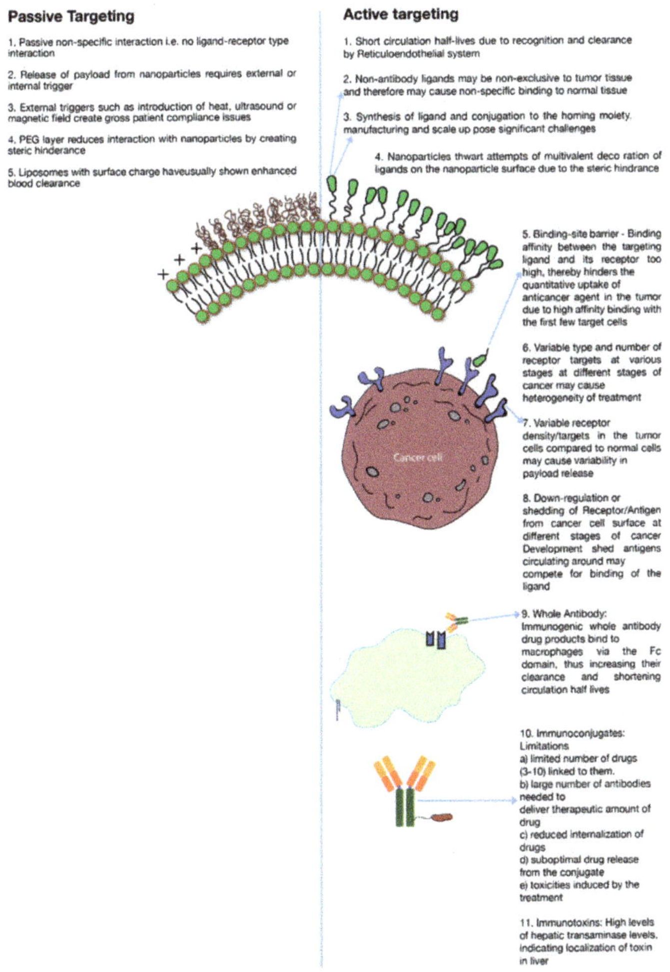

Figure 2. Limitations of active and passive targeting.

3.1.2. Immunotoxins and Immunoconjugates

Immunotoxins are either similar to antibodies or are antibodies conjugated to toxins to render them cytotoxic. However, the whole conjugated molecule induces moderate to severe adverse effects which limits their use. A couple of severe side effects include high internalization in liver indicated by higher expression of liver transaminase (Figure 2). Other notable side effects of immunotoxin therapy are vascular leak syndrome (VLS) and influenza-like symptoms [5]. Also, blocked ricin (toxin) conjugated to anti-B4 antibody has demonstrated anti-ricin and human anti-mouse antibody responses [5].

Immunoconjugates, on the other hand, are close analogues of Immunotoxins where instead of a toxin, an anticancer drug is conjugated to an antibody or protein. Antibody-drug conjugates (ADC's) also fall under this category. As a conjugate, the cytotoxic effect is imparted by the cytotoxic drug while the targeting is driven by the associated antibody or protein. There are several constraints of using immunoconjugates as a potent tool against tumor. Prominent among these are: (a) limited number of cytotoxic agents that can be conjugated to anchoring molecules without severely impacting its binding avidity towards target antigen. On an average, 3–10 molecules of cytotoxic drug are known to conjugated to the anchoring antibody [5] (Figure 2). (b) Due to limited number of drugs conjugated to each antibody, a high number of antibodies are required to deliver therapeutic levels of the drug. (c) Poor localization of actives; (d) suboptimal drug release from the conjugate; (e) ADC related toxicities e.g., gastro-intestinal (GI) toxicities caused by SGN-15 immunoconjugate [5,70] (Figure 2).

3.1.3. Immunoliposomes

Immunoliposomes are liposomes that carry targeting or anchoring ligands/antibodies on their surface. The conjugation of targeting ligands/antibodies is achieved either by bio-conjugation with exposed sulfhydryl groups attained after di-sulfide bond reduction [71] or through lysine functionalization using 2-Iminothiolane [72,73], N-succinimidyl 3-(2-pyridyldithio)propionate (SPDP) [74] or N-Succinimidyl-S-acetylthioacetate (SATA) [75]. Click chemistry of azide functionalized phospholipids with cyclooctyne modified antibodies is a most recent example [76].

Immunoliposomes usually have intravascular and extravascular targets. Intravascular targets are considered more accessible for intravascularly administered immunoliposomes. Anti-VEGFR2 and anti-VEGFR3 Dox loaded immunoliposomes are common examples that have resulted in greater reduction in tumor mass in animal studies using antibodies against vascular endothelial growth factor receptors for targeting tumor-associated neovascular endothelial cells [77]. Other immunoliposome targets include brain, uterus, red blood cells, and T lymphocytes among others. Anti-Transferrin receptor (TfR) immunoliposome is one example where anti-amyloid-β antibodies were targeted across the brain–blood barrier [78]. Anti-vascular cell adhesion molecule (anti-VCAM), anti-TfR and anti-intercellular adhesion molecule (anti-ICAM) immunoliposomes were screened for optimizing blood to brain drug delivery ratios [76]. Anti-oxytocin receptor (OTR) immunoliposomes were studied for drug delivery to the uterus [79]. Additionally, Moles E. et.al investigated anti-Glycophorin A (GPA) immunoliposomes for antimalarial drug delivery to malaria-parasitized RBCs [80,81]. Similarly, Ramana et al., attempted anti-HIV drugs loaded anti-CD4 immunoliposomes delivery to T lymphocytes [82].

Multiple immunoliposome targets have been discussed above and are also shown in Table 1. It is important to note that there are some fundamental challenges associated with immunoliposomes.

Although, immunoliposomes can carry a large payload of drug molecules in their lipid bilayer or their aqueous interior, and, therefore, have high drug to antibody ratio, on the flipside, immunoliposomes carry only limited number of antibody molecules on their surface due to steric hinderance. Also, the bulky and complex structure of these systems triggers an immunological response and, therefore, enhances their systemic clearance (Figure 2). Circulating plasma proteins form protein corona upon exposure of liposomes, thereby triggering opsonization by complement proteins. Immunoliposomes, therefore, are subsequently cleared from blood circulation by reticuloendothelial system (RES) in liver and spleen [83]. Furthermore, immunoliposomes need to be optimized to contain the effects of heterogenous tumor properties, else the efficacy may vary depending upon several histological and microenvironmental factors as mentioned previously. Potentially, Immunoliposomes can be decorated with two different antibody fragments to target multiple epitopes on tumor cells, or even different cells population on the tumor tissue [84]. However, the receptor/antigen density and the affinity of the antibody for a specific antigen or the 'binding-site barrier' issue (Figure 2) may still pose a barrier which may lead to poor tumor penetration and poor efficacy against cells with down-regulation of target antigens. Designing immunoliposomes are becoming increasingly valuable and highly challenging with the evolution of new therapeutic modalities such as like siRNA and mRNA etc., as payloads [85].

3.1.4. Manufacturing and Clinical Challenges of Active Targeting

A significant manufacturing challenge associated with active targeting, specifically immunoliposomes, is the scale up of nanomaterial manufacturing process. The issue is two pronged, firstly the large-scale manufacture of the constituent lipid–ligand conjugate (Figure 2) and secondly, the large-scale preparation of liposomes using the constituent lipids with consistent particle size distribution and lamellarity (Table 2). The conjugation of lipid–ligand conjugate is usually a multi-step synthesis process that involves use of organic solvents. This increases complexity and cost of production during cGMP (current-Good Manufacturing Practices) scale up of the conjugate and subsequent formulation preparation. It is important to note that the functional stability of the conjugate is important during various processing conditions as the incorporation of nanoconjugate alters the chemical makeup of the nano-formulation and leads to uncertainty in biodistribution, pharmacokinetic, and pharmacodynamic profiles [86]. Another problem is the differences in the heterogeneity in the cancer cell receptor expressions between small animals (rodents, rabbits) to humans. The optimization of the drug product to maximize its interaction with receptors on the cancer cell surface depends on the correlation of human vs. animal data and hence the translation of preclinical study results into clinical studies.

Table 2. Challenges common to both active and passive targeting.

	Active and Passive Targeting Challenges
1.	Scale up liposome preparation to reproducibly achieve target product profile including in vitro drug release rate, particle size distribution, lamellarity, stability, drug encapsulation efficiency, etc.
2.	Separation of raw lipids in a mixture of lipids and ability to analyze them
3.	Determination of complete stability and toxicity profile of novel lipids involved in formulations
4.	Stability of liposomes in solution
5.	Determination of biodistribution of liposomes appropriate PK/PD models to predict parameters in humans
6.	Immunogenic reactions such as CARPA upon IV administration of liposomes have resulted in additional layer of challenge

Abbreviations: PK, Pharmacokinetics; PD, Pharmacodynamics; CARPA, Complement activation-related pseudoallergy; IV, Intravenous.

3.2. Passive Tumor Targeting Approach

Passive targeting approach is distinct as it does not utilize a ligand/receptor or antibody/antigen interaction but rather exploits physiological characteristics of the tumor micro-environment. Passive targeting largely exploits the 'Enhanced Permeation and Retention' effect (Figure 3) for the localization of drugs in the tumor tissue. The enhanced permeation (localization) of nano drug delivery systems in the tumor occurs due to fenestrated tumor blood vasculature. Once permeated in the tumor environment nano drug delivery systems are retained at the target site due to poor lymphatic drainage.

It is worthwhile to note that while passive targeting eliminates some of the issues of active targeting (e.g., antigen heterogeneity, receptor density, etc.) it brings its own limitations to the cancer therapy. To cite a few examples: low drug release at target site, high systemic clearance of surface charged nano drug delivery systems (Figure 2) and the need for either external stimuli i.e., heat, light and/magnetic field at the tumor site or endogenous stimuli i.e., pH, hypoxia etc., to trigger drug release (Figure 2). Only liposomal drug delivery systems and their external drug release trigger mechanisms are discussed in detail in this review.

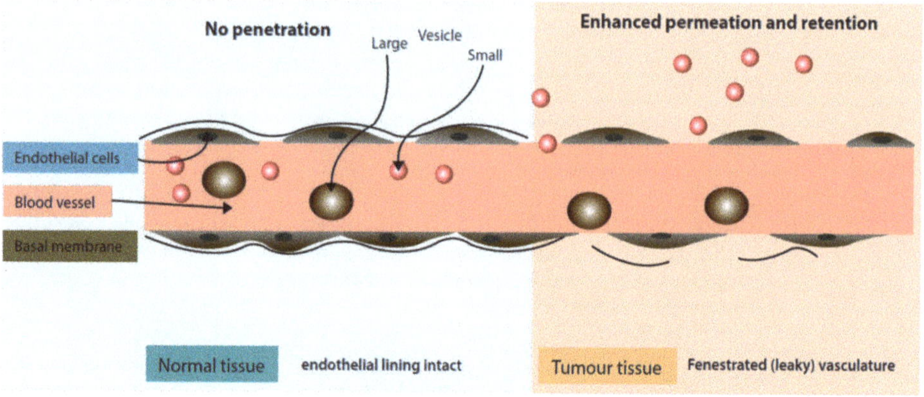

Figure 3. 'Enhanced Permeation and Retention' effect exhibiting enhanced permeability of liposomes in inter-tumoral space.

3.2.1. Traditional Liposomes

Historically, very early liposomes i.e., traditional liposomes introduced in the 1960s were devoid of any biocompatible polymer coating on their surface. Upon administration to systemic circulation, traditional liposomes trigger immune response by mononuclear phagocyte system (MPS). This activation of the immune system is indeed exploited in treatment of some bacterial/fungal infections of the immune system. A standard example is liposomal amphotericin B which is targeted to fungus-infected macrophages. This liposomal drug was primary line of treatment during recent SARS-COV-2 related fungal infections in India [87]. Beyond targeting the MPS system, traditional liposomes find little significance in targeting tumor cells due to rapid recognition and clearance by macrophages [88,89].

At the molecular level, cationic liposomes are more prone to recognition by MPS because of their affinity towards negatively charged serum proteins. Serum protein bound liposomes have tendencies to trigger the MPS system owing to their bigger size. As an example, cationic liposomes prepared with equimolar mixture of cationic lipid 1,2-dioleyl-3-N,N,N-trimethylaminopropane chloride (DOTMA) and neutral lipids i.e., DOPE or DOPC have propensity towards serum protein binding as depicted by their protein binding (PB) value 500g protein/mol or higher [90]. In a similar study, keeping DOTMA up to half of the total lipid composition of liposomes resulted in very strong plasma protein interactions that triggered formation of clots [91]. Moreover, liposome formulations prepared with another cationic lipid i.e., N-N-dioleoyl-N,N-dimethylammonium chloride (DODAC) and DOPE showed a very high PB value of 800g protein/mol and subsequently poor apparent half-life of only a few minutes [90]. Cationic liposomes even higher PB values of up to 1100 g proteins/mol have also been reported [90,92].

To enhance the circulation half-lives of liposomes various approaches have been implemented. One such approach is to alter the surface charge composition of liposomes by addition of a negatively charge lipid phosphatidyl inositol to the liposomal formulation which stabilizes the liposomes in vivo [93]. Liposomes prepared with hydrogenated phosphatidyl inositol/phosphatidyl choline/cholesterol (HPI/HPC/CH) exhibited an apparent half-life of 15.5 h of encapsulated doxorubicin as compared to 1 h of traditional liposomes prepared with egg-originated phosphatidyl glycerol (PG), phosphatidyl choline (PC) and cholesterol [93].

3.2.2. Stealth Liposome

Since high blood clearance of traditional liposomes was a major challenge, as a breakthrough to this problem, liposomes grafted with a biocompatible polymer that could evade immune recognition were introduced. Polyethylene Glycol (PEG) is one such example of a biocompatible polymer. Presence of the PEG–lipid conjugate allows for formation of a sterically stabilized hydrophilic aqueous shell that renders the liposomal system evasive to the immune system. Due to the steric stabilization imparted by the PEG layer, serum protein binding blood clearance of the liposomes is greatly reduced. The PEG coated liposomes are, therefore, called 'Stealth Liposomes' (SL) due to evasive nature of these systems.

A commercially available relevant example of a stealth liposome (SL) is 'Doxil' (Figure 4).

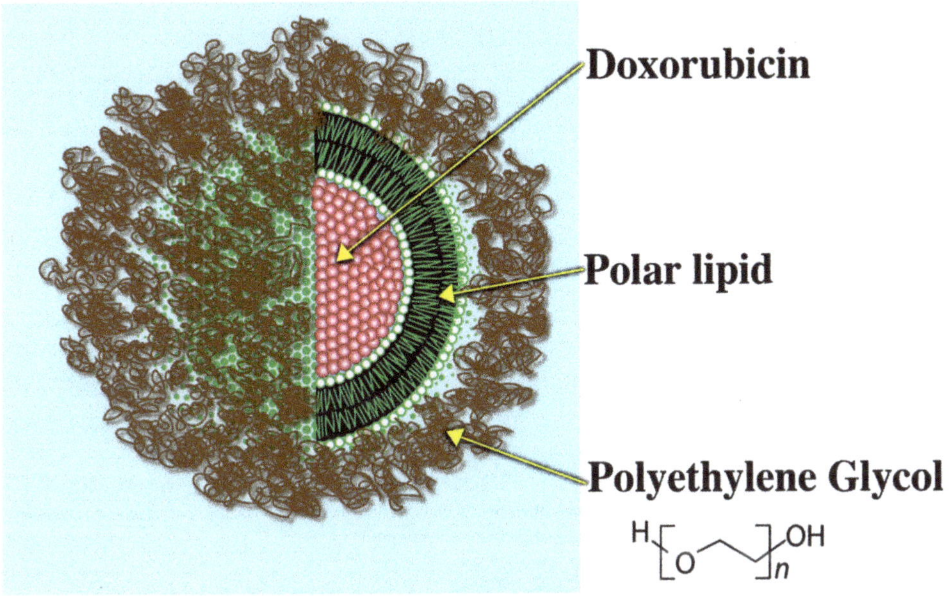

Figure 4. Doxil coated with Polyethylene Glycol.

An example of significant improvement in the performance of a drug using SL technology is Epirubicin. Administration of un-encapsulated Epirubicin causes rapid blood clearance of the drug yielding a very short half-life of only 14 min. On the contrary, the half-life of an encapsulated form of the drug was significantly higher i.e., 18 h [93]. This improvement was also reflected in the bioavailability of the drug where the AUC of encapsulated form showed more than 200X increase than the un-encapsulated form [93].

Other important marker of the immune system avoidance is the measure of PB. It has been reported that addition of a PEG layer markedly lowers the PB value [90,94]. To cite a few examples, traditional liposomes composed of egg-PC/CH/1,2-dioleoyl-sn-glycero-3-phosphate (EPC/CH/DOPA) and DSPC/CH in a mol ratio of 35:45:20 and 55:45, respectively, had PB values of 46 and 19, respectively. However, upon the addition of 5% of a PEGylated lipid i.e., 1, 2-Distearoyl-sn-glycero-3-phosphoethanolamine-Poly(ethylene glycol) (DSPE-PEG), to the respective formulations, reduced the PB values to 25 and 7, respectively [90]. Similarly, blood cell binding of glass coated DPPE/DSPE-PEG liposomes significantly reduced as the level of PEGylated lipid DSPE-PEG in the liposomes was raised from 0 to 1 mol% [94]. The rate of cell binding, however, reduced with higher levels of DSPE-PEG added to the liposome [94].

Although implementation of PEGylated lipids has largely improved the circulation half-life and localization of liposomes in target tissues, there are major drawbacks associated with the SL technology. Since the steric hinderance imparted by PEG limits liposomal binding to immune cells, equivalently, it also limits the binding and subsequent internalization to tumor cells once liposomes have extravasated to tumor environment (Figure 2). It was reported that a Te parameter i.e., AUC tumor/AUC plasma ratio was nearly three-fold lower for PEGylated liposomes (DSPC/CH/DSPE-PEG) as compared to traditional liposomes DSPC)/CH in C26 tumor bearing mice [95]. Similarly, in the Lewis lung model study using DSPC/CH and DSPC/CH/PEG-PE, Te values for the PEGylated liposomes were approximately half of the non-PEGylated liposomes [96].

Due to reduced internalization of liposomes by tumor cells, once reaching the tumor tissue, the drug release largely relies on passive diffusion of drug to extra-liposomal space, which is a slow process and leading to sub-optimal levels of an anticancer drug in tumor.

3.2.3. Requirements of Stimuli Induced Drug Release

To significantly increase drug release from liposomes accumulated in a tumoral space, endogenous triggers or external triggering mechanisms have been envisioned. Endogenous triggers in the tumor micro-environment are acidic pH, hypoxia, enzymatic degradation, etc. The major limitations of endogenous triggers are chemical instability of pH sensitive lipids [4,97], poor hypoxic heterogeneity in tumors [98,99] and less reliable enzyme heterogeneity in tumors [100]. Barring enzyme heterogeneity issue in the tumors, peptide-based supramolecular assembly/disassembly provides an interesting trigger mechanism that can retain the drug cargo in blood circulation and release upon enzymatic hydrolysis in the tumor environment [101,102]. One such study was performed by Kalafatovic et al. [103] where a peptide micelle was converted to fibrillar nanostructures to trigger drug release. The trigger for such conversions is change in the hydrophilic–lipophilic balance triggered by enzymatic hydrolysis. In an interesting approach, to avoid heterogeneity in tumor environment by utilizing all the above endogenous triggers (i.e., pH, redox potential and endogenous proteinase concentration), Zhang et al. [104] developed a protein based nanospheres for triggered release of encapsulated Chlorin e6.

External triggers, on the other hand, complicate the therapy by requiring external clinical intervention and thereby creating gross patient incompliance. In this review, external trigger mechanisms such as application of ultrasound, light and temperature to trigger drug release are discussed in detail.

Ultrasound Induced Triggered Release

Ultrasound (US) are mechanical longitudinal waves propagate due to pressure changes in the medium with a periodic vibration of frequencies higher than the human audible range of 20 kHz [105]. Drug release by US is due to different mechanisms such as cavitation, acoustics and hyperthermia [106]. Cavitation and acoustics related mechanisms are more widely used and discussed here. VanOsdol and colleagues utilized ultrasonic cavitation for DXR drug release by incorporating perfluoropentane gas (PFP5) in liposomes [107]. They observed that microbubble formation by using PFP5 was able to increase the drug concentration to target tissues to 1.4 times upon the use of high intensity focused ultrasound (HIFU). Another prominent drug release mechanism by acoustics and is well demonstrated by acoustically active liposomes (AAL). AAL's possess air pockets that may expand upon pressure change and upon exposure to US radiation. The expansion of air pockets leads disruption of liposomal membrane and, therefore, release of encapsulated contents. A significant benefit of this trigger mechanism is that it is a non-invasive technique which can be controlled. Besides triggering drug release from liposomes, this technique can also alter the permeability of cell membrane [108,109]. A prominent example of AAL's is calcein-loaded liposomes prepared from EPC/DPPE/1,2-Dipalmitoyl-sn-glycero-3-phosphoglycerol (DPPG)/CH at a molar ratio of 69:8:8:15 [108]. The calcein release was shown to be well controlled, however, encapsulation efficiency of these liposomes was very low ($\leq$ 20%) [108]. Additionally, such systems have not been tested for encapsulation and the release of hydrophobic drugs that localize in the lipid domains of the liposomes rather than aqueous interiors of liposomes.

Light Induced Triggered Release

Another important trigger is the application of light for drug release. A study conducted by Leung et al. [110] explored triggered release by light induced chemical changes in the lipid constituents of the liposomes. Broadly, these changes include photo-isomerization, photo-cleavage or photo-polymerization of photo-sensitive lipid constituents of the liposome membrane. A majority of photo-sensitive liposomes incorporate isomerizable lipids that can convert form one isomeric form to the other upon light activation. A prominent example of these liposome includes the ones that are prepared by azobenzene lipid. Azobenzene can isomerize to cis form upon exposure to UV-light and converts back to the transform upon exposure to visible (blue) light [110] (Figure 5).

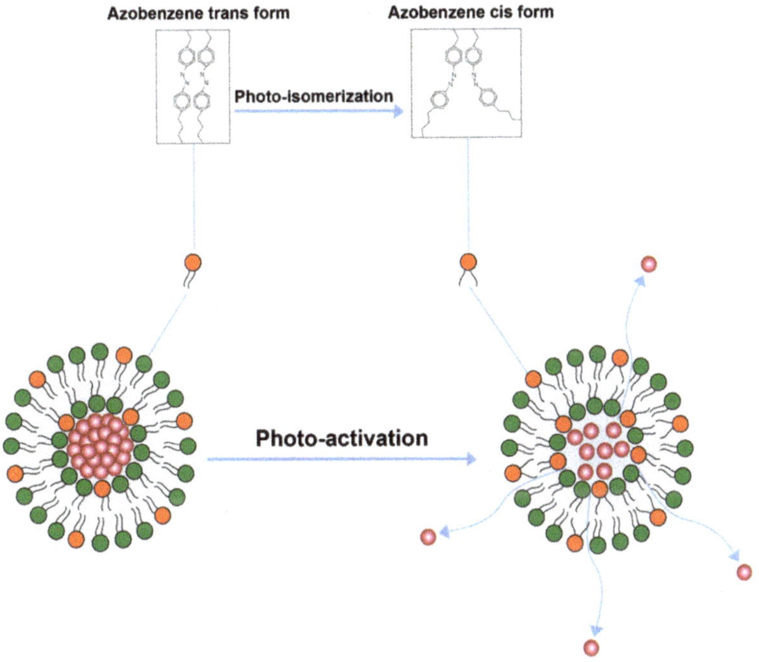

Figure 5. Drug release from liposomes by photo-isomerization of lipids.

This isomerization of lipids disrupts membrane structure and releases encapsulated contents. Besides azobenzene, light sensitive liposomes composed of retinoyl-phospholipids [111] and spiropyran, which converts to merocyanine at lower visible 365 nm, have also been tested [112]. The major challenge with photo-isomerization is that the wavelengths required to photo-isomerize the photosensitive lipids fall in lower visible spectrum which have poor penetration depth in the body.

Another trigger mechanism that uses light activation is inclusion of photo-cleavable lipid constituents in the liposomal membrane [110] (Figure 6). Photo-cleavable lipids essentially break-down upon exposure to lipid and thence disrupt the membrane structure. The cleavage upon light exposure causes changes in the hydrophilicity of the lipid constituents which are, therefore, not able to retain membrane structure and allow for drug release. Similar use of photocleavable lipids derived from plasmalogen have also been reported [113]. Effect of photo-cleavage may be assisted by use of photosensitizers molecules such as tin octabutoxyphthalocyanine, zinc phthalocyanine, or bacteriochlorophyll a. [114].

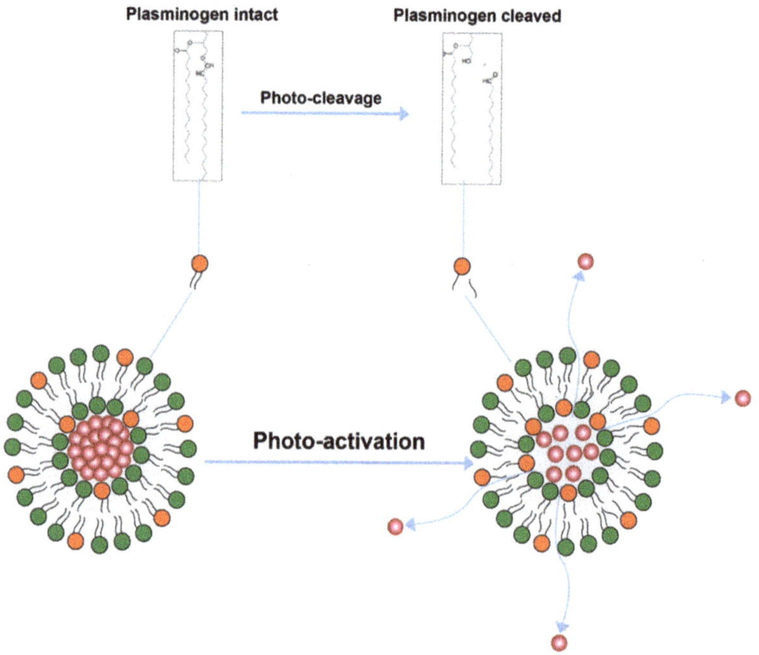

Figure 6. Drug release from liposomes by photo-cleavage of lipids.

The photosensitizer molecules, however, result in the formation of reactive oxygen species in the body which may compromise patient safety [4].

Furthermore, dithiane-based lipids have also been reported to increase the drug release from liposomes [115,116]. In an interesting report, a synthetic DOPE-based photocleavable lipid NVOC-DOPE was transformed to DOPE upon exposure to xenon lamp, causing subsequent liposome membrane disruption [117]. Yavlovich, et al., have also investigated the inclusion of 2-nitrobenzyl lipid derivate of PC, named NB-PC in liposomes for the photo-cleavage triggered release. Nile red was found to increase its release relative to the concentration of NB-PC in the liposome upon UV irradiation at 350 nm [118].

Photo-polymerization is another light triggered drug release mechanism [110,111] (Figure 7) where polymerization of lipids upon activation by light causes pairing of photo-polymerizable lipids on the liposome surface creating loose pockets on liposome surface from where drugs may escape the liposome interior. Formation of these loose pockets on liposome surface is also aptly illustrated by the polymerization of a lipid 1,2-bis [10-(2′,4′-hexadienoyloxy)-decanoyl]-sn-phosphatidylcholine (bis-SorbPC) after upon UV exposure which resulted in more than 100X increase overall release of a fluorescent molecule [111,119]. Similarly, Yavlovich and co-workers demonstrated much higher MCF-7 breast cancer cell inhibition using 514 nm light exposure after delivering by doxorubicin loaded in liposome containing photopolymerizable lipid 1,2-bis (tricosa-10,12-diynoyl) sn-glycer-3-phosphocholine (DC 8,9 PC) [120].

The UV wavelength required to trigger the release may be tuned by inclusion of photosensitizing dyes such as 1,1′-dioctadecyl-3,3,3′,3′- tetramethylindocarbocyanine iodide in liposomes towards the higher UV wavelengths that are considered biologically safe [111].

Photo-polymerization is an intriguing concept, however, there are a few limitations, such as the stability of polymerizable lipids in aqueous suspensions have not been tested yet [111], and more importantly, the penetration depth of UV light in human subjects remains a challenge.

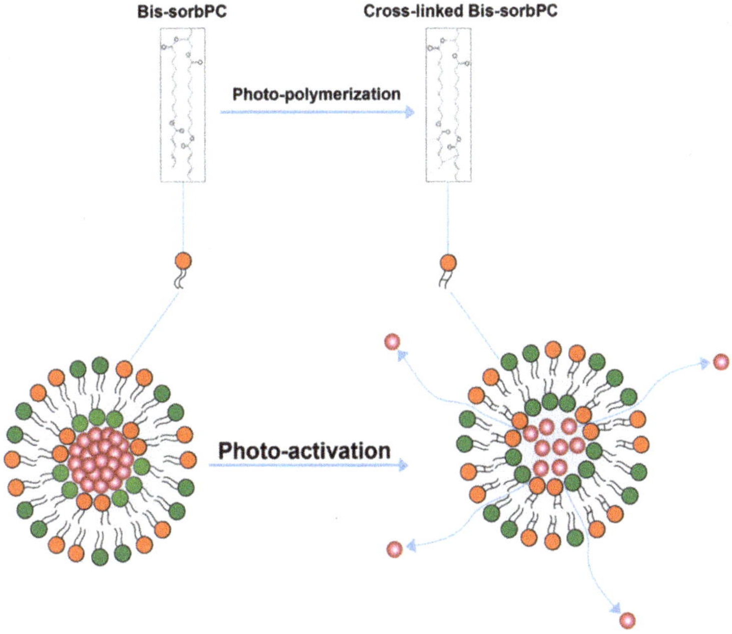

Figure 7. Drug release from liposomes by photo-polymerization of lipids.

Additionally, in an interesting photo-oxidation approach using Bacteriochlorophyll/ diplasmenylcholine (Bchl:DPPlsC) liposomes, it was reported that photo-oxidation induced drug release is severely impacted by hypoxic (low Po2) tumor environment [121]. Poor photo-oxidation leads to development of physiologically favorable atmosphere for growth of non-apoptotic cells [121]. Other such approach of utilizing photo-oxidation include the addition of photochemical agents such as Porphyrin-phospholipid (POP), talaporfin sodium (TPS) and Indocyanine green and octadecylamine (ICG-ODA) in combination of oxidation sensitive lipids containing liposomes such as DOPC, cholesterol and 1-(1z-octadecenyl) -2-oleoyl-sn-glycero-3-phosphocholine (PLsPC) and have reported in better cytotoxicity upon photo-exposure conditions. All the photo-oxidative approaches, nevertheless, require external stimuli imparted by near infra-red application [122,123].

Hyperthermia Induced Triggered Release

A different technique to trigger drug release after localization of liposomes in the tumor tissue is by application of heat. This approach is significant as it provides a variety of advantages. Firstly, the application of heat enhances the blood vessel permeability at the tumor site which causes enhanced extravasation of liposomes (Figure 8). Secondly, it triggers the drug release from liposomes in the vicinity of the tumor (Figure 8) and thirdly, it enhances the blood flow and increases the drug uptake. One such drug release mechanism was implemented for the release of Neomycin [124].

A common approach to enhance drug release using thermos-sensitive liposomes is the inclusion of lower melting lipids in the liposome composition. In some examples, the application of heat induces trans to a gauche conformational change of the constituent lipids at their transition temperature [125]. This transitions the gel phase of the lipid bilayer to the fluid phase and triggers the rate of drug diffusion and hence the drug release enhancement (Figure 9) [125]. It is, however, important to note that a homogenous or nearly homogenous composition of bilayer by inclusion of lower melting lipids such as 1,2-Dipalmitoyl-sn-Glycero-3-Phosphatidylcholine (DPPC) (MP = 41 °C) have resulted in a less than optimum drug release [125]. One challenge with having a low melting lipid is that the drug cargo is poorly retained during blood circulation due to a less rigid membrane structure. Furthermore, inclusion of lipids with different melting temperatures and carbon chain lengths results in the creation of membrane packing heterogeneity and, therefore, increases drug release. Such heterogeneity was depicted by the broadening of peaks in differential scanning calorimetry in liposomes composed of DSPC (MP = 53 °C) and DPPC lipids [126]. It should be, however, be noted that higher melting lipids would require higher temperatures to induce drug release (higher than 43 °C) which may cause necrosis to normal tissues in the vicinity of the tumor tissue [125]. According to one report necrosis on porcine muscle was initiated after 30 min. of heat application at 40–43 °C [127].

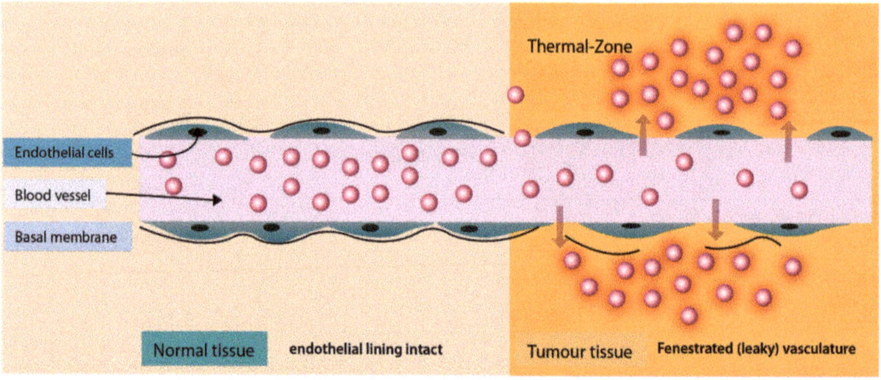

Figure 8. Enhanced liposomal extravasation and drug release at tumor site upon application of heat.

It, therefore, remains a challenge to fine tune the drug release at mild hyperthermia conditions (39–41 °C) for efficient drug cargo release.

Another heat triggered drug release approach is inclusion of lyso-lipids as lipid constituents of thermo-sensitive liposomes. Lyso-lipids have a heavier head group with a single carbon chain and due to this typical structure, these lipids would characteristically form micellar structures. When incorporated into liposomes these lipids gain translational movement upon heating to their transition temperature and form early melting pockets on the membrane surface. These pockets arrange into micelle-like curved structure at these pockets which essentially create for enhanced drug release (Figure 10) [125]. Provided that lyso-lipids are included in appropriate ratios, it has been shown that these lipids effectively lower the phase transition temperatures required for triggered release. Liposomes prepared with 10 mol % of the Mono Palmitoyl Phosphatidyl Choline (MPPC) (lyso-lipid) lead to change in phase transition temperature to 39–40 °C from 43 °C and subsequently a very fast drug release i.e., nearly 50% after 20 s of exposure at 42 °C [128]. The rapid drug release, therefore, enables shorter heat exposure times which subsequently decreases the possibility of initiation of necrosis in normal tissue in the vicinity of the tumor [125]. However, the challenge with lyso-lipid liposomes is their in vivo stability, lyso-lipids impart instability to liposomal structure due to desorption of lyso-lipid while liposomes are in blood circulation. It has been reported that after 1 h of injection up to 70% of the lyso-lipids were desorbed from the liposome surface [129,130] and the amount of drug released recovered from liposomes mice plasma after 4 h of injection was significantly low [129]. Although, in a 2020 study, a phase clinical data of ThermoDox® formulation of DPPC:MSPC:DSPE-PEG2000 (86:10:4 molar ratio) were announced but the in vivo stability in pigs suggest an estimated half-life of only 4.8 h. [131,132].

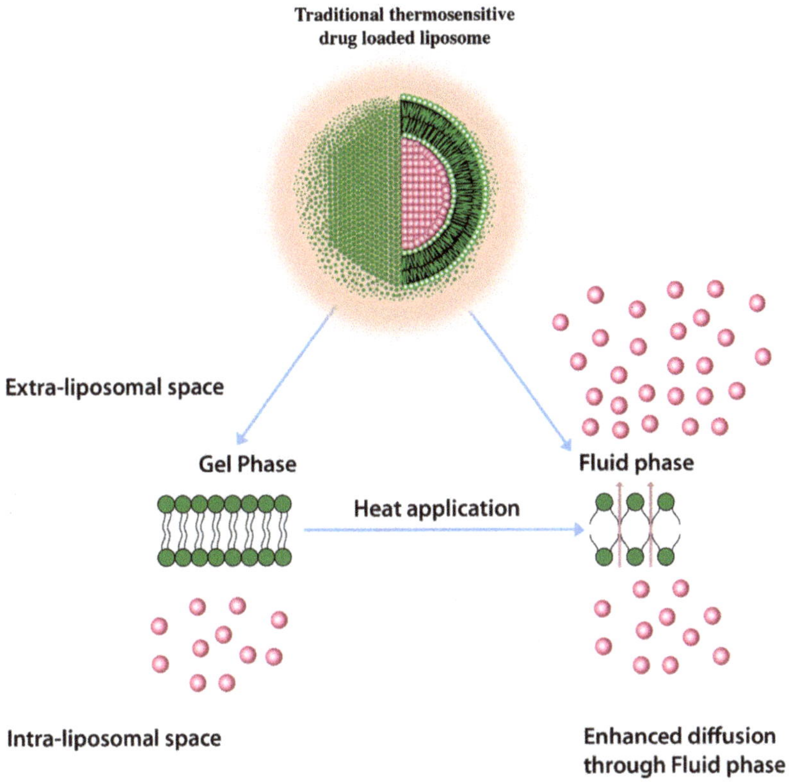

Figure 9. Traditional thermosensitive liposomes showing gel to fluid phase transition upon application of heat.

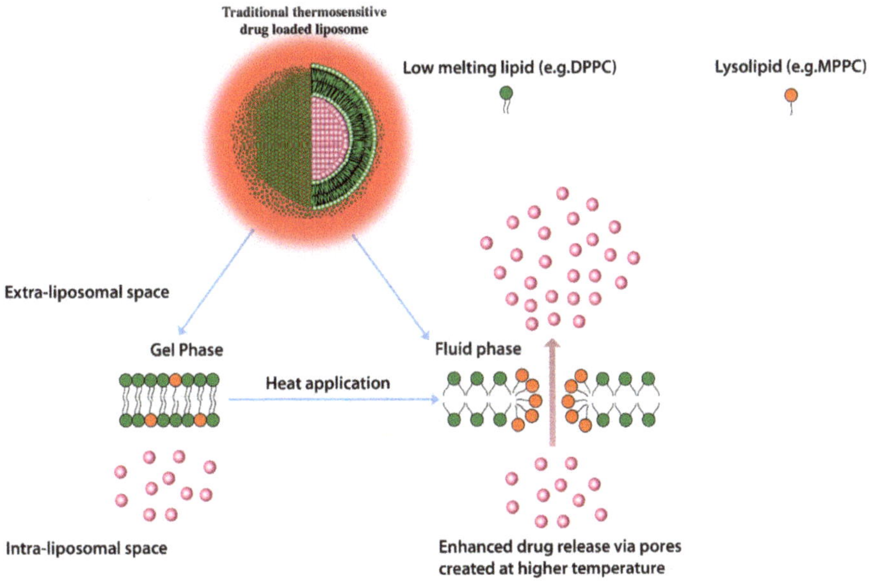

Figure 10. Traditional thermosensitive drug loaded liposomes showing formation of micellar pockets upon application of heat.

The instability of lyso-lipid based liposomes, therefore, significantly reduces the thermo-sensitive feature of these liposomes.

Another limitation with heat triggered release is that it can only impact tumors that are located close to the body surface as compared to deep seated tumors because of higher temperature requirements to reach the desired temperature differential. Attempts to insert electrodes (microwave and radiofrequency) to deep seated tumors remain impractical due to the insertion depth and invasive nature of these procedures [125]. As an alternative ultrasound with a controlled focal zone were developed but regardless, monitoring of temperature would still require temperature probes penetrated into the tumor environment [125].

Also, heat trigger imparted by microwave and radio wave applicators is limited due to the therapeutic depth of only up to 3 cm [128].

Triggered Release by Magnetic Field from Magnetic Liposomes

Magnetic field is another mechanism that can trigger drug release from liposomes. In one study drug release was triggered by including iron oxide in the liposome membrane bilayer (Figure 11), which catalyzed local heating upon application of the magnetitic field. The local heating led to membrane disruption and, therefore, drug release [133].

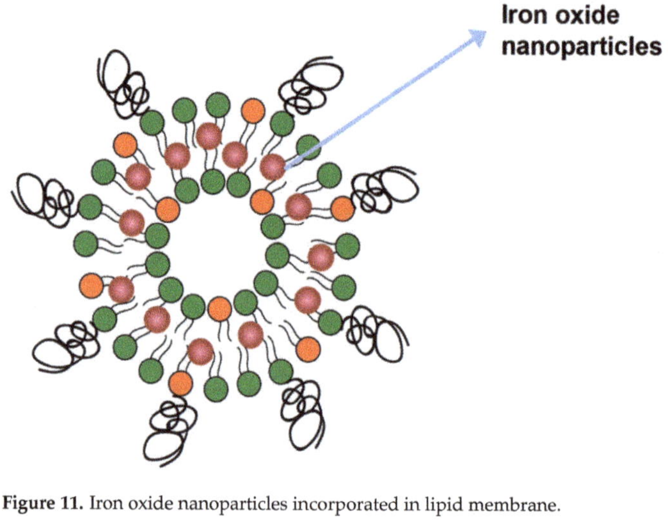

Figure 11. Iron oxide nanoparticles incorporated in lipid membrane.

Similarly, nearly 70 % of the drug Adriamycin was released when a ferromagnetic material was incorporated in liposome membrane bilayer at a ferro–colloid concentration of 1.2 mg Fe/mL [134].

In an interesting approach, liposomes were directed to tumor tissue by entrapping magnetite particles and then by applying a magnetic field on the target tissue [135].

In studies using Syrian male hamster limbs, under the influence of a study magnetic field in doxorubicin concentration increased 3X to 4X in tumor upon intravenous administration of magnetic liposomes [135]. Instead of having an externally placed magnetic field in the above examples, a non-magnetic alloy was rather placed directly in the tumor in another similar study using a limb tumor model [136]. A clear distinction between Adriamycin release with and without magnetic field was observed [136].

Additionally, a clear effect of the magnetic field on radiolabeled albumin loaded liposome was observed in rat models. Precisely, a samarium cobalt magnet was placed in the left kidney of rats and, therefore, showed a 25X increase in radioactivity in the left kidney compared to the right kidney which had no magnet [137].

In an interesting example, a 1.7X increase in cargo release at the tumor site was observed by using magnetic liposomes prepared with bacterial magnetic particles containing cis-diamminedichloroplatinum (II) as compared to magnetic liposomes prepared with synthetic magnetic materials [138].

Furthermore, in a unique dual targeting study, magnetic liposomes first targeted blood cells followed later magnetically directed to the brain for delivery of the cargo [139].

Although a variety of approaches have been employed, the application of the magnetic field has, until now, limited the use of magnetic liposomes due to gross patient incompliance.

3.3. Manufacturing and Clinical Challenges Common to Both Active and Passive Targeting

Besides requirements of triggered release and limited payload release at the site of action due to a multitude of reasons mentioned hitherto, active and passive targeting also presents manufacturing and clinical challenges (Table 2). The product related characteristics (in vitro drug release rate, particle size distribution, lamellarity, stability, drug encapsulation efficiency, etc.) obtained in a laboratory with a millimeter scale of the product should be reproducible when the product is scaled up in liters and should still maintain the same physicochemical properties and conform to the product release specifications. The manufacture, stability, degradation products, source and characterization of the lipidic components of the liposomes should be appropriately characterized prior to regulatory filing. In case of commercially available lipids, determining the positional specificity of acyl side chains is required and critical. In case of natural lipids (e.g., egg lecithin), the purification of the lipids is a challenge, and the composition of fatty acid requires robust analytical methods (Table 2). In addition, the analytical method should be qualified to distinguish and identify the lipid of interest in a mixture of lipids. Another crucial requirement is the determination of the amount of divalent cation and the counter ion content. The drug substance to lipid ratio at critical manufacturing unit operations is necessary and should be accurately and precisely determined to ensure consistent drug loading and drug release.

In addition, the approval of generic passively targeted liposomal products remains a challenge. The differences in the efficacy of lipodox which was launched a generic equivalent to Doxil has posed questions on the bioequivalence of the product in clinical trials [140]. The exact reason behind the difference although remains unknown.

Furthermore, the Pharmacokinetic/pharmacodynamic (PK/PD) profile of the liposome formulation is different from other conventional dosage forms. It is well known that the pharmacokinetic profile of liposomal amphotericin is different from the PK of amphotericin free drug [141]. It has been observed that the renal and fecal clearance of liposomal amphotericin is 10 times lower than the non-liposomal formulation [141]. The PK disposition of the drug depends on the PK of the liposomes which in turn depends on binding or fusion with plasma proteins and mononuclear phagocyte system (MPS), drug retention after dilution in the blood circulation and at low pH tumor environment [142–144]. Therefore, measuring the plasma concentration itself cannot be used to determined bioavailability. It should be noted that current FDA guidelines mandate that the bioanalytical method can determine both encapsulated and un-encapsulated drug content for product approval purposes. Early in the product development phase, radiolabeled liposomal products can be used for mass balance studies of plasma, urine and fecal samples to determine the PK profile. For liposomes not designed to be labeled, the quantitation of liposome accumulation in the tissue requires validated analytical methods that include tissue harvesting or organ isolation [145] and, therefore, pose a challenge in precise quantitative determination of liposomal accumulation and uptake by tumor tissues. This creates hurdles in translation from pre-clinical to clinical performance and, therefore, requires highly predictive models (Table 2).

In addition, formulation-based effects viz. size and method and level of drug loading on biodistribution of liposomes should also be considered, the release rate of drug using same lipid composition might provide different efficacy and safety profiles and mere more accumulation of liposomes at the tumor site cannot guarantee higher efficacy levels [146].

The rate of drug release and retention of the encapsulated drug depends on its physical state. When drug is precipitated inside the liposome carrier then the drug release is slower compared to when the drug is stored in solution form. The salt used to retain the drug also affects the encapsulation efficiency and drug release rate. Manganese sulfate has been known to be more effective in doxorubicin retention due to formation of complex rather than the ammonium sulfate salt [147].

As for the IV administration of liposomal formulation, the introduction of nanoparticles in the blood circulation stirs up stress reaction which is manifested in the form of activation related pseudo-allergy (CARPA) (Table 2). CARPA is caused as a result of nanoparticles entering the bloodstreams that are perceived as pathogenic organisms by the body. CARPA is managed by altering the rate of infusion, co-administering immune suppressants and employing less reactive infusion protocols [148–150]. CARPA has now gained attention by regulatory agencies and is perceived as safety risk in IV administration of liposomes [148]. European regulatory agency has now introduced CARPA test in pre-clinical test as a recommendation in development of generic liposomal formulations.

4. Need for Better Pre-Clinical and Clinical Strategies

Effectively translating preclinical research to clinical research is the need of the hour. Often, preclinical studies are conducted with a handful of liposome preparations; it is important to be able to perform high throughput screening of liposomes to comprehend biological and cellular interactions. Kelly et al. [151] have reported a number of cell interaction, toxicity and immune reactivity studies using high throughput methods. With the frequent use of well-developed high throughput techniques, correlation of biodistribution of liposomes and their PK/PD profile can be developed. The correlation of the PK/PD data, biodistribution and the efficacy data are of paramount importance. The determination of pharmacokinetic and tissue distribution profile is very critical for safety and efficacy determination of liposomes as the biodistribution is formulation specific and traditional bioequivalence studies may not interpret true biodistribution. The biodistribution profile of the liposomes is a key product of the formulation characteristics of a liposome. It has been known that the small size liposomes ($\leq$ 100 nm) can reach deeper into tumor spheroid models [152]. It has also been known that the PEG coated liposomes have limited interaction with cancer cells compared to liposomes without any steric (Figure 2). This is especially helpful in segregating the effectiveness of the carrier in reaching the target and penetrating the tumor with the anticancer efficacy of the encapsulated drug.

The efficacy data experimentally determined should be extrapolated to humans using predictive computational/mathematical modeling. High throughput techniques and physiologically based pharmacokinetic modeling can also be developed for experiments involving in situ whole organs to understand biodistribution kinetics and predict PK parameters in humans.

A lot of work at the pre-clinical stage is performed using pharmacokinetic modeling tools, however, validated pharmacodynamic concentration vs. effect modeling systems need to be developed and implemented.

5. Conclusions

In this review, challenges and limitations associated with conventional anticancer therapies viz. chemotherapy, radiotherapy and cancer surgery were reviewed. Cancer targeting (active or passive targeting) as an alternate and break-through to some of the problems associated with the non-specificity of conventional therapies were discussed. While there is a certain appeal to using active targeting, as it is directed to the tumor, nonetheless antigen and receptor heterogeneity, immunogenicity, drug encapsulation level, etc., remain a problem. Moreover, passive targeting resolves some of the problems such as immunogenicity, these systems rely heavily on drug release triggering mechanisms (either external or endogenous stimuli). External stimuli were discussed in detail and are considered as either poorly effective or generate gross patient compliance issues. Lastly, there are manufacturing and clinical challenges associated with both active and passively targeted liposomes. In this regard, the need for robust analytical methods to determine biodistribution, PK and PD profile of liposomes was highlighted in addition to a critical gap between efficient preclinical to clinical efficacy predictive modeling.

We believe that while presenting the issues with current anticancer therapies, we also highlight the potential opportunities that will encourage further research in this area.

Author Contributions: Conceptualization, V.G., J.C.H. and R.G.; writing—original draft preparation, V.G. and J.C.H.; writing—review and editing, V.G., J.C.H. and R.G.; visualization, V.G.; supervision, J.C.H. All authors have read and agreed to the published version of the manuscript.

Funding: This work received no external funding.

Institutional Review Board Statement: Not applicable.

Informed Consent Statement: Not applicable.

Data Availability Statement: Data sharing not applicable.

Acknowledgments: Authors would like to thank Khushboo Bali for their contribution towards the electronic artwork presented in this article.

Conflicts of Interest: The authors declare no conflict of interest.

References

1. Available online: https://web.archive.org/web/20210707200955/https://gicr.iarc.fr/public/docs/20120906-WorldCancerFactSheet.pdf (accessed on 7 July 2021).
2. Available online: https://web.archive.org/web/20210707201547/https://gco.iarc.fr/today/data/factsheets/cancers/39-All-cancers-fact-sheet.pdf (accessed on 7 July 2021).
3. Available online: https://web.archive.org/web/20210707201915/https://www.cancer.org/content/dam/cancer-org/research/cancer-facts-and-statistics/annual-cancer-facts-and-figures/2021/cancer-facts-and-figures-2021.pdf (accessed on 7 July 2021).
4. Gyanani, V. Turning Stealth Liposomes into Cationic Liposomes for Anticancer Drug Delivery. Ph.D. Thesis, University of the Pacific, Stockton, CA, USA, 2013.
5. Allen, T.M. Ligand-targeted therapeutics in anticancer therapy. *Nat. Rev. Cancer* **2002**, *2*, 750–763. [CrossRef]
6. Yao, X.; Panichpisal, K.; Kurtzman, N.; Nugent, K. Cisplatin nephrotoxicity: A review. *Am. J. Med. Sci.* **2007**, *334*, 115–124. [CrossRef] [PubMed]
7. Pfeffer, B.; Tziros, C.; Katz, R.J. Current concepts of anthracycline cardiotoxicity: Pathogenesis, diagnosis and prevention. *Br. J. Cardiol.* **2009**, *16*, 85–89.
8. Partridge, A.H.; Burstein, H.J.; Winer, E.P. Side effects of chemotherapy and combined chemohormonal therapy in women with early-stage breast cancer. *J. Natl. Cancer Inst. Monogr.* **2001**, *30*, 135–142. [CrossRef] [PubMed]
9. Fabbrocini, G.; Cameli, N.; Romano, M.C.; Mariano, M.; Panariello, L.; Bianca, D.; Giuseppe, M. Chemotherapy and skin reactions. *J. Exp. Clin. Cancer Res.* **2012**, *31*, 50. [CrossRef]
10. Gottesman, M.M.; Fojo, T.; Bates, S.E. Multidrug resistance in cancer: Role of ATP–dependent transporters. *Nat. Rev. Cancer* **2002**, *2*, 48–58. [CrossRef]
11. Bentzen, S.M. Preventing or reducing late side effects of radiation therapy: Radiobiology meets molecular pathology. *Nat. Rev. Cancer* **2006**, *6*, 702–713. [CrossRef]
12. Bosslet, K.; Straub, R.; Blumrich, M.; Czech, J.; Gerken, M.; Sperker, B.; Kroemer, H.K.; Gesson, J.P.; Koch, M.; Monneret, C. Elucidation of the mechanism enabling tumor selective prodrug monotherapy. *Cancer Res.* **1998**, *58*, 1195–1201.
13. Senzer, N.; Nemunaitis, J.; Nemunaitis, D.; Bedell, C.; Edelman, G.; Barve, M.; Nunan, R.; Pirollo, K.F.; Rait, A.; Chang, E.H. Results of a Phase I Trial of SGT-53: A Systemically Administered, Tumor-Targeting Immunoliposome Nanocomplex Incorporating a Plasmid Encoding wtp53. *Clin. Gene Cell Ther. Oral Abstr. Sess.* **2012**, *20*. [CrossRef]
14. Pirollo, K.F.; Nemunaitis, J.; Leung, P.K.; Nunan, R.; Adams, J.; Chang, E.H. Safety and Efficacy in Advanced Solid Tumors of a Targeted Nanocomplex Carrying the p53 Gene Used in Combination with Docetaxel: A Phase 1b Study. *Mol. Ther.* **2016**, *24*, 1697–1706. [CrossRef]
15. Kim, E.M.; Jeong, H.J. Liposomes: Biomedical Applications. *Chonnam. Med. J.* **2021**, *57*, 27–35. [CrossRef] [PubMed]
16. Available online: https://clinicaltrials.gov/ct2/show/NCT03076372 (accessed on 12 August 2021).
17. Moles, E.; Kavallaris, M. A potent targeted cancer nanotherapeutic. *Nat. Biomed. Eng.* **2019**, *3*, 248–250. [CrossRef] [PubMed]
18. Wang, D.; Sun, Y.; Liu, Y.; Meng, F.; Lee, R.J. Clinical translation of immunoliposomes for cancer therapy: Recent perspectives. *Expert Opin. Drug Deliv.* **2018**, *15*, 893–903. [CrossRef]

19. Yan, W.; Leung, S.S.; To, K.K. Updates on the use of liposomes for active tumor targeting in cancer therapy. *Nanomedicine* **2020**, *15*, 303–318. [CrossRef]
20. Available online: https://clinicaltrials.gov/ct2/show/NCT03603379 (accessed on 12 August 2021).
21. Paranthaman, S.; Goravinahalli Shivananjegowda, M.; Mahadev, M.; Moin, A.; Hagalavadi Nanjappa, S.; Nanjaiyah, N.; Chidambaram, S.B.; Gowda, D.V. Nanodelivery Systems Targeting Epidermal Growth Factor Receptors for Glioma Management. *Pharmaceutics* **2020**, *12*, 1198. [CrossRef]
22. Miller, K.; Cortes, J.; Hurvitz, S.A.; Krop, I.E.; Tripathy, D.; Verma, S.; Riahi, K.; Reynolds, J.G.; Wickham, T.J.; Molnar, I.; et al. HERMIONE: A randomized Phase 2 trial of MM-302 plus trastuzumab versus chemotherapy of physician's choice plus trastuzumab in patients with previously treated, anthracycline-naïve, HER2-positive, locally advanced/metastatic breast cancer. *BMC Cancer* **2016**, *16*, 352. [CrossRef]
23. Available online: https://www.clinicaltrials.gov/ct2/show/NCT01304797 (accessed on 12 August 2021).
24. Gargett, T.; Abbas, M.N.; Rolan, P.; Price, J.D.; Gosling, K.M.; Ferrante, A.; Ruszkiewicz, A.; Atmosukarto, I.I.C.; Altin, J.; Parish, C.R.; et al. Phase I trial of Lipovaxin-MM, a novel dendritic cell-targeted liposomal vaccine for malignant melanoma. *Cancer Immunol. Immunother.* **2018**, *67*, 1461–1472. [CrossRef] [PubMed]
25. Liu, C.; Zhang, L.; Zhu, W.; Guo, R.; Sun, H.; Chen, X.; Deng, N. Barriers and Strategies of Cationic Liposomes for Cancer Gene Therapy. *Mol. Ther.-Methods Clin. Dev.* **2020**, *18*, 751–764. [CrossRef]
26. Available online: https://www.clinicaltrials.gov/ct2/show/NCT01517464 (accessed on 12 August 2021).
27. Siefker-Radtke, A.; Zhang, X.Q.; Guo, C.C.; Shen, Y.; Pirollo, K.F.; Sabir, S.; Leung, C.; Leong-Wu, C.; Ling, C.M.; Chang, E.H.; et al. A Phase l Study of a Tumor-targeted Systemic Nanodelivery System, SGT-94, in Genitourinary Cancers. *Mol. Ther.* **2016**, *24*, 1484–1491. [CrossRef]
28. Available online: https://www.cancer.gov/publications/dictionaries/cancer-drug/def/748730 (accessed on 12 August 2021).
29. Available online: https://patents.justia.com/patent/20180334724 (accessed on 12 August 2021).
30. Song, X.L.; Liu, S.; Jiang, Y.; Gu, L.Y.; Xiao, Y.; Wang, X.; Cheng, L.; Li, X.T. Targeting vincristine plus tetrandrine liposomes modified with DSPE-PEG(2000)-transferrin in treatment of brain glioma. *Eur. J. Pharm. Sci.* **2017**, *96*, 129–140. [CrossRef]
31. Chiani, M.; Norouzian, D.; Shokrgozar, M.A.; Azadmanesh, K.; Najmafshar, A.; Mehrabi, M.R.; Akbarzadeh, A. Folic acid conjugated nanoliposomes as promising carriers for targeted delivery of bleomycin. *Artif. Cells Nanomed. Biotechnol.* **2018**, *46*, 757–763. [CrossRef] [PubMed]
32. Della Giovampaola, C.; Capone, A.; Ermini, L.; Lupetti, P.; Vannuccini, E.; Finetti, F.; Donnini, S.; Ziche, M.; Magnani, A.; Leone, G.; et al. Formulation of liposomes functionalized with Lotus lectin and effective in targeting highly proliferative cells. *Biochim Biophys. Acta Gen. Subj.* **2017**, *1861*, 860–870. [CrossRef] [PubMed]
33. Cristiano, M.C.; Cosco, D.; Celia, C.; Tudose, A.; Mare, R.; Paolino, D.; Fresta, M. Anticancer activity of all-trans retinoic acid-loaded liposomes on human thyroid carcinoma cells. *Colloids Surf. B Biointerfaces* **2017**, *150*, 408–416. [CrossRef]
34. Grace, V.M.; Viswanathan, S. Pharmacokinetics and therapeutic efficiency of a novel cationic liposome nano-formulated all trans retinoic acid in lung cancer mice model. *J. Drug Deliv. Sci. Technol.* **2017**, *39*, 223–236. [CrossRef]
35. Lancet, J.E.; Uy, G.L.; Cortes, J.E.; Newell, L.F.; Lin, T.L.; Ritchie, E.K.; Stuart, R.K.; Strickland, S.A.; Hogge, D.; Solomon, S.R.; et al. CPX-351 (cytarabine and daunorubicin) Liposome for Injection Versus Conventional Cytarabine Plus Daunorubicin in Older Patients with Newly Diagnosed Secondary Acute Myeloid Leukemia. *J. Clin. Oncol.* **2018**, *36*, 2684–2692. [CrossRef] [PubMed]
36. Pelzer, U.; Blanc, J.F.; Melisi, D.; Cubillo, A.; Von Hoff, D.D.; Wang-Gillam, A.; Chen, L.T.; Siveke, J.T.; Wan, Y.; Solem, C.T.; et al. Quality-adjusted survival with combination nal-IRI+5-FU/LV vs. 5-FU/LV alone in metastatic pancreatic cancer patients previously treated with gemcitabine-based therapy: A Q-TWiST analysis. *Br. J. Cancer* **2017**, *116*, 1247–1253. [CrossRef]
37. Tran, S.; DeGiovanni, P.J.; Piel, B.; Rai, P. Cancer nanomedicine: A review of recent success in drug delivery. *Clin. Transl. Med.* **2017**, *6*, 44. [CrossRef] [PubMed]
38. Bulbake, U.; Doppalapudi, S.; Kommineni, N.; Khan, W. Liposomal Formulations in Clinical Use: An Updated Review. *Pharmaceutics* **2017**, *9*, 12. [CrossRef]
39. Lamichhane, N.; Udayakumar, T.S.; D'Souza, W.D.; Simone, C.B., 2nd; Raghavan, S.R.; Polf, J.; Mahmood, J. Liposomes: Clinical Applications and Potential for Image-Guided Drug Delivery. *Molecules* **2018**, *23*, 288. [CrossRef] [PubMed]
40. Bozzuto, G.; Molinari, A. Liposomes as nanomedical devices. *Int. J. Nanomed.* **2015**, *10*, 975–999. [CrossRef]
41. Available online: http://web.archive.org/web/20210813002334/https://patents.google.com/patent/AU2013347990A1/en (accessed on 13 August 2021).
42. Available online: http://web.archive.org/web/20210813001653/http://www.druginformation.com/rxdrugs/V/VinCRIStine%20Sulfate%20LIPOSOME%20Injection.html (accessed on 13 August 2021).
43. Available online: http://web.archive.org/web/20210813003036/https://www.bausch.com/ecp/our-products/rx-pharmaceuticals/rx-pharmaceuticals/visudyne-verteporfin-for-injection (accessed on 13 August 2021).
44. Ghosh, S.; Carter, K.A.; Lovell, J.F. Liposomal formulations of photosensitizers. *Biomaterials* **2019**, *218*, 119341. [CrossRef] [PubMed]
45. Available online: https://web.archive.org/web/20210422023716/https://clinicaltrials.gov/ct2/show/NCT04590664 (accessed on 13 August 2021).
46. Available online: https://web.archive.org/web/20210813005341/https://clinicaltrials.gov/ct2/show/NCT00617981 (accessed on 13 August 2021).

47. Lombardo, D.; Calandra, P.; Barreca, D.; Magazù, S.; Kiselev, M.A. Soft Interaction in Liposome Nanocarriers for Therapeutic Drug Delivery. *Nanomaterials* **2016**, *6*, 125. [CrossRef] [PubMed]
48. Available online: http://web.archive.org/web/20210813010747/https://www.syncorebio.com/en/sb05pc-endotag-1-phase-iii-been-approved-in-china-by-nmpa/ (accessed on 13 August 2021).
49. Hong, D.S.; Kang, Y.-K.; Borad, M.; Sachdev, J.; Ejadi, S.; Lim, H.Y.; Brenner, A.J.; Park, K.; Lee, J.L.; Kim, T.Y.; et al. Phase 1 study of MRX34, a liposomal miR-34a mimic, in patients with advanced solid tumors. *Br. J. Cancer* **2020**, *122*, 1630–1637. [CrossRef] [PubMed]
50. Lin, X.; Chen, W.; Wei, F.; Zhou, B.P.; Hung, M.C.; Xie, X. Nanoparticle Delivery of miR-34a Eradicates Long-term-cultured Breast Cancer Stem Cells via Targeting C22ORF28 Directly. *Theranostics* **2017**, *7*, 4805–4824. [CrossRef]
51. Shi, J.; Kantoff, P.W.; Wooster, R.; Farokhzad, O.C. Cancer nanomedicine: Progress, challenges and opportunities. *Nat. Rev. Cancer* **2017**, *17*, 20–37. [CrossRef]
52. Available online: https://web.archive.org/web/20210813021139/https://www.onivyde.com/websites/onivyde_us_online/wp-content/uploads/sites/3/2018/12/14105740/ONIVYDE_USPI.pdf (accessed on 13 August 2021).
53. Available online: http://web.archive.org/web/20210225052514if_/https://www.curetoday.com/view/onivyde-shows-promise-in-patients-with-small-cell-lung-cancer-who-become-resistant-to-chemotherapy (accessed on 13 August 2021).
54. Gabizon, A.; Shmeeda, H.; Tahover, E.; Kornev, G.; Patil, Y.; Amitay, Y.; Ohana, P.; Sapir, E.; Zalipsky, S. Development of Promitil®, a lipidic prodrug of mitomycin c in PEGylated liposomes: From bench to bedside. *Adv. Drug Deliv. Rev.* **2020**, *154–155*, 13–26. [CrossRef]
55. Available online: http://lipomedix.com/Products/%C2%AEPromitil (accessed on 12 August 2021).
56. Available online: http://web.archive.org/web/20210813024839/https://www.globenewswire.com/news-release/2020/01/23/1974347/0/en/LipoMedix-Announces-Publication-of-Positive-Phase-1-Data-for-Promitil-PL-MLP-in-Research-Journal-Investigational-New-Drugs.html (accessed on 13 August 2021).
57. Available online: https://web.archive.org/web/20210813025653/https://www.genprex.com/technology/reqorsa/ (accessed on 13 August 2021).
58. Available online: https://web.archive.org/web/20210813030047/https://adisinsight.springer.com/drugs/800018766 (accessed on 13 August 2021).
59. Available online: https://web.archive.org/web/20210813030656/https://clinicaltrials.gov/ct2/show/NCT04078295 (accessed on 13 August 2021).
60. Available online: https://web.archive.org/web/20210813031053/https://ascopubs.or (accessed on 13 August 2021).
61. Chien, Y.C.; Chou, Y.H.; Wang, W.H.; Chen, J.C.; Chang, W.S.; Tsai, C.W.; Bau, D.T.; Hwang, J.J. Therapeutic Efficacy Evaluation of Pegylated Liposome Encapsulated with Vinorelbine Plus (111) in Repeated Treatments in Human Colorectal Carcinoma with Multimodalities of Molecular Imaging. *Cancer Genom. Proteom.* **2020**, *17*, 61–76. [CrossRef]
62. Greil, R.; Greil-Ressler, S.; Weiss, L.; Schönlieb, C.; Magnes, T.; Radl, B.; Bolger, G.T.; Vcelar, B.; Sordillo, P.P. A phase 1 dose-escalation study on the safety, tolerability and activity of liposomal curcumin (Lipocurc(™)) in patients with locally advanced or metastatic cancer. *Cancer Chemother. Pharmacol.* **2018**, *82*, 695–706. [CrossRef] [PubMed]
63. Bolger, G.T.; Licollari, A.; Tan, A.; Greil, R.; Vcelar, B.; Majeed, M.; Helson, L. Distribution and Metabolism of Lipocurc™ (Liposomal Curcumin) in Dog and Human Blood Cells: Species Selectivity and Pharmacokinetic Relevance. *Anticancer Res.* **2017**, *37*, 3483. [PubMed]
64. Available online: https://web.archive.org/web/20210813032817/https://apnews.com/press-release/pr-businesswire/eb9457dc9500491e918b53fdeeb75494 (accessed on 12 August 2021).
65. Graziani, S.R.; Vital, C.G.; Morikawa, A.T.; Van Eyll, B.M.; Fernandes Junior, H.J.; Kalil Filho, R.; Maranhão, R.C. Phase II study of paclitaxel associated with lipid core nanoparticles (LDE) as third-line treatment of patients with epithelial ovarian carcinoma. *Med. Oncol.* **2017**, *34*, 151. [CrossRef] [PubMed]
66. Occhiutto, M.L.; Freitas, F.R.; Lima, P.P.; Maranhão, R.C.; Costa, V.P. Paclitaxel Associated with Lipid Nanoparticles as a New Antiscarring Agent in Experimental Glaucoma Surgery. *Investig. Ophthalmol. Vis. Sci.* **2016**, *57*, 971–978. [CrossRef]
67. Gomes, F.L.T.; Maranhão, R.C.; Tavares, E.R.; Carvalho, P.O.; Higuchi, M.L.; Mattos, F.R.; Pitta, F.G.; Hatab, S.A.; Kalil-Filho, R.; Serrano, C.V., Jr. Regression of Atherosclerotic Plaques of Cholesterol-Fed Rabbits by Combined Chemotherapy with Paclitaxel and Methotrexate Carried in Lipid Core Nanoparticles. *J. Cardiovasc. Pharmacol. Ther.* **2018**, *23*, 561–569. [CrossRef] [PubMed]
68. Peer, D.; Karp, J.M.; Hong, S.; Farokhzad, O.C.; Margalit, R.; Langer, R. Nanocarriers as an emerging platform for cancer therapy. *Nat. Nanotechnol.* **2007**, *2*, 751–760. [CrossRef]
69. Adams, G.P.; Schier, R.; McCall, A.M.; Simmons, H.H.; Horak, E.M.; Alpaugh, R.K.; Marks, J.D.; Weiner, L.M. High affinity restricts the localization and tumor penetration of single-chain fv antibody molecules. *Cancer Res.* **2001**, *61*, 4750–4755. [PubMed]
70. Tolcher, A.W.; Sugarman, S.; Gelmon, K.A.; Cohen, R.; Saleh, M.; Isaacs, C.; Young, L.; Healey, D.; Onetto, N.; Slichenmyer, W. Randomized phase II study of BR96-doxorubicin conjugate in patients with metastatic breast cancer. *J. Clin. Oncol.* **1999**, *17*, 478–484. [CrossRef] [PubMed]
71. Kamoun, W.S.; Kirpotin, D.B.; Huang, Z.R.; Tipparaju, S.K.; Noble, C.O.; Hayes, M.E.; Luus, L.; Koshkaryev, A.; Kim, J.; Olivier, K.; et al. Antitumour activity and tolerability of an EphA2-targeted nanotherapeutic in multiple mouse models. *Nat. Biomed. Eng.* **2019**, *3*, 264–280. [CrossRef] [PubMed]

72. Matusewicz, L.; Filip-Psurska, B.; Psurski, M.; Tabaczar, S.; Podkalicka, J.; Wietrzyk, J.; Ziółkowski, P.; Czogalla, A.; Sikorski, A.F. EGFR-targeted immunoliposomes as a selective delivery system of simvastatin, with potential use in treatment of triple-negative breast cancers. *Int. J. Pharm.* **2019**, *569*, 118605. [CrossRef] [PubMed]
73. Khayrani, A.C.; Mahmud, H.; Oo, A.K.K.; Zahra, M.H.; Oze, M.; Du, J.; Alam, M.J.; Afify, S.M.; Quora, H.A.A.; Shigehiro, T.; et al. Targeting Ovarian Cancer Cells Overexpressing CD44 with Immunoliposomes Encapsulating Glycosylated Paclitaxel. *Int. J. Mol. Sci.* **2019**, *20*, 1042. [CrossRef] [PubMed]
74. Hua, S. Synthesis and in vitro characterization of oxytocin receptor targeted PEGylated immunoliposomes for drug delivery to the uterus. *J. Liposome Res.* **2019**, *29*, 357–367. [CrossRef] [PubMed]
75. Takahara, M.; Kamiya, N. Synthetic Strategies for Artificial Lipidation of Functional Proteins. *Chem.-A Eur. J.* **2020**, *26*, 4645–4655. [CrossRef] [PubMed]
76. Marcos-Contreras, O.A.; Greineder, C.F.; Kiseleva, R.Y.; Parhiz, H.; Walsh, L.R.; Zuluaga-Ramirez, V.; Myerson, J.W.; Hood, E.D.; Villa, C.H.; Tombacz, I.; et al. Selective targeting of nanomedicine to inflamed cerebral vasculature to enhance the blood–brain barrier. *Proc. Natl. Acad. Sci. USA* **2020**, *117*, 3405. [CrossRef] [PubMed]
77. Orleth, A.; Mamot, C.; Rochlitz, C.; Ritschard, R.; Alitalo, K.; Christofori, G.; Wicki, A. Simultaneous targeting of VEGF-receptors 2 and 3 with immunoliposomes enhances therapeutic efficacy. *J. Drug Target.* **2016**, *24*, 80–89. [CrossRef] [PubMed]
78. Loureiro, J.A.; Gomes, B.; Fricker, G.; Cardoso, I.; Ribeiro, C.A.; Gaiteiro, C.; Coelho, M.A.; Pereira Mdo, C.; Rocha, S. Dual ligand immunoliposomes for drug delivery to the brain. *Colloids Surf. B Biointerfaces* **2015**, *134*, 213–219. [CrossRef] [PubMed]
79. Paul, J.W.; Hua, S.; Ilicic, M.; Tolosa, J.M.; Butler, T.; Robertson, S.; Smith, R. Drug delivery to the human and mouse uterus using immunoliposomes targeted to the oxytocin receptor. *Am. J. Obstet. Gynecol.* **2017**, *216*, e1–e283. [CrossRef] [PubMed]
80. Moles, E.; Urbán, P.; Jiménez-Díaz, M.B.; Viera-Morilla, S.; Angulo-Barturen, I.; Busquets, M.A.; Fernàndez-Busquets, X. Immunoliposome-mediated drug delivery to Plasmodium-infected and non-infected red blood cells as a dual therapeutic/prophylactic antimalarial strategy. *J. Control. Release* **2015**, *210*, 217–229. [CrossRef] [PubMed]
81. Moles, E.; Galiano, S.; Gomes, A.; Quiliano, M.; Teixeira, C.; Aldana, I.; Gomes, P.; Fernàndez-Busquets, X. ImmunoPEGliposomes for the targeted delivery of novel lipophilic drugs to red blood cells in a falciparum malaria murine model. *Biomaterials* **2017**, *145*, 178–191. [CrossRef] [PubMed]
82. Ramana, L.N.; Sharma, S.; Sethuraman, S.; Ranga, U.; Krishnan, U.M. Stealth anti-CD4 conjugated immunoliposomes with dual antiretroviral drugs–modern Trojan horses to combat HIV. *Eur. J. Pharm. Biopharm.* **2015**, *89*, 300–311. [CrossRef] [PubMed]
83. Ding, T.; Guan, J.; Wang, M.; Long, Q.; Liu, X.; Qian, J.; Wei, X.; Lu, W.; Zhan, C. Natural IgM dominates in vivo performance of liposomes. *J. Control. Release* **2020**, *319*, 371–381. [CrossRef]
84. Rabenhold, M.; Steiniger, F.; Fahr, A.; Kontermann, R.E.; Rüger, R. Bispecific single-chain diabody-immunoliposomes targeting endoglin (CD105) and fibroblast activation protein (FAP) simultaneously. *J. Control. Release* **2015**, *201*, 56–67. [CrossRef] [PubMed]
85. Peng, J.; Chen, J.; Xie, F.; Bao, W.; Xu, H.; Wang, H.; Xu, Y.; Du, Z. Herceptin-conjugated paclitaxel loaded PCL-PEG worm-like nanocrystal micelles for the combinatorial treatment of HER2-positive breast cancer. *Biomaterials* **2019**, *222*, 119420. [CrossRef]
86. Kraft, J.C.; Freeling, J.P.; Wang, Z.; Ho, R.J.Y. Emerging research and clinical development trends of liposome and lipid nanoparticle drug delivery systems. *J. Pharm. Sci.* **2014**, *103*, 29–52. [CrossRef] [PubMed]
87. Available online: https://web.archive.org/web/20210728202637/https://www.sciencenews.org/article/coronavirus-covid-deadly-black-fungus-infection-india (accessed on 28 July 2021).
88. Immordino, M.L.; Dosio, F.; Cattel, L. Stealth liposomes: Review of the basic science, rationale, and clinical applications, existing and potential. *Int. J. Nanomed.* **2006**, *1*, 297–315.
89. Scherphof, G.L.; Dijkstra, J.; Spanjer, H.H.; Derksen, J.T.; Roerdink, F.H. Uptake and intracellular processing of targeted and nontargeted liposomes by rat Kupffer cells in vivo and in vitro. *Ann. N. Y. Acad. Sci.* **1985**, *446*, 368–384. [CrossRef]
90. Cullis, P.R.; Chonn, A.; Semple, S.C. Interactions of liposomes and lipid-based carrier systems with blood proteins: Relation to clearance behaviour in vivo. *Adv. Drug Deliv. Rev.* **1998**, *32*, 3–17.
91. Senior, J.H.; Trimble, K.R.; Maskiewicz, R. Interaction of positively-charged liposomes with blood: Implications for their application in vivo. *Biochim. Biophys. Acta* **1991**, *1070*, 173–179. [CrossRef]
92. Oku, N.; Tokudome, Y.; Namba, Y.; Saito, N.; Endo, M.; Hasegawa, Y.; Kawai, M.; Tsukada, H.; Okada, S. Effect of serum protein binding on real-time trafficking of liposomes with different charges analyzed by positron emission tomography. *Biochim. Biophys. Acta* **1996**, *1280*, 149–154. [CrossRef]
93. Philippot, J.R.; Schube, F. *Liposomes as Tools in Basic Research and Industry*, 1st ed.; CRC Press: Boca Raton, FL, USA, 1994; p. 181.
94. Du, H.; Chandaroy, P.; Hui, S.W. Grafted poly-(ethylene glycol) on lipid surfaces inhibits protein adsorption and cell adhesion. *Biochim. Biophys. Acta* **1997**, *1326*, 236–248. [CrossRef]
95. Hong, R.L.; Huang, C.J.; Tseng, Y.L.; Pang, V.F.; Chen, S.T.; Liu, J.J.; Chang, F.H. Direct comparison of liposomal doxorubicin with or without polyethylene glycol coating in C-26 tumor-bearing mice: Is surface coating with polyethylene glycol beneficial? *Clin. Cancer Res.* **1999**, *5*, 3645–3652.
96. Parr, M.J.; Masin, D.; Cullis, P.R.; Bally, M.B. Accumulation of liposomal lipid and encapsulated doxorubicin in murine Lewis lung carcinoma: The lack of beneficial effects by coating liposomes with poly(ethylene-glycol). *J. Pharmacol. Exp. Ther.* **1997**, *280*, 1319–1327.

97. Kale, A.A.; Torchilin, V.P. Design, Synthesis, and Characterization of pH-Sensitive PEG−PE Conjugates for Stimuli-Sensitive Pharmaceutical Nanocarriers: The Effect of Substitutes at the Hydrazone Linkage on the pH Stability of PEG−PE Conjugates. *Bioconjugate Chem.* **2007**, *18*, 363–370. [CrossRef] [PubMed]
98. Sun, Y.; Zhao, D.; Wang, G.; Wang, Y.; Cao, L.; Sun, J.; Jiang, Q.; He, Z. Recent progress of hypoxia-modulated multifunctional nanomedicines to enhance photodynamic therapy: Opportunities, challenges, and future development. *Acta Pharm. Sin. B* **2020**, *10*, 1382–1396. [CrossRef]
99. Sharma, A.; Arambula, J.F.; Koo, S.; Kumar, R.; Singh, H.; Sessler, J.L.; Kim, J.S. Hypoxia-targeted drug delivery. *Chem. Soc. Rev.* **2019**, *48*, 771–813. [CrossRef]
100. Andresen, T.L.; Thompson, D.H.; Kaasgaard, T. Enzyme-triggered nanomedicine: Drug release strategies in cancer therapy (Invited Review). *Mol. Membr. Biol.* **2010**, *27*, 353–363. [CrossRef] [PubMed]
101. Li, S.; Zou, Q.; Xing, R.; Govindaraju, T.; Fakhrullin, R.; Yan, X. Peptide-modulated self-assembly as a versatile strategy for tumor supramolecular nanotheranostics. *Theranostics* **2019**, *9*, 3249–3261. [CrossRef] [PubMed]
102. Horsman, M.R.; Vaupel, P. Pathophysiological Basis for the Formation of the Tumor Microenvironment. *Front. Oncol.* **2016**, *6*, 1–12. [CrossRef] [PubMed]
103. Kalafatovic, D.; Nobis, M.; Son, J.; Anderson, K.I.; Ulijn, R.V. MMP-9 triggered self-assembly of doxorubicin nanofiber depots halts tumor growth. *Biomaterials* **2016**, *98*, 192–202. [CrossRef] [PubMed]
104. Zhang, N.; Zhao, F.; Zou, Q.; Li, Y.; Ma, G.; Yan, X. Multitriggered Tumor-Responsive Drug Delivery Vehicles Based on Protein and Polypeptide Coassembly for Enhanced Photodynamic Tumor Ablation. *Small* **2016**, *12*, 5936–5943. [CrossRef]
105. Canavese, G.; Ancona, A.; Racca, L.; Canta, M.; Dumontel, B.; Barbaresco, F.; Limongi, T.; Cauda, V. Nanoparticle-assisted ultrasound: A special focus on sonodynamic therapy against cancer. *Chem. Eng. J.* **2018**, *340*, 155–172. [CrossRef]
106. Sirsi, S.R.; Borden, M.A. State-of-the-art materials for ultrasound-triggered drug delivery. *Adv. Drug Deliv. Rev.* **2014**, *72*, 3–14. [CrossRef]
107. VanOsdol, J.; Ektate, K.; Ramasamy, S.; Maples, D.; Collins, W.; Malayer, J.; Ranjan, A. Sequential HIFU heating and nanobubble encapsulation provide efficient drug penetration from stealth and temperature sensitive liposomes in colon cancer. *J. Control. Release* **2017**, *247*, 55–63. [CrossRef]
108. Huang, S.L.; MacDonald, R.C. Acoustically active liposomes for drug encapsulation and ultrasound-triggered release. *Biochim. Biophys. Acta* **2004**, *1665*, 134–141. [CrossRef]
109. Rapoport, N. Combined cancer therapy by micellar-encapsulated drug and ultrasound. *Int. J. Pharm.* **2004**, *277*, 155–162. [CrossRef] [PubMed]
110. Leung, S.J.; Romanowski, M. Light-Activated Content Release from Liposomes. *Theranostics* **2012**, *2*, 1020–1036. [CrossRef]
111. Pidgeon, C.; Hunt, C.A. Light sensitive liposomes. *Photochem. Photobiol.* **1983**, *37*, 491–494. [CrossRef]
112. Ohya, Y.; Okuyama, Y.; Fukunaga, A.; Ouchi, T. Photo-sensitive lipid membrane perturbation by a single chain lipid having terminal spiropyran group. *Supramol. Chem.* **1998**, *5*, 21–29. [CrossRef]
113. Anderson, V.C.; Thompson, D.H. Triggered release of hydrophilic agents from plasmalogen liposomes using visible light or acid. *Biochim. Biophys. Acta* **1992**, *1109*, 33–42. [CrossRef]
114. Thompson, D.H.; Gerasimov, O.V.; Wheeler, J.J.; Rui, Y.; Anderson, V.C. Triggerable plasmalogen liposomes: Improvement of system efficiency. *Biochim. Biophys. Acta* **1996**, *1279*, 25–34. [CrossRef]
115. Wan, Y.; Angleson, J.K.; Kutateladze, A.G. Liposomes from Novel Photolabile Phospholipids: Light-Induced Unloading of Small Molecules as Monitored by PFG NMR. *J. Am. Chem. Soc.* **2002**, *124*, 5610–5611. [CrossRef]
116. Li, Z.; Wan, Y.; Kutateladze, A.G. Dithiane-based photolabile amphiphiles: Toward photolabile liposomes. *Langmuir* **2003**, *19*, 6381–6391. [CrossRef]
117. Zhang, Z.; Smith, B.D. Synthesis and Characterization of NVOC-DOPE, a Caged Photoactivatable Derivative of Dioleoylphosphatidylethanolamine. *Bioconjugate Chem.* **1999**, *10*, 1150–1152. [CrossRef] [PubMed]
118. Bayer, A.M.; Alam, S.; Mattern-Schain, S.I.; Best, M.D. Triggered liposomal release through a synthetic phosphatidylcholine analogue bearing a photocleavable moiety embedded within the sn-2 acyl chain. *Chemistry* **2014**, *20*, 3350–3357. [CrossRef]
119. O'Brien, D.F.; Armitage, B.; Benedicto, A.; Bennett, D.E.; Lamparski, H.G.; Lee, Y.; Srisiri, W.; Sisson, T.M. Polymerization of Preformed Self-Organized Assemblies. *Acc. Chem. Res.* **1998**, *31*, 861–868. [CrossRef]
120. Yavlovich, A.; Singh, A.; Blumenthal, R.; Puri, A. A novel class of photo-triggerable liposomes containing DPPC:$DC_{8,9}$PC as vehicles for delivery of doxorubcin to cells. *Biochim. Biophys. Acta Biomembr.* **2011**, *1808*, 117–126. [CrossRef] [PubMed]
121. Gerasimov, O.V.; Boomer, J.A.; Qualls, M.M.; Thompson, D.H. Cytosolic drug delivery using pH- and light-sensitive liposomes. *Adv. Drug Deliv. Rev.* **1999**, *38*, 317–338. [CrossRef]
122. Fuse, T.; Tagami, T.; Tane, M.; Ozeki, T. Effective light-triggered contents release from helper lipid-incorporated liposomes co-encapsulating gemcitabine and a water-soluble photosensitizer. *Int. J. Pharm.* **2018**, *540*, 50–56. [CrossRef] [PubMed]
123. Li, Q.; Li, W.; Di, H.; Luo, L.; Zhu, C.; Yang, J.; Yin, X.; Yin, H.; Gao, J.; Du, Y.; et al. A photosensitive liposome with NIR light triggered doxorubicin release as a combined photodynamic-chemo therapy system. *J. Control. Release* **2018**, *277*, 114–125. [CrossRef]
124. Yatvin, M.B.; Weinstein, J.N.; Dennis, W.H.; Blumenthal, R. Design of liposomes for enhanced local release of drugs by hyperthermia. *Science* **1978**, *202*, 1290–1293. [CrossRef]

125. Ta, T.; Porter, T.M. Thermosensitive liposomes for localized delivery and triggered release of chemotherapy. *J. Control. Release* **2013**, *169*, 112–125. [CrossRef] [PubMed]
126. Nibu, Y.; Inoue, T.; Motoda, I. Effect of headgroup type on the miscibility of homologous phospholipids with different acyl chain lengths in hydrated bilayer. *Biophys. Chem.* **1995**, *56*, 273–280. [CrossRef]
127. Meshorer, A.; Prionas, S.D.; Fajardo, L.F.; Meyer, J.L.; Hahn, G.M.; Martinez, A.A. The effects of hyperthermia on normal mesenchymal tissues. Application of a histologic grading system. *Arch. Pathol. Lab. Med.* **1983**, *107*, 328–334. [PubMed]
128. Anyarambhatla, G.R.; Needham, D. Enhancement of the Phase Transition Permeability of DPPC Liposomes by Incorporation of MPPC: A New Temperature-Sensitive Liposome for use with Mild Hyperthermia. *J. Liposome Res.* **1999**, *9*, 491–506. [CrossRef]
129. Banno, B.; Ickenstein, L.M.; Chiu, G.N.C.; Bally, M.B.; Thewalt, J.; Brief, E.; Wasan, E.K. The functional roles of poly(ethylene glycol)-lipid and lysolipid in the drug retention and release from lysolipid-containing thermosensitive liposomes in vitro and in vivo. *J. Pharm. Sci.* **2010**, *99*, 2295–2308. [CrossRef] [PubMed]
130. Sandström, M.C.; Ickenstein, L.M.; Mayer, L.D.; Edwards, K. Effects of lipid segregation and lysolipid dissociation on drug release from thermosensitive liposomes. *J. Control. Release* **2005**, *107*, 131–142. [CrossRef] [PubMed]
131. Available online: https://web.archive.org/web/20210728223201/https://www.globenewswire.com/en/news-release/2020/04/15/2016425/0/en/Celsion-Reports-that-Sufficient-Events-Have-Been-Reached-for-the-Second-Interim-Analysis-of-the-Phase-III-OPTIMA-Study-of-ThermoDox-in-Primary-Liver-Cancer.html (accessed on 28 July 2021).
132. Swenson, C.E.; Haemmerich, D.; Maul, D.H.; Knox, B.; Ehrhart, N.; Reed, R.A. Increased Duration of Heating Boosts Local Drug Deposition during Radiofrequency Ablation in Combination with Thermally Sensitive Liposomes (ThermoDox) in a Porcine Model. *PLoS ONE* **2015**, *10*, e0139752. [CrossRef]
133. Amstad, E.; Kohlbrecher, J.; Müller, E.; Schweizer, T.; Textor, M.; Reimhult, E. Triggered Release from Liposomes through Magnetic Actuation of Iron Oxide Nanoparticle Containing Membranes. *Nano Lett.* **2011**, *11*, 1664–1670. [CrossRef]
134. Babincová, M.; Cicmanec, P.; Altanerová, V.; Altaner, C.; Babinec, P. AC-magnetic field controlled drug release from magnetoliposomes: Design of a method for site-specific chemotherapy. *Bioelectrochemistry* **2002**, *55*, 17–19. [CrossRef]
135. Nobuto, H.; Sugita, T.; Kubo, T.; Shimose, S.; Yasunaga, Y.; Murakami, T.; Ochi, M. Evaluation of systemic chemotherapy with magnetic liposomal doxorubicin and a dipole external electromagnet. *Int. J. Cancer* **2004**, *109*, 627–635. [CrossRef]
136. Kubo, T.; Sugita, T.; Shimose, S.; Nitta, Y.; Ikuta, Y.; Murakami, T. Targeted systemic chemotherapy using magnetic liposomes with incorporated adriamycin for osteosarcoma in hamsters. *Int. J. Oncol.* **2001**, *18*, 121–125. [CrossRef] [PubMed]
137. Babincová, M.; Altanerová, V.; Lampert, M.; Altaner, C.; Machová, E.; Srámka, M.; Babinec, P. Site-specific in vivo targeting of magnetoliposomes using externally applied magnetic field. *Z. Naturforsch. C J. Biosci.* **2000**, *55*, 278–281. [CrossRef]
138. Matsunaga, T.; Higashi, Y.; Tsujimura, N. Drug delivery by magnetoliposomes containing bacterial magnetic particles. *Cell Eng.* **1997**, *2*, 7–11.
139. Jain, S.; Mishra, V.; Singh, P.; Dubey, P.K.; Saraf, D.K.; Vyas, S.P. RGD-anchored magnetic liposomes for monocytes/neutrophils-mediated brain targeting. *Int. J. Pharm.* **2003**, *261*, 43–55. [CrossRef]
140. Smith, J.A.; Costales, A.B.; Jaffari, M.; Urbauer, D.L.; Frumovitz, M.; Kutac, C.K.; Tran, H.; Coleman, R.L. Is it equivalent? Evaluation of the clinical activity of single agent Lipodox® compared to single agent Doxil® in ovarian cancer treatment. *J. Oncol. Pharm. Pract.* **2016**, *22*, 599–604. [CrossRef]
141. Bekersky, I.; Fielding, R.M.; Dressler, D.E.; Lee, J.W.; Buell, D.N.; Walsh, T.J. Pharmacokinetics, excretion, and mass balance of liposomal amphotericin B (AmBisome) and amphotericin B deoxycholate in humans. *Antimicrob. Agents Chemother.* **2002**, *46*, 828–833. [CrossRef]
142. Charrois, G.J.R.; Allen, T.M. Drug release rate influences the pharmacokinetics, biodistribution, therapeutic activity, and toxicity of pegylated liposomal doxorubicin formulations in murine breast cancer. *Biochim. Biophys. Acta* **2004**, *1663*, 167–177. [CrossRef]
143. Boswell, G.W.; Buell, D.; Bekersky, I. AmBisome (liposomal amphotericin B): A comparative review. *J. Clin. Pharmacol.* **1998**, *38*, 583–592. [CrossRef]
144. Walsh, T.J.; Yeldandi, V.; McEvoy, M.; Gonzalez, C.; Chanock, S.; Freifeld, A.; Seibel, N.I.; Whitcomb, P.O.; Jarosinski, P.; Boswell, G.; et al. Safety, Tolerance, and Pharmacokinetics of a Small Unilamellar Liposomal Formulation of Amphotericin B (AmBisome) in Neutropenic Patients. *Antimicrob. Agents Chemother.* **1998**, *42*, 2391–2398. [CrossRef]
145. Paolo, D.D.; Ambrogio, C.; Pastorino, F.; Brignole, C.; Martinengo, C.; Carosio, R.; Loi, M.; Pagnan, G.; Emionite, L.; Cilli, M.; et al. Selective Therapeutic Targeting of the Anaplastic Lymphoma Kinase with Liposomal siRNA Induces Apoptosis and Inhibits Angiogenesis in Neuroblastoma. *Mol. Ther.* **2011**, *19*, 2201–2212. [CrossRef]
146. Cui, J.; Li, C.; Guo, W.; Li, Y.; Wang, C.; Zhang, L.; Zhang, L.; Hao, Y.; Wang, Y. Direct comparison of two pegylated liposomal doxorubicin formulations: Is AUC predictive for toxicity and efficacy? *J. Control. Release* **2007**, *118*, 204–215. [CrossRef]
147. Cheung, B.C.L.; Sun, T.H.T.; Leenhouts, J.M.; Cullis, P.R. Loading of doxorubicin into liposomes by forming Mn^{2+}-drug complexes. *Biochim. Biophys. Acta Biomembr.* **1998**, *1414*, 205–216. [CrossRef]
148. Szebeni, J.; Storm, G. Complement activation as a bioequivalence issue relevant to the development of generic liposomes and other nanoparticulate drugs. *Biochem. Biphys. Res. Commun.* **2015**, *468*, 490–497. [CrossRef]
149. Szebeni, J.; Fishbane, S.; Hedenus, M.; Howaldt, S.; Locatelli, F.; Patni, S.; Rampton, D.; Weiss, G.; Folkersen, J. Hypersensitivity to intravenous iron: Classification, terminology, mechanisms and management. *Br. J. Pharmacol.* **2015**, *172*, 5025–5036. [CrossRef]

150. Szebeni, J.; Muggia, F.; Barenholz, Y. Case Study: Complement Activation Related Hypersensitivity Reactions to PEGylated Liposomal Doxorubicin—Experimental and Clinical Evidence, Mechanisms and Approaches to Inhibition. In *Handbook of Immunological Properties of Engineered Nanomaterials*, 2nd ed.; Dobrovolskaia, M.A., McNeil, S.E., Eds.; World Scientific Publishing Co Pte Ltd.: Singapore, 2016; Volume 2, pp. 331–361.
151. Kelly, C.; Lawlor, C.; Burke, C.; Barlow, J.W.; Ramsey, J.M.; Jefferies, C.; Cryan, S. High-throughput methods for screening liposome-macrophage cell interaction. *J. Liposome Res.* **2015**, *25*, 211–221. [CrossRef] [PubMed]
152. Wientjes, M.G.; Yeung, B.Z.; Lu, Z.; Wientjes, M.G.; Au, J.L.S. Predicting diffusive transport of cationic liposomes in 3-dimensional tumor spheroids. *J. Control. Release* **2014**, *192*, 10–18. [CrossRef]

pharmaceuticals

MDPI

Review

Dermal Drug Delivery of Phytochemicals with Phenolic Structure via Lipid-Based Nanotechnologies

Viliana Gugleva *, Nadezhda Ivanova, Yoana Sotirova and Velichka Andonova

Department of Pharmaceutical Technologies, Faculty of Pharmacy, Medical University of Varna, 55 Marin Drinov Str., 9000 Varna, Bulgaria; nadejda.ivanova@mu-varna.bg (N.I.); Yoana.Sotirova@mu-varna.bg (Y.S.); Velichka.Andonova@mu-varna.bg (V.A.)

* Correspondence: viliana.gugleva@mu-varna.bg

Abstract: Phenolic compounds are a large, heterogeneous group of secondary metabolites found in various plants and herbal substances. From the perspective of dermatology, the most important benefits for human health are their pharmacological effects on oxidation processes, inflammation, vascular pathology, immune response, precancerous and oncological lesions or formations, and microbial growth. Because the nature of phenolic compounds is designed to fit the phytochemical needs of plants and not the biopharmaceutical requirements for a specific route of delivery (dermal or other), their utilization in cutaneous formulations sets challenges to drug development. These are encountered often due to insufficient water solubility, high molecular weight and low permeation and/or high reactivity (inherent for the set of representatives) and subsequent chemical/photochemical instability and ionizability. The inclusion of phenolic phytochemicals in lipid-based nanocarriers (such as nanoemulsions, liposomes and solid lipid nanoparticles) is so far recognized as a strategic physico-chemical approach to improve their in situ stability and introduction to the skin barriers, with a view to enhance bioavailability and therapeutic potency. This current review is focused on recent advances and achievements in this area.

Keywords: biologically active compounds; dermal drug delivery; liposomes; nanoemulsions; nanostructured lipid carriers; polyphenols; phytophenols; solid lipid nanoparticles; skin permeation

Citation: Gugleva, V.; Ivanova, N.; Sotirova, Y.; Andonova, V. Dermal Drug Delivery of Phytochemicals with Phenolic Structure via Lipid-Based Nanotechnologies. *Pharmaceuticals* **2021**, *14*, 837. https://doi.org/10.3390/ph14090837

Academic Editors: Ana Catarina Silva, João Nuno Moreira and José Manuel Sousa Lobo

Received: 30 July 2021
Accepted: 20 August 2021
Published: 24 August 2021

1. Introduction

Phenolics are a large group of secondary metabolites comprising one or more phenolic rings in their chemical composition [1]. The myriad structural variations determine an inherent diversity and heterogeneity in the group. The over 8000 identified representatives of herbal/vegetable origin differ in the number of phenolic rings and phenolic groups, the presence of other substitutes of the H-atom/s in the aromatic core, and the level of saturation/dehydration [2,3]. Subgroups are the simple phenols (phenolic acids, alcohols, and others), the flavonoids, anthraquinones, naphtoquinones, acetophenones, xanthones, stilbenes, tannins, phloroglucinols, and lignans [2,3]. Despite the structural variety, the majority of phenolics exhibit antioxidant, anti-inflammatory, and antimicrobial activity in vivo [4–6], to which they principally owe their therapeutical potential in the treatment of series of health disorders [7]. Furthermore, such a pharmacological profile justifies the increasing interest in the utilization of phenolic compounds in cosmetics for esthetic purposes (antiaging, antihyperpigmentation products, and others) [8–11]. From the clinical perspective of dermatology, the local or systemic application of phenolic compounds may contribute to the cure or prevention of many skin diseases. Among them are cancerous or precancerous conditions, acne vulgaris, allergies, rosacea, atopic dermatitis, psoriasis, vitiligo, wounds, and many more [12]. Widely explored members of the phytophenolics group in the therapy of dermatological problems include caffeic, ferulic, chlorogenic, coumaric and gallic acids, resveratrol, catechins, quercetin, rutin, kaempferol, curcumin, luteolin, hypericin, hyperforin [2,13–16]. Many other potent representatives, as well as herbal extracts rich in phenolic content, have fallen under the therapeutic focus of skin diseases/disorders. However, the main setbacks to the dermal delivery of phenolic compounds appear to be their chemical instability and potential discrepancy with the biopharmaceutical requirements for this route of application [17,18]. Dermal drug transport is dictated, to a large extent, by the physico-chemical particularities of the active ingredients. Extreme polarity or strict hydrophobicity, high molecular mass, the presence of ionizable functional groups and their dissociation at the physiological/pathophysiological pH of the skin layers are all prerequisites for limited cutaneous permeation of the drug [19,20]. Since one or more of them are intrinsic for the majority of phenolic compounds, they do not always represent the best candidates for dermal transport [21,22]. Another limitation is often set by insufficient chemical stability of particular representatives [23,24] (e.g., resveratrol [25–27], hypericin [28,29], hyperforin [30–32], quercetin [33–35], cathehin [36–38]), for which precise control over the selection of dermal vehicles and technological operations for drug introduction in preformulation stage is required. It is worth mentioning that physico-chemical properties, skin permeation, and chemical stability of phenolics are strongly affected by the presence of the glycoside part attached to the aglycone, and its type [39,40]. Most often, but not always, the phenolic aglycons are preferred for dermal delivery as a result of their higher permeability coefficient and skin deposition, unless pharmacological/toxicological reasons or stability considerations direct the choice of researchers in favor of a glycoside form [21,41–43].

The inclusion of active pharmaceutical ingredients in drug delivery systems is the contemporary approach to overcome problems such as poor solubility, stability, and permeation [44–46]. Indisputably, lipid-based nanoparticles are among the most attractive drug carriers in the field of dermal and transdermal drug delivery [47,48]. This is in compliance with their structural similarity to skin barriers and compatibility with the majority of dermal bases. The nanotechnologies in question are based on the physico-chemical interaction between liquid, soft or hard lipids (phospholipids, mono, di or triglycerides, fatty acids or alcohols, waxes, cholesterol) and surfactants, in the presence or not of other excipients under different type of processing [49]. Depending on the nature of the lipids, the experimental conditions, and the ingredients ratio, nanosized aggregates may occur with different morphology, from liquid core-elastic wall vesicles (liposomes, niosomes, ethosomes) to thermodynamically stable liquid-in-liquid systems (nanoemulsions) or variously structured solid or soft particles (solid lipid nanoparticles or other types of nanostructured lipid carriers). However, all of the above-mentioned lipid-based nanocarriers possess some universal features, such as the ability to modify drug release, encapsulate efficiently hydrophobic molecules (and some hydrophilic ones, as well), improve drug solubility and permeation, and increase drug stability by providing a protective microenvironment [47–49]. As the lipid-based nanotechnologies often involve steps in preparation at higher temperatures and/or sonication [50], the chemical stability of the active compounds under such conditions should be investigated and considered. This is highly relevant, although not widely discussed for the phenolic compounds and their introduction to lipid-based nanostructures.

2. Phenolic Compounds

The term 'phenolics' relates to all biologically active compounds having at least one phenolic ring in their structure. Being a major class of secondary metabolites with a vital role in growth regulation, defense, and signaling, they are widely distributed among the plant kingdom [51,52]. Phenolic compounds originate from the shikimic and acetic acid biosynthetic pathways. Besides being united by a common genesis, and, therefore, elements in the structure [53], the representatives of this group share similarities in their pharmacological activity, mechanism of action, and therapeutic effects. An essential quality of phenolics is the reduction of oxidative stress in vivo [4,5] by scavenging reactive oxygen and nitrogen species (ROS, RNS) and free radicals, inhibition of key enzymes (xanthine oxidase, lipoxygenases, cyclooxygenases, monoamine oxidase, nicotinamide adenine dinucleotide phosphate oxidase and other), suppressing ROS/RNS generation, activating natural antioxidant systems (as superoxide dismutase, catalase, glutathione peroxidase [13,54]) and chelating metal ions (well-known to act as catalysts of oxidation processes [55]) [13,56,57]. The antioxidant ability of phenolics is determined, in the utmost, by the presence of electron-donating phenolic group/s, whereas the electron-donation process is highly dependent on the electron-density distribution in the aromatic core and thus the nature of the other substitutes in the structure [58,59]. Phenolic compounds are known to build stable radicals after neutralizing reactive species and free radicals, and terminate the oxidative chain reactions by interaction with one another [60]. Since oxidative stress is a fundamental element in the genesis of inflammatory, allergic, oncogenic, and atherogenic pathologies [61–64], the emphatic antioxidant properties of phenolics are the underlying prerequisite for their numerous health benefits in humans. It is known that many molecular mechanisms other than antioxidant activity are involved and contribute to the anticancer, anti-inflammatory, antiallergic, immunomodulatory, antimicrobial, antiaging/regenerative, antiatherogenic, and vasoprotective potency of phenolics. However, they are particularly related to the individual structures, the presence, and the type of glycoside parts, which we discuss below by groups and members. More importantly, the mechanisms of action of phenolics suit the functional and structural deficiencies related to many skin diseases and conditions, wherefore they are widely investigated and applied in the field of dermatology.

3. Fields of Application of Phenolic Compounds in Dermatology

The prevalence of skin diseases has substantially increased in recent years (by almost 50% for the past three decades) [65,66]. Today, they represent the fourth most common cause of all human diseases and affect approximately one-third of the world population [67]. The need exists for new therapeutic alternatives to be sought, as the treatment of the most frequently encountered skin disorders often includes the local or systemic use of steroids and antibiotics, both known to exhibit explicit side effects and long-term health risks [68–71].

The majority of most common dermatological diseases are associated with oxidative stress (ROS/RNS generation) and activation of the immune-inflammatory cascade [61,62,72]; such diseases are referred as inflammatory skin diseases [73,74]. These include atopic dermatitis (eczema), acne vulgaris, psoriasis, allergic contact dermatitis, urticaria (hives), seborrheic dermatitis, lupus erythematosus [75,76], alopecia areata [77], rosacea [78], vitiligo [79], skin malignancies (for whose pathogenesis inflammation is a key mechanism) [80,81] and others. In this regard, the phenolics' antioxidant activity makes them suitable therapeutic agents for the local treatment of these pathologies. Furthermore, reduction of oxidative stress in the skin tissues is also important in the name of prevention against UV-radiation-mediated aging, loss of natural antioxidant capacity, DNA damage, and initialization of carcinogenesis. The most promising protective agencies, in this regard, are representatives of the anthocyanins and catechins (flavan-3-ols) [82,83], which, indeed, are among the strongest antioxidants in the flavonoid class [58]. Other molecular mechanisms of action, unrelated or indirectly related to antioxidant activity, are also established for the set of representatives, and they extend further the phytophenolics' therapeutic field. The most important of such effects, with relevance to skin diseases and dermal drug delivery, are described below.

3.1. Interaction with Bacterial Cell Walls, Cell Membranes, and Synergism with Antibiotics

The ability of some phenolic compounds to interact with bacterial cell walls and cell membranes is fundamental to their antibacterial activity [84]. In several studies, phenolic compounds (epigallocatechin gallate, epicatechin gallate, gallic and caffeic acids) have been demonstrated to interfere with bacterial cell wall integrity, causing damage in its structure and leakage of cellular constituents [85–87]. The interaction is attributed to a bonding of the active phenolic molecules with the peptidoglycan layer through hydrogen and/or covalent bonds (for Gram-positive bacteria) and/or the lipopolysaccharides (for Gram-negative bacteria) [84,85]. Furthermore, inhibitory actions on the penicillinase enzyme and the efflux pump are found to contribute to a decrease in antibiotic resistance and synergistic antibacterial activity of phenolics with antibiotics [88–91]. Much more of the phenolic group representatives are proven to owe their antibacterial potency to alteration of bacterial cell membrane permeability, fluidity, ion transport, and respiration [82]. Rigidification or fluidization may be observed depending on the chemical structure of the phenolic molecule (polarity, molecular mass, and conformation) and its positioning among the lipid bilayer [92,93]. For example, the flavonoids kaempferol, chrysin, quercetin, baicalein, luteolin, epigallocatechin gallate, gallocatechin, theaflavin, and theaflavin gallate, when in contact with the bacterial cell membrane, decrease its fluidity, while the isoflavonoids puerarin, ononin, daidzein, genistein, and the stilbene resveratrol have shown the opposite effect [90,91]. Destabilitization of the bacterial cell membranes could also result from phenolics stepping into reaction with enzymes responsible for cell membrane stability and integrity [68,94]. In addition, some phenolic acids (caffeic and gallic acids) acidify the bacterial membrane, leading to its disruption and changes in permeability and ion transport [95]. Membrane damage and subsequent potassium loss from the bacterial intercellular space are also reported for galangin [96], a flavonoid (flavanol) found in propolis, to which the antibacterial properties of the latter could be partially attributed [97].

3.2. Interaction with Microbial DNA/RNA Polymerases and Topoisomerases, Proteases, Transcriptases, Surface Proteins (Adhesins), and Other Virulence Factors

In general, the biologically active aglycons of phenolic compounds possess a structure rich in reactive functional groups, multiple phenolic groups, carbonyl groups (e.g., xanthones, anthraquinones, most flavonoids), free or esterified carboxylic groups (phenolic acids), among others. They easily step into hydrogen bonding with other biomolecules (nucleotides, proteins, including adhesins and receptors, enzymes as DNA/RNA polymerases and topoisomerases, transcriptases, proteases, and many others) [94,98,99] or complexation with metal ions (iron ions) [100] that are essential for the infectious cycle of pathogenic bacteria and viruses (adhesion, entry, replication and spread) [84,101]. This is a wide-ranging and nonspecific complex of potential interactions of phenolics that has led many researchers to understand their antiviral and antibacterial properties. Examples relevant to skin infections to support this theory include curcumin (diferuloylmethane), which exerts its antiviral activity against human herpesvirus -1 (and other DNA viruses) by blocking the histone-acetyltransferase activity of specific transcriptional coactivator proteins (p300 and the CREB-binding proteins) [102,103]. Curcumin, again, is also found to inhibit the adhesins-mediated adsorption and replication of human herpesvirus 1 and 2 [104,105]. Epigallocatechin gallate, which was previously mentioned to possess a destructive effect on bacterial cell walls, exhibits its antibacterial action against methicillin-resistant Staphylococcus aureus also by inhibiting multiple staphylococcal virulence factors [6,90]. Quercetin, kaempferol and other flavonoids inhibit staphylococcal topoisomerases [106–108].

Today, the antibacterial, antiviral, and antifungal activity of phenolic compounds is considered a fact after being a subject of study for decades [109,110]. They have shown activity against the most frequent causative agents of skin infections, such as bacteria of the genera Staphylococcus, Pseudomonas, Enterococcus, the Herpes virus 1 and 2, the dermatophytes genera Trichophyton, Epidermophyton, and Microsporum [2,95,111]. Therefore, their topical use is highly beneficial for the purposes of infectious skin diseases' healing (dermatophytosis, impetigo, herpes infections, infected wounds, and others). Special attention is dedicated to dermal products containing phenolic compounds in cases of antibiotic-resistant infections, which have become more and more commonly encountered problem [2,112]. However, the exact mechanism of antimicrobial activity of a given phenolic compound is not always thoroughly investigated and fully understood. Even so, the significance of many other phenolic representatives as antimicrobial agents, beyond the list of examples given above, needs to be acknowledged. Among them are the main active compounds in Hypericum perfuratum preparations: hypericin, pseudohypericin and hyperforin [113–116], resveratrol [117,118], vitexin and isovitexin [119], hesperidin [120,121], and eugenol [122].

3.3. Effects on Skin Renewal, Proliferation, Collagen, and Elastin Synthesis

Indisputably, the regenerative properties of the phenolic compounds are among their strengths and justify the role of this phytochemical group in the therapy of wounds, incised or chronic, burns, infected wounds, etc. (for which, of course, the antimicrobial properties also contribute) [123–126]. Skin regeneration is a complex process that involves a vascular response (hemostasis and coagulation), cellular response (inflammation), proliferation phase (re-epithelialization), neovascularization (angiogenesis), granulation tissue formation, and remodeling (strengthening by conversion of collagen type III to type I) [127]. The reduction of oxidative stress in the early stages of injury may facilitate physiological responses (swelling, redness, pain) because of the direct relationship of reactive species and free radicals with the inflammatory mediators' secretion [128] (vasoactive amines and proteins, cytokines, prostaglandins [128,129]). The late phases of wound healing are based primarily on the proliferation and migration of fibroblasts, keratinocytes, and endothelial cells, and the activation of collagen and fibronectin synthesis [130]. The signaling pathways responsible for these processes also include cytokines and growth factors release from epithelial and nonepithelial cells, and are dependent on oxidative balance and supported by antioxidant-acting molecules. It is clear now that many phenolic antioxidants favor skin regeneration and renewal by reducing inflammation, inhibiting matrix metalloproteases, collagenases, elastases, increasing the expression of endothelial growth factor and the transforming growth factor, and thereby promote re-epithelization, angiogenesis, maturation, and thus tissue regeneration. Such activity is also highly desirable in the fight against age-related changes of the skin [131] (wrinkles appearance, loss of elasticity, thinning). Examples of phenolic compounds or herbal preparations that have been demonstrated to exert these mechanisms in vitro and/or in vivo are luteolin [132], epigallocatechin gallate and extracts rich in it, and other tannins [133,134], crude grape pomace and its main constituent gallic acid [135], lignans in seedcake extract [126], other phenolic-rich content extracts from the cacao pod [136], Phyllanthus emblica, Manilkara zapota [137], Clausena excavate [138], Sphaeranthus amaranthoides [139], Meum athamanticum, Centella asiatica, Aegopodium podagraria [140] and many more. Despite the undeniable role of the antioxidant properties of phenolics for skin regeneration, other supplementary mechanisms are found to be involved in the healing/protective processes. For instance, several genes involved in skin renewal (Kruppel-like factor 10, E2F-4 transcription factor, and epidermal growth response factor) have been up-regulated in human dermal fibroblast cell cultures when treated with Populous nigra preparations (rich in caffeic, p-coumaric, cinnamic, isoferulic acids, pinocembrin, salicin, and other phenolic compounds) [141]. Similar modulatory effects on gene transcription have been established for ellagitannins from oak wood, caffeoyl- derivatives from mate leaf, and phenolic acids from benzoin resin [142].

3.4. Effects on Melanin Synthesis

Melanin is a term referring to a complex of natural pigments with a crucial role in skin coloring and photoprotection. It is deposed in the keratinocytes after migration from the melanocytes cells, where it is produced from tyrosine through multiple oxidation reactions catalyzed by the enzyme tyrosinase [143–145]. Many phenolic compounds have shown competitive inhibitory activity on tyrosinase due to a structural resemblance with its initial substrate tyrosine, and chelation of the copper ions present at the binding sites of the enzyme [10,146,147]. In this regard, phenolics have found their application as tyrosinase inhibitors in the treatment of hyperpigmentation skin disorders [10]. Furthermore, melanogenesis suppression is considered to be one of several mechanisms of the phenolics' anticancer activity in the therapy of melanoma-type skin tumors [2,148,149]. Among the strongest tyrosinase inhibitors from the phytophenolic group are isoliquiritigenin [150] (chalcone structure), galangin [151], kaempferol [152], luteolin [153], apigenin [153], resveratrol [154], isoeugenol [155], p-coumaric, caffeic and rosmarinic acid [156,157]. With respect to antimelanogenic activity, glycoside forms of some phenolic compounds have shown higher efficacy due to increased tyrosinase inhibitory capacity [158,159], and/or lower toxicity [160]. It should be noted that significant cytotoxicity on melanocytes and risk of leucodermia (induced vitiligo), ochronosis (diffuse skin bluish-black discoloration), and carcinogenesis are inherent for many skin-lightening substances, including those of the natural phenolics class [145,161,162]. The very potent whitening agent hydroquinone, for instance, has fallen into the list of forbidden substances in cosmetics as a result of confirmed relation between its topical use and the above-mentioned adverse reactions [160,163]. In general, the contemporary research in this area is focused on seeking synthetic or semisynthetic phenolic molecules that will inherit the natural compounds' high depigmentation activity with less toxicity and higher stability [10,164].

Paradoxically, in some cases, the application of phenolic compounds has shown beneficial effects in the therapy of vitiligo [165], an autoimmune-determined disturbance in melanogenesis manifesting itself as white patches on the skin [166]. Such cases occur when (1) phenolics are used as whitening agents in order simulate merging of the white vitiligo spots and lead to total whitening (depigmentation therapy; synthetic or semisynthetic phenolics), or (2) antioxidants protect the melanocytes and keratinocytes [167] (mostly natural or semisynthetic phenolics). Oxidative stress is considered one of the main inducers of auto-reactive T-cells against the epidermal melanocytes and the destruction of the latter [166]. Therefore, in terms of an ongoing oxidative stress-related autoimmune response against the melanocytes, phenolic compounds may exhibit a protective action toward melanogenesis [166,168] (e.g., curcumin and its metabolite tetrahydrocurcumin [169], quercetin [170,171], the green tea polyphenols, epicatechin, epicatechin-3-gallate, and epigallocatechin [170]).

3.5. Photosensitization

Photosensitization may occur due to a phototoxic reaction (an acute light-induced tissue response to a photoreactive chemical) or photoallergy (an immunologically mediated response to a chemical, initiated by the formation of photoproducts following a photochemical reaction). It is a concern for compounds that possess high molar absorptivity (>1000 L $mol^{-1}\cdot cm^{-1}$) at each wavelength within the range of natural sunlight (from 290 to 700 nm), generate reactive species after absorption of light, and distribute/accumulate in the skin [172]. Such properties among the phytophenolic group are characteristic for anthracene derivatives [173] (anthraquinones—aloin A, aloe-emodin, hypericin), lignans (in the composition of silymarin), and curcumin, and some of its derivatives [174]. They may cause photosensitization (sunburn-like symptomatic such as skin irritation, erythema, pruritis, edema [175]) after systemic, as well as dermal administration [172].

3.6. Antitumor Activity of Phenolics

Skin cancers, being the most serious group of skin diseases (incl. basal cell carcinoma, squamous cell carcinoma, malignant melanoma) [2], are among the most tempting research areas for scientists to explore the potency of alternative treatment options, and the therapeutic application of a promising group such as phenolic compounds makes no exception. The anticancer activity of phenolics is primarily due to their antioxidant properties and high reactivity (hydrogen and/or covalent bonding with essential biomolecules), whereas one or both of which lead to additional mechanisms determining their complex action and high efficiency. In particular, phenolic compounds are proven to interfere with the cancer cell life cycle by inducing caspases activity and apoptosis of cancer cells (curcumin [176–178], luteolin [179], vitexin [180], epicatechin gallate [177,181], gallic acid [182], eugenol [183]) and regulation of gene expression in cancer cells (for example, *eugenol* is found to induce down-regulation of c-Myc, H-ras and Bcl2 expression and up-regulation of p53); to inhibit epidermal growth factor-induced neoplastic transformations in cell lines (caffeic acid [184]); to inhibit tyrosinase and melanogenesis (a mechanism relevant to melanoma type of skin cancer; examples are given in a previous section); to inhibit the proteasome; an enzyme complex responsible for the degradation of essential proteins involved in cell development, and lead to subsequent suppression of cancer cell growth and spread (catechin-3-gallate and epigallocatechin gallate [185], gallic acid [186], apigenin [187], quercetin [187], curcumin [188]), and to destabilize lysosomal membrane through permeabilization and cause cancer cell death (pterostilbene, a dimethoxylated analog of resveratrol [189]). These examples are only a few concrete representatives chosen for subjects of specific investigation, whereas the whole complex of proposed mechanisms of action is potentially valid for a much larger sample of natural and modified phenolic compounds.

3.7. Phenolics as Pro-Oxidants

Amongst the abundance of scientific reports regarding the mechanisms of action of phenolic compounds (including those mentioned in this review), it is not hard to follow an apparent controversy. For example, some phenolic compounds are found to promote injured skin regeneration by inducing the epidermal growth factor and transforming growth factor, whereas the same or similar compounds are shown in different studies to suppress epithelial cancer cell development and spread due to opposing effects on growth regulation factors [190,191]. There is a theory based on the concept of a switch between anti-and pro-oxidant properties of phenolics as a function of microenvironmental factors. A decrease in antioxidant properties and switch to pro-oxidant activity of phenolic compounds is observed under conditions of decreased pH (intrinsic for cancer cell lines) and upon complexation in the presence of transition metals (Cu, Fe: $Cu^{2+} \rightarrow Cu^{+}$, $Fe^{3+} \rightarrow Fe^{2+}$; extracted from the herbal drugs, for example), which indeed stabilizes the phenoxyl radicals and enhances the production of reactive species [192]. Formation of metal-phenolic networks is more likely for 3-hydroxy-, 4-carbonyl flavonoids (flavonols—e.g., quercetin, kaempferol, galangin, morin, myricetin) [193]. The environment-determined switch to pro-oxidant properties is a matter of potential toxicity and is among the possible explanations for anticancer activity [194].

4. Dermal Drug Delivery of Phenolic Compounds

Despite the countless proofs for the multidirectional therapeutic potential of phenolic compounds in dermatology, a few simple facts must be acknowledged. (1) In order for them to exert their molecular mechanisms on targeted structures, they must reach the latter and accumulate in sufficient concentrations. (2) They must possess sufficient stability during storage and until deposition in the relevant skin layer, and hence be included in proper dosage forms by suitable technological operations with the aid or not of drug-delivery vehicles. (3) Additional factors, such as potential toxicity under certain conditions, should be considered.

4.1. Biopharmaceutical Considerations of the Dermal Drug Delivery

Absorption is not a primary physiological function of the skin; on the contrary, the epidermal layer, in particular, is an effective barrier for the intrusion of foreign matter (including potentially hazardous matter). Therefore, dermal drug delivery is challenging and sets numerous requirements for the chosen therapeutic agents and dermal bases/vehicles. The skin possesses a complex structure of multiple layers with different morphology and function, starting with the corneum, the outermost nonviable, keratinized epidermal stratum responsible for the limited permeability of the epidermis. Molecules can pervade in it either by paracellular transport (through the lipid matrix; preferable route for mostly lipophilic compounds, $\log P \geq 2$) or via the transcellular route (through the corneocytes, the constructive type of cells in stratum corneum, often compared with bricks walled up in the "mortar" of lipid milieu; alternative transportation for more hydrophilic molecules). At this stage of entry (referred as penetration), it is evident that lipophilic properties of the applied therapeutic agent are preferable. However, further transportation of the substrates to the viable epidermis and the derma (permeation), and/or their percutaneous absorption, requires sufficient water solubility (~0.5–1.0 mg/mL) otherwise, they are retained in the congenial surrounding of stratum corneum and not be able to overcome the amphiphilic nature of the underlying cutaneous stratums. Other possible, but rather supplementary mechanisms of drug permeation through the skin, are the transfollicular transport or passage across the sweat glands [195,196]. The pathophysiology of the most common skin diseases (impartially reviewed in the previous sections) suggests that the therapeutic targets for phenolic compounds are settled either in the viable epidermis or the derma, rarely in the hypodermis (e.g., keratinocytes, melanocytes, immune cells, mast cells, endothelium, hair follicles, etc.). Therefore, permeation is essential for a practical manifestation of their activity. Besides, a balanced hydrophilic-lipophilic profile (and a respective suitable partition coefficient, ideally in the range of log P 2–3 [197,198]) is only one of the desired qualities for successful skin permeation. Further limitations are set by the molecular weight (<500 Da, but often a lower limit is set with respect to the other molecular particularities of the active compound) and the potential for ionization [199].

4.2. Physico-Chemical Properties of Some Common Phenolic Compounds and Their Glycosides

The separate classes of phenolic compounds differ substantially in their physico-chemical properties and skin permeation. The simple phenols, including phenolic acids, for example, are characterized by lower molecular weight and higher water solubility compared to the majority of other phenolics [200] (Table 1). A limitation for their cutaneous permeation is the presence of multiple ionizable groups (alcohol and carboxyl groups). The flavonoid aglycons (e.g., quercetin, kaemferol, luteolin, apigenin) are distinguished with extreme hydrophobicity, with the exception of the class of catechins that cross the water solubility barrier of >1 mg/mL (needed for effective skin permeation). The same undesirable practical insolubility in water is also inherent for the majority of other polyphenols (xanthones, anthraquinones, stilbenes, lignans, tannins, phloroglucinols). Glycosylation, as a biosynthetically occurring metabolic process, leads to the formation of more hydrophilic derivatives. However, the water solubility improvement of the phenolics' glycoside forms is sometimes insufficient (e.g., apigenin→vitexin, hesperetin→hesperidin, Table 1). In general, many approaches involving chemical modification of the phenolic compounds (sulfonation, phosphorylation, complexation, incl. with metal ions, biomacromolecules or cyclodextrins [99,201–203]) are studied for their potential to obtain analogs or prodrugs with increased water solubility and bioavailability. On the other hand, the "blocking" of reactive groups by etherification, esterification, and other processes, is a well-known approach to improve skin permeation due to reduced ionizability [204], whereas such operations, depending on the substrates' nature, may lead to an increase or a decrease in water solubility [205]. Examples could be given for caffeic acid and chlorogenic acid, where the latter, being an ester of the former with quinic acid, despite its higher molecular mass has better skin permeation [206]. A few methoxylated quercetin derivatives were shown to possess increased skin permeation compared to the native quercetin by Lin et al. [40]. The same authors reported even better dermal penetration of rutin (quercetin-3-*O*-rutinoside; Mw 610.52) compared to quercetin (Mw 302.24), due to higher hydrophilicity, although these results contradict other research findings [207].

Table 1. Physico-chemical characteristics of selected phenolic compounds.

Phenolic Class	Phenolic Subclass	Phenolic Compound	Molecular Weight (g/mol)	Partition Coefficient (Log P)	Solubility in Water at 25 °C (mg/mL)	Ionizable Groups with Corresponding pKa Values
Simple phenols and derivatives	Phenolic acids (hydroxybenzoic acid derivatives)	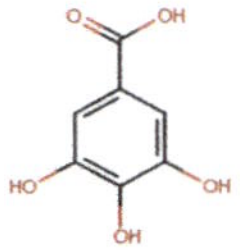 Gallic acid	170.12	−0.28 [208]	14.7 [209]	$pKa^1 = 4.51$ $pKa^2 = 8.7$ $pKa^3 = 11.4$ $pKa^4 > 13$ [210]
		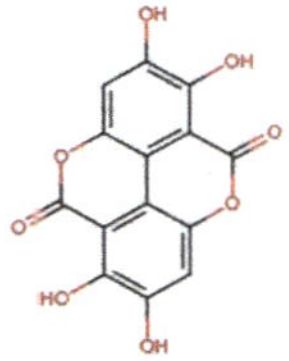 Ellagic acid (ellagitannin, dimer of gallic acid)	390.12	1.37 [211]	0.0097 [212,213] (at 37 °C)	$pKa^1 = 5.42$ $pKa^2 = 6.76$ [214]
	Phenolic acids (hydroxycinnamic acid derivatives)	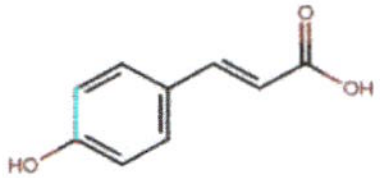 p-Coumaric acid	164.05	1.46 [215]	0.01 [216]	$pKa^1 = 4.92$ $pKa^2 = 9.28$ [217]
		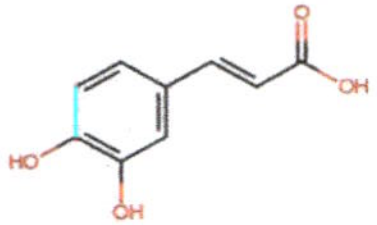 Caffeic acid	180.16	1.15 [218]	0.98 [209]	$pKa^1 = 4.83$ $pKa^2 = 8.90$ $pKa^3 = 10.28$ [217]

Table 1. *Cont.*

Phenolic Class	Phenolic Subclass	Phenolic Compound	Molecular Weight (g/mol)	Partition Coefficient (Log P)	Solubility in Water at 25 °C (mg/mL)	Ionizable Groups with Corresponding pKa Values
		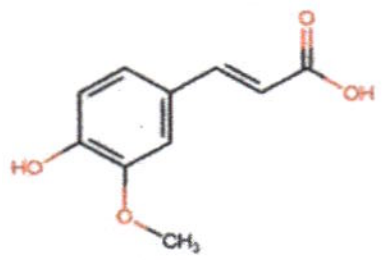 Ferulic acid	194.18	1.51 [219]	0.78 [209]	$pKa^1 = 4.66$ $pKa^2 = 9.09$ [217]
		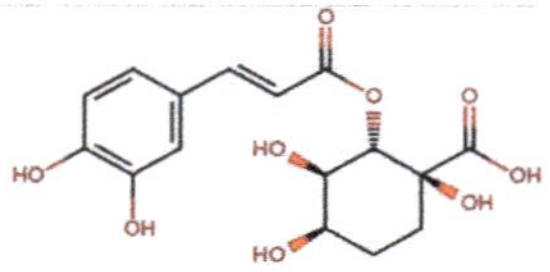 Chlorogenic acid	354.31	−0.75 [218]	3.44 * [220]	$pKa^1 = 3.50$ $pKa^2 = 8.42$ $pKa^3 = 11.00$ [221]
	Other simple phenols	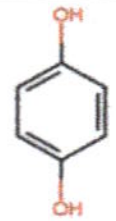 Hydroquinone	110.11	0.59 [222]	7.20 [223]	$pKa^1 = 9.85$ $pKa^2 = 11.40$ [224]
		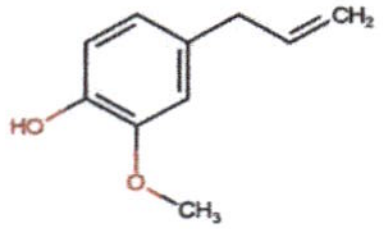 Eugenol	164.20	2.49 [225]	2.46 [226]	pKa = 10.19 [227]

Table 1. *Cont.*

Phenolic Class	Phenolic Subclass	Phenolic Compound	Molecular Weight (g/mol)	Partition Coefficient (Log P)	Solubility in Water at 25 °C (mg/mL)	Ionizable Groups with Corresponding pKa Values
Flavonoids	Flavones	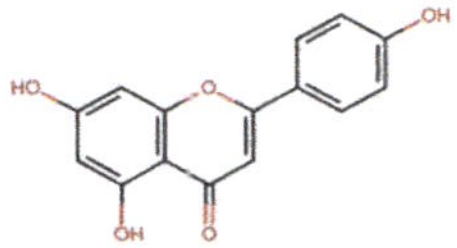 Apigenin	270.05	2.92 [228]	0.00135 [229]	$pKa^1 = 7.12$ $pKa^2 = 8.10$ [230]
		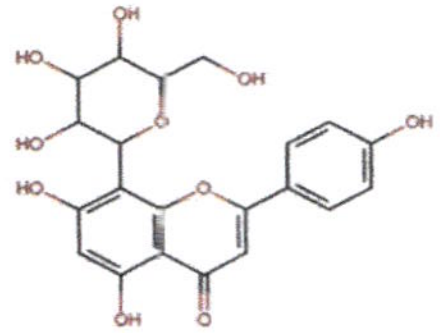 Vitexin (Apigenin-8-C-glucoside)	432.38	0.1 * [231]	0.0762 [232]	$pKa^1 = 6.27$ * [233] **
		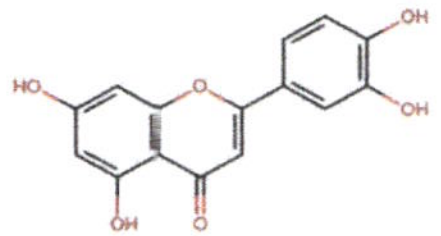 Luteolin	286.24	3.22 [228]	0.14 * [234]	$pKa^1 = 6.57$ * [234] **

Table 1. *Cont.*

Phenolic Class	Phenolic Subclass	Phenolic Compound	Molecular Weight (g/mol)	Partition Coefficient (Log P)	Solubility in Water at 25 °C (mg/mL)	Ionizable Groups with Corresponding pKa Values
	Flavonols	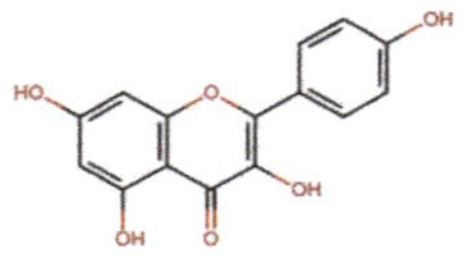 Kaemferol	286.23	3.11 [228]	0.113 [235] (at 30 °C)	$pKa^1 = 6.96$ $pKa^2 = 8.78$ $pKa^3 = 10.60$ [236]
		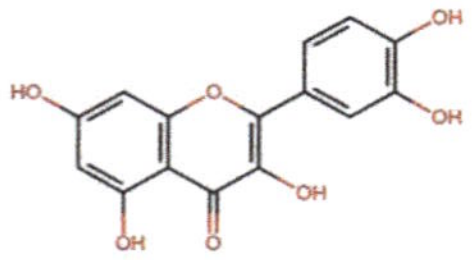 Quercetin	302.24	1.82 [228]	0.0004 [237] −0.002 [238]	$pKa^1 = 7.10$ $pKa^2 = 9.09$ $pKa^3 = 11.12$ [236]
		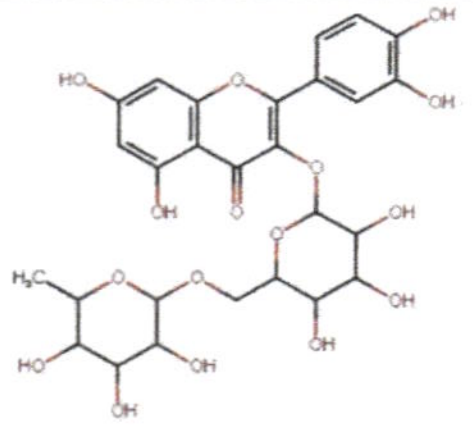 Rutin (Quercetin-3-O-rutinoside)	610.52	0.76 [22]	0.125 [239]	$pKa^1 = 2.92$ $pKa^2 = 6.72$ $pKa^3 = 8.26$ $pKa^4 = 12.57$ [240]

Table 1. *Cont.*

Phenolic Class	Phenolic Subclass	Phenolic Compound	Molecular Weight (g/mol)	Partition Coefficient (Log P)	Solubility in Water at 25 °C (mg/mL)	Ionizable Groups with Corresponding pKa Values
	Flavanones	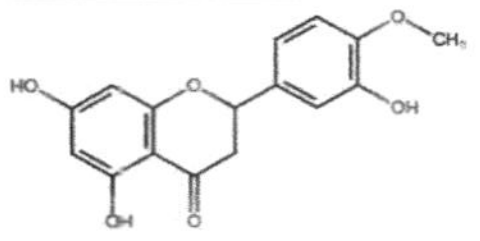 Hesperitin	302.27	2.9 [241]	0.01572 [241]	$pKa^1 = 7.55$ * $pKa^2 = 8.50$ * $pKa^3 = 9.65$ *
		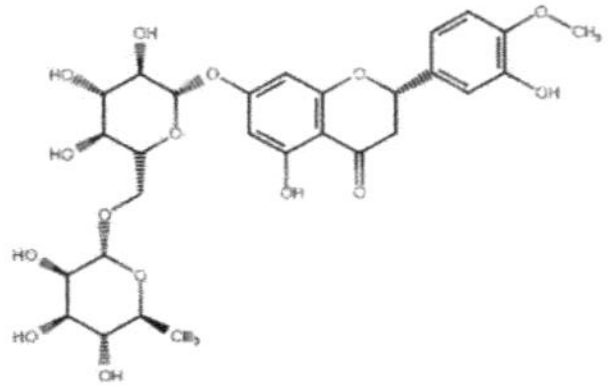 Hesperidin (Hesperitin-7-(6-*O*-(alpha-L-rhamnopyranosyl)-beta-D-glucopyranosyl)	610.19	1.78 [242]	0.00495 [242]	$pKa^1 = 10.0$ $pKa^2 > 11.5$ [243]
	Flavan-3-ols	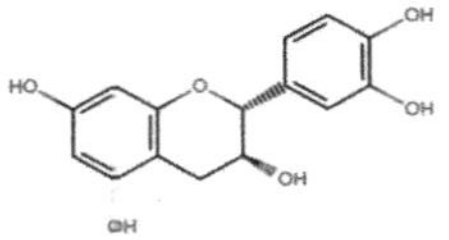 Catechin	290.26	0.41 [244]	7.66 [245]	$pKa^1 = 8.68$ $pKa^2 = 9.70$ $pKa^3 = 11.55$ [236]

Table 1. *Cont.*

Phenolic Class	Phenolic Subclass	Phenolic Compound	Molecular Weight (g/mol)	Partition Coefficient (Log P)	Solubility in Water at 25 °C (mg/mL)	Ionizable Groups with Corresponding pKa Values
		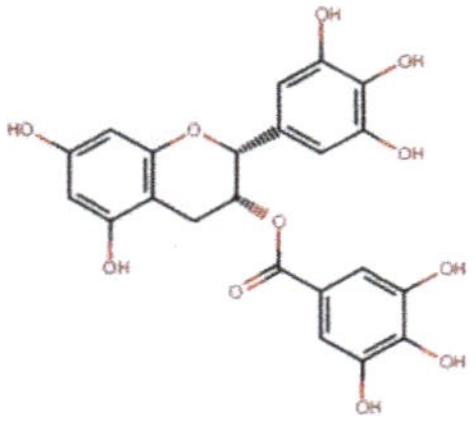 Epigallocatechin gallate	458.37	0.46 [246]	16.05 [247]	$pKa^1 = 7.75$ $pKa^2 = 8.00$ [248]
Curcuminoids		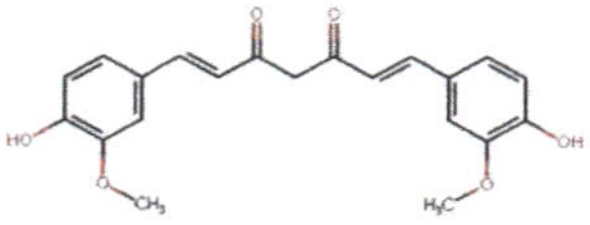 Curcumin (keto form)	368.38	3.0 [249]	0.0006 [250]	$pKa^1 = 7.7–8.5$ $pKa^2 = 8.5–10.4$ $pKa^3 = 9.5–10.7$ [249]
Stilbenes		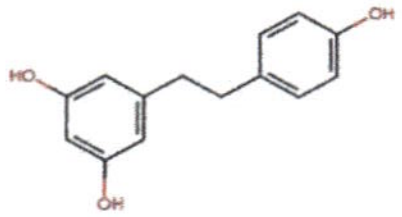 Resveratrol	228.25	3.09 * [251]	0.05 [252]	$pKa^1 = 8.8$ $pKa^2 = 9.8$ $pKa^3 = 11.4$ [253]
Anthraquinones		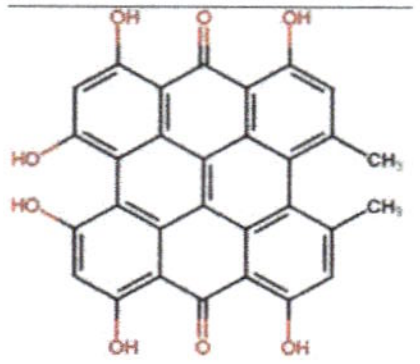 Hypericin	504.44	3.43 [254]	Practically insoluble in water [255] **	$pKa^1 = 2.00$ $pKa^2 = 11.00$ [256]

Table 1. *Cont.*

Phenolic Class	Phenolic Subclass	Phenolic Compound	Molecular Weight (g/mol)	Partition Coefficient (Log P)	Solubility in Water at 25 °C (mg/mL)	Ionizable Groups with Corresponding pKa Values
Phloroglucinols		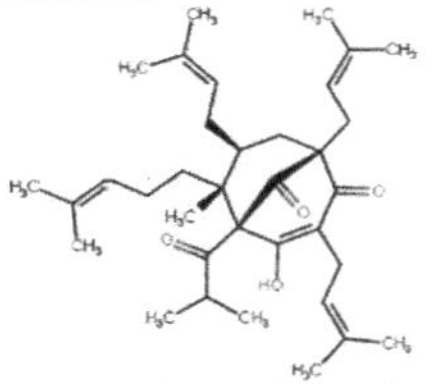 Hyperforin	536.78	13.17 [257]	2.34×10^{-12} [257]	pKa = 6.32 * [258]

* calculated value; ** information (or further information) was not found.

4.3. Stability of Phenolics

The chemical stability of phytophenolics is a priority concern since these highly reactive molecules take part in all types of degradation processes (incl. oxidation/autooxidation, hydrolysis, isomerization) and lose their therapeutical efficacy over time [34,259–261]. Furthermore, for the majority of chemically sensitive phenolics, light irradiation has been identified as a determining factor for decomposition process mechanisms and rates [259,262]. Therefore, many phenolic compounds are known to be susceptible to photodegradation (resveratrol [263], curcumin [264], hypericin [255], hyperforin [31], eugenol [265], quercetin [266], and many others) [267]. Furthermore, polymerization is another undesirable event for some simple phenols and polyphenols (catalyzed or not by oxidation processes) [259,268], which leads to substantial changes in their pharmacological activity, molecular mass, and skin permeation potential.

Considering this information, the choice of a dermal drug delivery vehicle (viz. the inclusion of permeation enhancers in the composition or the utilization of nanoparticulate delivery systems, the type of solvents, etc.) determines the penetration potential and stability of the chosen phenolic compound(s). Among the numerous investigated approaches with respect to improved skin permeation and stability (including chemical modification, prodrug development, complexation, solvent type optimization, inclusion of the therapeutic substrates in micro and nanosized carriers), the application of lipid-based nanotechnologies for the dermal delivery of phenolics has gained the most interest and practical significance. In favor of the lipid nanoparticulate systems are the ability to incorporate and stabilize sensitive molecules, "disguise" some of their unfavorable structural particularities for dermal transport, and the opportunity they provide for modified drug release. Another interesting aspect of dermal drug delivery of phytochemicals with a phenolic structure via lipid-based nanotechnologies is hidden in the fact that phenolic antioxidants inhibit lipid peroxidation in the corpus of these nanovehicles and provide longer endurance of the latter. Therefore, it can be stated that the relation between phenolic phytochemicals and lipid nanocarriers could, under some circumstances, be described as symbiotic.

5. Lipid-Based Nanotechnologies

Lipid-based nanosystems are the subject of great interest in dermal and transdermal drug delivery, as they provide a successful approach to overcome the limitations of conventional topical formulations, improving at the same time the characteristics of the loaded cargo (drugs and biologically active compounds), its skin permeation and consequently therapy efficacy [49]. The lipid nature of nanoscale drug delivery systems, such as solid lipid nanoparticles (SLNs), nanostructured lipid carriers (NLCs), liposomes, or nanoemulsions, ensures their excellent skin tolerability, biodegradability and, if necessary, allows their easily structural modification/optimization in the formulation process due to the great variety of lipid constituents. Furthermore, their salient characteristics, such as improved solubility, stability, and bioavailability of the incorporated active ingredients, as well the achieved controlled release profile, would be particularly beneficial for the inclusion of phytochemicals with phenolic structures, allowing them to fully deploy their favorable dermal effects [269]. In this regard, a summary of the specifics of the most commonly used lipid-based nanosystems, and their application as nanocarriers for encapsulation of phenolic compounds in dermal/transdermal delivery, is provided below.

5.1. Liposomes

Liposomes may be considered among the first lipid-based nanosystems. After their discovery in the 1960s by Bangham, they were initially proposed as a model for biological membranes due to their compositional similarity. However, later in the 1970s, thanks to their excellent biocompatibility properties and entrapment ability, they were studied as potential drug delivery platforms [270,271]. Structurally, liposomes are spherical vesicles consisting of one or more phospholipid bilayers surrounding an inner aqueous compartment [272,273]. The vesicular structure, resulting from the amphipathic properties of the bilayer forming lipids, provides the opportunity to encapsulate hydrophobic and hydrophilic molecules [274]. The origin of the phospholipids (from various natural or synthetic sources) and their chemical structure influence liposomal properties and membrane fluidity. In their study, Jacquot et al. [275] investigated the effect of marine (salmon) and plant (rapeseed) isolated phospholipids on membrane fluidity and the mechanical properties of liposomal bilayers compared to dioleylphosphatidylcholine and dipalmitoylphosphatidylcholine-based membranes as references. The authors reported that the membrane fluidity was influenced by the saturation of the fatty acid chains; the highest values were obtained in the membranes based on dioleylphosphatidylcholine (unsaturated acyl chains) and lowest in the bilayers formed from dipalmitoylphosphatidylcholine (saturated acyl chains). Regarding mechanical properties, phase segregation was reported for the rapeseed membranes, whereas the unsaturated salmon bilayer was characterized by a homogenous structure. The rigidity of the liposomal bilayer may be further increased by the inclusion of cholesterol, which can fill the cavities resulting from the loose packing of phospholipids, thus improving liposomal in vitro and in vivo stability [276,277]. Liposomal physicochemical parameters (size, surface charge), membrane characteristics, and interaction between the encapsulated active agent and liposomal constituents, influence the mechanism and extent of the drug delivery process [278,279]. The appropriate size of liposomes for topical application is below 300 nm to reach deeper skin layers. However, vesicles with a size below 70 nm are characterized with maximum deposition in the epidermis as well the dermis [280]. Several mechanisms are proposed to explain the active agent transfer from liposomes to the skin, such as vesicle fusion with lipids of stratum corneum as a result of their similar structure; a fluidizing effect, leading to impaired skin integrity; intact liposomal penetration into different dermal layers (associated with their flexibility; possible alterations in size and structure); improved drug delivery through hair follicles or sweat ducts facilitated by liposomal vesicular structure, and free active agent penetration after its release from liposomes (Figure 1) [271,281,282]. To evaluate the influence of zeta potential on transdermal delivery, Park et al. [283] investigated *resveratrol* permeation from conventional liposomes as well from vesicles coated with chitosan. According to the authors, higher resveratrol skin deposition was estimated from the chitosan-coated vesicles due to the repulsive electrostatic interaction between cationic chitosan vesicles and negatively charged epidermal lipids. The incorporation of phenolic compounds in liposomes, as well their interaction with phospholipids, has been studied by many researchers. In their study Malekar et al. [274] investigated the localization of five chemically diverse phenolic compounds (raloxifene, garcinol, quercetin, trans-resveratrol, bisphenol A) in dipalmitoylphosphatidylcholine-based liposomal bilayer and their influence on colloidal stability. As reported by the authors, the phenolic compounds, localized in the central regions of the bilayer (resveratrol and quercetin), negatively influenced liposomal colloidal stability due to decreased contact with phosphate head groups. Inversely, phytochemicals in the glycerol region of the acyl chains (raloxifene, garcinol, bisphenol A) contributed to better stability thanks to the enhanced exposure with phosphate head groups or electrostatic repulsion forces. Phan et al. [92] studied the interaction mechanism of two different classes of polyphenols (flavonoids and trans-stilbenes) with liposomal membranes. The flavonoids' gallate, galloyl, and hydroxyl groups are connected via hydrogen bonds with membrane lipids, leading to compact phospholipid assembly, reduced surface area, and forming a stiffer bilayer. The benzyl open ring structure of trans stilbenes, on the other site, determines its deeper intercalation into the hydrophobic bilayer, causing extension of the membrane area and enhancing its fluidity.

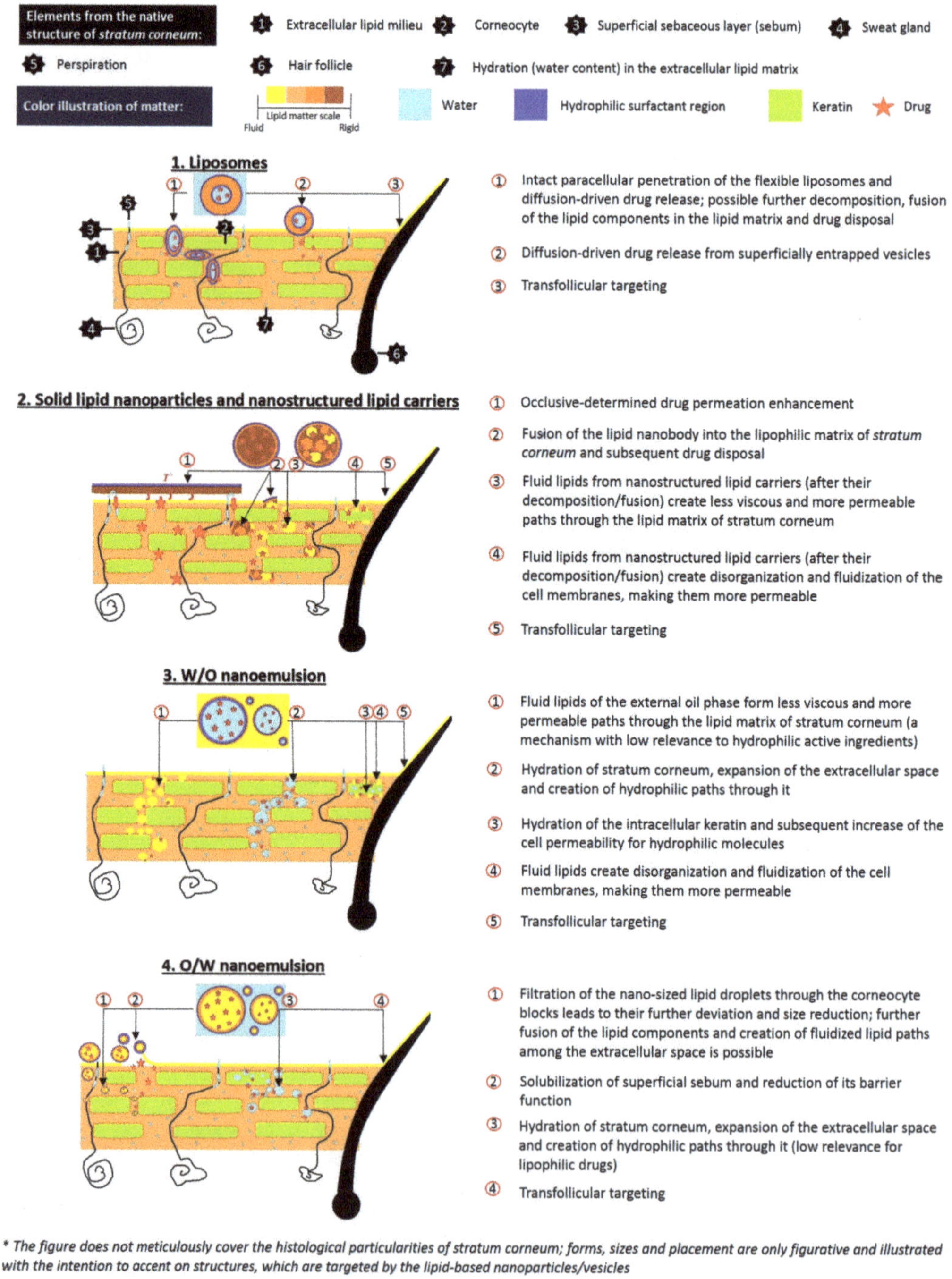

Figure 1. Possible mechanisms of drug permeation enhancement through *stratum corneum* by lipid-based nanoparticles/vesicles.

5.2. Solid Lipid Nanoparticles

Solid lipid nanoparticles, reported for the first time in the 1990s by Professor R.H. Müller and Professor M. Gasco, were proposed as an alternative approach to overcome the limitations associated with liposomes (e.g., phospholipid oxidation, costly materials, and production process, limited physical stability, difficulties in process scale-up) and polymeric nanoparticles (polymer toxic degradation process) [284,285]. As suggested by their name, SLNs are composed of individual or a mixture of lipids, solid at ambient and body temperature, dispersed in water or an aqueous phase containing surfactant [286]. Most commonly used lipids for SLNs preparation include triglycerides (trimyristin, tristearin), fatty acids (stearic, palmitic acid), waxes (beeswax, cetyl palmitate), and mono/di/triglycerides mixtures (glyceryl behenate—Compritol 888 ATO, glyceryl palmitostearate—Precirol ATO 5) [287]. Solid lipid nanoparticles can be suitable carriers for both hydrophobic and hydrophilic compounds. According to their structure and drug localization they can be classified as homogenous matrix models and core-shell models (drug-enriched shell and drug-enriched core) [288]. In the first case, the active agent is molecularly dispersed within the matrix or present as amorphous clusters. Homogenous matrix SLNs are obtained by cold or hot (when encapsulating highly lipophilic molecules) homogenization methods. In the second model, an outer shell containing the active agent surrounds a lipid core. The specific morphology of drug-enriched shell nanoparticles results from phase separation during the cooling phase; initially, the lipid in the center precipitates, shaping the inner, compound-free compartment. However, at the same time, drug concentration in the residual melted lipid increases and, after solidification, a drug-enriched shell is formed. In the third model SLNs, due to drug super-saturation in the lipid melt, a crystallization of the active agent is observed before the crystallization of the lipids, resulting in a drug-enriched core enclosed by a lipid (drug-free) shell [288–290]. The type of SLNs and their composition and physicochemical parameters affect their skin permeation. Due to the lipid nature of SLNs, as possible mechanisms of skin penetration (analogous to liposomes) the fusion of nanoparticles with lipids of stratum corneum, the lipid fluidizing properties of lipids, and transfollicular transfer are proposed. However, as a specific penetration mechanism, characteristic of SLNs may indicate their occlusive effect. Thanks to their large surface area and nanosized dimensions, they possess occlusive characteristics leading to improved skin hydration and enhanced penetration into dermal layers (Figure 1) [289,291]. In their study Kakkar et al. [292] used tetrahydrocurcumin-loaded SLNs characterized by sufficient occlusivity and anti-inflammatory effects. Their further incorporation in hydrogel formulation led to seventeen times higher skin permeation ability compared to plain tetrahydrocurcumin gel. Regarding their structure, suitable features for topical application include the drug-enriched shell nanoparticles, providing rapid drug release, which along with the occlusive effect is a favorable characteristic when increased drug penetration is necessary [288,293]. The disadvantages of SLNs, such as the tendency for drug expulsion or low drug loading capacity due to the ideal crystalline structure of the lipids, provide possibilities for further development, including the development of second-generation nanoparticles and structured lipid carriers (NLCs), which overcome the limitations mentioned above [284,294].

5.3. Nanostructured Lipid Carriers

Nanostructured lipid carriers are composed of solid and liquid lipids dispersed in the aqueous phase, stabilized by surfactants [295]. The inclusion of a liquid lipid in their composition disrupts the highly ordered crystalline structure characteristic of the SLNs. It leads to a less organized lipid matrix, providing space for more drug accumulation [296,297]. NLCs may be categorized into three types: imperfect crystal, amorphous and multiple types, by the lipid blending ratio and their method of preparation. Type I NLCs are prepared from lipids (predominantly solid, with small amount of oil phase), differing in their structure concerning chain length or saturation, leading to the formation of a disordered "imperfect" lipid matrix characterized by high encapsulation capacity. An amorphous structure, indicative of the second type of NLCs, is obtained by including specific lipids to the composition so the crystallization after cooling can be prevented. Consequently, leakage of the active agent also is minimized. The multiple model NLCs contain a significant amount of liquid oil phase in their composition, which facilitates a phase separation during the formulation process leading to nanosized liquid oil compartments among the solid lipid matrix. The solid matrix may be referred to as a barrier, providing a controlled release of the active agent, whereas the liquid lipids ensure better solubility of included lipophilic molecules and therefore determine higher drug encapsulation [284,293,298,299]. The effects of the included liquid lipid in the NLCs composition, as well as the selected oil phase on the encapsulation efficiency and antioxidant activity of the phenolic compound sesamol, was investigated by Puglia et al. [300]. The authors developed two different NLC formulations composed of the same solid lipid (Compritol®888 ATO) with varying liquid phases (Miglyol 812 or sesame oil), as well one model Compritol®888 ATO-based SLNs for reference. Sesamol encapsulation was higher in the NLCs formulations than the SLNs, with the highest entrapment efficiency values (>90%) and improved antioxidant activity for the formulation containing sesame oil as the liquid oil phase. The observed results may be attributed to the structural similarity between the active agent and selected oil phase, which determines the potent synergic effect. NLC composition also influences the occlusive effect and their dermal/transdermal delivery. In their study, Loo et al. [301] investigated the influence of lipid concentration (20% and 30%), solid lipid/oil ratio, and additives (lecithin, propylene glycol) on skin hydration and transepidermal water loss. According to the authors, NLCs with higher lipid content (30%), high solid lipid concentration (90%), and additives (slightly favorable outcomes in case of lecithin) were characterized with good occlusive properties and led to improved skin hydration and reduction of transepidermal water loss during the seven-day study period. Regarding particle size, another important factor determining the extent of skin permeation, both NLCs and SLNs may be prepared in the appropriate form for dermal application range (100–500 nm) via a high-pressure homogenization (hot and cold) method, which is also suitable for large scale production [289,298]. There is some controversial literature regarding the possibility of encapsulating temperature-sensitive compounds (such as some phenolic compounds) via the hot method. However, this technique is considered applicable due to the short heating time, except for highly temperature-sensitive, hydrophilic molecules, which might migrate to the aqueous phase during homogenization [288]. The mechanisms by which NLCs improve drug permeation through the skin are similar to those, discussed for SLNs (Figure 1).

5.4. Nanoemulsions

Nanoemulsions are isotropic colloidal dispersions composed of water and oil stabilized using surfactant/cosurfactant. One of the liquids is dispersed into nanosized droplets, usually between 20 and 200 nm [302]. The tiny droplet size causes their transparent/translucent appearance (analogical to microemulsions). However, differences between these two systems may result from the surfactant concentrations used (ca. 20% in microemulsions, vs. 3–10% in nanoemulsions), as well their dissimilar thermodynamic stability (nanoemulsions are thermodynamically unstable, while microemulsions are thermodynamically stable) [303,304]. Nanoemulsions are an attractive drug delivery system for topical application due to their miniature droplet size, homogenous size distribution, and large surface area, which ensure their uniform spreading onto the skin surface that facilitates drug penetration [305]. Similar to the other lipid-based nanosystems, an inverse relationship between the size of carriers and their transdermal penetration has been reported. According to Su et al. [306], who investigated transport through the skin of nanoemulsions loaded with environment-responsive and fluorescent dyes, formulations with droplets size of 80 nm can diffuse (but not penetrate) into the uncompromised epidermis and pass through canals of hair follicles, in contrast to larger (500 nm) sized formulations. The appropriate size of nanoemulsions is recommended to be below 50 nm to achieve an efficient transdermal delivery [307]. Other important factors affecting transdermal transportation of nanoemulsions are the formulation composition and type of emulsion (*w*/*o* or *o*/*w*). The oil phase of the systems may be composed of fatty acids (e.g., oleic acid), esters of fatty acids and alcohols oils (isopropyl myristate/GRAS certified), triglycerides (triacetin/GRAS certified), as well nonpolar essential oils or lipid-soluble vitamins, among others [304,308]. Liu et al. [309] investigated the influence of different oil phases (eutectic mixture of menthol and camphor or isopropyl myristate) on transdermal delivery of glabridin-loaded nanoemulsions. According to the performed skin permeation studies, the formulation composed of binary eutectic mixture led to three times higher skin permeation of glabridin (compared to isopropyl myristate nanoemulsion), which was seven times higher than the isoflavane solution. Depending on the type of nanoemulsion, different permeation mechanisms were discussed. In the case of encapsulation of hydrophilic molecules in *w*/*o* nanoemulsions, transdermal transportation may be facilitated as a result of the solubilizing properties of the included surfactants on stratum corneum, and delivery via the pore pathway/hair follicles canals for large molecules. Regarding transdermal delivery of hydrophobic molecules from *o*/*w* nanoemulsions, active agent permeation may be achieved due to disruption of the *stratum corneum* (by creating permeable pathways as a result of fluidization of cell membranes and extracellular spaces), or improved permeation characteristics due to skin hydration (Figure 1) [307,310].

Various examples supporting the beneficial effects of lipid-based nanosystems concerning their improved physicochemical properties, or overcoming technological/biopharmaceutical limitations of different phenolic compounds, are presented in Table 2.

Table 2. Phenolic compounds, encapsulated in lipid-based nanosystems for dermal. application.

Main Class	Active Agent	Technological/Biopharmaceutical Issue	Lipid-Based Nanosystem/ Lipid Carrier	Obtained Results	References
Simple phenols and derivatives	Hydroquinone	Tendency to oxidation; hydrophilic structure hindering its topical application; side-effects due to systemic absorption	SLNs/Precirol® ATO5	• High hydroquinone encapsulation (app.90%); • long-standing physico-chemical stability; • enhanced skin accumulation	[311]
	Arbutin	Highly hydrophilic compound; limited skin permeation	Liposomes/ Soybean phosphatidylcholine; cholesterol	• Increased skin whitening efficacy; • Improved arbutin deposition in epidermis/dermis	[312,313]
	Thymoquinone (benzo-quinone)	Thermo/photosensitivity; hydrophobicity	Liposomes/ Phospholipon 90H®; cholesterol	• Improved anti-inflammatory action compared to plain solution; • enhanced stability against degradation; • increased skin permeation	[314]
	Protocatechuic acid; Ethyl protocatechuate (phenolic acid and derivative)	Sparingly hydrosolubilty (1:50); skin irritating properties; photosensitivity	SLNs/ Precirol ATO®5; NLCs/ Miglyol®810 N: Precirol ATO®5 3:7	• NLCs are the superior nanosystem concerning PDI and cell viability results compared to SLNs; • minimized skin irritation potential of protocatechuic acid; ensured UVB protection; • controlled release profile of phenolic acids without systemic exposure	[315,316]
	Ferulic acid (phenolic acid)	Poor water solubility; low stability	Nanoemulsion/ Isostearyl isosearate	• Improved solubility and permeability of ferulic acid; • significant antioxidant effect	[317]

Table 2. *Cont.*

Main Class	Active Agent	Technological/Biopharmaceutical Issue	Lipid-Based Nanosystem/ Lipid Carrier	Obtained Results	References
	Caffeic acid (hydroxyl-cinnamic acid)	Limited skin permeation	Liposomes/ egg phosphatidyl-choline; cholesterol	• High entrapment efficiency values (70%); • improved penetration compared to free caffeic acid; • preserved antioxidant activity	[318]
	Eugenol (Clove oil); (phenylpropene)	Predisposition to oxidation	SLNs/Stearic acid, Compritol®	• Development of eugenol loaded SLNs incorporated in carbopol hydrogel; • improved eugenol deposition in epidermis, compared to reference formulation; • achieved controlled release profile; • sufficient occlusive properties	[319]
Flavanoids	Naringin (flavanone)	Limited aqueous solubility; poor oral bioavailability	Liposomes/ Epikuron-200; cholesterol, Tween 80	• Improved skin deposition; • high encapsulation efficiency (99%); • very good physical stability	[320]
	Hesperidin (flavanone glycoside)	Poor aqueous solubility and bioavailability	NLCs/ Cupuaçu butter, buriti oil	• High encapsulation efficiency (96%); • sufficient physical stability; • noncytotoxic effect on melanoma cell lines	[321]
	Isoflavone-aglycon-rich fraction (genistein, daidzein, glycitein)	Limited aqueous solubility	Nanoemulsion/ Egg lecithin (Lipoid E-80®), medium-chain triglycerides	• Improved aqueous solubility; • development of nanoemulsion/hydrogel; • achieved active agent deposition in stratum corneum, epidermis and dermis (highest)	[322]
Anthraquinones	Aloe -emodin	Hydrophobic compound, crystallizes in water	Liposomes/ Hydrogenated soybean phosphatidyl-choline, cholesterol	• Improved skin permeation; • low cytotoxicity	[323]

Table 2. *Cont.*

Main Class	Active Agent	Technological/Biopharmaceutical Issue	Lipid-Based Nanosystem/ Lipid Carrier	Obtained Results	References
Naphthoquinones	Vitamin K1 (phylloquinone)	Highly lipophilic compound; photosensitivity	Liposomes/ Soy phosphatidyl-choline, α-tocopherol	• Elaboration of liposomal aqueous dispersion applied by nebulization; • Improved aqueous solubility; • increased deposition in epidermis and dermis compared to ointment formulation	[324]
Xanthones	Mangiferin	Poor water solubility (0.111 mg/mL); low bioavailability	Nanoemulsion/ Almond oil, Lipoid ®S75	• Enhanced permeation; • anti-inflammatory effect; • reduced edema and leukocyte infiltration	[325]
Stilbenes	Resveratrol	Low aqueous solubility; photosensitivity	SLNs/ Compritol 888 ATO NLCs/ Compritol 888 ATO; Miglyol oil	• *Resveratrol* loaded NLCs were superior to SLNs with respect to entrapment efficiency values, skin penetration, accumulation in dermis	[326,327]
	Pterostilbene	None; favorable characteristics compared to *resveratrol* (i.e., increased lipophilicity, membrane permeability and bioavailability)	Liposomes/ Lecithin	• Effectively prevents UVB-radiation induced skin carcinogenesis in mice	[328]
Tannins	Ellagic acid	Low aqueous solubility and permeability	NLCs/ Tristearin, Miglyol oil	• Improved solubility; • high antioxidant activity	[329]

The beneficial effects observed after incorporating phenolic phytochemicals in lipid-based nanocarriers, such as improved solubility, stability and skin permeation/penetration, are a prerequisite for further research, development, and industrial application. In Table 3 are presented some cosmetic products based on lipid nanocarriers encapsulating various phenolic compounds. The observed favorable outcomes may be described as synergetic; on the one side they result from the well-known antioxidant, antiaging or skin whitening properties of the phenolic phytochemicals [330], and on the other side results may be attributed to the penetration-enhancing properties or occlusive effects of the lipid nanocarriers.

Table 3. Cosmetic products containing phenolic phytochemicals formulated via nanotechnological approach.

Brand	Product	Phenolic Compounds	Lipid-Based Nanosystem	Benefits
Sesderma [331]	Sodyses Repair gel	Resveratrol, quercetin	Liposomes	• Supports healing process and proper skin recovery, • reduced scar tissue formation
	Factor G Renew Rejuvenating serum	Quercetin, pterostilbene	Liposomes	• Promotes cell regeneration, • increased collagen and elastin synthesis • antiwrinkle effect
	Hidroquin Whitening gel	Ferulic acid, Arbutin	Liposomes	• Skin whitening properties; • prevention and treatment of different skin imperfections
	Reti Age Eye contour gel	Pterostilbene	Liposomes	• Provides skin rejuvenation
	Kojicol Plus (+Kojic acid) Skin lightener cream	α-Arbutin,	Liposomes	• Skin whitening properties
M.Y.R. [332]	Curcumin liposome Melasma and acne cream	Curcumin	Liposomes	• Diminishes melasma patches, freckles, dark spots, acne scars • Antiaging effect
Vitacos [333]	NanoVital Vitanics Whitening essence	Arbutin	Nanoemulsion	• Moisturizing and skin lightening properties
Dr. Theiss Medipharma Cosme-tics [298]	Olivenöl Anti Falten Pflege-konzentrat	Olea europaea oil	NLCs	• Promotes cell regeneration and skin rejuvenation

6. Conclusions

The numerous beneficial effects characteristic of phytochemicals with phenolic structures, such as anti-inflammatory, antioxidant, antiproliferative, and antiaging activities, determine their broad utilization potential in pharmaceutics and the cosmetic industry. However, these advantageous features cannot be fully exploited due to unfavorable physicochemical or pharmacokinetic characteristics (i.e., poor solubility, stability, bioavailability). Lipid-based nanosystems, such as liposomes, solid lipid nanoparticles, nanostructured lipid carriers and nanoemulsions, represent a successful approach to overcome these limitations and improve their dermal/transdermal delivery. This review thoroughly discusses the physicochemical properties and mechanism of actions of various classes of phenolic compounds regarding their dermal application. Examples of their incorporation in different lipid nanocarriers, as well a summary of the obtained results, are also provided. According to the data, encapsulation of phenolic compounds in lipid-based nanosystems for topical application leads to improved solubility, stability, skin permeation capability and therapeutic performance in general.

Author Contributions: Conceptualization, V.A. and N.I.; methodology, V.G. and N.I.; investigation, N.I., Y.S. and V.G.; writing—original draft preparation V.G. and N.I.; writing—review and editing, V.A.; visualization, Y.S.; supervision, V.A.; project administration, V.A.; funding acquisition, V.A. All authors have read and agreed to the published version of the manuscript.

Funding: This work was funded by Medical University of Varna, Fund "Nauka" Project № 18027.

Institutional Review Board Statement: Not applicable.

Informed Consent Statement: Not applicable.

Data Availability Statement: Data sharing not applicable.

Acknowledgments: The authors would like to express their acknowledgement to the supporters: The Medical University of Varna.

Conflicts of Interest: The authors declare no conflict of interest.

References

1. Del Rio, D.; Rodriguez-Mateos, A.; Spencer, J.P.E.; Tognolini, M.; Borges, G.; Crozier, A. Dietary (Poly)phenolics in Human Health: Structures, Bioavailability, and Evidence of Protective Effects Against Chronic Diseases. *Antioxid. Redox Signal.* **2013**, *18*, 1818–1892. [CrossRef]
2. Działo, M.; Mierziak, J.; Korzun, U.; Preisner, M.; Szopa, J.; Kulma, A. The Potential of Plant Phenolics in Prevention and Therapy of Skin Disorders. *Int. J. Mol. Sci.* **2016**, *17*, 160. [CrossRef] [PubMed]
3. Lorenzo, J.M.; Estévez, M.; Barba, F.J.; Thirumdas, R.; Franco, D.; Munekata, P.E.S. Polyphenols: Bioaccessibility and bioavailability of bioactive components. In *Innovative Thermal and Non-Thermal Processing, Bioaccessibility and Bioavailability of Nutrients and Bioactive Compounds*, 1st ed.; Barba, F., Saraiva, J.M.A., Cravotto, G., Lorenzo, J., Eds.; Elsevier: Amsterdam, The Netherlands, 2019; pp. 309–322.
4. Martins, N.; Barros, L.; Ferreira, I.C.F.R. In vivo antioxidant activity of phenolic compounds: Facts and gaps. *Trends Food Sci. Technol.* **2016**, *48*, 1–12. [CrossRef]
5. Mehta, J.P.; Parmar, P.H.; Vadia, S.H.; Patel, M.K.; Tripathi, C.B. In-vitro antioxidant and in-vivo anti-inflammatory activities of aerial parts of *Cassia* species. *Arab. J. Chem.* **2017**, *10*, S1654–S1662. [CrossRef]
6. Miklasińska-Majdanik, M.; Kępa, M.; Wojtyczka, R.D.; Idzik, D.; Wąsik, T. Phenolic Compounds Diminish Antibiotic Resistance of *Staphylococcus Aureus* Clinical Strains. *Int. J. Environ. Res. Public Health* **2018**, *15*, 2321. [CrossRef]
7. Tungmunnithum, D.; Thongboonyou, A.; Pholboon, A.; Yangsabai, A. Flavonoids and Other Phenolic Compounds from Medicinal Plants for Pharmaceutical and Medical Aspects: An Overview. *Medicines* **2018**, *5*, 93. [CrossRef]
8. Kaurinovic, B.; Vastag, G. Flavonoids and Phenolic Acids as Potential Natural Antioxidants. In *Antioxidants*; Shalaby, E., Ed.; IntechOpen: London, UK, 2019; pp. 1–20.
9. Zillich, O.V.; Schweiggert-Weisz, U.; Eisner, P.; Kerscher, M. Polyphenols as active ingredients for cosmetic products. *Int. J. Cosmet. Sci.* **2015**, *37*, 455–464. [CrossRef] [PubMed]
10. Panzella, L.; Napolitano, A. Natural and Bioinspired Phenolic Compounds as Tyrosinase Inhibitors for the Treatment of Skin Hyperpigmentation: Recent Advances. *Cosmetics* **2019**, *6*, 57. [CrossRef]
11. Przybylska-Balcerek, A.; Stuper-Szablewska, K. Phenolic acids used in the cosmetics industry as natural antioxidants. *Eur. J. Med. Technol.* **2019**, *4*, 24–32.
12. Panzella, L. Natural Phenolic Compounds for Health, Food and Cosmetic Applications. *Antioxidants* **2020**, *9*, 427. [CrossRef]
13. Boo, Y.C. Can Plant Phenolic Compounds Protect the Skin from Airborne Particulate Matter? *Antioxidants* **2019**, *8*, 379. [CrossRef]
14. Kumar, N.; Goel, N. Phenolic acids: Natural versatile molecules with promising therapeutic applications. *Biotechnol. Rep.* **2019**, *24*, e00370. [CrossRef] [PubMed]
15. Schempp, C.M.; Müller, K.A.; Winghofer, B.; Schöpf, E.; Simon, J.C. Johanniskraut (Hypericum perforatum L.) Eine Pflanze mit Relevanz für die Dermatologie. *Hautarzt* **2002**, *53*, 316–321. [CrossRef]
16. Arct, J.; Pytkowska, K. Flavonoids as components of biologically active cosmeceuticals. *Clin. Dermatol.* **2008**, *26*, 347–357. [CrossRef] [PubMed]
17. Cosme, P.; Rodríguez, A.B.; Espino, J.; Garrido, M. Plant Phenolics: Bioavailability as a Key Determinant of Their Potential Health-Promoting Applications. *Antioxidants* **2020**, *9*, 1263. [CrossRef] [PubMed]

18. Soto, M.; Falqué, E.; Domínguez, H. Relevance of Natural Phenolics from Grape and Derivative Products in the Formulation of Cosmetics. *Cosmetics* **2015**, *2*, 259–276. [CrossRef]
19. Naik, A.; Kalia, Y.N.; Guy, R.H. Transdermal drug delivery: Overcoming the skin's barrier function. *Pharm. Sci. Technol. Today* **2000**, *3*, 318–326. [CrossRef]
20. Arct, J.; Gronwald, M.; Kasiura, K. Possibilities for the prediction of an active substance penetration through epidermis. *IFSCC Mag.* **2001**, *4*, 179–183.
21. Arct, J.; Oborska, A.; Mojski, M.; Binkowska, A.; Świdzikowska, B. Common cosmetic hydrophilic ingredients as penetration modifiers of flavonoids. *Int. J. Cosmet. Sci.* **2002**, *24*, 357–366. [CrossRef]
22. Chuang, S.-Y.; Lin, Y.-K.; Lin, C.-F.; Wang, P.-W.; Chen, E.-L.; Fang, J.-Y. Elucidating the Skin Delivery of Aglycone and Glycoside Flavonoids: How the Structures Affect Cutaneous Absorption. *Nutrients* **2017**, *9*, 1304. [CrossRef]
23. Fang, Z.; Bhandari, B. Encapsulation of polyphenols—A review. *Trends Food Sci. Technol.* **2010**, *21*, 510–523. [CrossRef]
24. Mahdavi, S.A.; Jafari, S.M.; Ghorbani, M.; Assadpoor, E. Spray-drying Microencapsulation of Anthocyanins by Natural Biopolymers: A Review. *Dry. Technol.* **2014**, *32*, 509–518. [CrossRef]
25. Kosović, E.; Topiař, M.; Cuřínová, P.; Sajfrtová, M. Stability testing of resveratrol and viniferin obtained from *Vitis vinifera* L. by various extraction methods considering the industrial viewpoint. *Sci. Rep.* **2020**, *10*, 5564. [CrossRef]
26. Dai, L.; Li, Y.; Kong, F.; Liu, K.; Si, C.; Ni, Y. Lignin-Based Nanoparticles Stabilized Pickering Emulsion for Stability Improvement and Thermal-Controlled Release of trans-Resveratrol. *ACS Sustain. Chem. Eng.* **2019**, *7*, 13497–13504. [CrossRef]
27. Kumar, R.; Kaur, K.; Uppal, S.; Mehta, S.K. Ultrasound processed nanoemulsion: A comparative approach between resveratrol and resveratrol cyclodextrin inclusion complex to study its binding interactions, antioxidant activity and UV light stability. *Ultrason. Sonochem.* **2017**, *37*, 478–489. [CrossRef] [PubMed]
28. Lima, A.M.; Pizzol, C.D.; Monteiro, F.B.F.; Creczynski-Pasa, T.B.; Andrade, G.P.; Ribeiro, A.O.; Perrusi, J.R. Hypericin encapsulated in solid lipid nanoparticles: Phototoxicity and photodynamic efficiency. *J. Photochem. Photobiol. B Biol.* **2013**, *125*, 146–154. [CrossRef]
29. Youssef, T.; Fadel, M.; Fahmy, R.; Kassab, K. Evaluation of hypericin-loaded solid lipid nanoparticles: Physicochemical properties, photostability and phototoxicity. *Pharm. Dev. Technol.* **2012**, *17*, 177–186. [CrossRef]
30. Füller, J.; Kellner, T.; Gaid, M.; Beerhues, L.; Müller-Goymann, C.C. Stabilization of hyperforin dicyclohexylammonium salt with dissolved albumin and albumin nanoparticles for studying hyperforin effects on 2D cultivation of keratinocytes in vitro. *Eur. J. Pharm. Biopharm.* **2018**, *126*, 115–122. [CrossRef] [PubMed]
31. Orth, H.C.J.; Rentel, C.; Schmidt, P.C. Isolation, Purity Analysis and Stability of Hyperforin as a Standard Material from *Hypericum perforatum* L. *J. Pharm. Pharmacol.* **1999**, *51*, 193–200. [CrossRef] [PubMed]
32. Koyu, H.; Haznedaroglu, M.Z. Investigation of impact of storage conditions on *Hypericum perforatum* L. dried total extract. *J. Food Drug Anal.* **2015**, *23*, 545–551. [CrossRef]
33. Park, S.N.; Lee, M.H.; Kim, S.J.; Yu, E.R. Preparation of quercetin and rutin-loaded ceramide liposomes and drug-releasing effect in liposome-in-hydrogel complex system. *Biochem. Biophys. Res. Commun.* **2013**, *435*, 361–366. [CrossRef]
34. Kwon, H.-J.; Hwang, J.; Lee, J.; Chae, S.-K.; Lee, J.-H.; Kim, J.-H.; Hwang, K.-S.; Kim, E.-C.; Park, Y.-D. Analysis and investigation of chemical stability on phenolic compounds in *Zanthoxylum schinifolium*-containing dentifrices. *J. Liq. Chromatogr. Relat. Technol.* **2014**, *37*, 1685–1701. [CrossRef]
35. Ramešová, Š.; Sokolová, R.; Degano, I.; Bulíčková, J.; Žabka, J.; Gál, M. On the stability of the bioactive flavonoids quercetin and luteolin under oxygen-free conditions. *Anal. Bioanal. Chem.* **2012**, *402*, 975–982. [CrossRef] [PubMed]
36. Luo, X.; Guan, R.; Chen, X.; Liu, M.; Hao, Y.; Jiang, H. Optimized Preparation of Catechin Nanoliposomes by Orthogonal Design and Stability Study. *Adv. J. Food Sci. Technol.* **2014**, *6*, 921–925. [CrossRef]
37. Latos-Brozio, M.; Masek, A. Natural Polymeric Compound Based on High Thermal Stability Catechin from Green Tea. *Biomolecules* **2020**, *10*, 1191. [CrossRef] [PubMed]
38. Li, N.; Taylor, L.S.; Ferruzzi, M.G.; Mauer, L.J. Kinetic Study of Catechin Stability: Effects of pH, Concentration, and Temperature. *J. Agric. Food Chem.* **2012**, *60*, 12531–12539. [CrossRef]
39. Jensen, J.S.; Wertz, C.F.; O'Neill, V.A. Preformulation Stability of trans-Resveratrol and trans-Resveratrol Glucoside (Piceid). *J. Agric. Food Chem.* **2010**, *58*, 1685–1690. [CrossRef]
40. Lin, C.-F.; Leu, Y.-L.; Al-Suwayeh, S.A.; Ku, M.-C.; Hwang, T.-L.; Fang, J.-Y. Anti-inflammatory activity and percutaneous absorption of quercetin and its polymethoxylated compound and glycosides: The relationships to chemical structures. *Eur. J. Pharm. Sci.* **2012**, *47*, 857–864. [CrossRef] [PubMed]
41. Křen, V. Glycoside vs. Aglycon: The Role of Glycosidic Residue in Biological Activity. In *Glycoscience*, 2nd ed.; Fraser-Reid, B.O., Tatsuta, K., Thiem, J., Eds.; Springer: Berlin/Heidelberg, Germany, 2008; pp. 2589–2644.
42. Choi, S.-J.; Tai, B.H.; Cuong, N.M.; Kim, Y.-H.; Jang, H.-D. Antioxidative and anti-inflammatory effect of quercetin and its glycosides isolated from mampat (*Cratoxylum formosum*). *Food Sci. Biotechnol.* **2012**, *21*, 587–595. [CrossRef]
43. Rha, C.-S.; Jeong, H.W.; Park, S.; Lee, S.; Jung, Y.S.; Kim, D.-O. Antioxidative, Anti-Inflammatory, and Anticancer Effects of Purified Flavonol Glycosides and Aglycones in Green Tea. *Antioxidants* **2019**, *8*, 278. [CrossRef] [PubMed]
44. Munin, A.; Edwards-Lévy, F. Encapsulation of Natural Polyphenolic Compounds; A Review. *Pharmaceutics* **2011**, *3*, 793–829. [CrossRef]

45. Belščak-Cvitanović, A.; Stojanović, R.; Manojlović, V.; Komes, D.; Cindrić, I.J.; Nedović, V.; Bugarski, B. Encapsulation of polyphenolic antioxidants from medicinal plant extracts in alginate–chitosan system enhanced with ascorbic acid by electrostatic extrusion. *Food Res. Int.* **2011**, *44*, 1094–1101. [CrossRef]
46. Tylkowski, B.; Tsibranska, I. Polyphenols encapsulation—Application of innovation technologies to improve stability of natural products. In *Microencapsulation*; Giamberini, M., Prieto, S.F., Tylkowski, B., Eds.; De Gruyter: Berlin, Germany; Boston, MA, USA, 2015; pp. 97–114.
47. Kumar, R. Lipid-Based Nanoparticles for Drug-Delivery Systems. In *Nanocarriers for Drug Delivery*; Mohapatra, S.S., Ranjan, S., Dasgupta, N., Mishra, R.K., Thomas, S., Eds.; Elsevier: Amsterdam, The Netherlands, 2019; pp. 249–284.
48. Sengar, V.; Jyoti, K.; Jain, U.K.; Katare, O.P.; Chandra, R.; Madan, J. Lipid nanoparticles for topical and transdermal delivery of pharmaceuticals and cosmeceuticals. In *Lipid Nanocarriers for Drug Targeting*, 1st ed.; Grumezescu, A., Ed.; Elsevier: Amsterdam, The Netherlands, 2018; pp. 413–436.
49. Kakadia, P.; Conway, B. Lipid nanoparticles for dermal drug delivery. *Curr. Pharm. Des.* **2015**, *21*, 2823–2829. [CrossRef] [PubMed]
50. Ganesan, P.; Narayanasamy, D. Lipid nanoparticles: Different preparation techniques, characterization, hurdles, and strategies for the production of solid lipid nanoparticles and nanostructured lipid carriers for oral drug delivery. *Sustain. Chem. Pharm.* **2017**, *6*, 37–56. [CrossRef]
51. Bhattacharya, A.; Sood, P.; Citovsky, V. The roles of plant phenolics in defence and communication during *Agrobacterium* and *Rhizobium* infection. *Mol. Plant. Pathol.* **2010**, *11*, 705–719. [CrossRef]
52. Patil, V.M.; Masand, N. Anticancer Potential of Flavonoids: Chemistry, Biological Activities, and Future Perspectives. In *Studies in Natural Products Chemistry*, 1st ed.; Atta-ur-Rahman, Ed.; Elsevier: Amsterdam, The Netherlands, 2018; Volume 59, pp. 401–430.
53. Zuiter, A.S. Proanthocyanidin: Chemistry and Biology: From Phenolic Compounds to Proanthocyanidins. In *Reference Module in Chemistry, Molecular Sciences and Chemical Engineering*; Elsevier: Amsterdam, The Netherlands, 2014; pp. 1–29.
54. Santos-Sánchez, N.F.; Salas-Coronado, R.; Villanueva-Cañongo, C.; Hernández-Carlos, B. Antioxidant Compounds and Their Antioxidant Mechanism. In *Antioxidants*; Shalaby, E., Ed.; IntechOpen: London, UK, 2019; pp. 1–28.
55. Snezhkina, A.V.; Kudryavtseva, A.V.; Kardymon, O.L.; Savvateeva, M.V.; Melnikova, N.V.; Krasnov, G.S.; Dmitriev, A.A. ROS Generation and Antioxidant Defense Systems in Normal and Malignant Cells. *Oxid. Med. Cell. Longev.* **2019**, *2019*, 1–17. [CrossRef]
56. Cherrak, S.A.; Mokhtari-Soulimane, N.; Berroukeche, F.; Bensenane, B.; Cherbonnel, A.; Merzouk, H.; Elhabiri, M. In Vitro Antioxidant versus Metal Ion Chelating Properties of Flavonoids: A Structure-Activity Investigation. *PLoS ONE* **2016**, *11*, e0165575. [CrossRef]
57. Hussain, T.; Tan, B.; Yin, Y.; Blachier, F.; Tossou, M.C.B.; Rahu, N. Oxidative Stress and Inflammation: What Polyphenols Can Do for Us? *Oxid. Med. Cell. Longev.* **2016**, *2016*, 1–9. [CrossRef]
58. Heim, K.E.; Tagliaferro, A.R.; Bobilya, D.J. Flavonoid antioxidants: Chemistry, metabolism and structure-activity relationships. *J. Nutr. Biochem.* **2002**, *13*, 572–584. [CrossRef]
59. Kumar, S.; Pandey, A.K. Chemistry and Biological Activities of Flavonoids: An Overview. *Sci. World J.* **2013**, *2013*, 1–16. [CrossRef]
60. Gijsman, P. Polymer Stabilization. In *Handbook of Environmental Degradation of Materials*, 2nd ed.; Kutz, M., Ed.; Elsevier: Amsterdam, The Netherlands, 2012; pp. 673–714.
61. Okayama, Y. Oxidative Stress in Allergic and Inflammatory Skin Diseases. *Curr. Drug Targets Inflamm. Allergy* **2005**, *4*, 517–519. [CrossRef] [PubMed]
62. Yahfoufi, N.; Alsadi, N.; Jambi, M.; Matar, C. The Immunomodulatory and Anti-Inflammatory Role of Polyphenols. *Nutrients* **2018**, *10*, 1618. [CrossRef] [PubMed]
63. Havermann, S.; Büchter, C.; Koch, K.; Wätjen, W. Role of Oxidative Stress in the Process of Carcinogenesis. In *Studies on Experimental Toxicology and Pharmacology. Oxidative Stress in Applied Basic Research and Clinical Practice*, 1st ed.; Roberts, S.M., Kehrer, J.P., Klotz, L.-O., Eds.; Humana Press: Totowa, NJ, USA, 2015; pp. 173–198.
64. Harrison, D.; Griendling, K.K.; Landmesser, U.; Hornig, B.; Drexler, H. Role of oxidative stress in atherosclerosis. *Am. J. Cardiol.* **2003**, *91*, 7A–11A. [CrossRef]
65. Giesey, R.L.; Mehrmal, S.; Uppal, P.; Delost, G. The Global Burden of Skin and Subcutaneous Disease: A Longitudinal Analysis from the Global Burden of Disease Study From 1990–2017. *SKIN J. Cutan. Med.* **2021**, *5*, 125–136. [CrossRef]
66. Karimkhani, C.; Dellavalle, R.P.; Coffeng, L.E.; Flohr, C.; Hay, R.J.; Langan, S.M.; Nsoesie, E.O.; Ferrari, A.J.; Erskine, H.E.; Silverberg, J.I.; et al. Global Skin Disease Morbidity and Mortality: An Update From the Global Burden of Disease Study 2013. *JAMA Dermatol.* **2017**, *153*, 406–412. [CrossRef] [PubMed]
67. Flohr, C.; Hay, R. Putting the burden of skin diseases on the global map. *Br. J. Dermatol.* **2021**, *184*, 189–190. [CrossRef]
68. Cushnie, T.P.T.; Lamb, A.J. Antimicrobial activity of flavonoids. *Int. J. Antimicrob. Agents* **2005**, *26*, 343–356. [CrossRef]
69. Tabassum, N.; Hamdani, M. Plants used to treat skin diseases. *Pharmacogn. Rev.* **2014**, *8*, 52–60. [CrossRef]
70. Gottlieb, A.B. Therapeutic options in the treatment of psoriasis and atopic dermatitis. *J. Am. Acad. Dermatol.* **2005**, *53*, S3–S16. [CrossRef]
71. Hajar, T.; Gontijo, J.R.V.; Hanifin, J.M. New and developing therapies for atopic dermatitis. *An. Bras. Dermatol.* **2018**, *93*, 104–107. [CrossRef]
72. Richmond, J.M.; Harris, J.E. Immunology and Skin in Health and Disease. *Cold Spring Harb. Perspect. Med.* **2014**, *4*, a015339. [CrossRef] [PubMed]

73. Dainichi, T.; Hanakawa, S.; Kabashima, K. Classification of inflammatory skin diseases: A proposal based on the disorders of the three-layered defense systems, barrier, innate immunity and acquired immunity. *J. Dermatol. Sci.* **2014**, *76*, 81–89. [CrossRef] [PubMed]
74. Gunter, N.V.; Teh, S.S.; Lim, Y.M.; Mah, S.H. Natural Xanthones and Skin Inflammatory Diseases: Multitargeting Mechanisms of Action and Potential Application. *Front. Pharmacol.* **2020**, *11*, 594202. [CrossRef] [PubMed]
75. Schwingen, J.; Kaplan, M.; Kurschus, F.C. Review-Current Concepts in Inflammatory Skin Diseases Evolved by Transcriptome Analysis: In-Depth Analysis of Atopic Dermatitis and Psoriasis. *Int. J. Mol. Sci.* **2020**, *21*, 699. [CrossRef]
76. Giang, J.; Seelen, M.A.J.; van Doorn, M.B.A.; Rissmann, R.; Prens, E.P.; Damman, J. Complement Activation in Inflammatory Skin Diseases. *Front. Immunol.* **2018**, *9*, 639. [CrossRef]
77. Cetin, E.D.; Savk, E.; Uslu, M.; Eskin, M.; Karul, A. Investigation of the Inflammatory Mechanisms in Alopecia Areata. *Am. J. Dermatopathol.* **2009**, *31*, 53–60. [CrossRef]
78. Woo, Y.; Lim, J.; Cho, D.; Park, H. Rosacea: Molecular Mechanisms and Management of a Chronic Cutaneous Inflammatory Condition. *Int. J. Mol. Sci.* **2016**, *17*, 1562. [CrossRef]
79. Richmond, J.M.; Frisoli, M.L.; Harris, J.E. Innate immune mechanisms in vitiligo: Danger from within. *Curr. Opin. Immunol.* **2013**, *25*, 676–682. [CrossRef]
80. Neagu, M.; Constantin, C.; Caruntu, C.; Dumitru, C.; Surcel, M.; Zurac, S. Inflammation: A key process in skin tumorigenesis. *Oncol. Lett.* **2019**, *17*, 4068–4084. [CrossRef]
81. de Oliveira, R.G., Jr.; Ferraz, C.A.A.; e Silva, M.G.; de Lavor, É.M.; Rolim, L.A.; de Lima, J.T.; Fleury, A.; Picot, L.; de Souza Siqueira Quintans, J.; Quintans, L.J., Jr.; et al. Flavonoids: Promising Natural Products for Treatment of Skin Cancer (Melanoma). In *Natural Products and Cancer Drug Discovery*; Badria, F.A., Ed.; Humana Press: Totowa, NJ, USA, 2017; pp. 161–210.
82. Katiyar, S.K.; Afaq, F.; Perez, A.; Mukhtar, H. Green tea polyphenol (-)-epigallocatechin-3-gallate treatment of human skin inhibits ultraviolet radiation-induced oxidative stress. *Carcinogenesis* **2001**, *22*, 287–294. [CrossRef]
83. Afaq, F.; Syed, D.N.; Malik, A.; Hadi, N.; Sarfaraz, S.; Kweon, M.-H.; Khan, N.; Zaid, M.A.; Mukhtar, H. Delphinidin, an Anthocyanidin in Pigmented Fruits and Vegetables, Protects Human HaCaT Keratinocytes and Mouse Skin Against UVB-Mediated Oxidative Stress and Apoptosis. *J. Investig. Dermatol.* **2007**, *127*, 222–232. [CrossRef]
84. Papuc, C.; Goran, G.V.; Predescu, C.N.; Nicorescu, V.; Stefan, G. Plant Polyphenols as Antioxidant and Antibacterial Agents for Shelf-Life Extension of Meat and Meat Products: Classification, Structures, Sources, and Action Mechanisms. *Compr. Rev. Food Sci. Food Saf.* **2017**, *16*, 1243–1268. [CrossRef] [PubMed]
85. Borges, A.; Ferreira, C.; Saavedra, M.J.; Simões, M. Antibacterial Activity and Mode of Action of Ferulic and Gallic Acids Against Pathogenic Bacteria. *Microb. Drug Resist.* **2013**, *19*, 256–265. [CrossRef] [PubMed]
86. Anderson, J.C.; Headley, C.; Stapleton, P.D.; Taylor, P.W. Synthesis and antibacterial activity of hydrolytically stable (−)-epicatechin gallate analogues for the modulation of β-lactam resistance in *Staphylococcus aureus*. *Bioorganic Med. Chem. Lett.* **2005**, *15*, 2633–2635. [CrossRef] [PubMed]
87. Zhao, W.-H.; Hu, Z.-Q.; Okubo, S.; Hara, Y.; Shimamura, T. Mechanism of Synergy between Epigallocatechin Gallate and β-Lactams against Methicillin-Resistant *Staphylococcus aureus*. *Antimicrob. Agents Chemother.* **2001**, *45*, 1737–1742. [CrossRef] [PubMed]
88. Khameneh, B.; Iranshahy, M.; Soheili, V.; Fazly Bazzaz, B.S. Review on plant antimicrobials: A mechanistic viewpoint. *Antimicrob. Resist. Infect. Control.* **2019**, *8*, 118. [CrossRef]
89. Sudano Roccaro, A.; Blanco, A.R.; Giuliano, F.; Rusciano, D.; Enea, V. Epigallocatechin-Gallate Enhances the Activity of Tetracycline in Staphylococci by Inhibiting Its Efflux from Bacterial Cells. *Antimicrob. Agents Chemother.* **2004**, *48*, 1968–1973. [CrossRef]
90. Zhao, W.-H.; Hu, Z.-Q.; Hara, Y.; Shimamura, T. Inhibition of Penicillinase by Epigallocatechin Gallate Resulting in Restoration of Antibacterial Activity of Penicillin Against Penicillinase-Producing *Staphylococcus Aureus*. *Antimicrob. Agents Chemother.* **2002**, *46*, 2266–2268. [CrossRef]
91. Qin, R.; Xiao, K.; Li, B.; Jiang, W.; Peng, W.; Zheng, J.; Zhou, H. The Combination of Catechin and Epicatechin Gallate from Fructus Crataegi Potentiates β-Lactam Antibiotics Against *Methicillin-Resistant Staphylococcus Aureus* (Mrsa) In Vitro and In Vivo. *Int. J. Mol. Sci.* **2013**, *14*, 1802–1821. [CrossRef]
92. Phan, H.T.T.; Yoda, T.; Chahal, B.; Morita, M.; Takagi, M.; Vestergaard, M.C. Structure-dependent interactions of polyphenols with a biomimetic membrane system. *Biochim. Biophys. Acta Biomembr.* **2014**, *1838*, 2670–2677. [CrossRef] [PubMed]
93. Wu, T.; He, M.; Zang, X.; Zhou, Y.; Qiu, T.; Pan, S.; Xu, X. A structure–activity relationship study of flavonoids as inhibitors of *E. coli* by membrane interaction effect. *Biochim. Biophys. Acta Biomembr.* **2013**, *1828*, 2751–2756. [CrossRef]
94. Donadio, G.; Mensitieri, F.; Santoro, V.; Parisi, V.; Bellone, M.L.; De Tommasi, N.; Izzo, V.; Dal Piaz, F. Interactions with Microbial Proteins Driving the Antibacterial Activity of Flavonoids. *Pharmaceutics* **2021**, *13*, 660. [CrossRef] [PubMed]
95. Pinho, E.; Ferreira, I.C.F.R.; Barros, L.; Carvalho, A.M.; Soares, G.; Henriques, M. Antibacterial Potential of Northeastern Portugal Wild Plant Extracts and Respective Phenolic Compounds. *BioMed Res. Int.* **2014**, *2014*, 1–8. [CrossRef]
96. Cushnie, T.P.T.; Lamb, A.J. Assessment of the antibacterial activity of galangin against 4-quinolone resistant strains of *Staphylococcus aureus*. *Phytomedicine* **2006**, *13*, 187–191. [CrossRef] [PubMed]
97. Przybyłek, I.; Karpiński, T.M. Antibacterial Properties of Propolis. *Molecules* **2019**, *24*, 2047. [CrossRef] [PubMed]

98. Park, S.; Yi, Y.; Lim, M.H. Reactivity of Flavonoids Containing a Catechol or Pyrogallol Moiety with Metal-Free and Metal-Associated Amyloid-β. *Bull. Korean Chem. Soc.* **2020**, *42*, 17–24. [CrossRef]
99. Barvinchenko, V.M.; Lipkovska, N.O.; Fedyanina, T.V.; Pogorelyi, V.K. Physico-chemical Properties of Supramolecular Complexes of Natural Flavonoids with Biomacromolecules. In *Nanomaterials and Supramolecular Structures*; Shpak, A.P., Gorbyk, P.P., Eds.; Springer: Dordrecht, The Netherlands, 2009; pp. 281–291.
100. Uivarosi, V.; Munteanu, A.C.; Sharma, A.; Singh Tuli, H. Metal Complexation and Patent Studies of Flavonoid. In *Current Aspects of Flavonoids: Their Role in Cancer Treatment*; Singh Tuli, H., Ed.; Springer: Singapore, 2019; pp. 39–89.
101. Wang, S.-X.; Zhang, F.-J.; Feng, Q.-P.; Li, Y.-L. Synthesis, characterization, and antibacterial activity of transition metal complexes with 5-hydroxy-7,4-dimethoxyflavone. *J. Inorg. Biochem.* **1992**, *46*, 251–257. [CrossRef]
102. Kutluay, S.B.; Doroghazi, J.; Roemer, M.E.; Triezenberg, S.J. Curcumin inhibits herpes simplex virus immediate-early gene expression by a mechanism independent of p300/CBP histone acetyltransferase activity. *Virology* **2008**, *373*, 239–247. [CrossRef]
103. Balasubramanyam, K.; Varier, R.A.; Altaf, M.; Swaminathan, V.; Siddappa, N.B.; Ranga, U.; Kundu, T.K. Curcumin, a Novel p300/CREB-binding Protein-specific Inhibitor of Acetyltransferase, Represses the Acetylation of Histone/Nonhistone Proteins and Histone Acetyltransferase-dependent Chromatin Transcription. *J. Biol. Chem.* **2004**, *279*, 51163–51171. [CrossRef]
104. Šudomová, M.; Hassan, S.T.S. Nutraceutical Curcumin with Promising Protection against Herpesvirus Infections and Their Associated Inflammation: Mechanisms and Pathways. *Microorganisms* **2021**, *9*, 292. [CrossRef]
105. Flores, D.J.; Lee, L.H.; Adams, S.D. Inhibition of Curcumin-Treated Herpes Simplex Virus 1 and 2 in Vero Cells. *Adv. Microbiol.* **2016**, *6*, 276–287. [CrossRef]
106. Bernard, F.X.; Sablé, S.; Cameron, B.; Provost, J.; Desnottes, J.F.; Crouzet, J.; Blanche, F. Glycosylated flavones as selective inhibitors of topoisomerase IV. *Antimicrob. Agents Chemother.* **1997**, *41*, 992–998. [CrossRef] [PubMed]
107. Barbieri, R.; Coppo, E.; Marchese, A.; Daglia, M.; Sobarzo-Sánchez, E.; Nabavi, S.F.; Nabavi, S.M. Phytochemicals for human disease: An update on plant-derived compounds antibacterial activity. *Microbiol. Res.* **2017**, *196*, 44–68. [CrossRef] [PubMed]
108. Liu, M.-H.; Otsuka, N.; Noyori, K.; Shiota, S.; Ogawa, W.; Kuroda, T.; Hatano, T.; Tsuchiya, T. Synergistic Effect of Kaempferol Glycosides Purified from *Laurus nobilis* and Fluoroquinolones on Methicillin-Resistant *Staphylococcus aureus*. *Biol. Pharm. Bull.* **2009**, *32*, 489–492. [CrossRef]
109. Xie, Y.; Yang, W.; Tang, F.; Chen, X.; Ren, L. Antibacterial Activities of Flavonoids: Structure-Activity Relationship and Mechanism. *Curr. Med. Chem.* **2014**, *22*, 132–149. [CrossRef] [PubMed]
110. Ninfali, P.; Antonelli, A.; Magnani, M.; Scarpa, E.S. Antiviral Properties of Flavonoids and Delivery Strategies. *Nutrients* **2020**, *12*, 2534. [CrossRef]
111. Adamczak, A.; Ożarowski, M.; Karpiński, T.M. Antibacterial Activity of Some Flavonoids and Organic Acids Widely Distributed in Plants. *J. Clin. Med.* **2020**, *9*, 109. [CrossRef] [PubMed]
112. Anani, K.; Adjrah, Y.; Ameyapoh, Y.; Karou, S.D.; Agbonon, A.; de Souza, C.; Gbeassor, M. Effects of hydroethanolic extracts of Balanites aegyptiaca (L.) Delile (Balanitaceae) on some resistant pathogens bacteria isolated from wounds. *J. Ethnopharmacol.* **2015**, *164*, 16–21. [CrossRef]
113. Saddiqe, Z.; Naeem, I.; Maimoona, A. A review of the antibacterial activity of *Hypericum perforatum* L. *J. Ethnopharmacol.* **2010**, *131*, 511–521. [CrossRef]
114. Wölfle, U.; Seelinger, G.; Schempp, C. Topical Application of St. John's Wort (*Hypericum perforatum*). *Planta Med.* **2013**, *80*, 109–120. [CrossRef]
115. Feyzioğlu, B.; Demircili, M.E.; Özdemir, M.; Doğan, M.; Baykan, M.; Baysal, B. Antibacterial effect of hypericin. *Afr. J. Microbiol. Res.* **2013**, *7*, 979–982.
116. Fritz, D.; Venturi, C.R.; Cargnin, S.; Schripsema, J.; Roehe, P.M.; Montanha, J.A.; von Poser, G.L. Herpes virus inhibitory substances from *Hypericum connatum* Lam., a plant used in southern Brazil to treat oral lesions. *J. Ethnopharmacol.* **2007**, *113*, 517–520. [CrossRef] [PubMed]
117. Wen, S.; Zhang, J.; Yang, B.; Elias, P.M.; Man, M.-Q. Role of Resveratrol in Regulating Cutaneous Functions. *Evid. Based Complement. Altern. Med.* **2020**, *2020*, 1–20. [CrossRef]
118. Chan, M.M.-Y. Antimicrobial effect of resveratrol on dermatophytes and bacterial pathogens of the skin. *Biochem. Pharmacol.* **2002**, *63*, 99–104. [CrossRef]
119. He, M.; Min, J.-W.; Kong, W.-L.; He, X.-H.; Li, J.-X.; Peng, B.-W. A review on the pharmacological effects of vitexin and isovitexin. *Fitoterapia* **2016**, *115*, 74–85. [CrossRef]
120. Man, M.-Q.; Yang, B.; Elias, P.M. Benefits of Hesperidin for Cutaneous Functions. *Evid. Based Complement. Altern. Med.* **2019**, *2019*, 1–19. [CrossRef]
121. Köksal Karayıldırım, Ç. Characterization and in vitro Evolution of Antibacterial Efficacy of Novel Hesperidin Microemulsion. *CBUJOS* **2017**, *13*, 943–947. [CrossRef]
122. Yadav, M.K.; Chae, S.-W.; Im, G.J.; Chung, J.-W.; Song, J.-J. Eugenol: A Phyto-Compound Effective against Methicillin-Resistant and Methicillin-Sensitive *Staphylococcus aureus* Clinical Strain Biofilms. *PLoS ONE* **2015**, *10*, e0119564. [CrossRef]
123. Guimarães, I.; Baptista-Silva, S.; Pintado, M.; Oliveira, A.L. Polyphenols: A Promising Avenue in Therapeutic Solutions for Wound Care. *Appl. Sci.* **2021**, *11*, 1230. [CrossRef]

124. Thang, P.T.; Patrick, S.; Teik, L.S.; Yung, C.S. Anti-oxidant effects of the extracts from the leaves of *Chromolaena odorata* on human dermal fibroblasts and epidermal keratinocytes against hydrogen peroxide and hypoxanthine-xanthine oxidase induced damage. *Burns* **2001**, *27*, 319–327. [CrossRef]
125. Bahramsoltani, R.; Farzaei, M.H.; Rahimi, R. Medicinal plants and their natural components as future drugs for the treatment of burn wounds: An integrative review. *Arch. Dermatol. Res.* **2014**, *306*, 601–617. [CrossRef]
126. Skórkowska-Telichowska, K.; Kulma, A.; Żuk, M.; Czuj, T.; Szopa, J. The Effects of Newly Developed Linen Dressings on Decubitus Ulcers. *J. Palliat. Med.* **2012**, *15*, 146–148. [CrossRef]
127. Reinke, J.M.; Sorg, H. Wound Repair and Regeneration. *Eur. Surg. Res.* **2012**, *49*, 35–43. [CrossRef]
128. Mittal, M.; Siddiqui, M.R.; Tran, K.; Reddy, S.P.; Malik, A.B. Reactive Oxygen Species in Inflammation and Tissue Injury. *Antioxid. Redox Signal.* **2014**, *20*, 1126–1167. [CrossRef]
129. Abdulkhaleq, L.A.; Assi, M.A.; Abdullah, R.; Zamri-Saad, M.; Taufiq-Yap, Y.H.; Hezmee, M.N.M. The crucial roles of inflammatory mediators in inflammation: A review. *Vet. World* **2018**, *11*, 627–635. [CrossRef] [PubMed]
130. Chen, D.; Hou, Q.; Zhong, L.; Zhao, Y.; Li, M.; Fu, X. Bioactive Molecules for Skin Repair and Regeneration: Progress and Perspectives. *Stem Cells Int.* **2019**, *2019*, 1–13. [CrossRef] [PubMed]
131. Eun, C.-H.; Kang, M.-S.; Kim, I.-J. Elastase/Collagenase Inhibition Compositions of *Citrus unshiu* and Its Association with Phenolic Content and Anti-Oxidant Activity. *Appl. Sci.* **2020**, *10*, 4838. [CrossRef]
132. Chen, L.-Y.; Cheng, H.-L.; Kuan, Y.-H.; Liang, T.-J.; Chao, Y.-Y.; Lin, H.-C. Therapeutic Potential of Luteolin on Impaired Wound Healing in Streptozotocin-Induced Rats. *Biomedicines* **2021**, *9*, 761. [CrossRef]
133. Thring, T.S.; Hili, P.; Naughton, D.P. Anti-collagenase, anti-elastase and anti-oxidant activities of extracts from 21 plants. *BMC Complement. Altern. Med.* **2009**, *9*, 27. [CrossRef]
134. Fujii, T.; Wakaizumi, M.; Ikami, T.; Saito, M. Amla (*Emblica officinalis* Gaertn.) extract promotes procollagen production and inhibits matrix metalloproteinase-1 in human skin fibroblasts. *J. Ethnopharmacol.* **2008**, *119*, 53–57. [CrossRef]
135. Wittenauer, J.; Mäckle, S.; Sußmann, D.; Schweiggert-Weisz, U.; Carle, R. Inhibitory effects of polyphenols from grape pomace extract on collagenase and elastase activity. *Fitoterapia* **2015**, *101*, 179–187. [CrossRef]
136. Abdul Karim, A.; Azlan, A.; Ismail, A.; Hashim, P.; Abd Gani, S.S.; Zainudin, B.H.; Abdullah, N.A. Phenolic composition, antioxidant, anti-wrinkles and tyrosinase inhibitory activities of cocoa pod extract. *BMC Complement. Altern. Med.* **2014**, *14*, 381. [CrossRef] [PubMed]
137. Pientaweeratch, S.; Panapisal, V.; Tansirikongkol, A. Antioxidant, anti-collagenase and anti-elastase activities of *Phyllanthus emblica*, *Manilkara zapota* and silymarin: An in vitro comparative study for anti-aging applications. *Pharm. Biol.* **2016**, *54*, 1865–1872. [CrossRef] [PubMed]
138. Fadhel Abbas Albaayit, S.; Abba, Y.; Rasedee, A.; Abdullah, N. Effect of *Clausena excavata* Burm. f. (Rutaceae) leaf extract on wound healing and antioxidant activity in rats. *Drug Des. Dev. Ther.* **2015**, *9*, 3507–3518.
139. Geethalakshmi, R.; Sakravarthi, C.; Kritika, T.; Arul Kirubakaran, M.; Sarada, D.V.L. Evaluation of antioxidant and wound healing potentials of *Sphaeranthus amaranthoides* Burm.f. *Biomed. Res. Int.* **2013**, *2013*, 1–7. [CrossRef]
140. Zofia, N.-Ł.; Martyna, Z.-D.; Aleksandra, Z.; Tomasz, B. Comparison of the Antiaging and Protective Properties of Plants from the *Apiaceae* Family. *Oxid. Med. Cell. Longev.* **2020**, *2020*, 1–16. [CrossRef]
141. Dudonné, S.; Poupard, P.; Coutière, P.; Woillez, M.; Richard, T.; Mérillon, J.-M.; Vitrac, X. Phenolic Composition and Antioxidant Properties of Poplar Bud (*Populus nigra*) Extract: Individual Antioxidant Contribution of Phenolics and Transcriptional Effect on Skin Aging. *J. Agric. Food Chem.* **2011**, *59*, 4527–4536. [CrossRef]
142. Dudonné, S.; Coutière, P.; Woillez, M.; Merillon, J.-M.; Vitrac, X. DNA macroarray study of skin aging-related genes expression modulation by antioxidant plant extracts on a replicative senescence model of human dermal fibroblasts. *Phytother. Res.* **2011**, *25*, 686–693. [CrossRef]
143. Blom van Staden, A.; Lall, N. Medicinal Plants as Alternative Treatments for Progressive Macular Hypomelanosis. In *Medicinal Plants for Holistic Health and Well-Being*; Lall, N., Ed.; Elsevier: Amsterdam, The Netherlands, 2018; pp. 145–182.
144. Liu, W.-S.; Kuan, Y.-D.; Chiu, K.-H.; Wang, W.-K.; Chang, F.-H.; Liu, C.-H.; Lee, C.-H. The Extract of *Rhodobacter sphaeroides* Inhibits Melanogenesis through the MEK/ERK Signaling Pathway. *Mar. Drugs* **2013**, *11*, 1899–1908. [CrossRef]
145. Parvez, S.; Kang, M.; Chung, H.-S.; Cho, C.; Hong, M.-C.; Shin, M.-K.; Bae, H. Survey and mechanism of skin depigmenting and lightening agents. *Phytother. Res.* **2006**, *20*, 921–934. [CrossRef]
146. Chai, W.-M.; Lin, M.-Z.; Wang, Y.-X.; Xu, K.-L.; Huang, W.-Y.; Pan, D.-D.; Zou, Z.-R.; Peng, Y.-Y. Inhibition of tyrosinase by cherimoya pericarp proanthocyanidins: Structural characterization, inhibitory activity and mechanism. *Food Res. Int.* **2017**, *100*, 731–739. [CrossRef] [PubMed]
147. Song, W.; Zhu, X.-F.; Ding, X.-D.; Yang, H.-B.; Qin, S.-T.; Chen, H.; Wei, S.-D. Structural features, antioxidant and tyrosinase inhibitory activities of proanthocyanidins in leaves of two tea cultivars. *Int. J. Food Prop.* **2016**, *20*, 1348–1358. [CrossRef]
148. Li, H.-R.; Habasi, M.; Xie, L.-Z.; Aisa, H.A. Effect of Chlorogenic Acid on Melanogenesis of B16 Melanoma Cells. *Molecules* **2014**, *19*, 12940–12948. [CrossRef] [PubMed]
149. Hariharan, V.; Toole, T.; Klarquist, J.; Mosenson, J.; Longley, B.J.; Le Poole, I.C. Topical application of bleaching phenols; in-vivo studies and mechanism of action relevant to melanoma treatment. *Melanoma Res.* **2011**, *21*, 115–126. [CrossRef] [PubMed]
150. Morgan, A.M.A.; Jeon, M.N.; Jeong, M.H.; Yang, S.Y.; Kim, Y.H. Chemical Components from the Stems of *Pueraria lobata* and Their Tyrosinase Inhibitory Activity. *Nat. Prod. Sci.* **2016**, *22*, 111–116. [CrossRef]

151. Chung, K.W.; Jeong, H.O.; Lee, E.K.; Kim, S.J.; Chun, P.; Chung, H.Y.; Moon, H.R. Evaluation of Antimelanogenic Activity and Mechanism of Galangin In Silico and In Vivo. *Biol. Pharm. Bull.* **2018**, *41*, 73–79. [CrossRef]
152. Solimine, J.; Garo, E.; Wedler, J.; Rusanov, K.; Fertig, O.; Hamburger, M.; Atanassov, I.; Butterweck, V. Tyrosinase inhibitory constituents from a polyphenol enriched fraction of rose oil distillation wastewater. *Fitoterapia* **2016**, *108*, 13–19. [CrossRef]
153. Kim, D.H.; Lee, J.H. Comparative evaluation of phenolic phytochemicals from perilla seeds of diverse species and screening for their tyrosinase inhibitory and antioxidant properties. *S. Afr. J. Bot.* **2019**, *123*, 341–350. [CrossRef]
154. Tanaka, Y.; Suzuki, M.; Kodachi, Y.; Nihei, K. Molecular design of potent, hydrophilic tyrosinase inhibitors based on the natural dihydrooxyresveratrol skeleton. *Carbohydr. Res.* **2019**, *472*, 42–49. [CrossRef]
155. Zuo, A.-R.; Dong, H.-H.; Yu, Y.-Y.; Shu, Q.-L.; Zheng, L.-X.; Yu, X.-Y.; Cao, S.-W. The antityrosinase and antioxidant activities of flavonoids dominated by the number and location of phenolic hydroxyl groups. *Chin. Med.* **2018**, *13*, 51. [CrossRef] [PubMed]
156. Crespo, M.I.; Chabán, M.F.; Lanza, P.A.; Joray, M.B.; Palacios, S.M.; Vera, D.M.A.; Carpinella, M.C. Inhibitory effects of compounds isolated from *Lepechinia meyenii* on tyrosinase. *Food Chem. Toxicol.* **2019**, *125*, 383–391. [CrossRef]
157. Akaberi, M.; Emami, S.A.; Vatani, M.; Tayarani-Najaran, Z. Evaluation of Antioxidant and Anti-Melanogenic Activity of Different Extracts of Aerial Parts of *N. Sintenisii* in Murine Melanoma B16F10 Cells. *Iran. J. Pharm. Res.* **2018**, *17*, 225–235.
158. Demirkiran, O.; Sabudak, T.; Ozturk, M.; Topcu, G. Antioxidant and Tyrosinase Inhibitory Activities of Flavonoids from *Trifolium nigrescens* Subsp. *petrisavi. J. Agric. Food Chem.* **2013**, *61*, 12598–12603. [CrossRef]
159. Uesugi, D.; Hamada, H.; Shimoda, K.; Kubota, N.; Ozaki, S.; Nagatani, N. Synthesis, oxygen radical absorbance capacity, and tyrosinase inhibitory activity of glycosides of resveratrol, pterostilbene, and pinostilbene. *Biosci. Biotechnol. Biochem.* **2017**, *81*, 226–230. [CrossRef]
160. Hu, Z.-M.; Zhou, Q.; Lei, T.-C.; Ding, S.-F.; Xu, S.-Z. Effects of hydroquinone and its glucoside derivatives on melanogenesis and antioxidation: Biosafety as skin whitening agents. *J. Dermatol. Sci.* **2009**, *55*, 179–184. [CrossRef] [PubMed]
161. Kammeyer, A.; Willemsen, K.J.; Ouwerkerk, W.; Bakker, W.J.; Ratsma, D.; Pronk, S.D.; Smit, N.P.M.; Luiten, R.M. Mechanism of action of 4-substituted phenols to induce vitiligo and antimelanoma immunity. *Pigment. Cell Melanoma Res.* **2019**, *32*, 540–552. [CrossRef] [PubMed]
162. Draelos, Z.D.; Deliencourt-Godefroy, G.; Lopes, L. An effective hydroquinone alternative for topical skin lightening. *J. Cosmet. Dermatol.* **2020**, *19*, 3258–3261. [CrossRef] [PubMed]
163. Gandhi, V.; Verma, P.; Naik, G. Exogenous ochronosis After Prolonged Use of Topical Hydroquinone (2%) in a 50-Year-Old Indian Female. *Indian J. Dermatol.* **2012**, *57*, 394–395. [CrossRef]
164. Park, J.; Park, J.H.; Suh, H.-J.; Lee, I.C.; Koh, J.; Boo, Y.C. Effects of resveratrol, oxyresveratrol, and their acetylated derivatives on cellular melanogenesis. *Arch. Dermatol. Res.* **2014**, *306*, 475–487. [CrossRef]
165. Gianfaldoni, S.; Tchernev, G.; Lotti, J.; Wollina, U.; Satolli, F.; Rovesti, M.; França, K.; Lotti, T. Unconventional Treatments for Vitiligo: Are They (Un) Satisfactory? *Open Access Maced. J. Med. Sci.* **2018**, *6*, 170–175. [CrossRef]
166. Rashighi, M.; Harris, J.E. Vitiligo Pathogenesis and Emerging Treatments. *Dermatol. Clin.* **2017**, *35*, 257–265. [CrossRef] [PubMed]
167. Shivasaraun, U.V.; Sureshkumar, R.; Karthika, C.; Puttappa, N. Flavonoids as adjuvant in psoralen based photochemotherapy in the management of vitiligo/leucoderma. *Med. Hypotheses* **2018**, *121*, 26–30. [CrossRef]
168. Gianfaldoni, S.; Wollina, U.; Tirant, M.; Tchernev, G.; Lotti, J.; Satolli, F.; Rovesti, M.; França, K.; Lotti, T. Herbal Compounds for the Treatment of Vitiligo: A Review. *Open Access Maced. J. Med. Sci.* **2018**, *6*, 203–207. [CrossRef]
169. Asawanonda, P.; Klahan, S.O. Tetrahydrocurcuminoid Cream Plus Targeted Narrowband UVB Phototherapy for Vitiligo: A Preliminary Randomized Controlled Study. *Photomed. Laser Surg.* **2010**, *28*, 679–684. [CrossRef]
170. Jeong, Y.-M.; Choi, Y.-G.; Kim, D.-S.; Park, S.-H.; Yoon, J.-A.; Kwon, S.-B.; Park, E.-S.; Park, K.-C. Cytoprotective effect of green tea extract and quercetin against hydrogen peroxide-induced oxidative stress. *Arch. Pharm. Res.* **2005**, *28*, 1251–1256. [CrossRef] [PubMed]
171. Guan, C.; Xu, W.; Hong, W.; Zhou, M.; Lin, F.; Fu, L.; Liu, D.; Xu, A. Quercetin attenuates the effects of H2O2 on endoplasmic reticulum morphology and tyrosinase export from the endoplasmic reticulum in melanocytes. *Mol. Med. Rep.* **2015**, *11*, 4285–4290. [CrossRef]
172. ICH Harmonised Tripartite Guideline: Photosafety Evaluation of Pharmaceuticals S10. 2013. Available online: https://database.ich.org/sites/default/files/S10_Guideline.pdf (accessed on 14 June 2021).
173. Learn, D.B.; Donald, F.P.; Sambuco, C.P. Photosafety: Current Methods and Future Direction. In *A Comprehensive Guide to Toxicology in Preclinical Drug Development*; Faqi, A.S., Ed.; Elsevier: Amsterdam, The Netherlands, 2013; pp. 395–422.
174. Li, X.; An, R.; Liang, K.; Wang, X.; You, L. Phototoxicity of traditional chinese medicine (TCM). *Toxicol. Res.* **2018**, *7*, 1012–1019. [CrossRef] [PubMed]
175. Kim, K.; Park, H.; Lim, K.-M. Phototoxicity: Its Mechanism and Animal Alternative Test Methods. *Toxicol. Res.* **2015**, *31*, 97–104. [CrossRef] [PubMed]
176. Costa, A.; Bonner, M.Y.; Arbiser, J.L. Use of Polyphenolic Compounds in Dermatologic Oncology. *Am. J. Clin. Dermatol.* **2016**, *17*, 369–385. [CrossRef]
177. Jiang, A.-J.; Jiang, G.; Li, L.-T.; Zheng, J.-N. Curcumin induces apoptosis through mitochondrial pathway and caspases activation in human melanoma cells. *Mol. Biol. Rep.* **2015**, *42*, 267–275. [CrossRef]

178. Abusnina, A.; Keravis, T.; Yougbaré, I.; Bronner, C.; Lugnier, C. Anti-proliferative effect of curcumin on melanoma cells is mediated by PDE1A inhibition that regulates the epigenetic integrator UHRF1. *Mol. Nutr. Food Res.* **2011**, *55*, 1677–1689. [CrossRef]
179. Attoub, S.; Hassan, A.H.; Vanhoecke, B.; Iratni, R.; Takahashi, T.; Gaben, A.-M.; Bracke, M.; Awad, S.; John, A.; Kamalboor, H.A.; et al. Inhibition of cell survival, invasion, tumor growth and histone deacetylase activity by the dietary flavonoid luteolin in human epithelioid cancer cells. *Eur. J. Pharmacol.* **2011**, *651*, 18–25. [CrossRef] [PubMed]
180. Tan, Z.; Zhang, Y.; Deng, J.; Zeng, G.; Zhang, Y. Purified Vitexin Compound 1 Suppresses Tumor Growth and Induces Cell Apoptosis in a Mouse Model of Human Choriocarcinoma. *Int. J. Gynecol. Cancer* **2012**, *22*, 360–366. [CrossRef] [PubMed]
181. Lim, Y.C.; Lee, S.-H.; Song, M.H.; Yamaguchi, K.; Yoon, J.-H.; Choi, E.C.; Baek, S.J. Growth inhibition and apoptosis by (−)-epicatechin gallate are mediated by cyclin D1 suppression in head and neck squamous carcinoma cells. *Eur. J. Cancer* **2006**, *42*, 3260–3266. [CrossRef] [PubMed]
182. Ji, B.-C.; Hsu, W.-H.; Yang, J.-S.; Hsia, T.-C.; Lu, C.-C.; Chiang, J.-H.; Yang, J.-L.; Lin, C.-H.; Lin, J.-J.; Wu Suen, L.-J.; et al. Gallic Acid Induces Apoptosis via Caspase-3 and Mitochondrion-Dependent Pathways in Vitro and Suppresses Lung Xenograft Tumor Growth in Vivo. *J. Agric. Food Chem.* **2009**, *57*, 7596–7604. [CrossRef]
183. Kim, G.C.; Choi, D.S.; Lim, J.S.; Jeong, H.C.; Kim, I.R.; Lee, M.H.; Park, B.S. Caspases-dependent Apoptosis in Human Melanoma Cell by Eugenol. *Korean J. Anat.* **2006**, *39*, 245–253.
184. Yang, G.; Fu, Y.; Malakhova, M.; Kurinov, I.; Zhu, F.; Yao, K.; Li, H.; Chen, H.; Li, W.; Lim, D.Y.; et al. Caffeic Acid Directly Targets ERK1/2 to Attenuate Solar UV-Induced Skin Carcinogenesis. *Cancer Prev. Res.* **2014**, *7*, 1056–1066. [CrossRef]
185. Wan, S.B.; Chen, D.; Ping Dou, Q.; Hang Chan, T. Study of the green tea polyphenols catechin-3-gallate (CG) and epicatechin-3-gallate (ECG) as proteasome inhibitors. *Bioorg. Med. Chem.* **2004**, *12*, 3521–3527. [CrossRef]
186. Pettinari, A.; Amici, M.; Cuccioloni, M.; Angeletti, M.; Fioretti, E.; Eleuteri, A.M. Effect of Polyphenolic Compounds on the Proteolytic Activities of Constitutive and Immuno-Proteasomes. *Antioxid. Redox Signal.* **2006**, *8*, 121–129. [CrossRef] [PubMed]
187. Chen, D.; Daniel, K.G.; Chen, M.S.; Kuhn, D.J.; Landis-Piwowar, K.R.; Ping Dou, Q. Dietary flavonoids as proteasome inhibitors and apoptosis inducers in human leukemia cells. *Biochem. Pharmacol.* **2005**, *69*, 1421–1432. [CrossRef]
188. Dikshit, P.; Goswami, A.; Mishra, A.; Chatterjee, M.; Ranjan Jana, N. Curcumin induces stress response, neurite outgrowth and prevent NF-κB activation by inhibiting the proteasome function. *Neurotox. Res.* **2006**, *9*, 29–37. [CrossRef] [PubMed]
189. Mena, S.; Rodriguez, M.L.; Ponsoda, X.; Estrela, J.M.; Jäättela, M.; Ortega, A.L. Pterostilbene-Induced Tumor Cytotoxicity: A Lysosomal Membrane Permeabilization-Dependent Mechanism. *PLoS ONE* **2012**, *7*, e44524. [CrossRef] [PubMed]
190. Chen, C.-L.; Chen, Y.; Tai, M.-C.; Liang, C.-M.; Lu, D.-W.; Chen, J.-T. Resveratrol inhibits transforming growth factor-β2-induced epithelial-to-mesenchymal transition in human retinal pigment epithelial cells by suppressing the Smad pathway. *Drug Des. Dev. Ther.* **2017**, *11*, 163–173. [CrossRef] [PubMed]
191. Ren, Z.; Shen, J.; Mei, X.; Dong, H.; Li, J.; Yu, H. Hesperidin inhibits the epithelial to mesenchymal transition induced by transforming growth factor-β1 in A549 cells through Smad signaling in the cytoplasm. *Braz. J. Pharm. Sci.* **2019**, *55*, e18172. [CrossRef]
192. Kalinowska, M.; Gryko, K.; Wróblewska, A.M.; Jabłońska-Trypuć, A.; Karpowicz, D. Phenolic content, chemical composition and anti-/pro-oxidant activity of Gold Milenium and Papierowka apple peel extracts. *Sci. Rep.* **2020**, *10*, 14951. [CrossRef]
193. Jomová, K.; Hudecova, L.; Lauro, P.; Simunkova, M.; Alwasel, S.H.; Alhazza, I.M.; Valko, M. A Switch between Antioxidant and Prooxidant Properties of the Phenolic Compounds Myricetin, Morin, 3′,4′-Dihydroxyflavone, Taxifolin and 4-Hydroxy-Coumarin in the Presence of Copper(II) Ions: A Spectroscopic, Absorption Titration and DNA Damage Study. *Molecules* **2019**, *24*, 4335. [CrossRef]
194. Kyselova, Z. Toxicological aspects of the use of phenolic compounds in disease prevention. *Interdiscip. Toxicol.* **2011**, *4*, 173–183. [CrossRef]
195. Lein, A.; Oussoren, C. Dermal. In *Practical Pharmaceutics*; Bouwman-Boer, Y., Fenton-May, V., Le Brun, P., Eds.; Springer: Cham, Switzerland, 2015; pp. 229–263.
196. Block, L.H. Medicated topicals. In *The science and practice of Pharmacy*, 21st ed.; Troy, D., Ed.; Lippincott Williams & Wilkins: Philadelphia, PA, USA, 2005; pp. 871–888.
197. Makuch, E.; Nowak, A.; Günther, A.; Pełech, R.; Kucharski, Ł.; Duchnik, W.; Klimowicz, A. Enhancement of the antioxidant and skin permeation properties of eugenol by the esterification of eugenol to new derivatives. *AMB Express* **2020**, *10*, 187. [CrossRef]
198. Günther, A.; Makuch, E.; Nowak, A.; Duchnik, W.; Kucharski, Ł.; Pełech, R.; Klimowicz, A. Enhancement of the Antioxidant and Skin Permeation Properties of Betulin and Its Derivatives. *Molecules* **2021**, *26*, 3435. [CrossRef]
199. Walters, K.A.; Lane, M.E. Dermal and Transdermal Drug Delivery Systems. In *Dermal Drug Delivery, 1st ed*; Ghosh, T.K., Ed.; CRC Press: Boca Raton, FL, USA, 2020; pp. 1–60.
200. Chen, J.; Yang, J.; Ma, L.; Li, J.; Shahzad, N.; Kim, C.K. Structure-antioxidant activity relationship of methoxy, phenolic hydroxyl, and carboxylic acid groups of phenolic acids. *Sci. Rep.* **2020**, *10*, 2611. [CrossRef]
201. Zhang, C.L.; Fan, J. Application of Hypericin in Tumor Treatment and Diagnosis. *J. Int. Pharm. Res. Int.* **2012**, *39*, 402–408.
202. Intagliata, S.; Modica, M.N.; Santagati, L.M.; Montenegro, L. Strategies to Improve Resveratrol Systemic and Topical Bioavailability: An Update. *Antioxidants* **2019**, *8*, 244. [CrossRef] [PubMed]
203. Kozak, W.; Rachon, J.; Daśko, M.; Demkowicz, S. Selected Methods for the Chemical Phosphorylation and Thiophosphorylation of Phenols. *Asian J. Org. Chem.* **2018**, *7*, 314–323. [CrossRef]

204. N'Da, D. Prodrug Strategies for Enhancing the Percutaneous Absorption of Drugs. *Molecules* **2014**, *19*, 20780–20807. [CrossRef] [PubMed]
205. Williamson, G.; Plumb, G.W.; Garcia-Conesa, M.T. Glycosylation, Esterification, and Polymerization of Flavonoids and Hydroxycinnamates: Effects on Antioxidant Properties. In *Plant Polyphenols 2*, 1st ed.; Gross, G.G., Hemingway, R.W., Yoshida, T., Branham, S.J., Eds.; Springer: Boston, MA, USA, 1999; pp. 483–494.
206. Nowak, A.; Cybulska, K.; Makuch, E.; Kucharski, Ł.; Różewicka-Czabańska, M.; Prowans, P.; Czapla, N.; Bargiel, P.; Petriczko, J.; Klimowicz, A. In Vitro Human Skin Penetration, Antioxidant and Antimicrobial Activity of Ethanol-Water Extract of Fireweed (*Epilobium angustifolium* L.). *Molecules* **2021**, *26*, 329. [CrossRef] [PubMed]
207. Alonso, C.; Rubio, L.; Touriño, S.; Martí, M.; Barba, C.; Fernández-Campos, F.; Coderch, L.; Luís Parra, J. Antioxidative effects and percutaneous absorption of five polyphenols. *Free Radic. Biol. Med.* **2014**, *75*, 149–155. [CrossRef]
208. Ng, T.B.; Wong, J.H.; Tam, C.; Liu, F.; Cheung, C.F.; Ng, C.C.W.; Tse, R.; Tse, T.F.; Chan, H. Methyl Gallate as an Antioxidant and Anti-HIV Agent. In *HIV/AIDS: Oxidative Stress and Dietary Antioxidants*, 1st ed.; Preedy, V.R., Watson, R.R., Eds.; Elsevier: Amsterdam, The Netherlands, 2018; pp. 161–168.
209. Mota, F.L.; Queimada, A.J.; Pinho, S.P.; Macedo, E.A. Aqueous Solubility of Some Natural Phenolic Compounds. *Ind. Eng. Chem. Res.* **2008**, *47*, 5182–5189. [CrossRef]
210. Badhani, B.; Sharma, N.; Kakkar, R. Gallic acid: A versatile antioxidant with promising therapeutic and industrial applications. *RSC Adv.* **2015**, *5*, 27540–27557. [CrossRef]
211. ChemSpider. Search and Share Chemistry. Ellagic Acid. Available online: http://www.chemspider.com/Chemical-Structure.4445149.html (accessed on 10 July 2021).
212. Evtyugin, D.D.; Magina, S.; Evtuguin, D.V. Recent Advances in the Production and Applications of Ellagic Acid and Its Derivatives. A Review. *Molecules* **2020**, *25*, 2745. [CrossRef]
213. Bala, I.; Bhardwaj, V.; Hariharan, S.; Kumar, M.N.V.R. Analytical methods for assay of ellagic acid and its solubility studies. *J. Pharm. Biomed. Anal.* **2006**, *40*, 206–210. [CrossRef]
214. Simić, A.Z.; Verbić, T.Ž.; Sentić, M.N.; Vojić, M.P.; Juranić, I.O.; Manojlović, D.D. Study of ellagic acid electro-oxidation mechanism. *Monatsh. Chem.* **2012**, *144*, 121–128. [CrossRef]
215. National Library of Medicine. National Center for Biotechnology Information. PubChem. Compound Summary. 4-Hydroxycinnamic Acid. Available online: https://pubchem.ncbi.nlm.nih.gov/compound/4-Hydroxycinnamic-acid#section=LogP (accessed on 11 July 2021).
216. Yu, Z.; Wang, Y.; Zhu, M.; Zhou, L. Measurement and Correlation of Solubility and Thermodynamic Properties of Vinpocetine in Nine Pure Solvents and (Ethanol + Water) Binary Solvent. *J. Chem. Eng. Data* **2018**, *64*, 150–160. [CrossRef]
217. Beltrán, J.L.; Sanli, N.; Fonrodona, G.; Barrón, D.; Özkan, G.; Barbosa, J. Spectrophotometric, potentiometric and chromatographic pKa values of polyphenolic acids in water and acetonitrile–water media. *Anal. Chim. Acta* **2003**, *484*, 253–264. [CrossRef]
218. Paracatu, L.C.; Faria, C.M.Q.G.; Quinello, C.; Rennó, C.; Palmeira, P.; Zeraik, M.L.; de Fonseca, L.M.; Ximenes, V.F. Caffeic Acid Phenethyl Ester: Consequences of Its Hydrophobicity in the Oxidative Functions and Cytokine Release by Leukocytes. *Evid. Based Complement. Altern. Med.* **2014**, *2014*, 1–13. [CrossRef]
219. National Library of Medicine. National Center for Biotechnology Information. PubChem. Ferulic Acid. Available online: https://pubchem.ncbi.nlm.nih.gov/compound/Ferulic-acid#section=LogP0.0 (accessed on 14 July 2021).
220. FOODB. Showing Compound Chlorogenic acid (FDB002582). Available online: https://foodb.ca/compounds/FDB002582 (accessed on 14 July 2021).
221. Šeruga, M.; Tomac, I. Electrochemical Behaviour of Some Chlorogenic Acids and Their Characterization in Coffee by Square-Wave Voltammetry. *Int. J. Electrochem. Sci.* **2014**, *9*, 6134–6154.
222. Hansch, C.; Leo, A.; Hoekman, D.H. *Exploring QSAR—Hydrophobic, Electronic, and Steric Constants*, 1st ed.; American Chemical Society: Washington, DC, USA, 1995; Volume 2, p. 20.
223. Cavender, F.L.; O'Donohue, J. Phenol and Phenolics. In *Patty's Toxicology*, 6th ed.; Bingham, E., Cohrssen, B., Eds.; John Wiley & Sons: Hoboken, NJ, USA, 2012; pp. 243–349.
224. Zahid, M.; Grampp, G.; Mansha, A.; Bhatti, I.A.; Asim, S. Absorption and Fluorescence Emission Attributes of a Fluorescent dye: 2,3,5,6-Tetracyano-p-Hydroquinone. *J. Fluoresc.* **2013**, *23*, 829–837. [CrossRef] [PubMed]
225. Dias, N.C.; Nawas, M.I.; Poole, C.F. Evaluation of a reversed-phase column (Supelcosil LC-ABZ) under isocratic and gradient elution conditions for estimating octanol–water partition coefficients. *Analyst* **2003**, *128*, 427–433. [CrossRef] [PubMed]
226. Yalkowsky, S.H.; He, Y.; Jain, P. *Handbook of Aqueous Solubility Data*, 2nd ed.; CRC Press: Boca Raton, FL, USA, 2010; p. 687.
227. Kortum, G.; Vogel, W.; Andrussow, K. Disssociation constants of organic acids in aqueous solution. In *Pure and Applied Chemistry*; Burrows, H.D., Stohner, J., Eds.; De Gruyter: Berlin, Germany; Boston, MA, USA, 1960; Volume 1, pp. 187–536.
228. Rothwell, J.A.; Day, A.J.; Morgan, M.R.A. Experimental Determination of Octanol−Water Partition Coefficients of Quercetin and Related Flavonoids. *J. Agric. Food Chem.* **2005**, *53*, 4355–4360. [CrossRef]
229. Wang, M.; Firrman, J.; Liu, L.; Yam, K. A Review on Flavonoid Apigenin: Dietary Intake, ADME, Antimicrobial Effects, and Interactions with Human Gut Microbiota. *BioMed Res. Int.* **2019**, *2019*, 1–18. [CrossRef]
230. National Library of Medicine. National Center for Biotechnology Information. PubChem. Apigenin. Available online: https://pubchem.ncbi.nlm.nih.gov/compound/Apigenin (accessed on 15 July 2021).

231. de Matos, A.M.; Martins, A.; Man, T.; Evans, D.; Walter, M.; Oliveira, M.C.; López, Ó.; Fernandez-Bolaños, J.G.; Dätwyler, P.; Ernst, B.; et al. Design and Synthesis of CNS-targeted Flavones and Analogues with Neuroprotective Potential Against H2O2- and Aβ1-42-Induced Toxicity in SH-SY5Y Human Neuroblastoma Cells. *Pharmaceuticals* **2019**, *12*, 98. [CrossRef] [PubMed]
232. Costa, E.C.; Menezes, P.M.N.; de Almeida, R.L.; Silva, F.S.; de Araújo Ribeiro, L.A.; de Silva, J.A.; de Oliveira, A.P.; da Cruz Araújo, E.C.; Rolim, L.A.; Nunes, X.P. Inclusion of vitexin in β-cyclodextrin: Preparation, characterization and expectorant/antitussive activities. *Heliyon* **2020**, *6*, e05461. [CrossRef]
233. Chemical Book. Vitexin. Available online: https://www.chemicalbook.com/ChemicalProductProperty_EN_CB3119208.htm (accessed on 17 July 2021).
234. FOODB. Showing Compound Luteolin (FDB013255). Available online: https://foodb.ca/compounds/FDB013255 (accessed on 17 July 2021).
235. Deng, S.-P.; Yang, Y.-L.; Cheng, X.-X.; Li, W.-R.; Cai, J.-Y. Synthesis, Spectroscopic Study and Radical Scavenging Activity of Kaempferol Derivatives: Enhanced Water Solubility and Antioxidant Activity. *Int. J. Mol. Sci.* **2019**, *20*, 975. [CrossRef]
236. Herrero-Martínez, J.M.; Sanmartin, M.; Rosés, M.; Bosch, E.; Ràfols, C. Determination of dissociation constants of flavonoids by capillary electrophoresis. *Electrophoresis* **2005**, *26*, 1886–1895. [CrossRef]
237. Lončarić, A.; Lamas Castro, J.P.; Guerra, E.; Lores, M. Increasing water solubility of Quercetin by increasing the temperature. In Proceedings of the 15th Instrumental Analysis Conference/Expoquimia, Barcelona, Spain, 3–5 October 2017.
238. Srinivas, K.; King, J.W.; Howard, L.R.; Monrad, J.K. Solubility and solution thermodynamic properties of quercetin and quercetin dihydrate in subcritical water. *J. Food Eng.* **2010**, *100*, 208–218. [CrossRef]
239. Pedriali, C.A.; Fernandes, A.U.; de Cássia Bernusso, L.; Polakiewicz, B. The synthesis of a water-soluble derivative of rutin as an antiradical agent. *Quím. Nova* **2008**, *31*, 2147–2151. [CrossRef]
240. Topolewski, P.; Zommer-Urbańska, S. Spectrophotometric investigation of protolytic equilibria of rutin. *Microchim. Acta* **1989**, *97*, 75–80. [CrossRef]
241. Srirangam, R.; Majumdar, S. Passive asymmetric transport of hesperetin across isolated rabbit cornea. *Int. J. Pharm.* **2010**, *394*, 60–67. [CrossRef] [PubMed]
242. Majumdar, S.; Srirangam, R. Solubility, Stability, Physicochemical Characteristics and In Vitro Ocular Tissue Permeability of Hesperidin: A Natural Bioflavonoid. *Pharm. Res.* **2008**, *26*, 1217–1225. [CrossRef] [PubMed]
243. Serra, H.; Mendes, T.; Bronze, M.R.; Simplício, A.L. Prediction of intestinal absorption and metabolism of pharmacologically active flavones and flavanones. *Bioorg. Med. Chem.* **2008**, *16*, 4009–4018. [CrossRef] [PubMed]
244. Poaty, B.; Dumarçay, S.; Perrin, D. New lipophilic catechin derivatives by oxa-Pictet-Spengler reaction. *Eur. Food Res. Technol.* **2009**, *230*, 111–117. [CrossRef]
245. Matsubara, T.; Wataoka, I.; Urakawa, H.; Yasunaga, H. High-Efficient Chemical Preparation of Catechinone Hair Dyestuff by Oxidation of (+)-Catechin in Water/Ethanol Mixed Solution. *Sen'i Gakkaishi* **2014**, *70*, 19–22. [CrossRef]
246. Chen, J.; Zhang, L.; Li, C.; Chen, R.; Liu, C.; Chen, M. Lipophilized Epigallocatechin Gallate Derivative Exerts Anti-Proliferation Efficacy through Induction of Cell Cycle Arrest and Apoptosis on DU145 Human Prostate Cancer Cells. *Nutrients* **2020**, *12*, 92. [CrossRef] [PubMed]
247. Zhang, X.; Wang, J.; Hu, J.-M.; Huang, Y.-W.; Wu, X.-Y.; Zi, C.-T.; Wang, X.-J.; Sheng, J. Synthesis and Biological Testing of Novel Glucosylated Epigallocatechin Gallate (EGCG) Derivatives. *Molecules* **2016**, *21*, 620. [CrossRef] [PubMed]
248. Muzolf-Panek, M.; Gliszczyńska-Świgło, A.; Szymusiak, H.; Tyrakowska, B. The influence of stereochemistry on the antioxidant properties of catechin epimers. *Eur. Food Res. Technol.* **2012**, *235*, 1001–1009. [CrossRef]
249. Priyadarsini, K.I. The Chemistry of Curcumin: From Extraction to Therapeutic Agent. *Molecules* **2014**, *19*, 20091–20112. [CrossRef]
250. Shin, G.H.; Li, J.; Cho, J.H.; Kim, J.T.; Park, H.J. Enhancement of Curcumin Solubility by Phase Change from Crystalline to Amorphous in Cur-TPGS Nanosuspension. *J. Food Sci.* **2016**, *81*, N494–N501. [CrossRef] [PubMed]
251. Yang, S.-C.; Tseng, C.-H.; Wang, P.-W.; Lu, P.-L.; Weng, Y.-H.; Yen, F.-L.; Fang, J.-Y. Pterostilbene, a Methoxylated Resveratrol Derivative, Efficiently Eradicates Planktonic, Biofilm, and Intracellular MRSA by Topical Application. *Front. Microbiol.* **2017**, *8*, 1103. [CrossRef]
252. Robinson, K.; Mock, C.; Liang, D. Pre-formulation studies of resveratrol. *Drug Dev. Ind. Pharm.* **2015**, *41*, 1464–1469. [CrossRef] [PubMed]
253. López-Nicolás, J.M.; García-Carmona, F. Aggregation State and pKaValues of (E)-Resveratrol As Determined by Fluorescence Spectroscopy and UV−Visible Absorption. *J. Agric. Food Chem.* **2008**, *56*, 7600–7605. [CrossRef] [PubMed]
254. Jürgenliemk, G.; Nahrstedt, A. Dissolution, solubility and cooperativity of phenolic compounds from Hypericum perforatum L. in aqueous systems. *Pharmazie* **2008**, *58*, 200–203.
255. Zhang, J.; Gao, L.; Hu, J.; Wang, C.; Hagedoorn, P.-L.; Li, N.; Zhou, X. Hypericin: Source, Determination, Separation, and Properties. *Sep. Purif. Rev.* **2020**, 1–10. [CrossRef]
256. Leonhartsberger, J.G.; Falk, H. The Protonation and Deprotonation Equilibria of Hypericin Revisited. *Monatsh. Chem.* **2002**, *133*, 167–172. [CrossRef]
257. National Library of Medicine. National Center for Biotechnology Information. PubChem. Hyperforin. Available online: https://pubchem.ncbi.nlm.nih.gov/compound/Hyperforin (accessed on 19 July 2021).
258. Hadzhiiliev, V.; Dimov, D. Separate isolation of hyperforin from hypericum perforatum (St. John's Wort) pursuant to the coefficents LOG Kow, PKa and densities of the included compounds. *Trakia J. Sci.* **2015**, *13*, 19–23. [CrossRef]

259. Cao, H.; Saroglu, O.; Karadag, A.; Diaconeasa, Z.; Zoccatelli, G.; Conte-Junior, C.A.; Gonzalez-Aguilar, G.A.; Ou, J.; Bai, W.; Zamarioli, C.M.; et al. Available technologies on improving the stability of polyphenols in food processing. *Food Front.* **2021**, *2*, 109–139. [CrossRef]
260. Esparza, I.; Cimminelli, M.J.; Moler, J.A.; Jiménez-Moreno, N.; Ancín-Azpilicueta, C. Stability of Phenolic Compounds in Grape Stem Extracts. *Antioxidants* **2020**, *9*, 720. [CrossRef]
261. Nuutila, A.M.; Kammiovirta, K.; Oksman-Caldentey, K.-M. Comparison of methods for the hydrolysis of flavonoids and phenolic acids from onion and spinach for HPLC analysis. *Food Chem.* **2002**, *76*, 519–525. [CrossRef]
262. Ali, A.; Chong, C.H.; Mah, S.H.; Abdullah, L.C.; Choong, T.S.Y.; Chua, B.L. Impact of Storage Conditions on the Stability of Predominant Phenolic Constituents and Antioxidant Activity of Dried *Piper betle* Extracts. *Molecules* **2018**, *23*, 484. [CrossRef] [PubMed]
263. Pignatello, R.; Pecora, T.M.G.; Cutuli, G.G.; Catalfo, A.; De Guidi, G.; Ruozi, B.; Tosi, G.; Cianciolo, S.; Musumeci, T. Antioxidant activity and photostability assessment of trans-resveratrol acrylate microspheres. *Pharm. Dev. Technol.* **2018**, *24*, 222–234. [CrossRef]
264. Dodangeh, M.; Tang, R.-C.; Gharanjig, K. Improving the photostability of curcumin using functional star-shaped polyamidoamine dendrimer: Application on PET. *Mater. Today Commun.* **2019**, *21*, 100620. [CrossRef]
265. Mihara, S.; Shibamoto, T. Photochemical reactions of eugenol and related compounds: Synthesis of new flavor chemicals. *J. Agric. Food Chem.* **1982**, *30*, 1215–1218. [CrossRef]
266. Dall'Acqua, S.; Miolo, G.; Innocenti, G.; Caffieri, S. The Photodegradation of Quercetin: Relation to Oxidation. *Molecules* **2012**, *17*, 8898–8907. [CrossRef] [PubMed]
267. Chaaban, H.; Ioannou, I.; Paris, C.; Charbonnel, C.; Ghoul, M. The photostability of flavanones, flavonols and flavones and evolution of their antioxidant activity. *J. Photochem. Photobiol. A Chem.* **2017**, *336*, 131–139. [CrossRef]
268. Iglesias, J.; Pazos, M.; Lois, S.; Medina, I. Contribution of Galloylation and Polymerization to the Antioxidant Activity of Polyphenols in Fish Lipid Systems. *J. Agric. Food Chem.* **2010**, *58*, 7423–7431. [CrossRef] [PubMed]
269. Vinardell, M.P.; Mitjans, M. Nanocarriers for Delivery of Antioxidants on the Skin. *Cosmetics* **2015**, *2*, 342–354. [CrossRef]
270. Shade, C.W. Liposomes as Advanced Delivery Systems for Nutraceuticals. *Integr. Med.* **2016**, *15*, 33–36.
271. Pierre, M.B.R.; dos Santos Miranda Costa, I. Liposomal systems as drug delivery vehicles for dermal and transdermal applications. *Arch. Dermatol. Res.* **2011**, *303*, 607–621. [CrossRef]
272. Ibaraki, H.; Kanazawa, T.; Oogi, C.; Takashima, Y.; Seta, Y. Effects of surface charge and flexibility of liposomes on dermal drug delivery. *J. Drug Deliv. Sci. Technol.* **2019**, *50*, 155–162. [CrossRef]
273. Akbarzadeh, A.; Rezaei-Sadabady, R.; Davaran, S.; Joo, S.W.; Zarghami, N.; Hanifehpour, Y.; Samiei, M.; Kouhi, M.; Nejati-Koshki, K. Liposome: Classification, preparation, and applications. *Nanoscale Res. Lett.* **2013**, *8*, 102. [CrossRef] [PubMed]
274. Malekar, S.A.; Sarode, A.L.; Bach, A.C., II; Worthen, D.R. The Localization of Phenolic Compounds in Liposomal Bilayers and Their Effects on Surface Characteristics and Colloidal Stability. *AAPS PharmSciTech* **2016**, *17*, 1468–1476. [CrossRef] [PubMed]
275. Jacquot, A.; Francius, G.; Razafitianamaharavo, A.; Dehghani, F.; Tamayol, A.; Linder, M.; Arab-Tehrany, E. Morphological and Physical Analysis of Natural Phospholipids-Based Biomembranes. *PLoS ONE* **2014**, *9*, e107435. [CrossRef] [PubMed]
276. Bozzuto, G.; Molinari, A. Liposomes as nanomedical devices. *Int. J. Nanomed.* **2015**, *10*, 975–999. [CrossRef] [PubMed]
277. Zoabi, A.; Touitou, E.; Margulis, K. Recent Advances in Nanomaterials for Dermal and Transdermal Applications. *Colloids Interfaces* **2021**, *5*, 18. [CrossRef]
278. Figueroa-Robles, A.; Antunes-Ricardo, M.; Guajardo-Flores, D. Encapsulation of phenolic compounds with liposomal improvement in the cosmetic industry. *Int. J. Pharm.* **2021**, *593*, 120125. [CrossRef]
279. Chinnagounder Periyasamy, P.; Leijten, J.C.H.; Dijkstra, P.J.; Karperien, M.; Post, J.N. Nanomaterials for the Local and Targeted Delivery of Osteoarthritis Drugs. *J. Nanomater.* **2012**, *2012*, 1–13. [CrossRef]
280. Verma, D.D.; Verma, S.; Blume, G.; Fahr, A. Particle size of liposomes influences dermal delivery of substances into skin. *Int. J. Pharm.* **2003**, *258*, 141–151. [CrossRef]
281. Hua, S. Lipid-based nano-delivery systems for skin delivery of drugs and bioactives. *Front. Pharmacol.* **2015**, *6*, 219. [CrossRef]
282. Zeb, A.; Arif, S.T.; Malik, M.; Shah, F.A.; Din, F.U.; Qureshi, O.S.; Lee, E.-S.; Lee, G.-Y.; Kim, J.-K. Potential of nanoparticulate carriers for improved drug delivery via skin. *J. Pharm. Investig.* **2018**, *49*, 485–517. [CrossRef]
283. Park, S.N.; Jo, N.R.; Jeon, S.H. Chitosan-coated liposomes for enhanced skin permeation of resveratrol. *J. Ind. Eng. Chem.* **2014**, *20*, 1481–1485. [CrossRef]
284. Mishra, V.; Bansal, K.; Verma, A.; Yadav, N.; Thakur, S.; Sudhakar, K.; Rosenholm, J. Solid Lipid Nanoparticles: Emerging Colloidal Nano Drug Delivery Systems. *Pharmaceutics* **2018**, *10*, 191. [CrossRef] [PubMed]
285. Mohammadi-Samani, S.; Ghasemiyeh, P. Solid lipid nanoparticles and nanostructured lipid carriers as novel drug delivery systems: Applications, advantages and disadvantages. *Res. Pharm. Sci.* **2018**, *13*, 288–303. [CrossRef]
286. Czajkowska-Kośnik, A.; Szekalska, M.; Winnicka, K. Nanostructured lipid carriers: A potential use for skin drug delivery systems. *Pharmacol. Rep.* **2019**, *71*, 156–166. [CrossRef] [PubMed]
287. Attama, A.A.; Momoh, M.A.; Builders, P.F. Lipid Nanoparticulate Drug Delivery Systems: A Revolution in Dosage Form Design and Development. In *Recent Advances in Novel Drug Carrier Systems*; Sezer, A.D., Ed.; IntechOpen: London, UK, 2012; pp. 107–140.
288. Müller, R.H.; Radtke, M.; Wissing, S.A. Solid lipid nanoparticles (SLN) and nanostructured lipid carriers (NLC) in cosmetic and dermatological preparations. *Adv. Drug Deliv. Rev.* **2002**, *54*, S131–S155. [CrossRef]

289. Liu, M.; Wen, J.; Sharma, M. Solid Lipid Nanoparticles for Topical Drug Delivery: Mechanisms, Dosage Form Perspectives, and Translational Status. *Curr. Pharm. Des.* **2020**, *26*, 3203–3217. [CrossRef] [PubMed]
290. Balamurugan, K.; Chintamani, P. Lipid nano particulate drug delivery: An overview of the emerging trend. *Pharma Innov. J.* **2018**, *7*, 779–789.
291. Wissing, S.; Lippacher, A.; Müller, R. Investigations on the occlusive properties of solid lipid nanoparticles (SLN). *J. Cosmet. Sci.* **2001**, *52*, 313–324. [PubMed]
292. Kakkar, V.; Kaur, I.P.; Kaur, A.P.; Saini, K.; Singh, K.K. Topical delivery of tetrahydrocurcumin lipid nanoparticles effectively inhibits skin inflammation: In *vitro* and in vivo study. *Drug Dev. Ind. Pharm.* **2018**, *44*, 1701–1712. [CrossRef]
293. Borges, A.; de Freitas, V.; Mateus, N.; Fernandes, I.; Oliveira, J. Solid Lipid Nanoparticles as Carriers of Natural Phenolic Compounds. *Antioxidants* **2020**, *9*, 998. [CrossRef]
294. Costa, C.P.; Barreiro, S.; Moreira, J.N.; Silva, R.; Almeida, H.; Sousa Lobo, J.M.; Silva, A.C. In Vitro Studies on Nasal Formulations of Nanostructured Lipid Carriers (NLC) and Solid Lipid Nanoparticles (SLN). *Pharmaceuticals* **2021**, *14*, 711. [CrossRef]
295. Garcês, A.; Amaral, M.H.; Sousa Lobo, J.M.; Silva, A.C. Formulations based on solid lipid nanoparticles (SLN) and nanostructured lipid carriers (NLC) for cutaneous use: A review. *Eur. J. Pharm. Sci.* **2018**, *112*, 159–167. [CrossRef]
296. Bhise, K.; Kashaw, S.K.; Sau, S.; Iyer, A.K. Nanostructured lipid carriers employing polyphenols as promising anticancer agents: Quality by design (QbD) approach. *Int. J. Pharm.* **2017**, *526*, 506–515. [CrossRef] [PubMed]
297. Tichota, D.; Silva, A.C.; Sousa Lobo, J.M.; Amaral, M.H. Design, characterization, and clinical evaluation of argan oil nanostructured lipid carriers to improve skin hydration. *Int. J. Nanomedicine* **2014**, *9*, 3855–3864. [PubMed]
298. Battaglia, L.; Ugazio, E. Lipid Nano- and Microparticles: An Overview of Patent-Related Research. *J. Nanomater.* **2019**, *2019*, 1–22. [CrossRef]
299. Jaiswal, P.; Gidwani, B.; Vyas, A. Nanostructured lipid carriers and their current application in targeted drug delivery. *Artif. Cells Nanomed. Biotechnol.* **2016**, *44*, 27–40. [CrossRef]
300. Puglia, C.; Lauro, M.; Offerta, A.; Crascì, L.; Micicchè, L.; Panico, A.; Bonina, F.; Puglisi, G. Nanostructured Lipid Carriers (NLC) as Vehicles for Topical Administration of Sesamol: In Vitro Percutaneous Absorption Study and Evaluation of Antioxidant Activity. *Planta Med.* **2016**, *83*, 398–404. [CrossRef] [PubMed]
301. Loo, C.H.; Basri, M.; Ismail, R.; Lau, H.L.N.; Tejo, B.A.; Kanthimathi, M.S.; Hassan, H.A.; Choo, Y. Effect of compositions in nanostructured lipid carriers (NLC) on skin hydration and occlusion. *Int. J. Nanomedicine* **2013**, *8*, 13–22. [CrossRef]
302. Jaiswal, M.; Dudhe, R.; Sharma, P.K. Nanoemulsion: An advanced mode of drug delivery system. *3 Biotech.* **2014**, *5*, 123–127. [CrossRef] [PubMed]
303. Che Marzuki, N.H.; Wahab, R.A.; Abdul Hamid, M. An overview of nanoemulsion: Concepts of development and cosmeceutical applications. *Biotechnol. Biotechnol. Equip.* **2019**, *33*, 779–797. [CrossRef]
304. Nastiti, C.; Ponto, T.; Abd, E.; Grice, J.; Benson, H.; Roberts, M. Topical Nano and Microemulsions for Skin Delivery. *Pharmaceutics* **2017**, *9*, 37. [CrossRef]
305. Ugur Kaplan, A.B.; Cetin, M.; Orgul, D.; Taghizadehghalehjoughi, A.; Hacımuftuoglu, A.; Hekimoglu, S. Formulation and in vitro evaluation of topical nanoemulsion and nanoemulsion-based gels containing daidzein. *J. Drug Deliv. Sci. Technol.* **2019**, *52*, 189–203. [CrossRef]
306. Su, R.; Fan, W.; Yu, Q.; Dong, X.; Qi, J.; Zhu, Q.; Zhao, W.; Wu, W.; Chen, Z.; Li, Y.; et al. Size-dependent penetration of nanoemulsions into epidermis and hair follicles: Implications for transdermal delivery and immunization. *Oncotarget* **2017**, *8*, 38214–38226. [CrossRef]
307. Rai, V.K.; Mishra, N.; Yadav, K.S.; Yadav, N.P. Nanoemulsion as pharmaceutical carrier for dermal and transdermal drug delivery: Formulation, development, stability issues, basic considerations and applications. *J. Control. Release* **2018**, *270*, 203–225. [CrossRef] [PubMed]
308. Aswathanarayan, J.B.; Vittal, R.R. Nanoemulsions and Their Potential Applications in Food Industry. *Front. Sustain. Food Syst.* **2019**, *3*, 95. [CrossRef]
309. Liu, C.; Hu, J.; Sui, H.; Zhao, Q.; Zhang, X.; Wang, W. Enhanced skin permeation of glabridin using eutectic mixture-based nanoemulsion. *Drug Deliv. Transl. Res.* **2017**, *7*, 325–332. [CrossRef] [PubMed]
310. Shaker, D.S.; Ishak, R.A.H.; Ghoneim, A.; Elhuoni, M.A. Nanoemulsion: A Review on Mechanisms for the Transdermal Delivery of Hydrophobic and Hydrophilic Drugs. *Sci. Pharm.* **2019**, *87*, 17. [CrossRef]
311. Ghanbarzadeh, S.; Hariri, R.; Kouhsoltani, M.; Shokri, J.; Javadzadeh, Y.; Hamishehkar, H. Enhanced stability and dermal delivery of hydroquinone using solid lipid nanoparticles. *Colloids Surf. B. Biointerfaces* **2015**, *136*, 1004–1010. [CrossRef] [PubMed]
312. Wen, A.-H.; Choi, M.-K.; Kim, D.-D. Formulation of Liposome for topical delivery of arbutin. *Arch. Pharm. Res.* **2006**, *29*, 1187–1192. [CrossRef]
313. de Lourdes Reis Giada, M. Food Phenolic Compounds: Main Classes, Sources and Their Antioxidant Power. In *Oxidative Stress and Chronic Degenerative Diseases—A Role for Antioxidants*; Morales-Gonzalez, J.A., Ed.; IntechOpen: London, UK, 2013; pp. 87–112.
314. Mostafa, M.; Alaaeldin, E.; Aly, U.F.; Sarhan, H.A. Optimization and Characterization of Thymoquinone-Loaded Liposomes with Enhanced Topical Anti-inflammatory Activity. *AAPS PharmSciTech* **2018**, *19*, 3490–3500. [CrossRef]
315. Kakkar, S.; Bais, S. A Review on Protocatechuic Acid and Its Pharmacological Potential. *Int. Sch. Res. Notices* **2014**, *2014*, 1–9. [CrossRef]

316. Daré, R.G.; Costa, A.; Nakamura, C.V.; Truiti, M.C.T.; Ximenes, V.F.; Lautenschlager, S.O.S.; Sarmento, B. Evaluation of lipid nanoparticles for topical delivery of protocatechuic acid and ethyl protocatechuate as a new photoprotection strategy. *Int. J. Pharm.* **2020**, *582*, 119336. [CrossRef]
317. Harwansh, R.K.; Mukherjee, P.K.; Bahadur, S.; Biswas, R. Enhanced permeability of ferulic acid loaded nanoemulsion based gel through skin against UVA mediated oxidative stress. *Life Sci.* **2015**, *141*, 202–211. [CrossRef]
318. Katuwavila, N.P.; Perera, A.D.L.C.; Karunaratne, V.; Amaratunga, G.A.J.; Karunaratne, D.N. Improved Delivery of Caffeic Acid through Liposomal Encapsulation. *J. Nanomater.* **2016**, *2016*, 1–7. [CrossRef]
319. Garg, A.; Singh, S. Targeting of eugenol-loaded solid lipid nanoparticles to the epidermal layer of human skin. *Nanomedicine* **2014**, *9*, 1223–1238. [CrossRef]
320. Tsai, M.-J.; Huang, Y.-B.; Fang, J.-W.; Fu, Y.-S.; Wu, P.-C. Preparation and Characterization of Naringenin-Loaded Elastic Liposomes for Topical Application. *PLoS ONE* **2015**, *10*, e0131026. [CrossRef]
321. Durán, N.; Costa, A.F.; Stanisic, D.; Bernardes, J.S.; Tasic, L. Nanotoxicity and Dermal Application of Nanostructured Lipid Carrier Loaded with Hesperidin from Orange Residue. *J. Phys. Conf. Ser.* **2019**, *1323*, 012021. [CrossRef]
322. Nemitz, M.C.; von Poser, G.L.; Teixeira, H.F. In vitro skin permeation/retention of daidzein, genistein and glycitein from a soybean isoflavone rich fraction-loaded nanoemulsions and derived hydrogels. *J. Drug Deliv. Sci. Technol.* **2019**, *51*, 63–69. [CrossRef]
323. Chou, T.-H.; Liang, C.-H. The Molecular Effects of Aloe-Emodin (AE)/Liposome-AE on Human Nonmelanoma Skin Cancer Cells and Skin Permeation. *Chem. Res. Toxicol.* **2009**, *22*, 2017–2028. [CrossRef] [PubMed]
324. Campani, V.; Marchese, D.; Pitaro, M.T.; Pitaro, M.; Grieco, P.; De Rosa, G. Development of a liposome-based formulation for vitamin K1 nebulization on the skin. *Int. J. Nanomedicine* **2014**, *9*, 1823–1832. [PubMed]
325. Pleguezuelos-Villa, M.; Nácher, A.; Hernández, M.J.; Ofelia Vila Buso, M.A.; Ruiz Sauri, A.; Díez-Sales, O. Mangiferin nanoemulsions in treatment of inflammatory disorders and skin regeneration. *Int. J. Pharm.* **2019**, *564*, 299–307. [CrossRef] [PubMed]
326. Gugleva, V.; Zasheva, S.; Hristova, M.; Andonova, V. Topical use of resveratrol: Technological aspects. *Pharmacia* **2020**, *67*, 89–94. [CrossRef]
327. Gokce, E.; Korkmaz, E.; Dellera, E.; Sandri, G.; Bonferoni, M.C.; Ozer, O. Resveratrol-loaded solid lipid nanoparticles versus nanostructured lipid carriers: Evaluation of antioxidant potential for dermal applications. *Int. J. Nanomedicine* **2012**, *7*, 1841–1850. [CrossRef]
328. Sirerol, J.A.; Feddi, F.; Mena, S.; Rodriguez, M.L.; Sirera, P.; Aupí, M.; Pérez, S.; Asensi, M.; Ortega, A.; Estrela, J.M. Topical treatment with pterostilbene, a natural phytoalexin, effectively protects hairless mice against UVB radiation-induced skin damage and carcinogenesis. *Free Radic. Biol. Med.* **2015**, *85*, 1–11. [CrossRef] [PubMed]
329. Singh Hallan, S.; Sguizzato, M.; Pavoni, G.; Baldisserotto, A.; Drechsler, M.; Mariani, P.; Esposito, E.; Cortesi, R. Ellagic Acid Containing Nanostructured Lipid Carriers for Topical Application: A Preliminary Study. *Molecules* **2020**, *25*, 1449. [CrossRef] [PubMed]
330. Ferreira, M.S.; Magalhães, M.C.; Oliveira, R.; Sousa-Lobo, J.M.; Almeida, I.F. Trends in the Use of Botanicals in Anti-Aging Cosmetics. *Molecules* **2021**, *26*, 3584. [CrossRef] [PubMed]
331. SESDERMA Listening to Your Skin. Available online: https://www.sesderma.com/eu_en/home (accessed on 23 July 2021).
332. M.Y.R. COSMETICS SOLUTION Innovative Organization. Available online: https://www.myrcosmeticssolution.com/ (accessed on 23 July 2021).
333. VITACOS Corporation. Available online: http://www.vitacos.co.kr/english/main.php?m1=44&m2=46&m3=&board_mode=list&board_no=19&board_search_keyword=&board_page=1&board_search_head_word=&board_mode=view&board_no=20 (accessed on 23 July 2021).

pharmaceuticals

MDPI

Review

Lipid Nanoparticulate Drug Delivery Systems: Recent Advances in the Treatment of Skin Disorders

Stefan R. Stefanov * and **Velichka Y. Andonova**

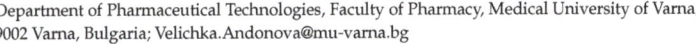

Department of Pharmaceutical Technologies, Faculty of Pharmacy, Medical University of Varna, 9002 Varna, Bulgaria; Velichka.Andonova@mu-varna.bg
* Correspondence: Stefan.Stefanov@mu-varna.bg

Abstract: The multifunctional role of the human skin is well known. It acts as a sensory and immune organ that protects the human body from harmful environmental impacts such as chemical, mechanical, and physical threats, reduces UV radiation effects, prevents moisture loss, and helps thermoregulation. In this regard, skin disorders related to skin integrity require adequate treatment. Lipid nanoparticles (LN) are recognized as promising drug delivery systems (DDS) in treating skin disorders. Solid lipid nanoparticles (SLN) together with nanostructured lipid carriers (NLC) exhibit excellent tolerability as these are produced from physiological and biodegradable lipids. Moreover, LN applied to the skin can improve stability, drug targeting, occlusion, penetration enhancement, and increased skin hydration compared with other drug nanocarriers. Furthermore, the features of LN can be enhanced by inclusion in suitable bases such as creams, ointments, gels (i.e., hydrogel, emulgel, bigel), lotions, etc. This review focuses on recent developments in lipid nanoparticle systems and their application to treating skin diseases. We point out and consider the reasons for their creation, pay attention to their advantages and disadvantages, list the main production techniques for obtaining them, and examine the place assigned to them in solving the problems caused by skin disorders.

Keywords: skin diseases; lipid-based nanosystems; solid lipid nanoparticles; nanostructured lipid carriers; cream; ointment; gel

Citation: Stefanov, S.R.; Andonova, V.Y. Lipid Nanoparticulate Drug Delivery Systems: Recent Advances in the Treatment of Skin Disorders. *Pharmaceuticals* **2021**, *14*, 1083. https://doi.org/10.3390/ph14111083

Academic Editors: Ana Catarina Silva, João Nuno Moreira, José Manuel Sousa Lobo and Jianping Qi

Received: 17 August 2021
Accepted: 21 October 2021
Published: 26 October 2021

1. Introduction

Skin diseases cause significant discomfort to millions of people around the world daily. Various studies show that between 30 and 70% of the world's population suffers from skin diseases [1]. In most cases, skin diseases are caused mainly by various infectious pathogens (bacteria, fungi, viruses) or inflammatory processes of various etiologies [2,3]. The majority of skin diseases are acute and have a significant psychological impact on individuals. Despite substantial advances in dermatological treatment, many infectious skin problems remain complex and persistent in treatment. These problems depend on the type of pathogen, the integrity of the skin layers, and especially on the patient's medical status [4]. A number skin diseases such as atopic dermatitis, allergic contact dermatitis, and psoriasis are chronic and represent a complex result of infiltration of inflammatory T cells and increased production of cytokines in the lesions [5]. The success of topical treatment of skin diseases requires a timely, accurate diagnosis, as well as an effective, simple, and not very invasive targeted topical treatment. In addition, it depends on the type of dosage form (the type of delivery system used to supply the drug to the skin) and the application method [6].

This review focuses on the recent advances of lipid-based nanosystems in the treatment of skin disorders. We discuss the most common types of lipid-based nanocarriers researched for dermal drug delivery and used for the treatment of skin disorders by incorporation into appropriate dosage forms, namely: Nanovesicular carriers, lipid nanoparticulate carriers, microemulsions, and nanoemulsions. The considered compositions are intended principally for local treatment and are an attempt to reflect the current picture of development in this field.

2. Skin

The skin is the largest metabolically active organ of the human body. Its vital functions include protection from external environmental threats, vitamin D synthesis, and the maintenance of the body's dynamic balance [7–9]. Moreover, the protective function is expressed by limiting the direct invasion of microorganisms as a physical barrier [10]. This defensive mechanism provides physical and immunological, metabolic, and UV protection [11]. Good knowledge of the barrier properties of the skin and the assessment of changes in the barrier functions as a result of skin diseases can be used to successfully develop new effective drug delivery systems, especially for the diseased skin and for the application of therapeutic agents such as drugs or vaccines [12,13]. Topical pharmaceuticals for the treatment of skin disorders can reach the problematic site without the risk of massive systemic absorption or other lateral effects [14].

In short, the skin consists of three main layers—epidermis, dermis, and hypodermis (subcutaneous fat tissue) [15].

The superficial part of the skin is called the epidermis. In essence, it is a laminar, squamous corneal epithelium composed mostly of two types of cells: Keratinocytes and dendritic cells (antigen-presenting cells) [16].

The epidermis consists of five layers—the stratum corneum, stratum lucidum, stratum granulosum (granular ply), stratum spinosum (spinous ply), and stratum germinativum (basal ply) [17]. No blood vessels were found in the epidermis [18]. The structure of the epidermis is schematically represented in Figure 1.

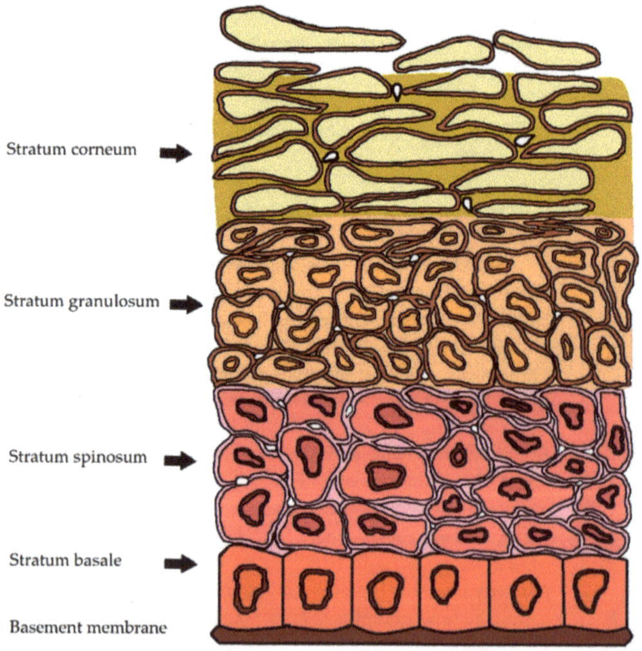

Figure 1. Schematic representation of the epidermis. Epidermis has a thickness of 0.1–0.2 mm. Stratum corneum (10–20 μm) and the viable epidermis (50–150 μm).

The outermost sublayer of the epidermis, named *stratum corneum* (SC) (10–20 μm), plays a fundamental role as the body's first and main physical skin barrier from external menaces [19–21]. It consists of corneocytes—specific cells that are the essential limiting factor for permeation through the skin, restricting the passage of molecules significantly larger than 500 Da [22]. The SC functions as a two-compartment system organized in a "brick and mortar" formation, with an extracellular matrix of lamellar membranes [23]. The structure of the stratum corneum is schematically represented in Figure 2.

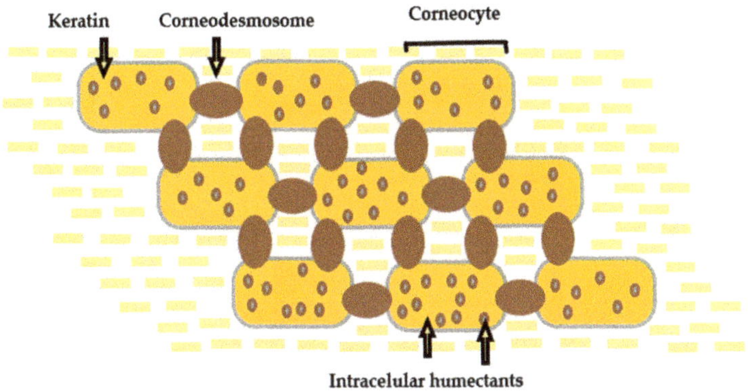

Figure 2. Structure of the *stratum corneum*—"brick and mortar" formation. The pathway between the stacked corneocytes is filled with "mortar" lipids.

The permeation of matter through the SC is possible primarily through passive diffusion in three ways: Transcellular (the bulk of flux), intercellular, and appendageal [24–26]. For all of the substances permeating the skin, diffusion through the SC is a rate-limiting stage [27]. In this regard, significant efforts are being made to establish and improve skin nanoparticle delivery systems that can supply and sustainably release active substances of varying lipophilicity and molecular weights to and through the skin, as well as ensure their protection against skin metabolism [28].

Keratinocytes, melanocytes (melanin producers), Merkel cells (sensory receptors), and Langerhans cells (immunocompetent cells) are epidermal formations—essential for the skin's vitality [29]. In addition, it is crucial to consider the barrier nature of the diseased skin, since there are substantial differences in barrier abilities between healthy and diseased skin. Therefore, we have reason to say that the skin reflects a person's health.

3. Skin Disorders

The skin can be affected by various pathological changes, i.e., inflammatory, neoplastic, traumatic, hormonal, degenerative, and even hereditarily determined [30]. Infectious skin diseases such as bacterial, fungal or viral affect people and cause various dermatological problems. Chronic inflammatory skin diseases such as atopic dermatitis, allergic contact dermatitis, psoriasis, etc., are a consequence of infiltration of inflammatory T cells [31]. The schematic representation of various skin disorders is shown in Figure 3 [32–43].

In practice, most of the skin disorders are complicated, polygenic, and multifactorial [44]. This indicates that multiple factors, lifestyle, and the environment play a fundamental role in the clinical picture of the diseases [45].

Treatment of Skin Disorders with Conventional Topical Delivery Systems

The human skin creates a vast opportunity for drug delivery application. In general, dermal (topical) and transdermal skin drug delivery can be differentiated. Dermal delivery is the application of the drug directly at the place of action—on the skin's surface. Transdermal drug delivery is an alternative, painless, and non-invasive approach used to deliver drugs for therapeutic use [46].

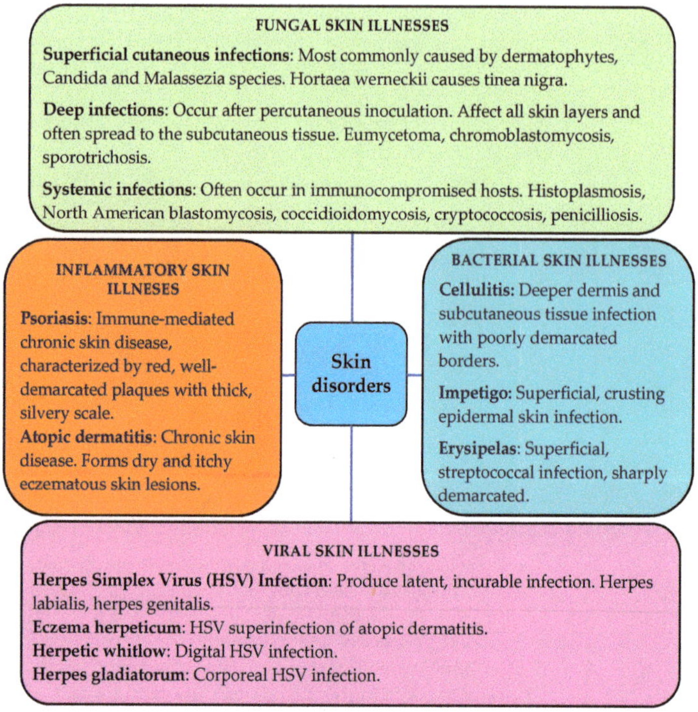

Figure 3. Representation of the most common skin disorders [32–43].

Many conventional topical preparations are intended for topical delivery of the drug and not for systemic action. This skin preparation delivers a concentrated amount of the active ingredient for absorption via the application layer [47]. In addition, the use of penetration enhancers in conventional formulations increases the delivery rate through the epidermis, but can also cause unwanted side effects [48].

Some of the commonly used therapeutic solutions are listed in Table 1.

Table 1. Mostly used therapeutic solutions for T cell-mediated skin disorders.

Drug Substance	Main Action	References
Corticosteroids	For local application. Manifests a slight immunosuppressive effect. Ineffectiveness in severe cases.	[49]
Retinoids	Retinoids can be synthetic or natural derivatives of vitamin A. Probable mechanisms of action: Facilitate the transport of cytoplasmic retinoid-binding proteins; influence angiogenesis; modulate T cell responses.	[50,51]
Vitamin D3 metabolites	Metabolites of vitamin D3 are included in ointments and creams for the treatment of psoriasis. Good effects in milder diseases. Not fully understood effects. The 1,25(OH)2D3 enhances the suppressive activity of CD4(+)CD25(+) cells in draining lymph nodes.	[52–54]
UVB treatment	Multiple effects and effectiveness for several T cell-mediated skin diseases. Not equally effective in the different disorders. Unspecific and generally immunosuppressive.	[55–57]
Methotrexate	Immunosuppressive effect. It does not target specific T cell groups. Still not a fully understood therapeutic effect.	[49,51]
Cyclosporine A	Affects IL-2 producing cells, in particular CD4(+) T cells. General immunosuppressive effect.	[49,51]

For chronic inflammatory skin diseases, a topical treatment is often not too efficient. Therefore, more efficacious medicinal products (MP) are given systemically, where they can be immunosuppressive, and their long-term usage is not recommended as they suppress the affected area [58].

A large part of therapeutic indications is treated by MP, which are intended for topical administration [59]. These MP feature different molecular structures, but retain some common physicochemical characteristics such as high lipophilicity and poor aqueous solubility. For them, the rate and extent of drug delivery have to be sufficient to achieve local therapeutic concentrations in an acceptable term and provide an effective pharmacological action [60].

The barrier function of the targeted biologic membrane provides a significant challenge for optimal therapy. The efficacy of drug delivery and the therapeutic effect depend mainly on the diffusion affinity of the drug substance and the interaction between the excipients of the formulation and the membrane components. Therefore, the conducive balance between potency and deliverability has to be ensured through the design and development of a delivery system to reach optimum therapeutic levels at the site of infection [60].

Biologics have become increasingly popular as a targeted treatment. Biologics are products composed of sugars, proteins, nucleic acids or complex combinations of these substances. Several biologics that target specific subgroups of cells in the skin have been tested [61].

Empirical experience shows that conventional topical preparations suffer from certain limitations and are compromised in patient compliance, safety, and efficacy of therapy [62]. Against this background, the need for advanced carriers that could effectively improve skin penetration and reduce drug-related side effects is more than necessary [63].

An inventive strategy for improving the penetration of molecules through the epidermal barrier is the application of nanocarriers due to the advantage of their lipophilicity, which mediates the passage through the intact lipid layer. The use of lipid nanoparticles in dermal formulations provides several benefits: Chemical protection of the incorporated drug molecules, application to the skin of labile drug substances, improved bioavailability of drugs, and the ability for better release by provision penetration and retention in the skin [64].

Lipid-based nanosystems have proven to be suitable for dermal carriers due to their biocompatibility, efficient delivery of active ingredients, and stability. In addition, their enhanced surface leads to the improved penetration of active ingredients [65].

4. Lipid-Based Drug Delivery Systems

Lipid-based drug delivery systems (LBDDS) are formulations containing a dissolved or suspended drug substance in lipidic excipients [66]. LBDDS are a progressive strategy to formulate pharmaceuticals for topical delivery [67]. Liposomes, which are "pioneers" among lipid DDS, have been used to improve drug solubility and traditionally for topical and transdermal drug delivery.

Table 2 presents a brief overview of lipid-based drug delivery systems.

Table 2. Presentation of some lipid-based delivery systems.

Lipid-Based Delivery System	Description	Advantages	Disadvantages
		Nanovesicular carriers	
Liposomes [68]	Conventional single or multilayer vesicles. Formed by contact of biodegradable lipids with an aqueous medium. Widely used as drug carriers for hydrophilic and lipophilic molecules.	Biocompatible and biodegradable lipids. Conventional production processes. Improved local delivery. Suitable for loading both hydrophobic and hydrophilic substances.	Insufficient chemical and physical stability. Short half-life. Inadequate penetration into the viable epidermis and dermis. High production costs. Difficulties in scalability.
Transfersomes [69–71]	Highly deformable, elastic or ultra-flexible liposomes. Vesicles, similar to conventional liposomes in terms of preparation and structure. Claimed to permeate as intact vesicles through the skin layers. Functionally deformed due to the presence of an edge activator.	Smaller vesicle size, higher elasticity. Compared with conventional liposomes—better penetration through the skin. High membrane hydrophilicity and elasticity allow them to avoid aggregation and fusion under osmotic stress, unlike the conventional liposomes.	Elasticity of these vesicles can be compromised by hydrophobic drug loading. Occlusive application and complete skin hydration limit transdermal delivery due to inhibition of transdermal hydration. Relatively high production costs. Absence of well-established regulatory guidance for skin delivery.
Ethosomes [72,73]	Lipid vesicles are composed of phospholipids, ethanol, and water. Similar to liposomes in terms of their preparation techniques and structure. Concentration of ethanol 20–45%. Their size decreases with an increase in the ethanol concentration. Exhibit high encapsulation efficiency.	Appropriate for both hydrophobic and hydrophilic drug loading. Enhanced skin delivery under both occlusive and nonocclusive conditions. Higher elasticity, smaller vesicle size, and higher entrapment efficiency than conventional liposomes.	High ethanol content can lead to skin irritation and toxicity. Possible structural and chemical instability during long-term storage. Need to optimize the concentration of lipids and ethanol for improved physicochemical properties and stability of ethosomes.
		Lipid nanoparticulate carriers	
Solid lipid nanoparticles [74,75]	Colloidal lipid nanoparticles are composed of a physiological biodegradable solid lipophilic matrix (solid at room temperature and body temperature), in which the drug molecules can be incorporated.	Increased drug stability. High drug payload. Incorporation of lipophilic and hydrophilic drugs. Avoidance of organic solvents. Lack of biotoxicity of the carrier. Relatively cost-effective.	SLN are incorporated into semisolid carriers such as ointments and gels due to the high water content. Potential expulsion of active compounds during storage. Cost-effective manufacturing process.
Nanostructure Lipid Carriers [76,77]	Colloidal lipid nanoparticles composed of physiological mixing liquid lipid (oils) with the solid lipids, in which the liquid lipid is incorporated into the solid matrix or localized at the surface of solid particles	Improved drug loading compared with SLN. Lower water content compared with SLN. Firmly incorporates the drug substance during storage. Biodegradable and biocompatible. Large-scale production is easily possible.	Tendency to unpredictable gelation. Polymorphic transition. Low drug incorporation due to the crystalline structure of solid lipids. Lack of long-term stability data.
Lipospheres [78–80]	Microspheres, composed of solid hydrophobic lipid core and stabilized by a monolayer of a phospholipid embedded on the surface.	Improved drug stability, especially for photo-labile drugs. Possibility for controlled drug release. Controlled particle size. High drug loading. Biodegradable and biocompatible.	Larger particle size and poor skin permeation compared with lipid-based vesicular carriers, SLN, and NLC. Poor drug loading for hydrophilic compounds.

5. Nanovesicular Carriers

Liposomes (further accepted as conventional liposomes) are considered to be the first generation of nanovesicular carriers. They are small artificial vesicles of the spherical shape created from cholesterol and natural, non-toxic phospholipids with an enclosed inner aqueous core [81]. There are several methods for liposome preparation such as thin-film hydration, reverse phase evaporation, and microfluidic mixing [82]. In 1980, Mezei and Gulasekharam reported the first generation of liposomes as drug delivery systems for topical administration [83]. Since then, liposomes are widely applied as dermal drug carriers [84].

The second generation of nanovesicular carriers—transfersomes were developed in 1992 by Cevc et al. They are modified liposomes with an average diameter below 300 nm and contain an edge activator that makes transfersomes nearly eight times more flexible than the conventional liposomes [85–87]. Edge activators can be sorbitan esters, sodium cholate, polysorbates, dipotassium glycyrrhizinate, etc. [88]. The competitive advantage of transfersomes is their ability to squeeze through tiny holes, five to ten times smaller than the vesicles dimensions [89–92]. In 1996, Touitou designed the ethosomes—the next step for improving permeation abilities [93]. These contain a fluid bilayer in their structure due to the high concentration of ethanol—20 to 45 wt%. Ethosomes potentiate the penetration effect through the clogged and unlocked skin and lead to drug penetration to a depth of about 200 μm [94]. Numerous studies have been devoted to the efficacy of ethosomes for dermal drug delivery in both occlusive and non-occlusive applications [95,96]. They demonstrate an excellent ability to improve the skin permeation of drugs, both highly lipophilic and highly hydrophilic active ingredients [97–101]. A certain number of studies are reported for the superior skin delivery of ethosomes compared with liposomes, transferosomes, and commercial formulations [102]. For example, psoralen-loaded ethosomes (an antipsoriasis drug) have shown 3.50 and 2.15 times higher permeation flux and skin deposition, respectively, compared with liposomes [103].

Table 3 summarizes some of the patents for the application of ethosomal drug delivery.

Table 3. Presentation of some of the patents for the application of ethosomes in skin formulations.

Application	Title/Inventors	Year	Results
CN103006562 (A)	Daptomycin ethosome preparation/ Li Chong, Liu Xia, Yin Qikun, Wang Xiaoying, Chen Zhangbao	2013	Stable translucent dispersion system with a small and uniform particle size. High entrapment efficiency. Excellent transdermal performance. Simple and convenient preparation method.
EP 2810642 A1	Chitosan-modified ethosome structure/ Chin-Tung Lee, Po-Liang Chen	2013	The chitosan-modified ethosome structure contains different active substances. Improved storage and transportation.
CN103800277 (A)	Leflunomide ethosome composition and its preparation method/ Zhang Tao, Ding Yanji, Deng Jie, Luo Jing, Zhong Xiaodong	2014	Improves the transdermal rate of leflunomide. Improves curative effects.
CN103536700 A	Chinese medicinal ethosome gel patch for treating herpes zoster and preparation method thereof/Bu Ping, Hu Rong, Chen Lin, Wei Rong, Wu Huanhuan, Huang Xiaoli	2014	Easy in medication. Convenient to use. Good therapeutic effect. Strong analgesic action. No adverse reaction.
CN 104706571 A	Preparation method of ethosome/ natural material/polyvinyl alcohol composite hydrogel/Yang Xingxing, Lynn, Chen Mengxia, Fanlin Peng	2015	Addition of the polyvinyl alcohol, which improves the properties of the hydrogel.
CN106474065A	A kind of tetracaine ethosome and its preparation technology/Zhu Xiaoliang, Wu Dongze, Ma Xiaodong	2017	Stable in terms of component and proportion. Preferable percutaneous permeation.

5.1. Emerging Lipid Nanovesicular Carriers

The usefulness of different lipid vesicles prompted researchers to experiment with modifications to give them specific structural or application properties [104]. However, the current research on these vesicles is somewhat limited, especially for topical drug delivery. Table 4 lists the emerging lipid vesicles developed for skin drug delivery, in the recent past.

Table 4. Emerging lipid nanovesicular carriers for skin drug delivery.

Emerging Lipid Vesicles	Description	Reference
Niosomes	Nonionic surfactant and cholesterol (or its derivatives)—based vesicle with improved stability (especially oxidative stability).	[105,106]
Cubosomes	Submicron, nanostructured particles, composed of bicontinuous cubic liquid crystalline phase.	[107–109]
Hexosomes	Constructed of hexagonal liquid crystalline phases dispersed in a continuous aqueous medium.	[110]
Aquasomes	Self-assembled nanovesicles, composed of three layers.	[111]
Colloidosomes	Hollow shell microcapsules composed of coagulated particles.	[112]
Sphingosomes	Contained sphingolipids such as sphingosine, ceramide, sphingomyelin or glycosphingolipid; and are concentric, bilayered nanovesicles with an acidic pH inside.	[113]
Ufasomes	Lipid carriers attach to the surface of the skin and support the lipid exchange between the outermost layers of the SC.	[114,115]
Archeosomes	Consisted of archebacteria lipids, chemically distinct from eukaryotic and prokaryotic species. Less sensitive to high temperature, alkaline pH, and oxidative stress.	[116,117]
Lipoplexes	Cationic lipid-DNA complexes. Efficient carriers for cell transfection. Toxic effects arising from either cationic lipids or nucleic acids.	[118]
Proliposomes	Dry, free-flowing particles that immediately form a liposomal dispersion in contact with water.	[119,120]

Another nanovesicular carrier widely used for dermal drug delivery is called niosomes, with an average particle size between 50 and 200 nm [106]. These are based on nonionic surfactants and cholesterol and are considered more stable and less expensive than liposomes. Several methods can be used for niosomes preparation such as high-pressure homogenization, extrusion or sonication. Due to the small size of these vesicles, the drug loading and stability decrease. The problem can be solved by adding a stabilizer [121] that can be specified, as well as other nanovesicular carriers that are being increasingly explored in recent years for dermal delivery such as cubosomes, hexasomes, aquasomes, colloidosomes, sphingosomes, ufasomes, archeosomes, lipoplexes, proliposomes, etc. [111,122]. Cubosomes are bicontinuous cubic liquid crystalline phases with two different hydrophilic areas separated by a lipid bilayer [123]. Their preparation requires the usage of high-energy dispersion techniques [124,125]. Hexosomes are built from hexagonal liquid crystalline phases dispersed in a continuous aqueous medium [126]. Cubosomes and hexosomes can incorporate hydrophilic, hydrophobic, and amphiphilic drugs, increased drug loading, and good stability. It has recently been shown that incorporating bile salt edge activators into hexosomes can significantly improve their skin penetration properties [127]. Aquasomes are composed of three layers: A solid nanocrystalline core, an oligomeric shell, and a layer of a bioactive substance absorbed onto the shell [111]. They are produced via colloidal precipitation, plasma condensation, and inverted magnetron sputtering. Aquasomes have high drug loading capacity and can protect fragile drug molecules from degradation [128]. Colloidosomes are typically used to encapsulate sensitive bioactive compounds and are hollow shell microcapsules created of coagulated particles [111]. Sphingosomes are comprised of sphingolipids (sphingosine, ceramide, etc.) and are concentric, bilayered nanovesicles with an acidic pH inside [113]. The resultant vesicular systems can be unilamellar, multilamellar, oligolamellar or multivesicular. Different preparation methods such as reverse phase evaporation, mechanical dispersion, solvent injection, sonication, and microfluidization can be used for the production of sphingosomes. They are characterized by the enhanced drug loading efficiency and stability [129]. Ufasomes are composed of lipid bilayers derived from unsaturated fatty acids and ionic surfactants [130]. In parallel with the conventional liposomes, they are more stable and have a better drug loading efficiency, but are more susceptible to oxidation [131].

5.2. *Nanovesicular Carriers in the Treatment of Skin Disorders*

5.2.1. Antipsoriatic Effect

Psoriasis is a skin disorder characterized by impaired epidermal differentiation, commonly treated by systemic methotrexate, an effective cytotoxic drug. Abdelbary and Abou Ghaly generated topical methotrexate-loaded niosomes for the influence on psoriasis [132]. A thin-film hydration technique is used for the preparation by the inclusion of a surfactant (Span 60) and cholesterol. In comparison with the free drug solution, an increased drug deposition in the skin of rats is monitored.

5.2.2. Antifungal Effect

Perez et al. prepared ultra-deformable liposomes containing amphotericin B to treat cutaneous fungal infections and leishmaniasis [133]. Liposomes containing Tween 80 as an edge activator had maximal deformability and the highest drug/phospholipid ratio. Amphotericin B was encapsulated at 75% encapsulation efficiency in their bilayer. However, drug-loaded liposomes were more toxic to fungal strains than to mammalian cells.

5.2.3. Anti-Vitiligo Effect

Garg et al. developed ethosome-based nanohydrogel formulations of methoxsalen to effectively treat vitiligo with enhanced topical delivery [134]. The formulation contained approximately 28% of ethanol. Ethosomes are incorporated into Carbopol gels and showed substantially skin permeation (on rats), accumulating in epidermal and dermal layers. In addition, there are observed erythema and reduced skin phototoxicity in comparison with a conventional cream.

5.2.4. Anti-Acne Effect

The two main processes that are typical for *acne vulgaris* include:

- The proliferation of *propionibacterium acnes* bacteria in pilosebaceous units of the skin;
- Local inflammation [135].

Traditional topical anti-acne compositions mainly cause burning, erythema, photosensitivity, scaling, and bacterial resistance [136]. In 2008, Touitou et al. developed an ethosomal gel system containing clindamycin phosphate and salicylic acid for an efficient acne treatment and enhanced topical tolerability [135]. Recently, Apriani et al. developed an azelaic acid ethosome-based cream against *propionibacterium acne* [137]. The ethosomal cream demonstrated a superior antibactericidal activity compared with the marketed cream Zelface®.

5.2.5. Antiviral Effect

Acyclovir has been investigated for the topical treatment of viral infections for more than four decades [138]. In 1999, Horwitz et al. reported an ethosomal cream system for acyclovir—commercial Zovirax® [139]. Recently, Shukla et al. designed an ethosomal gel with acyclovir, where the ethosomes were prepared by the cold method [140]. The survey shows the in vitro drug release of 82% over 8 h with a zero-order release profile.

5.2.6. Local Anesthetic Effect

In the experimental work, Babaie et al. prepared lidocaine-loaded nanoethosomes for penetration into the deep strata of the skin with a particle size around 100 nm [141]. Increased ethanol concentration from 10 to 40% leads to the production of ethosomes with four-times larger particle sizes.

5.2.7. Antibiotic Effect

In 2005, Godin et al. developed an ethosomal system for the dermal delivery of antibiotics to improve their penetration through the SC and the bacterial membrane/cell wall [142,143]. In addition, Zahid et al. formulated ethosomes containing clindamycin phosphate in a recently announced report using a cold method [144]. The optimized formulation demonstrated an excellent in vitro drug release.

5.2.8. Anticarcinogenic Effect

A report by Cosco et al. represented the formation of transfersomes for the combined delivery of resveratrol and 5-fluorouracil. The co-encapsulation of the drugs synergistically improved their anti-cancer activity on skin cancer cells [145].

Table 5 presents the practical implementation of nanovesicular carriers in dermal drug delivery systems.

Table 5. Application of nanovesicular carriers in dermal DDS for the treatment of skin disorders.

LNP Type	API/Drug	Application	Reference
Conventional liposomes	Licorice	Licorice-loaded liposomes included in the formulation for the treatment of oxidative stress injuries.	[146]
Conventional liposomes	Quercetin and resveratrol	Quercetin- and resveratrol-loaded liposomes for the treatment of inflammatory/oxidative responses associated with skin cancer.	[147]
Liposomes	Tretinoin	A tretinoin-loaded liposomal formulation for the treatment of acne.	[148]
Liposomes	Benzoyl peroxide	Benzoyl peroxide and chloramphenicol encapsulation in liposomes for the treatment of acne.	[149]
Liposomes	Benzoyl peroxide/Adapalene	Benzoyl peroxide- and adapalene-loaded modified liposomal gel for the treatment of acne.	[150]
Transfersomes	Indocyanine green	Indocyanine green-loaded transfersomes for the treatment of acne vulgaris.	[151]
Transfersomes	5-Fluorouracil	5-Fluorouracil-loaded transfersomes for the treatment of skin cancer.	[152]
Transfersomes	Resveratrol and 5-fluorouracil	Transfersomes containing resveratrol and 5-fluorouracil for the treatment of skin cancer.	[145]
Transfersomes	Amphotericin B	Development of amphotericin B-loaded transfersomes for antifungal and antileishmanial treatment.	[133]
Transfersomes	siRNA	Transfersomes containing siRNA developed for delivery to the human basal epidermis for the treatment of melanoma.	[153]
Transfersomes	RNAi	Transfersomes containing RNAi, formulated for the treatment of psoriasis.	[154]
Transfersomes	Indocyanine	Indocyanine-loaded transfersomes for the treatment of basal cell carcinoma.	[155]
Transfersomes	Clindamycin	Development of clindamycin-loaded transfersomes for the treatment of acne.	[156]

Table 5. *Cont.*

LNP Type	API/Drug	Application	Reference
Transfersomes	Paclitaxel	Paclitaxel containing transfersomes, modified by a cell-penetrating-peptide embedded in oligopeptide hydrogel for the topical treatment of melanoma.	[157]
Transfersomes	Sodium stibogluconate	Transfersomes loaded with sodium stibogluconate for the treatment of leishmaniasis.	[158]
Transfersomes	Lidocaine	Lidocaine transferosomal gel, containing permeation enhancers for local anesthetic action.	[159]
Transfersomes	Sulforaphane	Transfersomes comprising sulforaphane for the treatment of skin cancer.	[160]
Transfersomes	Miltefosine polyphenol	Formulation of miltefosine polyphenol-loaded transfersomes for the topical treatment of leishmaniasis.	[161]
Transfersome	N-acetylcysteine	N-acetylcysteine-loaded transfersomes for antioxidant activity in anti-aging therapy.	[162]
Ethosomes	Methoxsalen	Formulation of ethosomes containing methoxsalen for the topical treatment against vitiligo.	[134]
Ethosomes	Griseofulvin	Design of griseofulvin-loaded ethosomes for enhanced antifungal treatment.	[163]
Ethosomes	Cryptotanshinone	Cryptotanshinone-loaded ethosomes for anti-acne treatment.	[164]
Ethosomes	Epigallocatechin-3-gallate	Epigallocatechin-3-gallate-loaded ethosomes for the treatment of skin cancer.	[165]
Ethosomes	Thymoquinone	Thymoquinone-loaded ethosomes for the topical treatment of acne.	[166]
Ethosomes	Clobetasol propionate	Ethosomes of clobetasol propionate for the treatment of eczema.	[167]
Ethosomes	Tretinoin	Gel containing tretinoin-loaded ethosomes for anti-acne treatment.	[168]
Ethosomes	Azelaic acid	Azelaic acid-loaded ethosomes for anti-acne treatment.	[137]
Niosomes	Resveratrol	Resveratrol-loaded niosomes for the treatment of psoriasis.	[169]
Niosomes	Diacerein	Niosomes for the topical diacerein delivery and treatment of psoriasis.	[170]
Niosomes	Celastrol	Celastrol-loaded niosomes for the treatment of psoriasis.	[171]
Cubosomes	Paclitaxel	Paclitaxel-loaded cubosomes against skin cancer.	[172]
Cubosomes	Erythromycin	Erythromycin-loaded cubosomes for the treatment of acne.	[173]
Hexosomes, cubosomes	Ketoconazole	Ketoconazole-loaded hexosomes for antifungal treatment.	[174]
Ufasomes	Minoxidil	Minoxidil-loaded ufasomes for the treatment of hair loss.	[175]

6. Solid Lipid Nanoparticles and Nanostructured Lipid Carriers

Solid lipid nanoparticles (SLN), as well as nanostructured lipid carriers (NLC), are extensively employed in cutaneous delivery systems. Since their creation in the nineties, lipid nanoparticles (SLN and NLC) are well known by the research and pharma technology community. Easily available raw materials, relatively simple production methods, biocompatibility, and non-toxicity as their advantages over other colloidal carriers can be mentioned as the main reasons for this [67].

Therefore, these two types of lipid nanoparticles—SLN and NLC, are classified according to their structure. First, SLN are developed with a composition of solid lipids only. Then, to upgrade to SLN, NLC were created by representing a mixture of solid and liquid lipids, with a predominant solid lipid [176].

The dermal use of SLN and NLC is proving to be one of the most convenient for therapeutic and cosmetic purposes, despite various applications to date. Lipid nanoparticles are aqueous dispersions with low viscosity for successful direct application to the skin, which implies their incorporation in semisolid systems based on SLN or NLC. One of the first successful administered and marketed products based on NLC is Cutanova® from Dr. Rimpler GmbH (Wedemark, Germany) and Nanobase® from Yamanouchi (Tokyo, Japan) [64].

6.1. *Solid Lipid Nanoparticles*

Generally speaking, SLN are nanometric colloidal carriers composed of a solid lipid core with an incorporated active pharmaceutical ingredient(s) (API) and a surfactant-stabilized shell [177–179]. SLN are composed in the 1990s and have unique properties such as biodegradability, impressive toxicity profile, protection of the API against degradation, high load capacity, sterilization ability, and scalability [180,181]. The interaction between the lipid core of SLN and the waxy lipids in SC leads to a significant permeation enhancement of the encapsulated drug into the skin, which determines their successful cutaneous application [182].

6.2. *Nanostructured Lipid Carriers*

The second generation of lipid nanoparticles—NLC, are composed of a mixture of solid lipids and liquid lipids in the nanocore, usually in a ratio of 7:3 to 9:1 [183]. This leads to a more significant disorder of the core of the lipid matrix, and accordingly decreases the melting point to stop the recrystallization of solid lipids [184]. NLC are considered to be an improved variety of SLN, holding the same unique properties, but with an optimized core composition, resulting in a higher drug loading capacity, better stability, and ability to act at lower temperatures. Of note is the fact that NLCs are still solid at body temperature [185].

6.3. *Preparation of SLN and NLC*

The literature describes a significant number of production methods and many different combinations of lipids to obtain SLN and NLC. Nevertheless, the most common technique used today is high-pressure homogenization (HPH). The procedure is divided into two stages:

- Hot homogenization—the lipids are heated above their melting point;
- Cold homogenization—takes place at low temperatures and is suitable for hydrophilic and temperature-sensitive API [186,187].

Other commonly used techniques are: Sonication/ultra-sonication [188,189], membrane contactor technique [190], phase inversion [191], solvent injection [192], emulsification [193], the microemulsion method [194], etc.

6.4. *SLN and NLC in the Treatment of Skin Disorders*

In dermal applications, SLN and NLC create a thin hydrophobic monolayer during skin contact, which has a pointed occlusive effect that settles the API penetration and prevents water loss from the skin [195].

When applied topically, the lipid nanoparticles interact with the sebum and specific skin lipids, provoking a change in the natural arrangement of corneocytes. As a result of this interaction, the encapsulated molecules are released, and their penetration into the lower layers of the epidermis and dermis is potentiated, depending on their lipophilicity, of course [196].

6.4.1. Antioxidant Effect

Okonogi and Riangjanapatee formulated NLC loaded with lycopene through a hot HPH. It has been found that the NLC with the highest concentration of lycopene had the slowest release rate and better antioxidant activity [197].

In another study, Shrotriya et al. reported the development of SLN loaded with resveratrol (entrapment efficiency of 86–89%) to treat irritant contact dermatitis (chronic skin disorder with eczematous injuries). The composition was realized by incorporation into a Carbopol gel and showed increased antioxidant activity compared with a conventional resveratrol gel [198].

Furthermore, Montenegro et al. designed a novel Idebenone (IDE)-loaded NLC containing tocopheryl acetate (VitE) as a liquid component to obtain a synergic effect between IDE and VitE [199].

6.4.2. Anti-Inflammatory Effect

Pivetta et al. formulated NLC with thymol for the local treatment of inflammatory skin diseases (entrapment efficiency of 89%). The NLC were incorporated into a gel and showed anti-inflammatory activity and healing of induced psoriasis in mice [200].

Gad et al. reported the encapsulation of chamomile oil in SLN for the local treatment of wounds. The composition contained stearic acid and chamomile oil and was prepared by the method of hot homogenization. Wound reduction was shown in the topical application in rats [201].

6.4.3. Antifungal Effect

Butani et al. developed a stable SLN system, containing amphotericin B with an enhancing antifungal activity (entrapment efficiency of 94%). The formulation indicated higher drug permeation and drug accumulation in the skin than the conventional gel in rats. A solvent diffusion technique was used for the preparation of the SLN [202].

NLC, for the treatment of candidiasis with Mediterranean essential oils and clotrimazole, were designed by Carbone et al. As a result, they are obtained as a stable NLC, without an initial burst effect and with prolonged release of clotrimazole, as well as an enhanced antifungal activity [203].

6.4.4. Anti-Acne Effect

Tretinoin-loaded NLC with anti-aging and anti-acne activities were reported by Ghate et al. The hot melt probe sonication and hot melt microemulsion methods were used to prepare the NLC. The tretinoin-loaded NLC in Carbopol gels showed no irritation or erythema after the application in rats [204].

Malik and Kaur developed the azelaic acid-loaded NLC, prepared by the melt emulsification and ultra-sonication method (entrapment efficiencies greater than 80%). NLC were incorporated into aloe-vera-based Carbopol hydrogels and demonstrated a deeper skin penetration than the commercial product (Aziderm 10%). Furthermore, the in vivo experiment in mice showed a higher effect of NLC incorporated into a gel than the plain drug suspended in the gel [205].

Table 6 presents the practical implementation of SLN and NLC in dermal drug delivery systems.

Table 6. Application of SLN and NLC DDS for the treatment of skin disorders.

LNP Type	API/Drug	Application	Reference
SLN	Doxorubicin	Doxorubicin-loaded SLN for the treatment of skin cancer.	[206]
SLN	Adapalene	Adapalene-loaded SLN in the gel for anti-acne treatment.	[207]
SLN	Triamcinolone acetonide	Triamcinolone acetonide-loaded SLN for the topical treatment of psoriasis.	[208]
SLN	Resveratrol, vitamin E, and epigallocatechin gallate	SLN containing resveratrol, vitamin E, and epigallocatechin gallate for antioxidant benefits.	[209]
SLN	Silybin	Silybin-loaded SLN enriched gel for irritant contact dermatitis.	[210]
SLN	Fluconazole	Fluconazole-loaded SLN topical gel for the treatment of pityriasis versicolor.	[211]
SLN	Tazarotene	Tazarotene-loaded SLN for the treatment of psoriasis.	[212]
SLN	Miconazole nitrate	Miconazole nitrate-loaded SLN for antifungal activity.	[213]
SLN	Adapalene	Adapalene-loaded SLN for anti-acne therapy.	[214]
SLN	Isotretinoin and α-tocopherol	SLN loaded with retinoic acid and lauric acid for the topical treatment of acne vulgaris.	[215]
NLC	Spironolactone	Spironolactone-loaded NLC-based gel for the effective treatment of acne vulgaris.	[216]
NLC	Clobetasol propionate	NLC-based topical gel of clobetasol propionate for the treatment of eczema.	[217]
NLC	Tacrolimus and tumor necrosis factor α siRNA	NLC co-delivering tacrolimus and tumor necrosis factor α siRNA for the treatment of psoriasis.	[218]
NLC	Itraconazole	Topical NLC containing itraconazole for the treatment of fungal infections.	[219]
NLC	Apremilast	NLC for topical delivery of apremilast for the treatment of psoriasis.	[220]
NLC	Dithranol	Dithranol-loaded NLC-based gel for the treatment of psoriasis.	[221]
NLC	Voriconazole	Voriconazole-loaded NLC for antifungal applications.	[222]
NLC	Mometasone furoate	NLC-based hydrogel of mometasone furoate for the treatment of psoriasis.	[223]
NLC	Antimicrobial peptide nisin Z	Antimicrobial peptide nisin Z with conventional antibiotic-loaded NLC to enhance antimicrobial activity.	[224]
NLC	Adapalene and vitamin C	Adapalene- and vitamin C-loaded NLC for acne treatment.	[225]

7. Microemulsions and Nanoemulsions

In general, microemulsions and nanoemulsions are dispersion systems composed of two immiscible liquid phases that can penetrate deeper levels of the skin [226]. Evidence suggests that they may disrupt the SC lipid structural order, resulting in the loss of skin barrier properties [227]. Despite the apparent similarities between these two systems representing low-viscosity colloidal dispersions, they are classified as entirely different formulations [228].

7.1. Microemulsions

It has been found that microemulsions are spontaneously formed, transparent, and isotropic thermodynamically stable dispersion systems. The composition of the droplets is carried out by the precise mixing of volumes of immiscible liquids (usually oil and water) and the interfacial film of stabilizing surfactants at specific pressures and temperatures [229]. Short alkyl chain alcohols such as co-surfactants are typically chosen to potent the spontaneous formation of microemulsions. The isotropic and visually mono-phasic transparent system, in which the droplet size is usually below 100 nm, creates a flexible interfacial film characterized by ultra-low surface tension values [230]. The microemulsion as a formulation can improve the delivery of skin MP with both hydrophilic and lipophilic active substances compared with conventional carriers. In this regard, Patel et al. reported that the microemulsion with ketoconazole penetrated more efficiently than the saturated aqueous solution [231].

Three various structural types of microemulsions can be formed:

- Oil-in-water (O/W) microemulsion;
- Water-in-oil (W/O) microemulsion;
- Bicontinuous microemulsion [232].

7.2. *Nanoemulsions*

Nanoemulsions typically contain 20–500 nm large droplets and have a different appearance depending on their size. Traditionally, they are stabilized by surfactants and do not change in the long term [233]. However, they are non-equilibrium structures, and an energetic input has to be typically applied (often from an emulsion) to form the droplet size according to the nanoscale [234]. The basic methods for preparing nanoemulsions are high-energy emulsifying methods such as HPH, ultrasound, jet spraying, microfluidization, and low energy emulsifying methods such as solvent displacement, spontaneous emulsification, phase inversion [235].

7.3. *Microemulsions and Nanoemulsions in the Treatment of Skin Disorders*

7.3.1. Antipsoriatic Effect

The clobetasol propionate- and calcipotriol-loaded nanoemulsion gel for the topical treatment of psoriasis is reported, developed, and optimized by Kaur et al. The spontaneous emulsification method was used for the preparation. Compared with the other commercial MP [236], the nanoemulsion containing gel showed higher antipsoriatic activity in mice.

Recently, Rajitha et al. reported the preparation of loaded nanoemulsion based on chaulmoogra oil, which is based on the self-emulsification method. Compared with the conventional methotrexate solution, the nanoemulsion showed enhanced skin permeation and retention of methotrexate in the deep skin layers [237].

7.3.2. Antifungal Effect

In another study, Coneac et al. reported the development of microemulsion-loaded hydrogels for the topical delivery of fluconazole. Nonionic surfactants have been used to stabilize the microemulsions, which then were incorporated in Carbopol gels. Compared with the conventional hydrogel and Nizoral® cream, the optimized microemulsion-loaded hydrogels showed higher in vitro flux values, higher release rate, and higher in vitro antifungal activity against Candida albicans [238].

7.3.3. Anti-Inflammatory Effect

Two nanoemulsion systems for the dermal application of natural or synthetic mixtures of pentacyclic triterpenes, with an anti-inflammatory effect, were reported by Alvarado et al. [239]. Slightly different permeation profiles of natural and synthetic triterpene-containing formulations are stated. The nanoemulsion, containing a natural triterpene mixture, demonstrated a more significant anti-inflammatory activity due to the slower permeation through the mouse skin [239].

In another study, Goindi et al. reported an ionic liquid-in-water microemulsion formulation that can solubilize etodolac, a poorly water-soluble anti-inflammatory drug. An effective permeation profile, as well as anti-arthritic and anti-inflammatory activities are evaluated in vivo in different models compared with a marketed formulation of etodolac (Proxym gel®) [240].

7.3.4. Antioxidant Effect

Lv et al. reported the preparation of essential oil-based microemulsions for topical application in order to improve the solubility, photostability, and skin permeation of quercetin. First, self-micro emulsifying DDS were prepared and then formed microemulsions. The microemulsions protected quercetin from degradation in an alkaline environment and under UV radiation. In these formulations, the in vitro skin permeation study on rats showed 2.5–3 times enhanced permeation capacity of quercetin compared with the conventional aqueous solution [241].

7.3.5. Local Anesthetic Effect

To optimize the percutaneous absorption of lidocaine and prilocaine, Negi et al. formed nanoemulsions using the high-shear mixing method followed by the HPH. The optimized nanoemulsion systems showed higher permeation rates and permeability coefficient values in parallel with the marketed cream and were further incorporated into a Carbopol hydrogel. In addition, the nanoemulsions and the nanoemulsion gel had a stronger anesthetic effect in vivo than the commercial product [242].

7.3.6. Anticarcinogenic Effect

In the last few years, Pham et al. developed a nano-emulsification approach to optimize the incorporation of Tocomin® for the accompanying therapy of skin carcinomas. Different preparation methods were used. The technique, combining a single-phase in-version temperature homogenization method with ultrasonication, produced a stable Tocomin®-loaded nanoemulsion, which demonstrated an exceeding cytotoxic profile against two human cutaneous carcinoma cell models [243].

Table 7 presents the practical implementation of microemulsions and nanoemulsions in dermal drug delivery systems.

Table 7. Application of microemulsions and nanoemulsions DDS for the treatment of skin disorders.

Type	API/Drug	Application	Reference
Microemulsion	Tazarotene	Tazarotene-loaded microemulsion for the treatment of psoriasis.	[244]
Microemulsion	Methotrexate	Methotrexate-loaded microemulsion for the treatment of psoriasis.	[245]
Microemulsion	Retinoid	Retinoid-loaded microemulsion for the treatment of psoriasis.	[246]
Microemulsion	Clotrimazole	Microemulsion coated with chitosan and containing clotrimazole for antifungal activity.	[247]
Microemulsion	Griseofulvin	Griseofulvin-loaded microemulsion for the antifungal treatment.	[248]
Microemulsion	Boswellia carterii oleo-gum-resin	Boswellia carterii oleo-gum resin-loaded microemulsion for the treatment of acne and eczema.	[249]
Microemulsion	Indian pennywort, walnut, and turmeric	Topical dosage microemulsion of Indian pennywort, walnut, and turmeric for the treatment of eczema.	[250]
Microemulsion	Triamcinolone	Microemulsion containing triamcinolone for transdermal delivery for the treatment of eczema.	[251]
Microemulsion	Retinyl palmitate	Microemulsion containing retinyl palmitate for the treatment of acne, aging, and psoriasis.	[252]
Nanoemulsion	Triptolide	Triptolide nanoemulsion gels for the treatment of eczema.	[253]
Nanoemulsion	Ivermectin	Nanoemulsion containing ivermectin for the treatment of different types of parasite infestations.	[254]
Nanoemulsion	Cyclosporine	Cyclosporine-loaded nanoemulsion for the treatment of psoriasis.	[255]

Table 7. *Cont.*

Type	API/Drug	Application	Reference
Nanoemulsion	Coumestrol /Hydroxyethylcellulose	Nanoemulsion containing coumestrol and hydroxyethylcellulose for the treatment of antiherpes.	[256]
Nanoemulsion	8-Methoxypsoralen	8-Methoxypsoralenloaded nanoemulsion for the treatment of vitiligo and psoriasis.	[257]
Nanoemulsion	Coenzyme Q10	Coenzyme Q10-loaded nanoemulsion as an antioxidant agent.	[258]
Nanoemulsion	Psoralen	Psoralen-loaded nanoemulsion for the treatment of psoriasis and vitiligo.	[259]
Nanoemulsion	Isotretinoin	Isotretinoin-loaded nanoemulsion for the treatment of acne.	[260]
Nanoemulsion	Amphotericin B	Amphotericin B-loaded nanoemulsion for the antifungal treatment.	[261]
Nanoemulsion	Zinc phthalocyanine	Zinc phthalocyanine-loaded nanoemulsion for use in photodynamic therapy for leishmaniasis.	[262]

8. Topical Dosage Forms with Lipid Nanoparticulate DDS for the Treatment of Skin Disorders

The size of Global Topical Drug Delivery Market was estimated at USD 95.08 billion in 2020 and expected to reach USD 101.10 billion in 2021 and USD 140.01 billion by 2026. The current market situation (USA, EUR, JP, AUS) for the topical skin products, shows domination of generic products—about 74% of all the approved topical products are generic equivalents of reference medicines (RLD). According to the collected data, gels, creams, ointments, lotions, and solutions dominate the market for both topical reference and topical generic products. The available semi-solid, solid, and liquid topical products contain different combinations of surfactants, oils, water, colloidal, and solid ingredients in solutions or dispersions [263].

Specific needs of skin, affected by inflammation, acne, or infections require adequate drug therapy with appropriate topical dosage forms. For example, the adhesive patch can provide a sustained and controlled release, while the gel can provide a faster and more intense action. On the other hand, some topical dosage forms may not be most suitable for application to certain areas of the skin, around the eyes, for example [264].

One of the most important considerations in the development of the topical dosage forms is the patient need. The second consideration is the drug's physicochemical properties. In general, regulatory procedures for the registration of topical products are slow, as clinical equivalence studies (clinical trials) involve a high number of participants, require time and significant costs to ensure a sufficiently objective assessment of the final therapeutic effect. Technological or cost problems are among the reasons for additional difficulties in the implementation of promising dermatological products [265].

Table 8 summarizes some of the literature available on topical nano-based topical dosage forms for skin diseases.

Table 8. Topical nanoformulations used in the treatment of various skin conditions.

Type	API/Drug	Disease	Reference
Nanoemulsion gel	Clobetasol propionate	Treatments of psoriasis.	[266]
Nanoethogel	Amphotericin B	Dermatophytes and fungal infections.	[236]
Nanoemulsion gel	5-Fluorouracil	Non-melanoma skin cancers.	[267]
Hydrogel	Zinc oxide	Wound healing effect on fibroblast cells.	[268]
Nanoemulgel, NLC	Vitamin E	Skin hydration.	[269]
Hydrogel	Cyclosporine and calcipotriol	Treatments of psoriasis.	[270]

9. Future Prospects of Lipid Nanoparticulate DDS for the Treatment of Skin Disorders

It can be generalized that the main challenges in the development of cutaneous lipid nanometric delivery systems include:

- Precise delivery across the skin and to certain skin strata, depending on the final target;
- Successful elimination of lipid nanomaterial toxicity threats in topical medical formulations and cosmetics;
- Ensuring improved permeation and low skin irritability as a result of the use of lipid nanocarriers;
- Improved cutaneous release of incorporated API with a broad spectrum of physiological and physicochemical properties.

Lipid nanoparticulate DDS can be employed intensively for the delivery of phytomedicines intended for topical administration. The approach can be promising in this regard, considering the difficulties in their delivery which is caused by their physicochemical properties.

The formulation of phytopreparations with lipid nanoparticles would find a useful application in nanomedicine at the desired targeted delivery, for example, in cancer treatments.

10. Conclusions

Skin disorders represent a progressively emerging clinical public health problem. Treatment strategies based on conventional formulations are non-specific and can lead to considerable systemic toxicity. The progressive approach of the use of lipid nanoformulations as skin drug delivery systems can provide an incomparable prospect for the application of highly competent and safe treatments with the improved benefit-risk ratio.

The use of lipid nanoparticlulate DDS is favored recently due to the GRAS status of the excipients. Lipid nanocarriers can effectively protect the API from degradation on the skin's surface, increase their concentration gradient in the upper skin layers, and enable gradual release. Lipid nanoparticles for topical application could be formulated with the high content of lipid matrix or dispersed in different foundations.

Lipid nanosystems provide a promising, flexible platform for the safe, effective, and biocompatible topical delivery of the API, as they do not cause cytotoxicity or morphological changes in the skin layers. The interest shown by pharmaceutical scientists, in the development of lipid nanoparticle delivery systems, may offer a future that provides sufficiently efficient lipid nanoparticle products for needy users.

Author Contributions: Conceptualization, V.Y.A. and S.R.S.; writing—original draft preparation, S.R.S.; writing—review and editing, V.Y.A. and S.R.S.; visualization, S.R.S.; supervision, V.Y.A.; project administration, V.Y.A. All authors have read and agreed to the published version of the manuscript.

Funding: This work was funded by the Medical University of Varna "Prof. Dr. Paraskev Stoyanov," Fund "Nauka" Project No. 18027.

Institutional Review Board Statement: Not applicable.

Informed Consent Statement: Not applicable.

Data Availability Statement: Data is contained within the article.

Acknowledgments: The authors would like to express their acknowledgement to the supporters—the Medical University of Varna "Paraskev Stoyanov," Varna, Bulgaria.

Conflicts of Interest: The authors declare no conflict of interest.

References

1. Sanclemente, G.; Burgos, C.; Nova, J.; Hernández, F.; González, C.; Reyes, M.I.; Córdoba, N.; Arévalo, Á.; Meléndez, E.; Colmenares, J.; et al. The impact of skin diseases on quality of life: A multicenter study. *Actas Dermosifiliogr.* **2017**, *108*, 244–252, (In English, Spanish). [CrossRef] [PubMed]
2. Seth, D.; Cheldize, K.; Brown, D.; Freeman, E.F. Global burden of skin disease: Inequities and innovations. *Curr. Dermatol. Rep.* **2017**, *6*, 204–210. [CrossRef] [PubMed]
3. Jain, S.; Barambhe, M.S.; Jain, J.; Jajoo, U.N.; Pandey, N. Prevalence of skin diseases in rural Central India: A community-based, cross-sectional, observational study. *J. Mahatma Gandhi Inst. Med. Sci.* **2016**, *21*, 111–115. [CrossRef]
4. Yew, Y.W.; Kuan, A.H.Y.; Ge, L.; Yap, C.W.; Heng, B.H. Psychosocial impact of skin diseases: A population-based study. *PLoS ONE* **2020**, *15*, e0244765. [CrossRef] [PubMed]
5. Jee, M.H.; Mraz, V.; Geisler, C.; Bonefeld, C.M. $\gamma\delta$ T cells and inflammatory skin diseases. *Immunol. Rev.* **2020**, *298*, 61–73. [CrossRef]
6. Akhtar, N.; Singh, V.; Yusuf, M.; Khan, R.A. Non-invasive drug delivery technology: Development and current status of transdermal drug delivery devices, techniques and biomedical applications. *Biomed. Eng. Biomed. Tech.* **2020**, *65*, 243–272. [CrossRef]
7. Holick, M.F. Photobiology of vitamin D. In *Vitamin D*, 4th ed.; Feldman, D., Ed.; Academic Press: London, UK, 2018; pp. 45–55.
8. Graham, H.K.; Eckersley, A.; Ozols, M.; Mellody, K.T.; Sherratt, M.J. Human Skin: Composition, structure and visualisation methods. In *Skin Biophysics*, 1st ed.; Limbert, G., Ed.; Springer: Cham, Switzerland, 2019; pp. 1–18.
9. Lundborg, M.; Narangifard, A.; Wennberg, C.L.; Lindahl, E.; Daneholt, B.; Norlén, L. Human skin barrier structure and function analyzed by cryo-EM and molecular dynamics simulation. *J. Struct. Biol.* **2018**, *203*, 149–161. [CrossRef] [PubMed]
10. Sguizzato, M.; Esposito, E.; Cortesi, R. Lipid-based nanosystems as a tool to overcome skin barrier. *Int. J. Mol. Sci.* **2021**, *22*, 8319. [CrossRef]
11. Woodby, B.; Penta, K.; Pecorelli, A.; Lila, M.A.; Valacchi, G. Skin health from the inside out. *Annu. Rev. Food Sci. Technol.* **2020**, *11*, 235–254. [CrossRef] [PubMed]
12. Lademann, J.; Schanzer, S.; Richter, H.; Meinke, M.C.; Weigmann, H.J.; Patzelt, A. Stripping procedures for penetration measurements of topically applied substances. In *Percutaneous Penetration Enhancers Drug Penetration into/through the Skin: Methodology and General Considerations*, 1st ed.; Dragicevic, N., Maibach, H., Eds.; Springer: Berlin, Germany, 2017; pp. 205–214.
13. Gorzelanny, C.; Mess, C.; Schneider, S.W.; Huck, V.; Brandner, J.M. Skin Barriers in Dermal Drug Delivery: Which Barriers Have to Be Overcome and How Can We Measure Them? *Pharmaceutics* **2020**, *12*, 684. [CrossRef]
14. Wohlrab, J. Topical preparations and their use in dermatology. *J. Dtsch. Dermatol. Ges.* **2016**, *14*, 1061–1069. [CrossRef]
15. Ribeiro, C.S.; Leal, F.; Jeunon, T. Skin anatomy, histology, and physiology. In *Daily Routine in Cosmetic Dermatology. Clinical Approaches and Procedures in Cosmetic Dermatology*; Issa, M., Tamura, B., Eds.; Springer: Cham, Switzerland, 2017; pp. 1–12.
16. Lavers, I. Exploring skin anatomy, function and site-specific treatment options. *J. Aesthet. Nurs.* **2017**, *6*, 172–180. [CrossRef]
17. Nafisi, S.; Maibach, H.I. Chapter 3—Skin penetration of nanoparticles. In *Micro and Nano Technologies, Emerging Nanotechnologies in Immunology*; Shegokar, R., Souto, E.B., Eds.; Elsevier: Amsterdam, The Netherlands, 2018; pp. 47–88.
18. Montagna, W.; Ebling, F.J.G. Human Skin. Encyclopedia Britannica. 2021. Available online: https://www.britannica.com/science/human-skin (accessed on 19 October 2021).
19. Osseiran, S.; Dela Cruz, J.; Jeong, S.; Wang, H.; Fthenakis, C.; Evans, C. Characterizing stratum corneum structure, barrier function, and chemical content of human skin with coherent Raman scattering imaging. *Biomed. Opt. Express.* **2018**, *9*, 6425–6443. [CrossRef] [PubMed]
20. Yokose, U.; Ishikawa, J.; Morokuma, Y.; Naoe, A.; Inoue, Y.; Yasuda, Y.; Tsujimura, H.; Fujimura, T.; Murase, T.; Hatamochi, A. The ceramide [NP]/[NS] ratio in the stratum corneum is a potential marker for skin properties and epidermal differentiation. *BMC Dermatol.* **2020**, *20*, 1–12. [CrossRef]
21. Desmet, E.; van Gele, M.; Lambert, J. Topically applied lipid- and surfactant-based nanoparticles in the treatment of skin disorders. *Expert Opin. Drug Del.* **2017**, *14*, 109–122. [CrossRef] [PubMed]
22. Das, C.; Olmsted, P.D. The physics of stratum corneum lipid membranes. *Phil. Trans. R. Soc. A* **2016**, *374*, 1–16. [CrossRef] [PubMed]
23. Matsui, T.; Amagai, M. Dissecting the formation, structure and barrier function of the stratum corneum. *Int. Immunol.* **2017**, *29*, 243–244. [CrossRef] [PubMed]
24. Ezati, N.; Roberts, M.S.; Zhang, Q.; Moghimi, H.R. Measurement of Hansen Solubility Parameters of Human Stratum Corneum. *Iran. J. Pharm. Res.* **2020**, *19*, 572–578. [PubMed]
25. Ruela, A.L.M.; Perissinato, A.G.; Lino, M.E.; Mudrik, P.S.; Pereira, G.R. Evaluation of skin absorption of drugs from topical and transdermal formulations. *Braz. J. Pharm. Sci.* **2016**, *52*, 527–544. [CrossRef]
26. Zsikó, S.; Csányi, E.; Kovács, A.; Budai-Szűcs, M.; Gácsi, A.; Berkó, S. Methods to Evaluate Skin Penetration in Vitro. *Sci. Pharm.* **2019**, *87*, 19. [CrossRef]
27. Walicka, A.; Iwanowska-Chomiak, B. Drug Diffusion Transport Through Human Skin. *Int. J. Appl. Mech. Eng.* **2018**, *23*, 977–988. [CrossRef]
28. Sala, M.; Diab, R.; Elaissari, A.; Fessi, H. Lipid nanocarriers as skin drug delivery systems: Properties, mechanisms of skin interactions and medical applications. *Int. J. Pharm.* **2018**, *535*, 1–17. [CrossRef] [PubMed]

29. Abd, E.; Yousef, S.A.; Pastore, M.N.; Telaprolu, K.; Mohammed, Y.H.; Namjoshi, S.; Grice, J.E.; Roberts, M.S. Skin models for the testing of transdermal drugs. *Clin. Pharmacol.* **2016**, *8*, 163–176. [CrossRef]
30. Tabassum, N.; Hamdani, M. Plants used to treat skin diseases. *Pharmacogn. Rev.* **2014**, *8*, 52–60. [CrossRef] [PubMed]
31. Ferreira, K.C.B.; Valle, A.B.C.d.S.; Paes, C.Q.; Tavares, G.D.; Pittella, F. Nanostructured Lipid Carriers for the Formulation of Topical Anti-Inflammatory Nanomedicines Based on Natural Substances. *Pharmaceutics* **2021**, *13*, 1454. [CrossRef]
32. Wolff, K.; Johnson, R.A.; Saavedra, A.P.; Roh, E.K. *Fitzpatrick's Color Atlas and Synopsis of Clinical Dermatology*, 8th ed.; McGraw-Hill Education: New York, NY, USA, 2017; pp. 693–759. Available online: https://accessmedicine.mhmedical.com/content.aspx?bookid=2043&sectionid=154893575 (accessed on 19 October 2021).
33. Urban, K.; Chu, S.; Scheufele, C.; Giesey, R.L.; Mehrmal, S.; Uppal, P.; Delost, G.R. The global, regional, and national burden of fungal skin diseases in 195 countries and territories: A cross-sectional analysis from the Global Burden of Disease Study 2017. *JAAD Int.* **2020**, *2*, 22–27. [CrossRef]
34. Craddock, L.N.; Schieke, S.M. Superficial fungal infection. In *Fitzpatrick's Dermatology*, 9th ed.; Kang, S., Amagai, M., Bruckner, A.L., Enk, A.H., Margolis, D.J., McMichael, A.J., Orringer, J.S., Eds.; McGraw-Hill: New York, NY, USA, 2019; Chapter 160; pp. 1–48. Available online: https://accessmedicine.mhmedical.com/content.aspx?sectionid=210432218&bookid=2570&Resultclick=2 (accessed on 19 October 2021).
35. Silverberg, B. A Structured Approach to Skin and Soft Tissue Infections (SSTIs) in an Ambulatory Setting. *Clin. Pract.* **2021**, *11*, 65–74. [CrossRef] [PubMed]
36. Pearson, D.R.; Margolis, D.J. Cellulitis and erysipelas. In *Fitzpatrick's Dermatology*, 9th ed.; Kang, S., Amagai, M., Bruckner, A.L., Enk, A.H., Margolis, D.J., McMichael, A.J., Orringer, J.S., Eds.; McGraw-Hill: New York, NY, USA, 2019; Chapter 151; pp. 1–19. Available online: https://accessmedicine.mhmedical.com/content.aspx?bookid=2570&sectionid=210413306 (accessed on 19 October 2021).
37. Sartelli, M.; Guirao, X.; Hardcastle, T.; Kluger, Y.; Boermeester, M.A.; Rasa, K.; Ansaloni, L.; Coccolini, F.; Montravers, P.; Abu-Zidan, F.M.; et al. 2018 WSES/SIS-E consensus conference: Recommendations for the management of skin and soft tissue infections. *World J. Emerg. Surg.* **2018**, *13*, 58. [CrossRef]
38. Falcone, M.; Concia, E.; Giusti, M.; Mazzone, A.; Santini, C.; Stefani, S.; Violi, F. Acute bacterial skin and skin structure infections in internal medicine wards: Old and new drugs. *Inter. Emerg. Med.* **2016**, *11*, 637–648. [CrossRef] [PubMed]
39. Khadr, L.; Harfouche, M.; Omori, R.; Schwarzer, G.; Chemaitelly, H.; Abu-Raddad, L.J. The Epidemiology of Herpes Simplex Virus Type 1 in Asia: Systematic Review, Meta-analyses, and Meta-regressions. *Clin. Infect. Dis.* **2019**, *68*, 757–772. [CrossRef]
40. Poole, C.L.; Kimberlin, D.W. Antiviral Approaches for the Treatment of Herpes Simplex Virus Infections in Newborn Infants. *Annu. Rev. Virol.* **2018**, *5*, 407–425. [CrossRef] [PubMed]
41. Mustafa, M.; Illzam, E.M.; Muniandy, R.K.; Sharifah, A.M.; Nang, M.K.; Ramesh, B. Herpes simplex virus infections, Pathophysiology and Management. *IOSR J. Dent. Med. Sci.* **2016**, *15*, 85–91. [CrossRef]
42. Schwingen, J.; Kaplan, M.; Kurschus, F.C. Review-Current Concepts in Inflammatory Skin Diseases Evolved by Transcriptome Analysis: In-Depth Analysis of Atopic Dermatitis and Psoriasis. *Int. J. Mol. Sci.* **2020**, *21*, 699. [CrossRef] [PubMed]
43. Ho, A.W.; Kupper, T.S. T cells and the skin: From protective immunity to inflammatory skin disorders. *Nat. Rev. Immunol.* **2019**, *19*, 490–502. [CrossRef]
44. Golan, Y. Current Treatment Options for Acute Skin and Skin-structure Infections. *Clin. Infect. Dis.* **2019**, *68*, 206–212. [CrossRef] [PubMed]
45. Aktas, E.; Esin, M.N. Skin disease symptoms and related risk factors among young workers in high-risk jobs. *Contact Dermat.* **2016**, *75*, 96–105. [CrossRef]
46. Münch, S.; Wohlrab, J.; Neubert, R.H.H. Dermal and transdermal delivery of pharmaceutically relevant macromolecules. *Eur. J. Pharm. Biopharm.* **2017**, *119*, 235–242. [CrossRef] [PubMed]
47. Jain, K.K. *Transdermal Drug Delivery-Technologies, Markets and Companies*; Jain PharmaBiotech: Basel, Switzerland, 2021; pp. 1–302.
48. Alany, R. Topical and Transdermal Formulation and Drug Delivery. *Pharm. Dev. Technol.* **2017**, *22*, 457. [CrossRef]
49. Brunaugh, A.D.; Smyth, H.D.C.; Williams, R.O., III. Topical and transdermal drug delivery. In *Essential Pharmaceutics*; AAPS Introductions in the Pharmaceutical Sciences; Springer: Cham, Switzerland, 2019; pp. 131–147.
50. Zasada, M.; Budzisz, E. Retinoids: Active molecules influencing skin structure formation in cosmetic and dermatological treatments. *Postep. Derm. Alergol.* **2019**, *36*, 392–397. [CrossRef] [PubMed]
51. Chien, A. Retinoids in Acne Management: Review of Current Understanding, Future Considerations, and Focus on Topical Treatments. *J. Drugs Dermatol.* **2018**, *17*, 51–55.
52. Temova Rakuša, Ž.; Pišlar, M.; Kristl, A.; Roškar, R. Comprehensive Stability Study of Vitamin D3 in Aqueous Solutions and Liquid Commercial Products. *Pharmaceutics* **2021**, *13*, 617. [CrossRef] [PubMed]
53. Arita, R.; Kawashima, M.; Ito, M.; Tsubota, K. Clinical safety and efficacy of vitamin D3 analog ointment for treatment of obstructive meibomian gland dysfunction. *BMC Ophthalmol.* **2017**, *17*, 84. [CrossRef]
54. Mahajan, H.; Deshmukh, G.; Dhoot, D.; Mamadi, R.; Barkate, H. Comparative Clinical Assessment of Effectiveness and Safety of Calcitriol and Calcipotriol in Mild Plaque Psoriasis. *Int. J. Clin. Dermatol.* **2020**, *3*, 28–31.
55. Singh, R.K.; Lee, K.M.; Jose, M.V.; Nakamura, M.; Ucmak, D.; Farahnik, B.; Abrouk, M.; Zhu, T.H.; Bhutani, T.; Liao, W. The Patient's Guide to Psoriasis Treatment. Part 1: UVB Phototherapy. *Dermatol. Ther.* **2016**, *6*, 307–313. [CrossRef] [PubMed]

56. Rossi, M.; Rovati, C.; Arisi, M.; Tomasi, C.; Calzavara-Pinton, I.; Venturini, M.; Calzavara-Pinton, P. A Short Cycle of Narrow-Band UVB Phototherapy in the Early Phase of Dupilumab Therapy Can Provide a Quicker Improvement of Severe Atopic Dermatitis. *Dermatology* **2021**, *237*, 407–415. [CrossRef]
57. Lossius, A.H.; Sundnes, O.; Ingham, A.C.; Edslev, S.M.; Bjørnholt, J.V.; Lilje, B.; Bradley, M.; Asad, S.; Haraldsen, G.; Skytt-Andersen, P.; et al. Shifts in the Skin Microbiota after UVB Treatment in Adult Atopic Dermatitis. *Dermatology* **2021**, 1–12. [CrossRef]
58. Eicher, L.; Knop, M.; Aszodi, N.; Senner, S.; French, L.; Wollenberg, A. A systematic review of factors influencing treatment adherence in chronic inflammatory skin disease-strategies for optimizing treatment outcome. *J. Eur. Acad. Dermatol. Venereol.* **2019**, *33*, 2253–2263. [CrossRef]
59. Leppert, W.; Malec–Milewska, M.; Zajaczkowska, R.; Wordliczek, J. Transdermal and Topical Drug Administration in the Treatment of Pain. *Molecules* **2018**, *23*, 681. [CrossRef]
60. Ray, P.; Singh, S.; Gupta, S. Topical antimicrobial therapy: Current status and challenges. *Indian J. Med. Microbiol.* **2019**, *37*, 299–308. [CrossRef]
61. Wohlrab, J. Neue Entwicklungen bei Topika. *Hautarzt* **2019**, *70*, 953–959. [CrossRef] [PubMed]
62. Garg, A.; Sharma, G.S.; Goyal, A.K.; Ghosh, G.; Si, S.C.; Rath, G. Recent advances in topical carriers of anti-fungal agents. *Heliyon* **2020**, *6*, e04663. [CrossRef] [PubMed]
63. Elmowafy, M. Skin penetration/permeation success determinants of nanocarriers: Pursuit of a perfect formulation. *Colloids Surf. B.* **2021**, *203*, 111748. [CrossRef] [PubMed]
64. Chella, N.; Shastri, N.R. Lipid Carriers: Role and Applications in Nano Drug Delivery. In *Particulate Technology for Delivery of Therapeutics*; Jana, S., Jana, S., Eds.; Springer: Singapore, 2017; pp. 253–289.
65. Garcês, A.; Amaral, M.H.; Sousa Lobo, J.M.; Silva, A.C. Formulations based on solid lipid nanoparticles (SLN) and nanostructured lipid carriers (NLC) for cutaneous use: A review. *Eur. J. Pharm. Sci.* **2018**, *112*, 159–167. [CrossRef] [PubMed]
66. Filipczak, N.; Yalamarty, S.S.K.; Li, X.; Khan, M.M.; Parveen, F.; Torchilin, V. Lipid-Based Drug Delivery Systems in Regenerative Medicine. *Materials* **2021**, *14*, 5371. [CrossRef] [PubMed]
67. LePree, J.M. Lipid based delivery—Are lipid-based drug delivery systems in your formulation toolbox? *Drug Dev. Deliv.* **2017**, *17*, 20–25. Available online: https://drug-dev.com/lipid-based-delivery-are-lipid-based-drug-delivery-systems-in-your-formulation-toolbox/ (accessed on 19 October 2021).
68. Carita, A.C.; Eloy, J.O.; Chorilli, M.; Lee, R.J.; Leonardi, G.R. Recent Advances and Perspectives in Liposomes for Cutaneous Drug Delivery. *Curr. Med. Chem.* **2018**, *25*, 606–635. [CrossRef]
69. Garg, V.; Singh, H.; Bimbrawh, S.; Singh, S.K.; Gulati, M.; Vaidya, Y.; Kaur, P. Ethosomes and Transfersomes: Principles, Perspectives and Practices. *Curr. Drug. Deliv.* **2017**, *14*, 613–633. [CrossRef] [PubMed]
70. Opatha, S.A.T.; Titapiwatanakun, V.; Chutoprapat, R. Transfersomes: A Promising Nanoencapsulation Technique for Transdermal Drug Delivery. *Pharmaceutics* **2020**, *12*, 855. [CrossRef]
71. Chaurasiya, P.; Ganju, E.; Upmanyu, N.; Ray, S.K.; Jain, P. Transfersomes: A novel technique for transdermal drug delivery. *J. Drug Deliv. Ther.* **2019**, *9*, 279–285. [CrossRef]
72. Nainwal, N.; Jawla, S.; Singh, R.; Saharan, V.A. Transdermal applications of ethosomes—A detailed review. *J. Liposome Res.* **2019**, *29*, 103–113. [CrossRef] [PubMed]
73. Natsheh, H.; Vettorato, E.; Touitou, E. Ethosomes for Dermal Administration of Natural Active Molecules. *Curr. Pharm. Des.* **2019**, *25*, 2338–2348. [CrossRef]
74. Paliwal, R.; Paliwal, S.R.; Kenwat, R.; Kurmi, B.D.; Sahu, M.K. Solid lipid nanoparticles: A review on recent perspectives and patents. *Expert Opin. Ther. Pat.* **2020**, *30*, 179–194. [CrossRef]
75. Liu, M.; Wen, J.; Sharma, M. Solid Lipid Nanoparticles for Topical Drug Delivery: Mechanisms, Dosage Form Perspectives, and Translational Status. *Curr. Pharm. Des.* **2020**, *26*, 3203–3217. [CrossRef] [PubMed]
76. Geng, Q.; Zhao, Y.; Wang, L.; Xu, L.; Chen, X.; Han, J. Development and Evaluation of Astaxanthin as Nanostructure Lipid Carriers in Topical Delivery. *AAPS Pharm. Sci. Tech.* **2020**, *21*, 318. [CrossRef] [PubMed]
77. Araujo, V.H.S.; Delello Di Filippo, L.; Duarte, J.L.; Spósito, L.; de Camargo, B.A.F.; da Silva, P.B.; Chorilli, M. Exploiting solid lipid nanoparticles and nanostructured lipid carriers for drug delivery against cutaneous fungal infections. *Crit. Rev. Microbiol.* **2020**, *47*, 79–90. [CrossRef]
78. Jain, A.; Pooladanda, V.; Bulbake, U.; Doppalapudi, S.; Rafeeqi, T.A.; Godugu, C.; Khan, W. Liposphere mediated topical delivery of thymoquinone in the treatment of psoriasis. *Nanomedicine* **2017**, *13*, 2251–2262. [CrossRef] [PubMed]
79. Esposito, E.; Sguizzato, M.; Bories, C.; Nastruzzi, C.; Cortesi, R. Production and Characterization of a Clotrimazole Liposphere Gel for Candidiasis Treatment. *Polymers* **2018**, *10*, 160. [CrossRef]
80. Waghule, T.; Gorantla, S.; Rapalli, V.K.; Shah, P.; Dubey, S.K.; Saha, R.N.; Singhvi, G. Emerging Trends in Topical Delivery of Curcumin Through Lipid Nanocarriers: Effectiveness in Skin Disorders. *AAPS Pharm. Sci. Tech.* **2020**, *21*, 284. [CrossRef]
81. Abu Lila, A.S.; Ishida, T. Liposomal Delivery Systems: Design Optimization and Current Applications. *Biol. Pharm. Bull.* **2017**, *40*, 1–10. [CrossRef] [PubMed]
82. Has, C.; Sunthar, P. A comprehensive review on recent preparation techniques of liposomes. *J. Liposome Res.* **2020**, *30*, 336–365. [CrossRef]

83. Mezei, M.; Gulasekharam, V. Liposomes—A selective drug delivery system for the topical route of administration I. Lotion dosage form. *Life Sci.* **1980**, *26*, 1473–1477. [CrossRef]
84. Lucia, M. Lipid-Based Nanoparticles as Carriers for Dermal Delivery of Antioxidants. *Curr. Drug. Metab.* **2017**, *18*, 469–480. [PubMed]
85. Yang, M.; Gu, Y.; Tang, X.; Wang, T.; Liu, J. Advancement of Lipid-Based Nanocarriers and Combination Application with Physical Penetration Technique. *Curr. Drug. Deliv.* **2019**, *16*, 312–324. [CrossRef]
86. Rai, S.; Pandey, V.; Rai, G. Transfersomes as versatile and flexible nano-vesicular carriers in skin cancer therapy: The state of the art. *Nano Rev. Exp.* **2017**, *8*, 1325708. [CrossRef] [PubMed]
87. Matos, C.; Lobão, P. Non-Steroidal Anti-Inflammatory Drugs Loaded Liposomes for Topical Treatment of Inflammatory and Degenerative Conditions. *Curr. Med. Chem.* **2020**, *27*, 3809–3829. [CrossRef] [PubMed]
88. Natsheh, H.; Touitou, E. Phospholipid Vesicles for Dermal/Transdermal and Nasal Administration of Active Molecules: The Effect of Surfactants and Alcohols on the Fluidity of Their Lipid Bilayers and Penetration Enhancement Properties. *Molecules* **2020**, *25*, 2959. [CrossRef] [PubMed]
89. Avadhani, K.S.; Manikkath, J.; Tiwari, M.; Chandrasekhar, M.; Godavarthi, A.; Vidya, S.M.; Hariharapura, R.C.; Kalthur, G.; Udupa, N.; Mutalik, S. Skin delivery of epigallocatechin-3-gallate (EGCG) and hyaluronic acid loaded nano-transfersomes for antioxidant and anti-aging effects in UV radiation induced skin damage. *Drug Deliv.* **2017**, *24*, 61–74. [CrossRef]
90. Chacko, I.A.; Ghate, V.M.; Dsouza, L.; Lewis, S.A. Lipid vesicles: A versatile drug delivery platform for dermal and transdermal applications. *Colloids Surf. B Biointerfaces* **2020**, *195*, 111262. [CrossRef]
91. Lai, F.; Caddeo, C.; Manca, M.L.; Manconi, M.; Sinico, C.; Fadda, A.M. What's new in the field of phospholipid vesicular nanocarriers for skin drug delivery. *Int. J. Pharm.* **2020**, *583*, 119398. [CrossRef]
92. Bnyan, R.; Khan, I.; Ehtezazi, T.; Saleem, I.; Gordon, S.; O'Neill, F.; Roberts, M. Formulation and optimisation of novel transfersomes for sustained release of local anaesthetic. *J. Pharm. Pharmacol.* **2019**, *71*, 1508–1519. [CrossRef]
93. Touitou, E. Compositions for Applying Active Substances to or through the Skin. US Patent 5,716,638, 10 February 1998.
94. Ita, K. Current Status of Ethosomes and Elastic Liposomes in Dermal and Transdermal Drug Delivery. *Curr. Pharm. Des.* **2016**, *22*, 5120–5126. [CrossRef]
95. Lin, H.; Lin, L.; Choi, Y.; Michniak-Kohn, B. Development and in-vitro evaluation of co-loaded berberine chloride and evodiamine ethosomes for treatment of melanoma. *Int. J. Pharm.* **2020**, *15*, 119278. [CrossRef] [PubMed]
96. Arora, D.; Nanda, S. Quality by design driven development of resveratrol loaded ethosomal hydrogel for improved dermatological benefits via enhanced skin permeation and retention. *Int. J. Pharm.* **2019**, *567*, 118448. [CrossRef]
97. Moolakkadath, T.; Aqil, M.; Ahad, A.; Imam, S.S.; Praveen, A.; Sultana, Y.; Mujeeb, M.; Iqbal, Z. Fisetin loaded binary ethosomes for management of skin cancer by dermal application on UV exposed mice. *Int. J. Pharm.* **2019**, *560*, 78–91. [CrossRef]
98. Lalotra, A.S.; Singh, V.; Khurana, B.; Agrawal, S.; Shrestha, S.; Arora, D. A Comprehensive Review on Nanotechnology-Based Innovations in Topical Drug Delivery for the Treatment of Skin Cancer. *Curr. Pharm. Des.* **2020**, *26*, 5720–5731. [CrossRef]
99. Pandey, K. An Overview on Promising Nanotechnological Approaches for the Treatment of Psoriasis. *Recent Pat. Nanotechnol.* **2020**, *14*, 102–118. [CrossRef] [PubMed]
100. Iqbal, B.; Ali, J.; Baboota, S. Recent advances and development in epidermal and dermal drug deposition enhancement technology. *Int. J. Dermatol.* **2018**, *57*, 646–660. [CrossRef] [PubMed]
101. Pathak, K.; Vaidya, A.; Sharma, V. Confronting Penetration Threshold via Fluidic Terpenoid Nanovesicles. *Curr. Drug. Deliv.* **2018**, *15*, 765–776. [CrossRef] [PubMed]
102. Kumar, L.; Verma, S.; Singh, M.; Chalotra, T.; Utreja, P. Advanced Drug Delivery Systems for Transdermal Delivery of Non-Steroidal Anti-Inflammatory Drugs: A Review. *Curr. Drug. Deliv.* **2018**, *15*, 1087–1099. [CrossRef]
103. Zhang, Y.T.; Shen, L.N.; Wu, Z.H.; Zhao, J.H.; Feng, N.P. Comparison of ethosomes and liposomes for skin delivery of psoralen for psoriasis therapy. *Int. J. Pharm.* **2014**, *471*, 449–452. [CrossRef] [PubMed]
104. Shabbir, M.; Nagra, U.; Zaman, M.; Mahmood, A.; Barkat, K. Lipid Vesicles and Nanoparticles for Non-invasive Topical and Transdermal Drug Delivery. *Curr. Pharm. Des.* **2020**, *26*, 2149–2166. [CrossRef] [PubMed]
105. Sun, M.C.; Xu, X.L.; Lou, X.F.; Du, Y.Z. Recent Progress and Future Directions: The Nano-Drug Delivery System for the Treatment of Vitiligo. *Int. J. Nanomed.* **2020**, *15*, 3267–3279. [CrossRef] [PubMed]
106. Soleymani, S.; Iranpanah, A.; Najafi, F.; Belwal, T.; Ramola, S.; Abbasabadi, Z.; Momtaz, S.; Farzaei, M.H. Implications of grape extract and its nanoformulated bioactive agent resveratrol against skin disorders. *Arch. Dermatol. Res.* **2019**, *311*, 577–588. [CrossRef]
107. Boge, L.; Hallstensson, K.; Ringstad, L.; Johansson, J.; Andersson, T.; Davoudi, M.; Larsson, P.T.; Mahlapuu, M.; Håkansson, J.; Andersson, M. Cubosomes for topical delivery of the antimicrobial peptide LL-37. *Eur. J. Pharm. Biopharm.* **2019**, *134*, 60–67. [CrossRef] [PubMed]
108. Baveloni, F.G.; Riccio, B.V.F.; Di Filippo, L.D.; Fernandes, M.A.; Meneguin, A.B.; Chorilli, M. Nanotechnology-based Drug Delivery Systems as Potential for Skin Application: A Review. *Curr. Med. Chem.* **2021**, *28*, 3216–3248. [CrossRef]
109. Kurangi, B.; Jalalpure, S.; Jagwani, S. Formulation and Evaluation of Resveratrol Loaded Cubosomal Nanoformulation for Topical Delivery. *Curr. Drug. Deliv.* **2021**, *18*, 607–619. [CrossRef] [PubMed]
110. Badie, H.; Abbas, H. Novel small self-assembled resveratrol-bearing cubosomes and hexosomes: Preparation, charachterization, and ex vivo permeation. *Drug Dev. Ind. Pharm.* **2018**, *44*, 2013–2025. [CrossRef] [PubMed]

111. Ahmad, U.; Ahmad, Z.; Khan, A.A.; Akhtar, J.; Singh, S.P.; Ahmad, F.J. Strategies in Development and Delivery of Nanotechnology Based Cosmetic Products. *Drug Res.* **2018**, *68*, 545–552. [CrossRef]
112. Sun, Q.; Chen, J.F.; Routh, A.F. Coated colloidosomes as novel drug delivery carriers. *Exp. Opin. Drug Del.* **2019**, *16*, 903–906. [CrossRef]
113. Bieberich, E. Sphingolipids and lipid rafts: Novel concepts and methods of analysis. *Chem. Phys. Lipids* **2018**, *216*, 114–131. [CrossRef]
114. Neupane, Y.R.; Mahtab, A.; Siddiqui, L.; Singh, A.; Gautam, N.; Rabbani, S.A.; Goel, H.; Talegaonkar, S. Biocompatible Nanovesicular Drug Delivery Systems with Targeting Potential for Autoimmune Diseases. *Curr. Pharm. Des.* **2020**, *26*, 5488–5502. [CrossRef] [PubMed]
115. Shetty, K.; Sherje, A.P. Nano intervention in topical delivery of corticosteroid for psoriasis and atopic dermatitis-a systematic review. *J. Mat. Sci. Mater. Med.* **2021**, *32*, 88. [CrossRef] [PubMed]
116. Vazzana, M.; Fangueiro, J.F.; Faggio, C.; Santini, A.; Souto, E.B. Archaeosomes for Skin Injuries. In *Carrier-Mediated Dermal Delivery: Applications in the Prevention and Treatment of Skin Disorders*; Ascenso, A., Ribeiro, H., Simões, S., Eds.; Pan Stanford Publishing: Singapore, 2017; pp. 323–355.
117. Sallam, M.A.; Prakash, S.; Kumbhojkar, N.; Shields, C.W.; Mitragotri, S. Formulation-based approaches for dermal delivery of vaccines and therapeutic nucleic acids: Recent advances and future perspectives. *Bioeng. Transl. Med.* **2021**, *6*, e10215. [CrossRef]
118. Lin, Y.L.; Chen, C.H.; Wu, H.Y.; Tsai, N.M.; Jian, T.Y.; Chang, Y.C.; Lin, C.H.; Wu, C.H.; Hsu, F.T.; Leung, T.K.; et al. Inhibition of breast cancer with transdermal tamoxifen-encapsulated lipoplex. *J. Nanobiotechnol.* **2016**, *14*, 11. [CrossRef]
119. Singh, N.; Kushwaha, P.; Ahmad, U.; Abdullah, M. Proliposomes: An Approach for the Development of Stable Liposome. *Ars. Pharm.* **2019**, *60*, 231–240.
120. Hiremath, N.; Gowda, D.V.; Anusha, R.; Shamant, B.S.; Srivastava, A.; Moin, A. Proliposomes: A novel approach to carrier drug delivery system. *J. Chem. Pharm. Res.* **2016**, *8*, 348–354.
121. Aziz, D.E.; Abdelbary, A.A.; Elassasy, A.I. Investigating superiority of novel bilosomes over niosomes in the transdermal delivery of diacerein: In vitro characterization, ex vivo permeation and in vivo skin deposition study. *J. Liposome Res.* **2019**, *29*, 73–85. [CrossRef]
122. Kotla, N.G.; Chandrasekar, B.; Rooney, P.; Sivaraman, G.; Larrañaga, A.; Krishna, K.V.; Pandit, A.; Rochev, Y. Biomimetic Lipid-Based Nanosystems for Enhanced Dermal Delivery of Drugs and Bioactive Agents. *ACS Biomater. Sci. Eng.* **2017**, *3*, 1262–1272. [CrossRef]
123. Karami, Z.; Hamidi, M. Cubosomes: Remarkable drug delivery potential. *Drug Discov. Today* **2016**, *21*, 789–801. [CrossRef]
124. Duarah, S.; Durai, R.D.; Narayanan, V.B. Nanoparticle-in-gel system for delivery of vitamin C for topical application. *Drug Deliv. Transl. Res.* **2017**, *7*, 750–760. [CrossRef]
125. Sureka, S.; Gupta, G.; Agarwal, M.; Mishra, A.; Singh, S.K.; Singh, R.P.; Sah, S.K.; de Jesus, A.; Pinto, T.; Dua, K. Formulation, In-Vitro and Ex-Vivo Evaluation of Tretinoin Loaded Cubosomal Gel for the Treatment of Acne. *Recent Pat. Drug Deliv. Formul.* **2018**, *12*, 121–129. [CrossRef] [PubMed]
126. Magana, J.R.; Esquena, J.; Solans, C.; Rodriguez-Abreu, C. Deconstruction of technical grade diglycerol isostearate enables the controlled preparation of hexosomes and liposomes. *J. Molec. Liq.* **2021**, *343*, 117594. [CrossRef]
127. Fornasier, M.; Pireddu, R.; Del Giudice, A.; Sinico, C.; Nylander, T.; Schillén, K.; Galantini, L.; Murgia, S. Tuning lipid structure by bile salts: Hexosomes for topical administration of catechin. *Colloids Surf. B. Biointerfaces* **2021**, *199*, 111564. [CrossRef] [PubMed]
128. Gururaj, S.S.; Ashok, V.B.; Swati, S.M.; Nilesh, R.B.; Prashant, H.K.; Nishant, P.K.; Sagar, T. An overview on nanocarrier technology Aquasomes. *J. Pharm. Res.* **2009**, *2*, 1174–1177.
129. Lopez, C.; Mériadec, C.; David-Briand, E.; Dupont, A.; Bizien, T.; Artzner, F.; Riaublanc, A.; Anton, M. Loading of lutein in egg-sphingomyelin vesicles as lipid carriers: Thermotropic phase behaviour, structure of sphingosome membranes and lutein crystals. *Food Res Int.* **2020**, *138*, 109770. [CrossRef]
130. Cristiano, M.C.; Froiio, F.; Mancuso, A.; Cosco, D.; Dini, L.; Di Marzio, L.; Fresta, M.; Paolino, D. Oleuropein-Laded Ufasomes Improve the Nutraceutical Efficacy. *Nanomaterials* **2021**, *11*, 105. [CrossRef] [PubMed]
131. Fan, Y.; Fang, Y.; Ma, L. The self-crosslinked ufasome of conjugated linoleic acid: Investigation of morphology, bilayer membrane and stability. *Colloids Surf. B. Biointerfaces* **2014**, *123*, 8–14. [CrossRef]
132. Abdelbary, A.A.; AbouGhaly, M.H. Design and optimization of topical methotrexate loaded niosomes for enhanced management of psoriasis: Application of Box–Behnken design, in-vitro evaluation and in-vivo skin deposition study. *Int. J. Pharm.* **2015**, *485*, 235–243. [CrossRef]
133. Perez, A.P.; Altube, M.J.; Schilrreff, P.; Apezteguia, G.; Celes, F.S.; Zacchino, S.; de Oliveira, C.I.; Romero, E.L.; Morilla, M.J. Topical amphotericin B inultradeformable liposomes: Formulation, skin penetration study, antifungal and antileishmanial activity in vitro. *Colloids Surf. B Biointerfaces* **2016**, *139*, 190–198. [CrossRef] [PubMed]
134. Garg, B.J.; Garg, N.K.; Beg, S.; Singh, B.; Katare, O.P. Nanosized ethosomes-based hydrogel formulations of methoxsalen for enhanced topical delivery against vitiligo: Formulation optimization, in vitro evaluation and preclinical assessment. *J. Drug Target.* **2016**, *24*, 233–246. [CrossRef]
135. Oge, L.K.; Broussard, A.; Marshall, M.D. Acne Vulgaris: Diagnosis and Treatment. *Am. Fam. Physician* **2019**, *100*, 475–484.
136. Sevimli Dikicier, B. Topical treatment of acne vulgaris: Efficiency, side effects, and adherence rate. *J. Int. Med. Res.* **2019**, *47*, 2987–2992. [CrossRef] [PubMed]

137. Apriani, E.F.; Rosana, Y.; Iskandarsyah, I. Formulation, characterization, and in vitro testing of azelaic acid ethosome-based cream against Propionibacterium acnes for the treatment of acne. *J. Adv. Pharm. Technol. Res.* **2019**, *10*, 75.
138. Schaeffer, H.J.; Beauchamp, L.; de Miranda, P.; Elion, G.B.; Bauer, D.J.; Collins, P. 9-(2-Hydroxyethoxymethyl) guanine activity against viruses of the herpes group. *Nature* **1978**, *272*, 583–585. [CrossRef] [PubMed]
139. Horwitz, E.; Pisanty, S.; Czerninski, R.; Helser, M.; Eliav, E.; Touitou, E. A clinical evaluation of a novel liposomal carrier for acyclovir in the topical treatment of recurrent herpes labialis. *Oral Surg. Oral Med. Oral Pathol. Oral Radiol. Endodontol.* **1999**, *87*, 700–705. [CrossRef]
140. Shukla, K.V.; Sharma, A.; Yadav, M. Formulation development and evaluation of ethosomal gel of acyclovir for the treatment of herpes zoster. *J. Nanosci. Nanotechnol.* **2019**, *9* (Suppl. 2), 664–668.
141. Babaie, S.; Ghanbarzadeh, S.; Davaran, S.; Kouhsoltani, M.; Hamishehkar, H. Nanoethosomes for Dermal Delivery of Lidocaine. *Adv. Pharm. Bull.* **2015**, *5*, 549–556. [CrossRef] [PubMed]
142. Godin, B.; Touitou, E.; Rubinstein, E.; Athamna, A.; Athamna, M. A new approach for treatment of deep skin infections by an ethosomal antibiotic preparation: An in vivo study. *J. Antimicrob. Chemother.* **2005**, *55*, 989–994. [CrossRef] [PubMed]
143. Godin, B.; Touitou, E. Erythromycin ethosomal systems: Physicochemical characterization and enhanced antibacterial activity. *Curr. Drug Deliv.* **2005**, *2*, 269–275. [CrossRef]
144. Zahid, S.R.; Dangi, S.; Shende, S.M.; Upmanyu, N. Formulation and evaluation of clindamycin phosphate ethosomal gel. *World J. Pharm. Pharm. Sci.* **2020**, *9*, 1804–1813.
145. Cosco, D.; Paolino, D.; Maiuolo, J.; Di Marzio, L.; Carafa, M.; Ventura, C.A.; Fresta, M. Ultradeformable liposomes as multidrug carrier of resveratrol and 5-fluorouracil for their topical delivery. *Int. J. Pharm.* **2015**, *489*, 1–10. [CrossRef]
146. Castangia, I.; Caddeo, C.; Manca, M.L.; Casu, L.; Latorre, A.C.; Diez-Sales, O.; Ruiz-Sauri, A.; Bacchetta, G.; Fadda, A.M.; Manconi, M. Delivery of liquorice extract by liposomes and hyalurosomes to protect the skin against oxidative stress injuries. *Carbohydr. Polym.* **2015**, *134*, 657–663. [CrossRef]
147. Caddeo, C.; Nacher, A.; Vassallo, A.; Armentano, M.F.; Pons, R.; Fernandez-Busquets, X.; Carbone, C.; Valenti, D.; Fadda, A.M.; Manconi, M. Effect of quercetin and resveratrol co-incorporated in liposomes against inflammatory/oxidative response associated with skin cancer. *Int. J. Pharm.* **2016**, *513*, 153–163. [CrossRef] [PubMed]
148. Rahman, S.A.; Abdelmalak, N.S.; Badawi, A.; Elbayoumy, T.; Sabry, N.; El Ramly, A. Tretinoin-loaded liposomal formulations: From lab to comparative clinical study in acne patients. *Drug Deliv.* **2016**, *23*, 1184–1193. [CrossRef] [PubMed]
149. Ingebrigtsen, S.G.; Škalko-Basnet, N.; Jacobsen, C.d.A.C.; Holsæter, A.M. Successful co-encapsulation of benzoyl peroxide and chloramphenicol in liposomes by a novel manufacturing method-dual asymmetric centrifugation. *Eur. J. Pharm. Sci.* **2017**, *97*, 192–199. [CrossRef] [PubMed]
150. Jain, S.; Kale, D.P.; Swami, R.; Katiyar, S.S. Codelivery of benzoyl peroxide & adapalene using modified liposomal gel for improved acne therapy. *Nanomedicine* **2018**, *13*, 1481–1493. [PubMed]
151. Sarwa, K.K.; Mazumder, B.; Rudrapal, M.; Verma, V.K. Potential of capsaicin-loaded transfersomes in arthritic rats. *Drug Deliv.* **2015**, *22*, 638–646. [CrossRef]
152. Khan, M.A.; Pandit, J.; Sultana, Y.; Sultana, S.; Ali, A.; Aqil, M.; Chauhan, M. Novel carbopol-based transfersomal gel of 5-fluorouracil for skin cancer treatment: In vitro characterization and in vivo study. *Drug Deliv.* **2015**, *22*, 795–802. [CrossRef]
153. Dorrani, M.; Garbuzenko, O.B.; Minko, T.; Michniak-Kohn, B. Development of edge-activated liposomes for siRNA delivery to human basal epidermis for melanoma therapy. *J. Control Release* **2016**, *228*, 150–158. [CrossRef]
154. Desmet, E.; Bracke, S.; Forier, K.; Taevernier, L.; Stuart, M.C.A.; De Spiegeleer, B.; Raemdonck, K.; Van Gele, M.; Lambert, J. An elastic liposomal formulation for RNAi-based topical treatment of skin disorders: Proof-of-concept in the treatment of psoriasis. *Int. J. Pharm.* **2016**, *500*, 268–274. [CrossRef] [PubMed]
155. Fadel, M.; Samy, N.; Nasr, M.; Alyoussef, A.A. Topical colloidal indocyanine green-mediated photodynamic therapy for treatment of basal cell carcinoma. *Pharm. Dev. Technol.* **2017**, *22*, 545–550. [CrossRef]
156. Gupta, M.; Prajapati, R.N.; Irchhaiya, R.; Singh, N.; Prajapati, S.K. Novel clindamycin loaded transfersomes formulation for effective management of acne. *World J. Pharm. Res.* **2017**, *6*, 765–773. [CrossRef]
157. Jiang, T.; Wang, T.; Li, T.; Ma, Y.; Shen, S.; He, B.; Mo, R. Enhanced Transdermal Drug Delivery by Transfer-some-Embedded Oligopeptide Hydrogel for Topical Chemotherapy of Melanoma. *ACS Nano* **2018**, *12*, 9693–9701. [CrossRef] [PubMed]
158. Dar, M.J.; Din, F.U.; Khan, G.M. Sodium stibogluconate loaded nano-deformable liposomes for topical treatment of leishmaniasis: Macrophage as a target cell. *Drug Deliv.* **2018**, *25*, 1595–1606. [CrossRef] [PubMed]
159. Omar, M.M.; Hasan, O.A.; El Sisi, A.M. Preparation and optimization of lidocaine transferosomal gel containing permeation enhancers: A promising approach for enhancement of skin permeation. *Int. J. Nanomed.* **2019**, *14*, 1551–1562. [CrossRef]
160. Cristiano, M.C.; Froiio, F.; Spaccapelo, R.; Mancuso, A.; Nisticò, S.P.; Udongo, B.P.; Fresta, M.; Paolino, D. Sulforaphane-Loaded Ultradeformable Vesicles as A Potential Natural Nanomedicine for the Treatment of Skin Cancer Diseases. *Pharmaceutics* **2020**, *12*, 6. [CrossRef]
161. Dar, M.J.; McElroy, C.A.; Khan, M.I.; Satoskar, A.R.; Khan, G.M. Development and evaluation of novel miltefosine-polyphenol co-loaded second generation nano-transfersomes for the topical treatment of cutaneous leishmaniasis. *Expert Opin. Drug Deliv.* **2020**, *17*, 97–110. [CrossRef]
162. Harmita, H.; Iskandarsyah, I.; Afifah, S.F. Effect of transfersome formulation on the stability and antioxidant activity of N-acetylcysteine in anti-aging cream. *Int. J. Appl. Pharm.* **2020**, *12*, 156–162. [CrossRef]

163. Marto, J.; Vitor, C.; Guerreiro, A.; Severino, C.; Eleuterio, C.; Ascenso, A.; Simoes, S. Ethosomes for enhanced skin delivery of griseofulvin. *Colloids Surf. B Biointerfaces* **2016**, *146*, 616–623. [CrossRef]
164. Yu, Z.; Lv, H.; Han, G.; Ma, K. Ethosomes loaded with cryptotanshinone for acne treatment through topical gel formulation. *PLoS ONE* **2016**, *11*, e0159967. [CrossRef]
165. El-Kayal, M.; Nasr, M.; Elkheshen, S.; Mortada, N. Colloidal (-)-epigallocatechin-3-gallate vesicular systems for prevention and treatment of skin cancer: A comprehensive experimental study with preclinical investigation. *Eur. J. Pharm. Sci.* **2019**, *137*, 104972. [CrossRef] [PubMed]
166. Kausar, H.; Mujeeb, M.; Ahad, A.; Moolakkadath, T.; Aqil, M.; Ahmad, A.; Akhter, H.M. Optimization of ethosomes for topical thymoquinone delivery for the treatment of skin acne. *J. Drug Deliv. Sci. Technol.* **2019**, *49*, 177–187. [CrossRef]
167. Richa, P.; Kumar, S.D.; Kumar, S.A. Formulation and evaluation of ethosomes of clobetasol propionate. *World J. Pharm. Res.* **2016**, *5*, 1183–1197.
168. Mishra, R.; Shende, S.; Jain, P.K.; Jain, V. Formulation and evaluation of gel containing ethosomes entrapped with tretinoin. *J. Drug Deliv. Ther.* **2018**, *8*, 315–321. [CrossRef]
169. Pando, D.; Matos, M.; Gutierrez, G.; Pazos, C. Formulation of resveratrol entrapped niosomes for topical use. *Colloids Surf. B Biointerfaces* **2015**, *128*, 398–404. [CrossRef] [PubMed]
170. Moghddam, S.R.M.; Ahad, A.; Aqil, M.; Imam, S.S.; Sultana, Y. Formulation and optimization of niosomes for topical diacerein delivery using 3-factor, 3-level Box-Behnken design for the management of psoriasis. *Mater. Sci. Eng. C* **2016**, *69*, 789–797. [CrossRef] [PubMed]
171. Meng, S.; Sun, L.; Wang, L.; Lin, Z.; Liu, Z.; Xi, L.; Wang, Z.; Zheng, Y. Loading of water-insoluble celastrol into niosome hydrogels for improved topical permeation and anti-psoriasis activity. *Colloids Surf. B Biointerfaces* **2019**, *182*, 110352. [CrossRef] [PubMed]
172. Zhai, J.; Tan, F.H.; Luwor, R.B.; Srinivasa Reddy, T.; Ahmed, N.; Drummond, C.J.; Tran, N. In Vitro and in Vivo Toxicity and Biodistribution of Paclitaxel-Loaded Cubosomes as a Drug Delivery Nanocarrier: A Case Study Using an A431 Skin Cancer Xenograft Model. *ACS Appl. Biol. Mater.* **2020**, *3*, 4198–4207. [CrossRef]
173. Khan, S.; Jain, P.; Jain, S.; Jain, R.; Bhargava, S.; Jain, A. Topical Delivery of Erythromycin through Cubosomes for Acne. *Pharm. Nanotechnol.* **2018**, *6*, 38–47. [CrossRef]
174. Rapalli, V.K.; Banerjee, S.; Khan, S.; Jha, P.N.; Gupta, G.; Dua, K.; Hasnain, M.S.; Nayak, A.K.; Dubey, S.K.; Singhvi, G. QbD-driven formulation development and evaluation of topical hydrogel containing ketoconazole loaded cubosomes. *Mater. Sci. Eng. C* **2021**, *119*, 111548. [CrossRef]
175. Kumar, P.; Singh, S.K.; Handa, V.; Kathuria, H. Oleic Acid Nanovesicles of Minoxidil for Enhanced Follicular Delivery. *Medicines* **2018**, *5*, 103. [CrossRef] [PubMed]
176. Silva, A.C.; Amaral, M.H.; Lobo, J.M.; Lopes, C.M. Lipid nanoparticles for the delivery of biopharmaceuticals. *Curr. Pharm. Biotechnol.* **2015**, *16*, 291–302. [CrossRef] [PubMed]
177. Trombino, S.; Mellace, S.; Cassano, R. Solid lipid nanoparticles for antifungal drugs delivery for topical applications. *Ther. Deliv.* **2016**, *7*, 639–647. [CrossRef] [PubMed]
178. Xing, H.; Wang, H.; Wu, B.; Zhang, X. Lipid nanoparticles for the delivery of active natural medicines. *Curr. Pharm. Des.* **2017**, *23*, 6705–6713. [CrossRef]
179. De Souza, M.L.; Dos Santos, W.M.; de Sousa, A.L.M.D.; de Albuquerque Wanderley Sales, V.; Nóbrega, F.P.; de Oliveira, M.V.G.; Rolim-Neto, P.J. Lipid Nanoparticles as a Skin Wound Healing Drug Delivery System: Discoveries and Advances. *Curr. Pharm. Des.* **2020**, *26*, 4536–4550. [CrossRef] [PubMed]
180. Naseri, N.; Valizadeh, H.; Zakeri-Milani, P. Solid Lipid Nanoparticles and Nanostructured Lipid Carriers: Structure, Preparation and Application. *Adv. Pharm. Bull.* **2015**, *5*, 305–313. [CrossRef]
181. Gratieri, T.; Krawczyk-Santos, A.P.; da Rocha, P.B.; Gelfuso, G.M.; Marreto, R.N.; Taveira, S.F. SLN- and NLC-Encapsulating Antifungal Agents: Skin Drug Delivery and their Unexplored Potential for Treating Onychomycosis. *Curr. Pharm. Des.* **2017**, *23*, 6684–6695. [CrossRef]
182. Pham, D.T.T.; Tran, P.H.L.; Tran, T.T.D. Development of solid dispersion lipid nanoparticles for improving skin delivery. *Saudi Pharm. J.* **2019**, *27*, 1019–1024. [CrossRef] [PubMed]
183. Waghule, T.; Rapalli, V.K.; Gorantla, S.; Saha, R.N.; Dubey, S.K.; Puri, A.; Singhvi, G. Nanostructured Lipid Carriers as Potential Drug Delivery Systems for Skin Disorders. *Curr. Pharm. Des.* **2020**, *26*, 4569–4579. [CrossRef]
184. Czajkowska-Kośnik, A.; Szekalska, M.; Winnicka, K. Nanostructured lipid carriers: A potential use for skin drug delivery systems. *Pharmacol. Rep.* **2019**, *71*, 156–166. [CrossRef]
185. Gordillo-Galeano, A.; Mora-Huertas, C.E. Solid lipid nanoparticles and nanostructured lipid carriers: A review emphasizing on particle structure and drug release. *Eur. J. Pharm. Biopharm.* **2018**, *133*, 285–308. [CrossRef] [PubMed]
186. Rajpoot, K. Solid Lipid Nanoparticles: A Promising Nanomaterial in Drug Delivery. *Curr. Pharm. Des.* **2019**, *25*, 3943–3959. [CrossRef] [PubMed]
187. Ganesan, P.; Narayanasamy, D. Lipid nanoparticles: Different preparation techniques, characterization, hurdles, and strategies for the production of solid lipid nanoparticles and nanostructured lipid carriers for oral drug delivery. *Sustain. Chem. Pharm.* **2017**, *6*, 37–56. [CrossRef]
188. Trivino, A.; Gumireddy, A.; Chauhan, H. Drug-Lipid-Surfactant Miscibility for the Development of Solid Lipid Nanoparticles. *AAPS Pharm. Sci. Tech.* **2019**, *20*, 46. [CrossRef]

189. Soleimanian, Y.; Goli, S.A.H.; Varshosaz, J.; Sahafi, S.M. Formulation and characterization of novel nanostructured lipid carriers made from beeswax, propolis wax and pomegranate seed oil. *Food Chem.* **2018**, *244*, 83–92. [CrossRef]
190. Sebaaly, C.; Charcosset, C.; Stainmesse, S.; Fessi, H.; Greige-Gerges, H. Clove essential oil-in-cyclodextrin-in-liposomes in the aqueous and lyophilized states: From laboratory to large scale using a membrane contactor. *Carbohydr. Polym.* **2016**, *138*, 75–85. [CrossRef]
191. Shah, M.K.; Khatri, P.; Vora, N.; Patel, N.K.; Jain, S.; Lin, S. Lipid nanocarriers: Preparation, characterization and absorption mechanism and applications to improve oral bioavailability of poorly water-soluble drugs. In *Biomedical Applications of Nanoparticles;* Grumezescu, A.M., Ed.; William Andrew Publishing: Norwich, NY, USA, 2019; pp. 117–147.
192. Duong, V.-A.; Nguyen, T.-T.-L.; Maeng, H.-J. Preparation of Solid Lipid Nanoparticles and Nanostructured Lipid Carriers for Drug Delivery and the Effects of Preparation Parameters of Solvent Injection Method. *Molecules* **2020**, *25*, 4781. [CrossRef] [PubMed]
193. Chaudhary, S.A.; Patel, D.M.; Patel, J.K.; Patel, D.H. Solvent Emulsification Evaporation and Solvent Emulsification Diffusion Techniques for Nanoparticles. In *Emerging Technologies for Nanoparticle Manufacturing;* Patel, J.K., Pathak, Y.V., Eds.; Springer: Cham, Switzerland, 2021; pp. 287–300.
194. Singh, D.; Tiwary, A.K.; Bedi, N. Self-microemulsifying Drug Delivery System for Problematic Molecules: An Update. *Recent Pat. Nanotech.* **2019**, *13*, 92–113. [CrossRef]
195. Desai, P.; Patlolla, R.R.; Singh, M. Interaction of nanoparticles and cell-penetrating peptides with skin for transdermal drug delivery. *Mol. Membr. Biol.* **2010**, *27*, 247–259. [CrossRef] [PubMed]
196. Jensen, L.B.; Petersson, K.; Nielsen, H.M. In vitro penetration properties of solid lipid nanoparticles in intact and barrier-impaired skin. *Eur. J. Pharm. Biopharm.* **2011**, *79*, 68–75. [CrossRef]
197. Okonogi, S.; Riangjanapatee, P. Physicochemical characterization of lycopene-loaded nanostructured lipid carrier formula-tions for topical administration. *Int. J. Pharm.* **2015**, *478*, 726–735. [CrossRef] [PubMed]
198. Shrotriya, S.N.; Ranpise, N.S.; Vidhate, B.V. Skin targeting of resveratrol utilizing solid lipid nanoparticle-engrossed gel for chemically induced irritant contact dermatitis. *Drug Deliv. Transl. Res.* **2017**, *7*, 37–52. [CrossRef] [PubMed]
199. Montenegro, L.; Messina, C.M.; Manuguerra, S.; Santagati, L.M.; Pasquinucci, L.; Turnaturi, R.; Parenti, C.; Arena, R.; Santulli, A. In Vitro Antioxidant Activity and In Vivo Topical Efficacy of Lipid Nanoparticles Co-Loading Idebenone and Tocopheryl Acetate. *Appl. Sci.* **2019**, *9*, 845. [CrossRef]
200. Pivetta, T.P.; Simões, S.; Araújo, M.M.; Carvalho, T.; Arruda, C.; Marcato, P.D. Development of nanoparticles from natural lipids for topical delivery of thymol: Investigation of its anti-inflammatory properties. *Colloids Surf. B Biointerfaces* **2018**, *164*, 281–290. [CrossRef]
201. Gad, H.A.; El-Rahman, F.A.A.; Hamdy, G.M. Chamomile oil loaded solid lipid nanoparticles: A naturally formulated remedy to enhance the wound healing. *J. Drug Deliv. Sci. Technol.* **2019**, *50*, 329–338. [CrossRef]
202. Butani, D.; Yewale, C.; Misra, A. Topical Amphotericin B solid lipid nanoparticles: Design and development. *Colloids Surf. B Biointerfaces* **2016**, *139*, 17–24. [CrossRef] [PubMed]
203. Carbone, C.; do Céu Teixeira, M.; do Céu Sousa, M.; Martins-Gomes, C.; Silva, A.M.; Souto, E.M.B.; Musumeci, T. Clotrimazole-Loaded Mediterranean Essential Oils NLC: A Synergic Treatment of Candida Skin Infections. *Pharmaceutics* **2019**, *11*, 231. [CrossRef]
204. Ghate, V.M.; Lewis, S.A.; Prabhu, P.; Dubey, A.; Patel, N. Nanostructured lipid carriers for the topical delivery of tretinoin. *Eur. J. Pharm. Biopharm.* **2016**, *108*, 253–261. [CrossRef]
205. Malik, D.S.; Kaur, G. Exploring therapeutic potential of azelaic acid loaded NLCs for the treatment of acne vulgaris. *J. Drug Deliv. Sci. Technol.* **2020**, *55*, 101418. [CrossRef]
206. Tupal, A.; Sabzichi, M.; Ramezani, F.; Kouhsoltani, M.; Hamishehkar, H. Dermal delivery of doxorubicin-loaded solid lipid nanoparticles for the treatment of skin cancer. *J. Microencapsul.* **2016**, *33*, 372–380. [CrossRef]
207. Harde, H.; Agrawal, A.K.; Katariya, M.; Kale, D.; Jain, S. Development of a topical adapalene-solid lipid nanoparticle load-ed gel with enhanced efficacy and improved skin tolerability. *RSC Adv.* **2015**, *5*, 43917–43929. [CrossRef]
208. Pradhan, M.; Singh, D.; Singh, M.R. Influence of selected variables on fabrication of Triamcinolone acetonide loaded solid lipid nanoparticles for topical treatment of dermal disorders. *Artif. Cells Nanomed. Biotechnol.* **2016**, *44*, 392–400. [CrossRef] [PubMed]
209. Wang, W.; Chen, L.; Huang, X.; Shao, A. Preparation and Characterization of Minoxidil Loaded Nanostructured Lipid Car-riers. *AAPS Pharm. Sci. Tech.* **2017**, *18*, 509–516. [CrossRef]
210. Shrotriya, S.N.; Vidhate, B.V.; Shukla, M.S. Formulation and development of Silybin loaded solid lipid nanoparticle enriched gel for irritant contact dermatitis. *J. Drug Deliv. Sci. Technol.* **2017**, *41*, 164–173. [CrossRef]
211. El-Housiny, S.; Shams Eldeen, M.A.; El-Attar, Y.A.; Salem, H.A.; Attia, D.; Bendas, E.R.; El-Nabarawi, M.A. Flucona-zole-loaded solid lipid nanoparticles topical gel for treatment of pityriasis versicolor: Formulation and clinical study. *Drug Deliv.* **2018**, *25*, 78–90. [CrossRef]
212. Aland, R.; Ganesan, M.; Rajeswara, R.P. Development and optimization of tazarotene loaded solid lipid nanoparticles for topical delivery. *Asian J. Pharm. Clin. Res.* **2019**, *12*, 63–77. [CrossRef]
213. Al-Maghrabi, P.M.; Khafagy, E.-S.; Ghorab, M.M.; Gad, S. Influence of formulation variables on miconazole nitrate-loaded lipid based nanocarrier for topical delivery. *Colloids Surf. B Biointerfaces* **2020**, *193*, 111046. [CrossRef]

214. Bhalekar, M.; Upadhaya, P.; Madgulkar, A. Formulation and evaluation of Adapalene-loaded nanoparticulates for epidermal localization. *Drug Deliv. Transl. Res.* **2015**, *5*, 585–595. [CrossRef]
215. Gupta, S.; Wairkar, S.; Bhatt, L.K. Isotretinoin and α-tocopherol acetate-loaded solid lipid nanoparticle topical gel for the treatment of acne. *J. Microencapsul.* **2020**, *37*, 1–9. [CrossRef] [PubMed]
216. Kelidari, H.R.; Saeedi, M.; Hajheydari, Z.; Akbari, J.; Morteza-Semnani, K.; Akhtari, J.; Valizadeh, H.; Asare-Addo, K.; Nokhodchi, A. Spironolactone loaded nanostructured lipid carrier gel for effective treatment of mild and moderate ac-ne vulgaris: A randomized, double-blind, prospective trial. *Colloids Surf. B Biointerfaces* **2016**, *146*, 47–53. [CrossRef]
217. Nagaich, U.; Gulati, N. Nanostructured lipid carriers (NLC) based controlled release topical gel of clobetasol propionate: Design and in vivo characterization. *Drug Deliv. Transl. Res.* **2016**, *6*, 289–298. [CrossRef]
218. Viegas, J.S.R.; Praça, F.G.; Caron, A.L.; Suzuki, I.; Silvestrini, A.V.P.; Medina, W.S.G.; Del Ciampo, J.O.; Kravicz, M.; Bentley, M.V.L.B. Nanostructured lipid carrier co-delivering tacrolimus and TNF-α siRNA as an innovate approach to psoriasis. *Drug Deliv. Transl. Res.* **2020**, *10*, 646–660. [CrossRef] [PubMed]
219. Passos, J.S.; De Martino, L.C.; Dartora, V.F.C.; De Araujo, G.L.B.; Ishida, K.; Lopes, L.B. Development, skin targeting and antifungal efficacy of topical lipid nanoparticles containing itraconazole. *Eur. J. Pharm. Sci.* **2020**, *149*, 105296. [CrossRef]
220. Madan, J.R.; Khobaragade, S.; Dua, K.; Awasthi, R. Formulation, optimization, and in vitro evaluation of nanostructured lipid carriers for topical delivery of Apremilast. *Dermatol. Ther.* **2020**, *33*, e13370. [CrossRef]
221. Sathe, P.; Saka, R.; Kommineni, N.; Raza, K.; Khan, W. Dithranol-loaded nanostructured lipid carrier-based gel ameliorate psoriasis in imiquimod-induced mice psoriatic plaque model. *Drug Dev. Ind. Pharm.* **2019**, *45*, 826–838. [CrossRef]
222. Waghule, T.; Rapalli, V.K.; Singhvi, G.; Manchanda, P.; Hans, N.; Dubey, S.K.; Hasnain, M.S.; Nayak, A.K. Voriconazole loaded nanostructured lipid carriers based topical delivery system: QbD based designing, characterization, in-vitro and ex-vivo evaluation. *J. Drug Deliv. Sci. Technol.* **2019**, *52*, 303–315. [CrossRef]
223. Kaur, N.; Sharma, K.; Bedi, N. Topical Nanostructured Lipid Carrier Based Hydrogel of Mometasone Furoate for the Treatment of Psoriasis. *Pharm. Nanotechnol.* **2018**, *6*, 133–143. [CrossRef]
224. Lewies, A.; Wentzel, J.F.; Jordaan, A.; Bezuidenhout, C.; Du Plessis, L.H. Interactions of the antimicrobial peptide nisin Z with conventional antibiotics and the use of nanostructured lipid carriers to enhance antimicrobial activity. *Int. J. Pharm.* **2017**, *526*, 244–253. [CrossRef] [PubMed]
225. Jain, A.; Garg, N.K.; Jain, A.; Kesharwani, P.; Jain, A.K.; Nirbhavane, P.; Tyagi, R.K. A synergistic approach of adapalene-loaded nanostructured lipid carriers, and vitamin C co-administration for treating acne. *Drug Dev. Ind. Pharm.* **2016**, *42*, 897–905. [CrossRef]
226. Baroli, B. Penetration of nanoparticles and nanomaterials in the skin: Fiction or reality? *J. Pharm. Sci.* **2009**, *99*, 21–50. [CrossRef] [PubMed]
227. Basavaraj, K.H. Nanotechnology in medicine and relevance to dermatology: Present concepts. *Indian J. Dermatol.* **2012**, *57*, 169–174. [CrossRef] [PubMed]
228. Tadros, T.; Izquierdo, P.; Esquena, J.; Solans, C. Formation and stability of nano-emulsions. *Adv. Colloid Interface Sci.* **2004**, *108–109*, 303–318. [CrossRef] [PubMed]
229. Lee, V.H.L. Nanotechnology: Challenging the limit of creativity in targeted drug delivery. *Adv. Drug Deliv. Rev.* **2004**, *56*, 1527–1528. [CrossRef]
230. Heuschkel, S.; Goebel, A.; Neubert, R.H.H. Microemulsions-modern colloidal carrier for dermal and transdermal drug delivery. *J. Pharm. Sci.* **2007**, *97*, 603–631. [CrossRef]
231. Patel, M.R.; Patel, R.B.; Parikh, J.R.; Solanki, A.B.; Patel, B.G. Investigating effect of microemulsion components: In vitro permeation of ketoconazole. *Pharm. Dev. Technol.* **2011**, *16*, 250–258. [CrossRef] [PubMed]
232. Kogan, A.; Garti, N. Microemulsions as transdermal drug delivery vehicles. *Adv. Colloid Interface Sci.* **2006**, *123–126*, 369–385. [CrossRef]
233. Anton, N.; Benoit, J.-P.; Saulnier, P. Design and production of nanoparticles formulated from nanoemulsion templates—A review. *J. Control Release* **2008**, *128*, 185–199. [CrossRef] [PubMed]
234. McClements, D.J. Nanoemulsions versus microemulsions: Terminology, differences, and similarities. *Soft Matter* **2012**, *8*, 1719–1729. [CrossRef]
235. Badnjevic, A. *CMBEBIH 2017: Proceedings of the International Conference on Medical and Biological Engineering 2017*; Springer: New York, NY, USA, 2017; p. 825.
236. Kaur, A.; Katiyar, S.S.; Kushwah, V.; Jain, S. Nanoemulsion loaded gel for topical co-delivery of clobitasol propionate and calcipotriol in psoriasis. *Nanomedicine* **2017**, *13*, 1473–1482. [CrossRef] [PubMed]
237. Rajitha, P.; Shammika, P.; Aiswarya, S.; Gopikrishnan, A.; Jayakumar, R.; Sabitha, M. Chaulmoogra oil based methotrexate loaded topical nanoemulsion for the treatment of psoriasis. *J. Drug Deliv. Sci. Technol.* **2019**, *49*, 463–476. [CrossRef]
238. Coneac, G.; Vlaia, V.; Olariu, I.; Mut, A.M.; Anghel, D.F.; Ilie, C.; Popoiu, C.; Lupuleasa, D.; Vlaia, L. Development and Evaluation of New Microemulsion-Based Hydrogel Formulations for Topical Delivery of Fluconazole. *AAPS PharmSciTech* **2015**, *16*, 889–904. [CrossRef] [PubMed]
239. Alvarado, H.L.; Abrego, G.; Souto, E.B.; Garduno-Ramirez, M.L.; Clares, B.; Garcia, M.L.; Calpena, A.C. Nanoemulsions for dermal controlled release of oleanolic and ursolic acids: In vitro, ex vivo and in vivo characterization. *Colloids Surf. B Biointerfaces* **2015**, *130*, 40–47. [CrossRef] [PubMed]

240. Goindi, S.; Kaur, R.; Kaur, R. An ionic liquid-in-water microemulsion as a potential carrier for topical delivery of poorly water soluble drug: Development, ex-vivo and in-vivo evaluation. *Int. J. Pharm.* **2015**, *495*, 913–923. [CrossRef]
241. Lv, X.; Liu, T.; Ma, H.; Tian, Y.; Li, L.; Li, Z.; Gao, M.; Zhang, J.; Tang, Z. Preparation of Essential Oil-Based Microemulsions for Improving the Solubility, pH Stability, Photostability, and Skin Permeation of Quercetin. *AAPS PharmSciTech* **2017**, *18*, 3097–3104. [CrossRef] [PubMed]
242. Negi, P.; Singh, B.; Sharma, G.; Beg, S.; Katare, O.P. Biocompatible lidocaine and prilocaine loaded-nanoemulsion system for enhanced percutaneous absorption: QbD-based optimisation, dermatokinetics and in vivo evaluation. *J. Microencapsul.* **2015**, *32*, 419–431. [CrossRef]
243. Pham, J.; Nayel, A.; Hoang, C.; Elbayoumi, T. Enhanced effectiveness of tocotrienol-based nano-emulsified system for topical delivery against skin carcinomas. *Drug Deliv.* **2016**, *23*, 1514–1524. [CrossRef]
244. Nasr, M.; Abdel-Hamid, S. Optimizing the dermal accumulation of a tazarotene microemulsion using skin deposition modeling. *Drug Dev. Ind. Pharm.* **2016**, *42*, 636–643. [CrossRef]
245. Amarji, B.; Garg, N.K.; Singh, B.; Katare, O.P. Microemulsions mediated effective delivery of methotrexate hydrogel: More than a tour de force in psoriasis therapeutics. *J. Drug Target.* **2016**, *24*, 147–160. [CrossRef] [PubMed]
246. Nasr, M.; Abdel-Hamid, S.; Moftah, N.H.; Fadel, M.; Alyoussef, A.A. Jojoba Oil Soft Colloidal Nanocarrier of a Synthetic Retinoid: Preparation, Characterization and Clinical Efficacy in Psoriatic Patients. *Curr. Drug Deliv.* **2017**, *14*, 426–432. [CrossRef]
247. Kumari, B.; Kesavan, K. Effect of chitosan coating on microemulsion for effective dermal clotrimazole delivery. *Pharm. Dev. Technol.* **2017**, *22*, 617–626. [CrossRef] [PubMed]
248. Moghimipour, E.; Salimi, A.; Changizi, S. Preparation and microstructural characterization of Griseofulvin microemulsions using different experimental methods: SAXS and DSC. *Adv. Pharm. Bull.* **2017**, *7*, 281–289. [CrossRef] [PubMed]
249. Omar, A.M.; Ammar, N.M.; Hussein, R.A.; Mostafa, D.M.; Basha, M.; Abdel Hamid, M.F. Boswellia carterii Birdwood topical microemulsion for the treatment of inflammatory dermatological conditions; a prospective study. *Trop. J. Nat. Prod. Res.* **2020**, *4*, 372–377.
250. Khiljee, S.; Ur Rehman, N.; Khiljee, T.; Loebenberg, R.; Ahmad, R.S. Formulation and clinical evaluation of topical dosage forms of Indian Penny Wort, walnut and turmeric in eczema. *Pak. J. Pharm. Sci.* **2015**, *28*, 2001–2007.
251. Jagdale, S.; Chaudhari, B. Optimization of microemulsion based transdermal gel of triamcinolone. *Recent Pat. Anti-Infect. Drug Discov.* **2017**, *12*, 61–78. [CrossRef]
252. Algahtani, M.S.; Ahmad, M.Z.; Ahmad, J. Nanoemulgel for improved topical delivery of retinyl palmitate: Formulation design and stability evaluation. *Nanomaterials* **2020**, *10*, 848. [CrossRef]
253. Yang, M.; Gu, Y.; Yang, D.; Tang, X.; Liu, J. Development of triptolide-nanoemulsion gels for percutaneous administration: Physicochemical, transport, pharmacokinetic and pharmacodynamic characteristics. *J. Nano Biotechnol.* **2017**, *15*, 88. [CrossRef]
254. Das, S.; Lee, S.H.; Chia, V.D.; Chow, P.S.; MacBeath, C.; Liu, Y.; Shlieout, G. Development of microemulsion based topical ivermectin formulations: Pre-formulation and formulation studies. *Colloids Surf. B Biointerfaces* **2020**, *189*, 110823. [CrossRef] [PubMed]
255. Pandey, S.S.; Maulvi, F.A.; Patel, P.S.; Shukla, M.R.; Shah, K.M.; Gupta, A.R.; Joshi, S.V.; Shah, D.O. Cyclosporine laden tailored microemulsion-gel depot for effective treatment of psoriasis: In vitro and in vivo studies. *Colloids Surf. B Biointerfaces* **2020**, *186*, 110681. [CrossRef] [PubMed]
256. Argenta, D.F.; Bidone, J.; Koester, L.S.; Bassani, V.L.; Simoes, C.M.O.; Teixeira, H.F. Topical Delivery of Coumestrol from Lipid Nanoemulsions Thickened with Hydroxyethylcellulose for Antiherpes Treatment. *AAPS PharmSciTech* **2018**, *19*, 192–200. [CrossRef]
257. Barradas, T.N.; Senna, J.P.; Cardoso, S.A.; de Holanda e Silva, K.G.; Elias Mansur, C.R. Formulation characterization and in vitro drug release of hydrogel-thickened nanoemulsions for topical delivery of 8-methoxypsoralen. *Mater Sci. Eng. C* **2018**, *92*, 245–253. [CrossRef]
258. Kaci, M.; Belhaffef, A.; Meziane, S.; Dostert, G.; Menu, P.; Velot, E.; Desobry, S.; Arab-Tehrany, E. Nanoemulsions and topical creams for the safe and effective delivery of lipophilic antioxidant coenzyme Q10. *Colloids Surf. B Biointerfaces* **2018**, *167*, 165–175. [CrossRef]
259. Barradas, T.N.; Senna, J.P.; Cardoso, S.A.; Nicoli, S.; Padula, C.; Santi, P.; Rossi, F.; de Holanda e Silva, K.G.; Mansur, C.R.E. Hydrogel-thickened nanoemulsions based on essential oils for topical delivery of psoralen: Permeation and stability studies. *Eur. J. Pharm. Sci.* **2017**, *116*, 38–50. [CrossRef] [PubMed]
260. Miastkowska, M.; Sikora, E.; Ogonowski, J.; Zielina, M.; Ludzik, A. The kinetic study of isotretinoin release from nanoemulsion. *Colloids Surf. A Physicochem. Eng. Asp.* **2016**, *510*, 63–68. [CrossRef]
261. Hussain, A.; Samad, A.; Singh, S.K.; Ahsan, M.N.; Haque, M.W.; Faruk, A.; Ahmed, F.J. Nanoemulsion gel-based topical delivery of an antifungal drug: In vitro activity and in vivo evaluation. *Drug Deliv.* **2016**, *23*, 642–657. [CrossRef] [PubMed]
262. Betzler de Oliveira de Siqueira, L.; da Silva Cardoso, V.; Rodrigues, I.A.; Vazquez-Villa, A.L.; Pereira dos Santos, E.; da Costa Leal Ribeiro Guimaraes, B.; dos Santos Cerqueira Coutinho, C.; Vermelho, A.B.; Ricci, E., Jr. Development and evaluation of zinc phthalocyanine nanoemulsions for use in photodynamic therapy for *Leishmania* spp. *Nanotechnology* **2017**, *28*, 65101. [CrossRef] [PubMed]

263. Topical Drug Delivery Market Research Report by Product (Liquid Formulations, Semi-Solid Formulations, and Solid Formulations), by Rout to Administration (Dermal Drug Delivery, Nasal Drug Delivery, and Ophthalmic Drug Delivery), by End-User, by Region (Americas, Asia-Pacific, and Europe, Middle East & Africa)—Global Forecast to 2026—Cumulative Impact of COVID-19. In *Global Topical Drug Delivery Industry*; GLOBE NEWSWIRE: New York, NY, USA, 2021. Available online: https://www.reportlinker.com/p06033143/?utm_source=GNW (accessed on 19 October 2021).
264. Proksch, E.; Berardesca, E.; Misery, L.; Engblom, J.; Bouwstra, J. Dry skin management: Practical approach in light of latest research on skin structure and function. *J. Dermatolog. Treat.* **2020**, *31*, 716–722. [CrossRef] [PubMed]
265. Roberts, M.S.; Mohammed, Y.; Pastore, M.N.; Namjoshi, S.; Yousef, S.; Alinaghi, A.; Haridass, I.N.; Abd, E.; Leite-Silva, V.R.; Benson, H.A.E.; et al. Topical and cutaneous delivery using nanosystems. *J. Control Release* **2017**, *247*, 86–105. [CrossRef]
266. Kaur, L.; Singh, K.; Paul, S.; Singh, S.; Singh, S.; Jain, S.K. A Mechanistic Study to Determine the Structural Similarities between Artificial Membrane Strat-M™ and Biological Membranes and Its Application to Carry Out Skin Permeation Study of Amphotericin B Nanoformulations. *AAPS PharmSciTech* **2018**, *19*, 1606–1624. [CrossRef] [PubMed]
267. Ahmad, N.; Ahmad, R.; Buheazaha, T.M.; AlHomoud, H.S.; Al-Nasif, H.A.; Sarafroz, M. A comparative ex vivo permeation evaluation of a novel 5-Fluorocuracil nanoemulsion-gel by topically applied in the different excised rat, goat, and cow skin. *Saudi J. Biol. Sci.* **2020**, *27*, 1024–1040. [CrossRef]
268. Raguvaran, R.; Manuja, B.K.; Chopra, M.; Thakur, R.; Anand, T.; Kalia, A.; Manuja, A. Sodium alginate and gum acacia hydrogels of ZnO nanoparticles show wound healing effect on fibroblast cells. *Int. J. Biol. Macromol.* **2017**, *96*, 185–191. [CrossRef]
269. Eiras, F.; Amaral, M.H.; Silva, R.; Martins, E.; Sousa Lobo, J.M.; Silva, A.C. Characterization and biocompatibility evaluation of cutaneous formulations containing lipid nanoparticles. *Int. J. Pharm.* **2017**, *519*, 373–380. [CrossRef] [PubMed]
270. Arora, R.; Katiyar, S.S.; Kushwah, V.; Jain, S. Solid lipid nanoparticles and nanostructured lipid carrier-based nanotherapeutics in treatment of psoriasis: A comparative study. *Expert Opin. Drug Deliv.* **2017**, *14*, 165–177. [CrossRef] [PubMed]

pharmaceuticals

Review

The Future of Tissue-Targeted Lipid Nanoparticle-Mediated Nucleic Acid Delivery

Ruvanthi N. Kularatne, Rachael M. Crist and Stephan T. Stern *

Nanotechnology Characterization Laboratory, Cancer Research Technology Program, Leidos Biomedical Research, Inc., Frederick National Laboratory for Cancer Research Sponsored by the National Cancer Institute, Frederick, MD 21702, USA; ruvanthinilanga.kularatne@nih.gov (R.N.K.); cristr@mail.nih.gov (R.M.C.)
* Correspondence: sternstephan@mail.nih.com

Abstract: The earliest example of in vivo expression of exogenous mRNA is by direct intramuscular injection in mice without the aid of a delivery vehicle. The current state of the art for therapeutic nucleic acid delivery is lipid nanoparticles (LNP), which are composed of cholesterol, a helper lipid, a PEGylated lipid and an ionizable amine-containing lipid. The liver is the primary organ of LNP accumulation following intravenous administration and is also observed to varying degrees following intramuscular and subcutaneous routes. Delivery of nucleic acid to hepatocytes by LNP has therapeutic potential, but there are many disease indications that would benefit from non-hepatic LNP tissue and cell population targeting, such as cancer, and neurological, cardiovascular and infectious diseases. This review will concentrate on the current efforts to develop the next generation of tissue-targeted LNP constructs for therapeutic nucleic acids.

Keywords: lipid nanoparticles; drug delivery; therapeutic nucleic acids

Citation: Kularatne, R.N.; Crist, R.M.; Stern, S.T. The Future of Tissue-Targeted Lipid Nanoparticle-Mediated Nucleic Acid Delivery. *Pharmaceuticals* **2022**, *15*, 897. https://doi.org/10.3390/ph15070897

Academic Editors: Ana Catarina Silva, João Nuno Moreira and José Manuel Sousa Lobo

Received: 15 June 2022
Accepted: 15 July 2022
Published: 20 July 2022

1. Introduction

The earliest example of in vivo expression of exogenous mRNA was by direct intramuscular injection in mice without the aid of a delivery vehicle [1]. This appears to defy what is known about nucleic acids, being that they are large, polar and metabolically unstable drugs that do not cross cell membranes. However, since cytoplasmic delivery is essential for mRNA transcription and efficacy, clearly "naked" mRNA at a sufficient dose can be taken up by cells and expressed in vivo, at least to some degree. Later investigations identified saturable, nucleotide-specific uptake mechanisms that involve intracellular vesicles [2]. Regardless of existing mechanisms for direct nucleotide cellular uptake, delivery platforms offer stability, suppression of immunogenicity and dramatically improved cellular transfection.

2. LNP Chemistry, Formulation and Background

Formulating therapeutic nucleic acids into nanoparticles is of utmost importance to prevent degradation by nucleases upon administration and to enhance cellular uptake of these negatively charged entities. The current state of the art for therapeutic nucleic acid delivery is lipid nanoparticles (LNP), which are composed of cholesterol, a helper lipid, a PEGylated lipid and an ionizable amine-containing lipid (Figure 1) [3]. The cholesterol and helper lipids are important for the integrity of the LNP, while the PEGylated lipid provides colloidal stability as well as stealth properties to limit accumulation in the reticuloendothelial system (RES). The most important ingredient in this recipe is the ionizable amine-containing lipid, which is responsible for the complexation of nucleic acid. Importantly, this ionizable lipid is only protonated at non-physiological pH, pKa 6–7, which means the lipid is not charged in the circulation [4], which is important as cationic nanoparticles are notoriously toxic [5]. Upon cell uptake and lysosomal localization, the ionizable lipid is again charged at the low lysosomal pH, which, together with the unique conical features of the component lipids, assists in lysosomal escape and mRNA expression or siRNA gene silencing [4].

Alcohol dilution is the most commonly used method for LNP formulation, in which the nucleic acid payload is dispersed in an aqueous buffer (e.g., citrate, acetate, HEPES, malic acid buffers) at an acidic pH (pH ~ 3–5) and the excipients are dissolved in alcohol, ethanol being predominantly used, but *t*-BuOH is also used occasionally [6]. The ionic strength of the buffer varies from 10 mM to 100 mM, where lower ionic strength buffers are used for smaller RNA and pDNA and a higher concentration is used for larger RNA. During formulation, the aqueous and organic phases are generally combined at a volume ratio of 3:1 by either rapid mixing with a pipette or using microfluidic mixing. Downstream processing consists of either dialysis, tangential flow filtration or centrifuge filtration against PBS to remove ethanol and for buffer exchange.

Tissue targeting LNP can be obtained by introducing targeting ligands directly to the formulation in ethanol, chemically conjugating to the LNP surface, or by modifying the composition of the lipids in the formulation. Herein, active targeting refers to LNPs that contains a target-specific ligand in the formulation, whereas passive targeting refers to constructs lacking chemically conjugated targeting moieties.

Active targeting of LNP using antibodies was adopted by several groups, where a functionalized DSPE-PEG was introduced during LNP formulation at 12.5–25 mol% of total PEG, followed by chemically grafting the antibody [7–9]. For example, a simple amidation was used to conjugate αCD34 antibody to DSPE-PEG-carboxyl [8], and thiol-maleimide conjugation was employed to attach anti-CD4 antibody [9,10] and mAb specific for PECAM-1 [11] to DSPE-PEG-maleimide containing LNP. Caveolae targeted delivery to the lungs was achieved by conjugating Fab-C4 to DSPE-PEG-maleimide via a Diels-Alder reaction, where the Fab-C4 contains a cyclopentadiene lysine derivative to allow the Diels-Alder transformation [7]. A different strategy was utilized by Goswani et al. where the targeting ligand was attached to cholesterol instead of PEG-lipid. Here, α-mannose containing an aminopropyl succinate spacer was conjugated to cholesterol via an amide bond and formulated into LNP to deliver saRNA to dendritic cells [12]. An example of introducing a targeting ligand directly into the formulation is whereby DSPE-PEG2000-mannose was incorporated into the formulation at 2.5 mol% (at 3 mol% total PEG-lipid) to allow selective delivery of LNP to liver sinusoidal endothelial cells [13].

Passive targeting is governed primarily by the size and charge of the LNP, which is acquired through changes in the molar compositions of the four types of lipids used in the formulation. One such example is the use of increasing amounts of DMG-PEG2000 from 0.004 μmol to 0.12 μmol to reduce the LNP size from 200 nm to 30 nm. The latter was shown to have enhanced cellular uptake by CD+ dendritic cells in lymph nodes [14]. The same report showed the use of CHEMS at ~20 mol% to obtain negatively charged LNP to further enhance cellular uptake. Replacing traditional linear PEG-lipids with 3% Tween 20, which contains three PEG chains and a single lipid chain, Zukancic et al. was able to demonstrate targeted delivery of pDNA LNP to draining lymph nodes, however at the expense of reduced encapsulation efficiency, ~50% [15]. On occasion, an additional lipid is introduced to achieve passive targeting, which has been termed selective organ targeting (SORT) lipids [16,17]. These SORT lipids are introduced to the LNP formulation by dissolution in THF or ethanol at different molar ratios before mixing with the RNA to obtain liver, spleen and lung targeting [17–20]. Lipid composition and the type of ionizable lipid used in the formulation have a greater impact on pDNA LNP transfection, with different ratios of DODAP and DOPE in the formulation [21] and changing the ionizable lipid from DLin-MC3-DMA to DLin-KC2-DMA [22] increasing transfection in the spleen, while uptake of these LNP was greatest in the liver [21,22].

Although many LNPs are currently in preclinical and clinical development, only three have been approved/authorized by the US Food and Drug Administration (FDA) for clinical use. These are Comirnaty® SARS-CoV-2 mRNA vaccine by BioNTech/Pfizer, mRNA-1273 SARS-CoV-2 mRNA vaccine by Moderna and Onpattro® transthyretin siRNA for hereditary amyloidosis by Alnylam [23]. By way of their rapid regulatory review and enormous clinical impact, the market approval of the LNP-based mRNA vaccines, in particular, will facilitate the translation of future nanomedicine products [23]. This truth has already been recognized by the savvy financial markets, with record investment flowing into nanomedicine startups [24], especially vaccine companies.

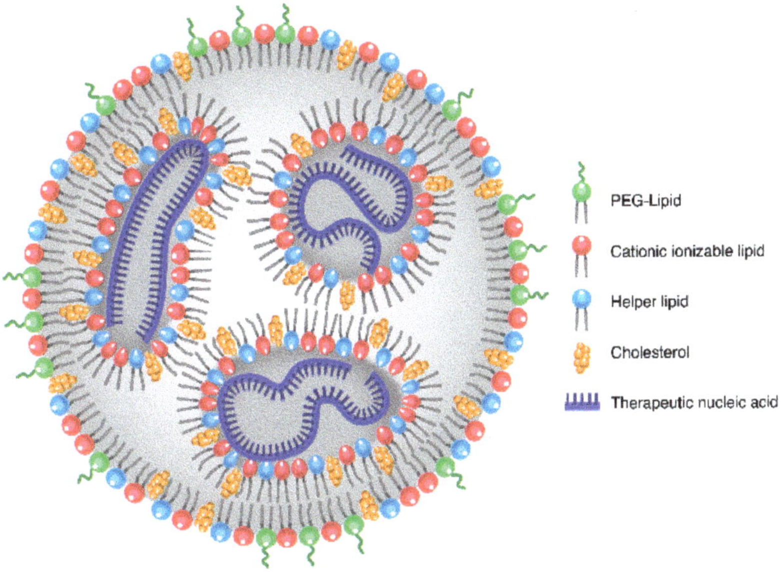

Figure 1. LNP Structure. The LNP interior contains electrostatically neutral inverted micelles, in which the negatively charged nucleic acid is surrounded by the ionizable lipid and other lipid components. The surface of the LNP is composed of a hydrophilic shell containing the PEG-lipid. (Figure adapted from Evers et al. [25]).

3. Inherent LNP Liver Tropism

The liver is the primary organ of LNP accumulation following intravenous administration and is also observed to varying degrees following intramuscular and subcutaneous routes, with larger LNP having less liver uptake [26]. For example, after intramuscular administration of an mRNA LNP vaccine to mice, branched DNA analysis of tissue mRNA identified muscle > lymph node > liver > spleen > testis as the primary organs of LNP accumulation in descending order [27]. Interestingly, mRNA LNP uptake does not necessarily correlate with mRNA protein expression [26]. The cell populations involved in liver uptake are dependent upon the underlying uptake mechanism. A common mechanism of uptake for most nanoparticles, including LNP, is scavenger receptor-mediated uptake into the hepatic Kupffer cells and sinusoidal endothelium following opsonization by non-specific absorption of plasma proteins [28]. Alternatively, Akinc et al. discovered that adsorption of endogenous apolipoprotein E (ApoE) can direct the uptake of LNP to hepatocytes through interaction with the low-density lipoprotein receptor (LDLR) located in these cells [29]. These researchers characterized this uptake mechanism by using LDLR knockout mice and hepatocytes in vitro and went on to show that the *N*-acetylgalactosamine (GalNAc) ligand covalently attached to LNP could also target hepatocytes through the asialoglycoprotein receptor (Table 1). The utility of GalNAc-mediated hepatocyte targeting of LNP is demonstrated by the recent approval of Onpattro transthyretin siRNA for hereditary amyloidosis mentioned above. Clearly, delivery of nucleic acid to hepatocytes by LNP has therapeutic potential, but there are many disease indications that would benefit from non-hepatic LNP tissue and cell population targeting, such as cancer and neurological and cardiovascular disease.

Although reducing hepatic uptake of parenterally administered LNP has been a challenge, alterations in LNP composition and physicochemical characteristics have been shown to influence liver distribution (Table 1). The LNP surface charge has been shown to influence the liver accumulation of intramuscularly administered LNP, with negatively charged LNP having greater liver uptake [4]. Similarly, the inclusion of neutral lipids to LNP resulted in liver tropism following intravenous injection, while the addition of cationic lipids to net neutral LNP resulted in a shift to lung uptake and the addition of negatively charged lipids to net neutral LNP resulted in splenic uptake [17]. The addition of oxidized cholesterol to LNP shifted liver uptake away from hepatocytes and into the hepatic microenvironment, including Kupffer cells and hepatic endothelial cells [30]. The inclusion of constrained lipids in LNP, such as adamantyl phospholipids, has also been shown to target hepatic Kupffer cells [31]. Apart from charge and composition, size can also influence hepatocyte transfection, presumably due to the hepatic architecture, with narrow sinusoidal fenestration pores of ~100 nm [32]; LNP > ~200 nm dramatically diminishes hepatocyte transfection [33].

Alternatives to LNP modification have also been attempted to prevent liver accumulation. In one example, a liposome termed a "nanoprimer" was used to saturate Kupffer cell-mediated clearance 10 min prior to administration of LNP containing Cy5.5 labeled human erythropoietin mRNA or factor VII siRNA, resulting in increased systemic fluorescence at 1 h post-dose and increased erythropoietin or decreased factor VII protein expression at 48 h post-dose, respectively [34]. Clever mRNA modifications have also been made in an attempt to reduce off-target liver expression by the design of hepatic-selective, suppressive micro-RNA (miRNA) binding sites into the untranslated regions of the mRNA [35]. This would decrease hepatic translation regardless of hepatic LNP uptake. The incorporation of suppressive miRNA elements can also be used to limit mRNA expression to a certain cell type. Magadum et al. utilized a miRNA responsive expression scheme they named 'specific modRNA translation system' or SMRT, to limit mRNA LNP expression to cardiomyocytes. In the SMRT scheme, a suppressive cardiomyocyte-specific miRNA binding site for miR1-208 was incorporated into the untranslated region of an mRNA coding for a negative-regulating protein, L7AE. Upon expression, the negative-regulating L7AE protein prevents the translation of the second mRNA of interest. However, in the case of cardiomyocyte-specific miRNA binding to the L7AE mRNA, the L7AE expression is suppressed and the second mRNA is translated [36].

Table 1. Tissue-targeted LNP. (DLS, dynamic light scattering; i.m., intramuscular; i.v., intravenous; s.c., subcutaneous; i.d., intradermal; i.p., intraperitoneal; r.o., retroorbital; PDI, polydispersity index; ZP, zeta potential).

LNP Targeting Components or Properties	Physicochemical Properties (DLS Size, PDI and Zeta Potential)	Route of Administration	Payload and Indication	Model	Tissue/Cell Type Specificity	Ref.
50 mol% 1,2-dioleoyl-3-trimethylammonium-propane (DOTAP)	113 nm 0.22 PDI −0.52 mV	i.v.	human Erythropoietin, mouse Interleukin-10, mouse Klotho, Luciferase and Cre mRNA, and Cas9 mRNA/sgTom1 *	18–20 g male C57BL/6 mice; (age and sex not specified) B6.Cg-Gt(ROSA)$^{26Sortm9(CAG\text{-}tdTomato)Hze}$/J mice (also known as Ai9 or Ai9(RCL-tdT) mice	hepatocyte uptake	[17]
30 molar% 1,2-dioleoyl-*sn*-glycero-3-phosphate (18PA)	142 nm 0.13 PDI −2.11 mV	i.v.	human Erythropoietin, mouse Interleukin-10, mouse Klotho, Luciferase and Cre mRNA, and Cas9 mRNA/sgPTEN and Cas9 mRNA/sgTom1 *	18–20 g male C57BL/6 mice; (age and sex not specified) B6.Cg-Gt(ROSA)$^{26Sortm9(CAG\text{-}tdTomato)Hze}$/J mice (also known as Ai9 or Ai9(RCL-tdT) mice	hepatocyte uptake	[17]
20 molar% 1,2-dioleoyl-3-dimethylammonium-propane (DODAP)	12 nm 0.18 PDI (ZP not specified)	i.v.	human Erythropoietin, mouse Interleukin-10, mouse Klotho, Luciferase and Cre mRNA, and Cas9 mRNA/sgPCSK9 and Cas9 mRNA/sgTom1 *	18–20 g male C57BL/6 mice; (age and sex not specified) B6.Cg-Gt(ROSA)$^{26Sortm9(CAG\text{-}tdTomato)Hze}$/J mice (also known as Ai9 or Ai9(RCL-tdT) mice	hepatocyte uptake	[17]
50:10:38.5:1.5% mole ratios DLin-KC2 DMA:DSPC:Cholesterol: DMG-PEG2000, with N:P molar ratio = 2, imparting negative charge	75 nm (PDI not specified) −10 mV	i.m.	Luciferase mRNA *	8-week-old female Balb/c mice	greater hepatic distribution following i.m. administration	[4]
50:23.5:6.5:20% mole ratios 7C1 **:C14PEG2K:18:1 Lyso PC 60:10:25:5% mole ratios 7C1 **:C14PEG2K:DOPE	20–200 nm (PDI not specified) (ZP not specified)	i.v.	ICAM-2 siRNA, Cre mRNA, CRISPR-Cas9 mRNA and ICAM-2 sgRNA *	5–12-week-old (sex not specified) LSL-Tomato, C57BL/6J, and constitutive SpCas9 mice	lung, spleen, liver and kidney endothelial cell uptake	[37]

Table 1. *Cont.*

LNP Targeting Components or Properties	Physicochemical Properties (DLS Size, PDI and Zeta Potential)	Route of Administration	Payload and Indication	Model	Tissue/Cell Type Specificity	Ref.
Endogenous absorption of apoE to neutral LNP	64.5 nm (PDI not specified) (ZP not specified)	i.v.	Factor VII siRNA *	6–8-week-old female C57Bl/6, ApoE−/− and LDLR−/− mice	hepatocyte uptake	[29]
N-acetylgalactosamine (GalNAc) ligand	69.4 nm (PDI not specified) (ZP not specified)	i.v.	Factor VII siRNA *	6–8-week-old female C57Bl/6 and ASGR2−/− mice	hepatocyte uptake	[29]
Plasmalemma vesicle-associated protein (PV1)	70 nm, 0.104 PDI and 160 nm, 0.150–0.240 PDI (ZP not specified)	i.v.	Luciferase mRNA, Cy5-mRNA *	5-week-old female Balb-c mice	lung uptake	[7]
Anti-Ly6c mAbs	70 nm (PDI not specified) (ZP not specified)	i.v.	Luciferase or IL-10 mRNA; treatment of inflammatory bowel disease	Colitis was induced in: 12-week-old female C57BL/6 mice using dextran sodium sulfate	leukocyte uptake	[38]
15–20 mol% C18PEG2000:80 mol% 7C1 **:0.1–10 mol% cholesterol	45–50 nm <0.2 PDI (ZP not specified)	i.v.	ICAM-2 siRNA, ICAM-2 targeting sgRNA *	5–12-week-old (sex not specified) C57BL6/j and constitutive SpCas9 mice	bone marrow endothelial cell	[39]
Anti-CD4 antibody	129 nm 0.12 PDI −10 mV	i.v.	Cy5-labeled siRNA and CD45 siRNA *	6–8-week-old (sex not specified) C57BL6/j mice	T cells	[9]
Anti-CD4 antibody	88 nm 0.1 PDI (ZP not specified)	i.v.	Cre recombinase-encoding mRNA *	(age not specified) (sex not specified) Ai6 (RCL-ZsGreen) mice on C57BL/6J	Splenic and lymph node T cells	[10]
Adamantane-constrained lipid	20–200 nm 0.20–0.23 PID (ZP not specified)	i.v.	GFP siRNA *	5–8-week-old female C57BL/6-Tg(UBC-GFP)30Scha/J, 'GFP mice'	splenic T cells	[40]

Table 1. *Cont.*

LNP Targeting Components or Properties	Physicochemical Properties (DLS Size, PDI and Zeta Potential)	Route of Administration	Payload and Indication	Model	Tissue/Cell Type Specificity	Ref.
Anti-CD29 antibody	66–75 nm 0.10–0.16 PDI (ZP not specified)	i.v.	PLK1 siRNA; treatment of disseminated bone marrow mantle cell lymphoma xenograft	8-week-old female C.B-17/IcrHsd-Prkdc scid mice	mantle cell lymphoma	[8]
Cholesterol oleate	22–115 nm (PDI not specified) (ZP not specified)	i.v.	ICAM-2 siRNA, GFP-targeted sgRNA *	5–8-week-old female C57BL/6J and C57BL/6-Tg(UBC-GFP)30Scha/J, 'GFP mice'	hepatic endothelial cells	[41]
~30 nm, negatively charged LNP	34 nm 0.242 PDI −12 mV	s.c.	DiD-labeled LNP (no nucleic acid) *	7–9-week-old female C57BL/6J mice	CD8+ dendritic cells/lymph node	[14]
35:5:55:5% mole ratios 7C1 **:Choles-terol:C14PEG2000:DOTAP	40 nm (PDI not specified) (ZP not specified)	nebulization	Therapeutic membrane-anchored FI6 antibody mRNA, H1N1 influenza model	6–8-week-old female BALBc mice	lung	[42]
~150 nm size, ~0.5% PEG density	150 nm <0.1 PD (ZP not specified)	intravitreal and subretinal injection	Cre, mCherry, luciferase mRNA *	1–6 months old male and female Albino BALB/c, Ai9, apoE−/−, Mertk−/− and C57BL6 mice	optic nerve, trabecular meshwork, retinal pigment epithelium, Muller glia	[43]
Ionizable lipids with low pKa and unsaturated hydrocarbon chains	83–229 nm 0.09–0.28 PDI (ZP not specified)	subretinal injection	Luciferase, EGFP, mCherry mRNA *	1–4 months old male and female Albino BALB/c mice	retinal pigment epithelium	[44]
Oxidized cholesterol	~80 nm 0.16 PDI (ZP not specified)	i.v.	Cre mRNA *	5–8-week-old (sex not specified) Ai14 Lox-Stop-Lox-tdTomato and C57BL/6J mice	hepatic endothelial and Kupffer cells	[30]

Table 1. *Cont.*

LNP Targeting Components or Properties	Physicochemical Properties (DLS Size, PDI and Zeta Potential)	Route of Administration	Payload and Indication	Model	Tissue/Cell Type Specificity	Ref.
Anti PECAM-1 antibody	103 nm 0.195 PDI −4.1 mV	i.v.	Luciferase mRNA *	(age not specified) (sex not specified) C57BL/6 mice	lung vascular endothelial and immune cells	[11]
Adamantyl-constrained lipid	100 nm (PDI not specified) (ZP not specified)	i.v.	Cre mRNA *	(age not specified) (sex not specified) Ai14 Lox-Stop-Lox-tdTomato mice	hepatic Kupffer cells	[31]
ApoE opsonization	55 nm 0.058 PDI (ZP not specified)	intracranial	PTEN, luciferase and GRIN1 siRNA *	26–30-day-old (sex not specified) Sprague Dawley rats	CNS neurons	[45]
CH6 osteoblast-specific aptamer	84 nm (PDI not specified) (ZP not specified)	i.v.	osteogenic pleckstrin homology domain-containing family O member 1 (*Plekho1*) siRNA; treatment of impaired bone formation (e.g., osteoporosis)	6-month-old female Sprague Dawley rats	osteoblasts	[46]
Mannose-cholesterol	~140 nm >0.2 PDI (ZP not specified)	i.d.	Influenze hemagglutanin saRNA; H1N1 influenza vaccine	6−8-week-old female BALB/c mice	dendritic cells	[12]
Mannose-PEG-DSPE	~100 nm (PDI not specified) (ZP not specified)	i.v.	Cre mRNA and FVIII siRNA *	7–10-week-old female C57BL/6 mice; 8-week-old (sex not specified) Lox-Stop-Lox-tdTomato	hepatic endothelial cells	[13]
EGFR-antibody	79 nm 0.085 PDI 7.7 mV	i.p.	Cas9 mRNA, (polo-like kinase) PLK1 sgRNA; disseminated ovarian cancer	8-week-old female Hsd: Athymic Nude-Foxn1nu mice with OV8 ovarian cancer peritoneal xenograft	disseminated ovarian cancer	[47]

Table 1. *Cont.*

LNP Targeting Components or Properties	Physicochemical Properties (DLS Size, PDI and Zeta Potential)	Route of Administration	Payload and Indication	Model	Tissue/Cell Type Specificity	Ref.
DEC205-antibody	90–130 nm 0.12–0.20 PDI (ZP not specified)	r.o.	CD40, CD80 and CD86 siRNA	6–12-week-old (sex not specified) C57BL/6 mice, inhibition of mixed lymphocyte response to LPS	CD8 alpha+ dendritic cells	[48]
CD4-antibody	88 nm 0.1 PDI (ZP not specified)	i.v.	Luciferase and Cre mRNA *	(age not specified) male and female C57BL/6 and Ai6 (RCL-ZsGreen) mice on C57BL/6J background	CD4+ T cells	[10]
CD5-antibody	80 nm 0.02–0.06 PDI (ZP not specified)	i.v.	CAR mRNA against fibroblast activation protein and Cre mRNA, cardiac fibrosis prevention	(age not specified) (sex not specified) C57BL/6NAi6 Cre-reporter mice ($Rosa26^{CAG-LSL-ZsGreen}$)	CD5+ T cells	[49]

* Experimental system, no therapeutic indication evaluated. ** 7C1 is a novel ionizable lipid; refer to publication for structure.

4. Non-Hepatic LNP Targeting

Several groups have used in vivo screening systems to select LNP compositions that target-specific tissues/cells without the use of targeting ligands. In particular, Dahlman's laboratory at the Georgia Institute of Technology has pioneered the use of an in vivo screen that correlates a unique LNP "DNA barcode" with siRNA delivery and function [39]. The technique identifies reduced protein expression resulting from siRNA knockdown in the tissue of interest by flow cytometry and then sequences the cells to identify the corresponding DNA barcode of the LNP responsible. Utilizing this method, over 100 LNP of varying composition were screened simultaneously for bone marrow endothelial cell (BMEC) transfection with an ICAM-2 siRNA payload, identifying LNP with 15–20 mol% C18PEG2000/80 mol% 7C1 helper lipid/0.1–10 mol% cholesterol as BMEC targeted. They then went on to show that an example of this BMEC-targeting LNP, 'BM1', could also deliver sgRNA in a constitutively expressed SpCas9 model, demonstrating the flexibility of this delivery platform.

LNP targeting of immune cell populations is of particular interest for the purposes of immunomodulation and vaccine delivery. While intramuscular injection of untargeted mRNA LNP vaccines results in significant accumulation in antigen-presenting cell (APC) populations at local lymph nodes, there is substantial accumulation in the muscle itself, as well as other tissues such as liver, spleen, bone marrow and testes [27]. The potential negative consequences of this off-target distribution are presently unknown. In order to increase vaccine efficacy as well as decrease potential risks of off-target distribution, researchers have tried to improve LNP distribution to lymph nodes and APC. As an example, Nakamura et al. evaluated the effect of size and charge on lipid nanoparticle lymph node tropism of LNP prepared by the popular microfluidic mixing technique [41]. They identified small (~30 nm), negatively charged LNP as having greatly superior lymph node dendritic cell distribution in comparison to larger (100–200 nm), neutral or cationic LNP [14]. This agrees with liposome studies by Kranz et al., who identified negatively charged liposomes as having greater lymphatic dendritic cell tropism [50]. Active targeting has also been utilized to target vaccines to APC. Incorporation of mannose conjugated cholesterol in an influenza hemagglutinin saRNA LNP to target the APC mannose receptor (CD206) resulted in enhanced dendritic primary cell uptake in vitro and a more rapid immune response in vivo following i.d. administration, with higher antibody titers and greater antigen-specific splenic CD4+ and CD8+ T cells [12]. The incorporation of a mannose targeting ligand has also been shown to target LNP to hepatic sinusoidal endothelial cells [13].

LNP has been targeted to T cells with surface conjugated anti-CD4 antibodies, resulting in uptake by T cells in the blood and lymphatic system following intravenous administration [9,10]. The LNP with conformationally constrained lipids was also found to target splenic T cells following intravenous administration [40]. Coating of antibodies on the surface of LNP incorporating an Fc binding lipid allowed for in vivo targeting of various immune cells, including macrophages, Treg, T helper, CTL, B cells and monocytes, corresponding to coating with anti-CD45, -CD25, -CD4, -CD8, -CD19 and -CD11b antibodies, respectively [8].

Lung delivery of nucleic acids has the potential for the treatment of a wide range of respiratory diseases, such as genetic defects such as cystic fibrosis and infectious diseases such as the common flu. In addition to systemic administration of lung-targeted LNP, direct inhalation of nebulized LNP has been attempted [7,17,42]. In the case of nebulization, researchers found high molar percentages of both PEG and cationic helper lipid improved lung transfection [42]. Administration of a nebulized 40 nm LNP with 55 and 5 molar% C14PEG2000 and DOTAP, respectively, delivered a payload of membrane-anchored FI6 antibody mRNA and protected against a lethal dose of influenza H1N1 in a murine model. Systemically administered LNP has also been targeted to the lung vasculature by conjugation of platelet endothelial cell adhesion molecule-1 (PECAM-1) antibodies to the LNP surface [11].

The eye is also of interest for LNP delivery for the treatment of such conditions as retinal degeneration. The eye benefits from being accessible for direct administration by topical, subretinal, intravitreal and suprachoroidal administration routes [51]. At this time, only viral vector-based oligonucleotide therapies are approved for the treatment of ocular diseases, such as Luxturna for inherited retinal dystrophy [51], but advancements are being made in LNP oligonucleotide delivery systems. Patel et al. identified LNP containing ionizable lipids with low pKa and unsaturated hydrocarbon chains as having the greatest retinal pigment epithelium (RPE) transfection following subretinal injection [44]. These researchers went on to discover that larger LNP, ~150 nm, having a lower PEG density of 0.5 mol% had greater transfection of the RPE following subretinal administration, and following intravitreal administration, had greater transfection of Muller glia, optic nerve and trabecular meshwork [43]. ApoE absorption and subsequent LDLR-mediated uptake, as well as phagocytosis, were not involved in the observed LNP RPE transfection.

LNP targeting of oligonucleotides to the CNS has potential for the treatment of neurological diseases as well as providing a tool for understanding brain function through manipulation of protein expression. Since ApoE is produced by astroglia and LDLR is found on neurons, LNP can be used to target neurons in the CNS, similar to how hepatocytes are targeted systemically in an ApoE-dependent fashion [52]. Back in 2013, Rungta et al. demonstrated that intracranial administration of siRNA-LNP constructs to the brain could silence neuronal *N*-methyl-D-aspartate (NMDA) receptors locally or regionally when administered by intracortical or intracerebroventricular injection, respectively [45]. They demonstrated that neuronal LNP uptake was ApoE-dependent by observing that LNP uptake into rat primary neurons only occurred upon supplementation of the culture media with ApoE. The primary issue for LNP-mediated CNS delivery, however, is overcoming the blood–brain barrier (BBB). The only example we found in our literature review for a BBB-targeted LNP utilized an RNA aptamer targeting the C-C chemokine receptor type 5 (CCR5), and this construct was only evaluated in an in vitro model of the BBB, not in vivo.

5. Oncology and Immuno-Oncology

An area of great promise for the future of LNP is cancer, in particular vaccine immunotherapy [53,54]. In fact, both Moderna and BioNTech, developers of the FDA-approved SARS-CoV-2 vaccines, are investing in immuno-oncology to further utilize their mRNA delivery technologies. BioNTech has several mRNA cancer vaccine candidates in clinical trials, including BNT111, in phase 2 clinical trials for melanoma (NCT04526899), BNT113, in phase 2 for HPV16-positive head and neck cancers (NCT04534205), and BNT112 in phase 1/2 for prostate cancer (NCT04382898). These mRNA vaccines are being explored in combination with anti-PD-1 immune checkpoint inhibitors such as cemiplimab and pembrolizumab [55]. Though, these formulations use BioNTech's FixVac platform technology (RNA-lipoplex delivery vehicles), not the LNP architecture as shown in Figure 1. Lipoplexes were one of the early delivery vehicles for mRNA targeting, although with the advantages lipid nanoparticles offer, such as increased stability and protection of the nucleic acid cargo, lipid nanoparticles are becoming a popular choice for the exploration of novel treatment strategies [53]. Additionally, in a recent interview, BioNTech CEO Uğur Şahin stressed the company's commitment to developing strategies to combat cancer with its mRNA cancer vaccine technology [56].

Moderna is using its LNP technology for the delivery of mRNA cancer vaccines as well as immuno-oncology therapeutics [57]. The following two cancer vaccine candidates are currently in clinical trials: mRNA-4157, a personalized cancer vaccine in phase 2 clinical trials for the treatment of melanoma (NCT03897881), and mRNA-5671, a KRAS vaccine in phase 1 clinical trials for the treatment of pancreatic, colorectal and non-small cell lung cancers (NCT03948763) [58]. Both vaccines are being tested in combination with pembrolizumab. In the immuno-oncology space, Moderna has the following two formulations in Phase 1 clinical trials: mRNA-2752, an LNP encapsulating mRNA encoding OX40L,

IL-23 and IL-36γ (NCT03739931, NCT02872025) and MEDI1191, an LNP encapsulating mRNA for IL-12 (NCT03946800) [58]. These formulations are being tested in combination with pembrolizumab and durvalumab, respectively.

Recently, Pfizer entered into an agreement with Acuitas Therapeutics to license their LNP technology for the development of several therapeutic and vaccine concepts [59]. There are already dozens of strategies in clinical trials for both cancers as well as infectious disease treatment and vaccine development [54]. Further, there are countless strategies in various phases of preclinical development. Oberli et al. have described a lipid nanoparticle-based mRNA vaccine that showed promise when tested in a B16F10 melanoma model in mice [60]. The vaccine, encoding for TRP2 and gp100 tumor-associated antigens, induced strong CD8 T cell activation and showed decreased tumor volume with increased animal survival in the highly aggressive cancer. In another example, Lee et al. used LNP for the delivery of tri-palmitoyl-S-glyceryl cysteine linked to a pentapeptide (termed Pam3), which is a known adjuvant of TLR1 and TLR2 [61]. In addition to enhanced CD8 T cell response, the Pam3-LNP showed superior tumor prevention in a mouse lymphoma model. Novel LNP-mRNA vaccines and treatments hold tremendous potential for future development, and with improved targeting strategies as described herein, the number of both preclinical and clinical studies is sure to multiply in the coming years.

6. Conclusions and Future Directions

There are surprisingly few examples of tissue-targeted LNP, apart from targeting of the liver, lung and the immune system, as well as a few examples of actively targeted concepts (Figure 2). One of the primary obstacles to tissue targeting is the natural physiological barrier to tissue accumulation presented by the vascular endothelium, as most tissues apart from the liver and spleen are not fenestrated, having a continuous endothelium [62]. While tumor vasculature often contains openings in the endothelium, the passive accumulation of nanoparticles through these pores into the tumor tissue has been found to be highly variable and inefficient, largely due to inconsistent pore size and density and extracellular matrix and lymphatic blockage that creates back pressure that counters convective and diffusive movement into the pore [63]. Additionally, animal cancer models, primarily mice, are often not representative of the clinical case and this has resulted in a poor correlation between preclinical and clinical efficacy of nanomedicine formulations [64]. Studies reviewing nanomedicine tumor uptake in the preclinical literature have identified both poor absolute tumor uptake, averaging ~0.7% of the total dose, but also greater tumor vs. systemic drug exposure in comparison to conventional drug formulations [65,66]; these data would support the reduced toxicity of nanomedicines, which generally correlates with systemic exposure, but also reduced efficacy, which correlates to tumor exposure.

With this in mind, it is of interest for future targeted LNP research to concentrate on active targeting of the vascular endothelium itself, not only the tissue of interest, utilizing strategies such as receptor-mediated transcytosis and paracellular transport to breach the vascular barrier [67,68]. Selectivity of this endothelial targeting strategy must rely on tissue-selective receptor expression that may benefit from modern ligand-receptor identification techniques such as phage display. Phage display is a versatile tool that can be used to screen proteins, peptides or antibodies for interaction with cells, tissues or biomarkers, conducted in vitro, ex vivo, as well as in vivo [69,70]. In addition to the identification of more selective targeting ligands, there is also the requirement to simultaneously optimize transfection efficiency, which as mentioned above is also tissue-dependent [26].

An alternative to tissue targeting using LNP composition or the addition of a targeting ligand is the incorporation of cell membrane-derived components into LNP. Addition of cell membrane-derived components to make biological hybrid LNP constructs can utilize the cell membrane's innate-stealth qualities to evade immune system recognition and homotypic features to target tissues and cells [71]. Common cell membrane-derived coatings used for stealth and tissue targeting are red blood cell (RBC) membranes, and cancer and platelet cell membranes, respectively [72–75]. This powerful targeting technique has been applied to patient-derived cancer cells (PDCC), with PDCC membrane-coated nanoparticles demonstrating PDCC-specific targeting preclinically in their respective xenograft models [73]. Similarly, cancer cell membrane-coated siRNA formulations have also been shown to selectively target in a homotypic fashion, in which only cancer cells of the membrane origin are targeted [76]. There is also the possibility of using a combination of active and biomimetic targeting approaches. For example, a cRGD-targeted, RBC membrane-coated polyplex was utilized for siRNA delivery to melanoma, with the RBC coating preventing opsonization and increasing circulation time [77]. Targeting ligands can also be engineered directly into the coating membrane. Park et al., for example, coated an mRNA polyplex with a mouse melanoma membrane engineered to express a viral fusion protein that enhances endosomal escape, dramatically improving transfection efficiency both in vitro and in vivo [78]. A more general targeting approach than cancer cell membrane homotypic targeting and active targeting are utilizing platelet membrane coatings, which have been shown to target a variety of disease states, including vascular disease, infections and cancer [75]. Utilizing this disease agnostic targeting approach, Zhuang et al. demonstrated the ability of a platelet membrane-coated survivan siRNA metallic nanoparticle to accumulate in and suppress the growth of an SK-BR-3 breast cancer xenograft [79].

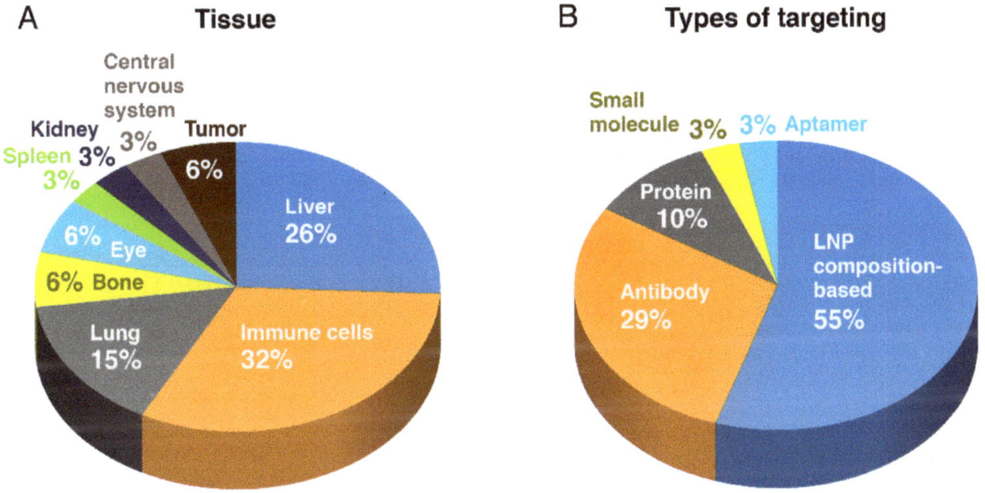

Figure 2. Trends in targeted LNP. The trends in LNP tissue target (**A**) and targeting mechanism (**B**) are displayed (from references in Table 1).

Another potentially impactful application of LNP technology is modification to exploit stimuli-responsive properties. Internal (e.g., pH, enzyme and redox) and external (e.g., temperature, light, ultrasound and magnetic fields) stimuli have been explored for a variety of nanoparticle platforms [80–84], with Celsion Corporation's ThermoDox arguably the most well-known example [85–87]. There are several reports in the literature using internal and external stimuli to afford the release of nucleic acid cargos. Miller et al. synthesized cationic lipoplexes incorporating matrix metalloproteinase-2 (MMP-2) and human leukocyte elastase (HLE) sensitive linkers, both of which are known to be upregulated in the tumor matrix, to demonstrate the targeted release of siRNA in vitro in several cell lines using luciferase knockdown experiments [88]. PEGylated lipids were modified to include the MMP-2 and HLE linkers, which when cleaved, effectively de-shield the nanoparticles of the PEG layer, promoting cellular uptake. In another example, Rabbitts et al. used external acoustic shock waves to enhance cellular uptake of mRNA lipoplex particles [89]. The lipoplex particle was engineered to take advantage of unique phase transitions that are triggered by the shock waves to promote cellular entry. Using fluorescently labeled GFP-modified mRNA, the lipoplexes were transfected into several cell lines and the fluorescence from the translated mRNA was quantified, with cells receiving the shock wave treatment showing a greater transfection efficiency. With appropriate modifications to either the lipid components or the nucleic acid cargo, LNP can also potentially take advantage of these internal and external release triggers to enhance tumor targeting.

Author Contributions: Conceptualization, S.T.S.; writing—original draft preparation, R.N.K., R.M.C. and S.T.S.; writing—review and editing, R.N.K., R.M.C. and S.T.S. All authors have read and agreed to the published version of the manuscript.

Funding: This project has been funded in whole or in part with Federal funds from the National Cancer Institute, National Institutes of Health, under Contract No. 75N91019D00024. The content of this publication does not necessarily reflect the views or policies of the Department of Health and Human Services, nor does mention of trade names, commercial products, or organizations imply endorsement by the U.S. Government.

Institutional Review Board Statement: Not applicable.

Informed Consent Statement: Not applicable.

Data Availability Statement: Data sharing not applicable.

Conflicts of Interest: The authors declare no conflict of interest.

References

1. Wolff, J.A.; Malone, R.W.; Williams, P.; Chong, W.; Acsadi, G.; Jani, A.; Felgner, P.L. Direct gene transfer into mouse muscle in vivo. *Science* **1990**, *247*, 1465–1468. [CrossRef] [PubMed]
2. Probst, J.; Weide, B.; Scheel, B.; Pichler, B.J.; Hoerr, I.; Rammensee, H.G.; Pascolo, S. Spontaneous cellular uptake of exogenous messenger RNA in vivo is nucleic acid-specific, saturable and ion dependent. *Gene Therapy* **2007**, *14*, 1175–1180. [CrossRef] [PubMed]
3. Eygeris, Y.; Gupta, M.; Kim, J.; Sahay, G. Chemistry of Lipid Nanoparticles for RNA Delivery. *Acc. Chem. Res.* **2022**, *55*, 2–12. [CrossRef] [PubMed]
4. Carrasco, M.J.; Alishetty, S.; Alameh, M.G.; Said, H.; Wright, L.; Paige, M.; Soliman, O.; Weissman, D.; Cleveland, T.E.T.; Grishaev, A.; et al. Ionization and structural properties of mRNA lipid nanoparticles influence expression in intramuscular and intravascular administration. *Commun. Biol.* **2021**, *4*, 956. [CrossRef]
5. Stern, S.T.; McNeil, S.E. Nanotechnology safety concerns revisited. *Toxicol. Sci.* **2008**, *101*, 4–21. [CrossRef]
6. Shobaki, N.; Sato, Y.; Harashima, H. Mixing lipids to manipulate the ionization status of lipid nanoparticles for specific tissue targeting. *Int. J. Nanomed.* **2018**, *13*, 8395–8410. [CrossRef]
7. Li, Q.; Chan, C.; Peterson, N.; Hanna, R.N.; Alfaro, A.; Allen, K.L.; Wu, H.; Dall'Acqua, W.F.; Borrok, M.J.; Santos, J.L. Engineering Caveolae-Targeted Lipid Nanoparticles To Deliver mRNA to the Lungs. *ACS Chem. Biol.* **2020**, *15*, 830–836. [CrossRef]
8. Kedmi, R.; Veiga, N.; Ramishetti, S.; Goldsmith, M.; Rosenblum, D.; Dammes, N.; Hazan-Halevy, I.; Nahary, L.; Leviatan-Ben-Arye, S.; Harlev, M.; et al. A modular platform for targeted RNAi therapeutics. *Nat. Nanotechnol.* **2018**, *13*, 214–219. [CrossRef]
9. Ramishetti, S.; Kedmi, R.; Goldsmith, M.; Leonard, F.; Sprague, A.G.; Godin, B.; Gozin, M.; Cullis, P.R.; Dykxhoorn, D.M.; Peer, D. Systemic Gene Silencing in Primary T Lymphocytes Using Targeted Lipid Nanoparticles. *ACS Nano* **2015**, *9*, 6706–6716. [CrossRef]
10. Tombacz, I.; Laczko, D.; Shahnawaz, H.; Muramatsu, H.; Natesan, A.; Yadegari, A.; Papp, T.E.; Alameh, M.G.; Shuvaev, V.; Mui, B.L.; et al. Highly efficient CD4+ T cell targeting and genetic recombination using engineered CD4+ cell-homing mRNA-LNPs. *Mol. Therapy* **2021**, *29*, 3293–3304. [CrossRef]
11. Parhiz, H.; Shuvaev, V.V.; Pardi, N.; Khoshnejad, M.; Kiseleva, R.Y.; Brenner, J.S.; Uhler, T.; Tuyishime, S.; Mui, B.L.; Tam, Y.K.; et al. PECAM-1 directed re-targeting of exogenous mRNA providing two orders of magnitude enhancement of vascular delivery and expression in lungs independent of apolipoprotein E-mediated uptake. *J. Control. Release* **2018**, *291*, 106–115. [CrossRef] [PubMed]
12. Goswami, R.; Chatzikleanthous, D.; Lou, G.; Giusti, F.; Bonci, A.; Taccone, M.; Brazzoli, M.; Gallorini, S.; Ferlenghi, I.; Berti, F.; et al. Mannosylation of LNP Results in Improved Potency for Self-Amplifying RNA (SAM) Vaccines. *ACS Infect. Dis.* **2019**, *5*, 1546–1558. [CrossRef] [PubMed]
13. Kim, M.; Jeong, M.; Hur, S.; Cho, Y.; Park, J.; Jung, H.; Seo, Y.; Woo, H.A.; Nam, K.T.; Lee, K.; et al. Engineered ionizable lipid nanoparticles for targeted delivery of RNA therapeutics into different types of cells in the liver. *Sci Adv.* **2021**, *7*, eabf4398. [CrossRef] [PubMed]
14. Nakamura, T.; Kawai, M.; Sato, Y.; Maeki, M.; Tokeshi, M.; Harashima, H. The Effect of Size and Charge of Lipid Nanoparticles Prepared by Microfluidic Mixing on Their Lymph Node Transitivity and Distribution. *Mol. Pharm.* **2020**, *17*, 944–953. [CrossRef]
15. Zukancic, D.; Suys, E.J.A.; Pilkington, E.H.; Algarni, A.; Al-Wassiti, H.; Truong, N.P. The Importance of Poly(ethylene glycol) and Lipid Structure in Targeted Gene Delivery to Lymph Nodes by Lipid Nanoparticles. *Pharmaceutics* **2020**, *12*, 1068. [CrossRef]

16. Dilliard, S.A.; Cheng, Q.; Siegwart, D.J. On the mechanism of tissue-specific mRNA delivery by selective organ targeting nanoparticles. *Proc. Natl. Acad. Sci. USA* **2021**, *118*, e2109256118. [CrossRef]
17. Cheng, Q.; Wei, T.; Farbiak, L.; Johnson, L.T.; Dilliard, S.A.; Siegwart, D.J. Selective organ targeting (SORT) nanoparticles for tissue-specific mRNA delivery and CRISPR-Cas gene editing. *Nat. Nanotechnol.* **2020**, *15*, 313–320. [CrossRef]
18. Liu, S.; Cheng, Q.; Wei, T.; Yu, X.; Johnson, L.T.; Farbiak, L.; Siegwart, D.J. Membrane-destabilizing ionizable phospholipids for organ-selective mRNA delivery and CRISPR-Cas gene editing. *Nat. Mater.* **2021**, *20*, 701–710. [CrossRef]
19. Alvarez-Benedicto, E.; Farbiak, L.; Marquez Ramirez, M.; Wang, X.; Johnson, L.T.; Mian, O.; Guerrero, E.D.; Siegwart, D.J. Optimization of phospholipid chemistry for improved lipid nanoparticle (LNP) delivery of messenger RNA (mRNA). *Biomater. Sci.* **2022**, *10*, 549–559. [CrossRef]
20. Lee, S.M.; Cheng, Q.; Yu, X.; Liu, S.; Johnson, L.T.; Siegwart, D.J. A Systematic Study of Unsaturation in Lipid Nanoparticles Leads to Improved mRNA Transfection In Vivo. *Angew. Chem. Int. Ed. Engl.* **2021**, *60*, 5848–5853. [CrossRef]
21. Kimura, S.; Khalil, I.A.; Elewa, Y.H.A.; Harashima, H. Novel lipid combination for delivery of plasmid DNA to immune cells in the spleen. *J. Control. Release* **2021**, *330*, 753–764. [CrossRef] [PubMed]
22. Algarni, A.; Pilkington, E.H.; Suys, E.J.A.; Al-Wassiti, H.; Pouton, C.W.; Truong, N.P. In vivo delivery of plasmid DNA by lipid nanoparticles: The influence of ionizable cationic lipids on organ-selective gene expression. *Biomater. Sci.* **2022**, *10*, 2940–2952. [CrossRef] [PubMed]
23. Milane, L.; Amiji, M. Clinical approval of nanotechnology-based SARS-CoV-2 mRNA vaccines: Impact on translational nanomedicine. *Drug Deliv. Transl. Res.* **2021**, *11*, 1309–1315. [CrossRef] [PubMed]
24. Surging Nanomedicine Investments Improve Global Healthcare and Pandemic Protection. *Global Health & Pharma*. Available online: https://www.ghp-news.com/surging-nanomedicine-investments-improve-global-healthcare-and-pandemic-protection/ (accessed on 13 June 2022).
25. Evers, M.J.W.; Kulkarni, J.A.; van der Meel, R.; Cullis, P.R.; Vader, P.; Schiffelers, R.M. State-of-the-Art Design and Rapid-Mixing Production Techniques of Lipid Nanoparticles for Nucleic Acid Delivery. *Small Methods* **2018**, *2*, 1700375. [CrossRef]
26. Di, J.; Du, Z.; Wu, K.; Jin, S.; Wang, X.; Li, T.; Xu, Y. Biodistribution and Non-linear Gene Expression of mRNA LNPs Affected by Delivery Route and Particle Size. *Pharm. Res.* **2022**, *39*, 105–114. [CrossRef]
27. Bahl, K.; Senn, J.J.; Yuzhakov, O.; Bulychev, A.; Brito, L.A.; Hassett, K.J.; Laska, M.E.; Smith, M.; Almarsson, O.; Thompson, J.; et al. Preclinical and Clinical Demonstration of Immunogenicity by mRNA Vaccines against H10N8 and H7N9 Influenza Viruses. *Mol. Therapy* **2017**, *25*, 1316–1327. [CrossRef]
28. Shi, B.; Keough, E.; Matter, A.; Leander, K.; Young, S.; Carlini, E.; Sachs, A.B.; Tao, W.; Abrams, M.; Howell, B.; et al. Biodistribution of small interfering RNA at the organ and cellular levels after lipid nanoparticle-mediated delivery. *J. Histochem. Cytochem.* **2011**, *59*, 727–740. [CrossRef]
29. Akinc, A.; Querbes, W.; De, S.; Qin, J.; Frank-Kamenetsky, M.; Jayaprakash, K.N.; Jayaraman, M.; Rajeev, K.G.; Cantley, W.L.; Dorkin, J.R.; et al. Targeted delivery of RNAi therapeutics with endogenous and exogenous ligand-based mechanisms. *Mol. Therapy* **2010**, *18*, 1357–1364. [CrossRef]
30. Paunovska, K.; Da Silva Sanchez, A.J.; Sago, C.D.; Gan, Z.; Lokugamage, M.P.; Islam, F.Z.; Kalathoor, S.; Krupczak, B.R.; Dahlman, J.E. Nanoparticles Containing Oxidized Cholesterol Deliver mRNA to the Liver Microenvironment at Clinically Relevant Doses. *Adv. Mater.* **2019**, *31*, e1807748. [CrossRef]
31. Gan, Z.; Lokugamage, M.P.; Hatit, M.Z.C.; Loughrey, D.; Paunovska, K.; Sato, M.; Cristian, A.; Dahlman, J.E. Nanoparticles containing constrained phospholipids deliver mRNA to liver immune cells in vivo without targeting ligands. *Bioeng. Transl. Med.* **2020**, *5*, e10161. [CrossRef]
32. Desjardins, M.; Griffiths, G. Phagocytosis: Latex leads the way. *Curr. Opin. Cell Biol.* **2003**, *15*, 498–503. [CrossRef]
33. Basha, G.; Novobrantseva, T.I.; Rosin, N.; Tam, Y.Y.; Hafez, I.M.; Wong, M.K.; Sugo, T.; Ruda, V.M.; Qin, J.; Klebanov, B.; et al. Influence of cationic lipid composition on gene silencing properties of lipid nanoparticle formulations of siRNA in antigen-presenting cells. *Mol. Therapy* **2011**, *19*, 2186–2200. [CrossRef] [PubMed]
34. Saunders, N.R.M.; Paolini, M.S.; Fenton, O.S.; Poul, L.; Devalliere, J.; Mpambani, F.; Darmon, A.; Bergere, M.; Jibault, O.; Germain, M.; et al. A Nanoprimer To Improve the Systemic Delivery of siRNA and mRNA. *Nano Lett.* **2020**, *20*, 4264–4269. [CrossRef]
35. Jain, R.; Frederick, J.P.; Huang, E.Y.; Burke, K.E.; Mauger, D.M.; Andrianova, E.A.; Farlow, S.J.; Siddiqui, S.; Pimentel, J.; Cheung-Ong, K.; et al. MicroRNAs Enable mRNA Therapeutics to Selectively Program Cancer Cells to Self-Destruct. *Nucleic Acid Ther.* **2018**, *28*, 285–296. [CrossRef]
36. Magadum, A.; Kurian, A.A.; Chepurko, E.; Sassi, Y.; Hajjar, R.J.; Zangi, L. Specific Modified mRNA Translation System. *Circulation* **2020**, *142*, 2485–2488. [CrossRef] [PubMed]
37. Sago, C.D.; Lokugamage, M.P.; Paunovska, K.; Vanover, D.A.; Monaco, C.M.; Shah, N.N.; Gamboa Castro, M.; Anderson, S.E.; Rudoltz, T.G.; Lando, G.N.; et al. High-throughput in vivo screen of functional mRNA delivery identifies nanoparticles for endothelial cell gene editing. *Proc. Natl. Acad. Sci. USA* **2018**, *115*, E9944–E9952. [CrossRef] [PubMed]
38. Veiga, N.; Goldsmith, M.; Granot, Y.; Rosenblum, D.; Dammes, N.; Kedmi, R.; Ramishetti, S.; Peer, D. Cell specific delivery of modified mRNA expressing therapeutic proteins to leukocytes. *Nat. Commun.* **2018**, *9*, 4493. [CrossRef]
39. Sago, C.D.; Lokugamage, M.P.; Islam, F.Z.; Krupczak, B.R.; Sato, M.; Dahlman, J.E. Nanoparticles That Deliver RNA to Bone Marrow Identified by in Vivo Directed Evolution. *J. Am. Chem. Soc.* **2018**, *140*, 17095–17105. [CrossRef]

40. Lokugamage, M.P.; Sago, C.D.; Gan, Z.; Krupczak, B.R.; Dahlman, J.E. Constrained Nanoparticles Deliver siRNA and sgRNA to T Cells In Vivo without Targeting Ligands. *Adv. Mater.* **2019**, *31*, e1902251. [CrossRef]
41. Paunovska, K.; Gil, C.J.; Lokugamage, M.P.; Sago, C.D.; Sato, M.; Lando, G.N.; Gamboa Castro, M.; Bryksin, A.V.; Dahlman, J.E. Analyzing 2000 in Vivo Drug Delivery Data Points Reveals Cholesterol Structure Impacts Nanoparticle Delivery. *ACS Nano* **2018**, *12*, 8341–8349. [CrossRef]
42. Lokugamage, M.P.; Vanover, D.; Beyersdorf, J.; Hatit, M.Z.C.; Rotolo, L.; Echeverri, E.S.; Peck, H.E.; Ni, H.; Yoon, J.K.; Kim, Y.; et al. Optimization of lipid nanoparticles for the delivery of nebulized therapeutic mRNA to the lungs. *Nat. Biomed. Eng.* **2021**, *5*, 1059–1068. [CrossRef]
43. Ryals, R.C.; Patel, S.; Acosta, C.; McKinney, M.; Pennesi, M.E.; Sahay, G. The effects of PEGylation on LNP based mRNA delivery to the eye. *PLoS ONE* **2020**, *15*, e0241006. [CrossRef] [PubMed]
44. Patel, S.; Ryals, R.C.; Weller, K.K.; Pennesi, M.E.; Sahay, G. Lipid nanoparticles for delivery of messenger RNA to the back of the eye. *J. Control. Release* **2019**, *303*, 91–100. [CrossRef] [PubMed]
45. Rungta, R.L.; Choi, H.B.; Lin, P.J.; Ko, R.W.; Ashby, D.; Nair, J.; Manoharan, M.; Cullis, P.R.; Macvicar, B.A. Lipid Nanoparticle Delivery of siRNA to Silence Neuronal Gene Expression in the Brain. *Mol. Therapy Nucleic Acids* **2013**, *2*, e136. [CrossRef] [PubMed]
46. Liang, C.; Guo, B.; Wu, H.; Shao, N.; Li, D.; Liu, J.; Dang, L.; Wang, C.; Li, H.; Li, S.; et al. Aptamer-functionalized lipid nanoparticles targeting osteoblasts as a novel RNA interference-based bone anabolic strategy. *Nat. Med.* **2015**, *21*, 288–294. [CrossRef] [PubMed]
47. Rosenblum, D.; Gutkin, A.; Kedmi, R.; Ramishetti, S.; Veiga, N.; Jacobi, A.M.; Schubert, M.S.; Friedmann-Morvinski, D.; Cohen, Z.R.; Behlke, M.A.; et al. CRISPR-Cas9 genome editing using targeted lipid nanoparticles for cancer therapy. *Sci. Adv.* **2020**, *6*, eabc9450. [CrossRef]
48. Katakowski, J.A.; Mukherjee, G.; Wilner, S.E.; Maier, K.E.; Harrison, M.T.; DiLorenzo, T.P.; Levy, M.; Palliser, D. Delivery of siRNAs to Dendritic Cells Using DEC205-Targeted Lipid Nanoparticles to Inhibit Immune Responses. *Mol. Therapy* **2016**, *24*, 146–155. [CrossRef]
49. Rurik, J.G.; Tombacz, I.; Yadegari, A.; Mendez Fernandez, P.O.; Shewale, S.V.; Li, L.; Kimura, T.; Soliman, O.Y.; Papp, T.E.; Tam, Y.K.; et al. CAR T cells produced in vivo to treat cardiac injury. *Science* **2022**, *375*, 91–96. [CrossRef]
50. Kranz, L.M.; Diken, M.; Haas, H.; Kreiter, S.; Loquai, C.; Reuter, K.C.; Meng, M.; Fritz, D.; Vascotto, F.; Hefesha, H.; et al. Systemic RNA delivery to dendritic cells exploits antiviral defence for cancer immunotherapy. *Nature* **2016**, *534*, 396–401. [CrossRef]
51. Khanani, A.M.; Thomas, M.J.; Aziz, A.A.; Weng, C.Y.; Danzig, C.J.; Yiu, G.; Kiss, S.; Waheed, N.K.; Kaiser, P.K. Review of gene therapies for age-related macular degeneration. *Eye* **2022**, *36*, 303–311. [CrossRef]
52. Vance, J.E.; Hayashi, H. Formation and function of apolipoprotein E-containing lipoproteins in the nervous system. *Biochim. Biophys. Acta* **2010**, *1801*, 806–818. [CrossRef] [PubMed]
53. Guevara, M.L.; Persano, F.; Persano, S. Advances in Lipid Nanoparticles for mRNA-Based Cancer Immunotherapy. *Front. Chem.* **2020**, *8*, 589959. [CrossRef] [PubMed]
54. Hou, X.; Zaks, T.; Langer, R.; Dong, Y. Lipid nanoparticles for mRNA delivery. *Nat. Rev. Mater.* **2021**, *6*, 1078–1094. [CrossRef] [PubMed]
55. BioNTech SE. Available online: https://www.biontech.com/int/en/home/pipeline-and-products/pipeline.html (accessed on 3 June 2022).
56. BioNTech's Second Act: Can it Transform the Fight against Cancer? *Financial Times*. Available online: https://www.ft.com/content/12ef99d4-063a-4a45-ae4d-e8115a9c3bb1 (accessed on 15 June 2022).
57. Miao, L.; Zhang, Y.; Huang, L. mRNA vaccine for cancer immunotherapy. *Mol. Cancer* **2021**, *20*, 41. [CrossRef] [PubMed]
58. Moderna Inc. Available online: https://www.modernatx.com/research/product-pipeline (accessed on 3 June 2022).
59. Pfizer Enters into Agreement with Acuitas Therapeutics for Lipid Nanoparticle Delivery System for Use in mRNA Vaccines and Therapeutics. Available online: https://www.pfizer.com/news/press-release/press-release-detail/pfizer-enters-agreement-acuitas-therapeutics-lipid (accessed on 13 June 2022).
60. Oberli, M.A.; Reichmuth, A.M.; Dorkin, J.R.; Mitchell, M.J.; Fenton, O.S.; Jaklenec, A.; Anderson, D.G.; Langer, R.; Blankschtein, D. Lipid Nanoparticle Assisted mRNA Delivery for Potent Cancer Immunotherapy. *Nano Lett.* **2017**, *17*, 1326–1335. [CrossRef]
61. Lee, K.; Kim, S.Y.; Seo, Y.; Kim, M.H.; Chang, J.; Lee, H. Adjuvant incorporated lipid nanoparticles for enhanced mRNA-mediated cancer immunotherapy. *Biomater. Sci.* **2020**, *8*, 1101–1105. [CrossRef]
62. Sarin, H. Physiologic upper limits of pore size of different blood capillary types and another perspective on the dual pore theory of microvascular permeability. *J. Angiogenes Res.* **2010**, *2*, 14. [CrossRef]
63. Nichols, J.W.; Bae, Y.H. EPR: Evidence and fallacy. *J. Control. Release* **2014**, *190*, 451–464. [CrossRef]
64. Petersen, G.H.; Alzghari, S.K.; Chee, W.; Sankari, S.S.; La-Beck, N.M. Meta-analysis of clinical and preclinical studies comparing the anticancer efficacy of liposomal versus conventional non-liposomal doxorubicin. *J. Control. Release* **2016**, *232*, 255–264. [CrossRef]
65. Price, L.S.L.; Stern, S.T.; Deal, A.M.; Kabanov, A.V.; Zamboni, W.C. A reanalysis of nanoparticle tumor delivery using classical pharmacokinetic metrics. *Sci. Adv.* **2020**, *6*, eaay9249. [CrossRef]
66. Wilhelm, S.; Tavares, A.J.; Dai, Q.; Ohta, S.; Audet, J.; Dvorak, H.F.; Chan, W.C.W. Analysis of nanoparticle delivery to tumours. *Nat. Rev. Mater.* **2016**, *1*, 16014. [CrossRef]

67. Han, L.; Jiang, C. Evolution of blood-brain barrier in brain diseases and related systemic nanoscale brain-targeting drug delivery strategies. *Acta Pharm. Sin. B* **2021**, *11*, 2306–2325. [CrossRef] [PubMed]
68. Zhou, Q.; Dong, C.; Fan, W.; Jiang, H.; Xiang, J.; Qiu, N.; Piao, Y.; Xie, T.; Luo, Y.; Li, Z.; et al. Tumor extravasation and infiltration as barriers of nanomedicine for high efficacy: The current status and transcytosis strategy. *Biomaterials* **2020**, *240*, 119902. [CrossRef] [PubMed]
69. Cochran, R.; Cochran, F. Phage display and molecular imaging: Expanding fields of vision in living subjects. *Biotechnol. Genet. Eng. Rev.* **2010**, *27*, 57–94. [CrossRef]
70. Deramchia, K.; Jacobin-Valat, M.J.; Vallet, A.; Bazin, H.; Santarelli, X.; Sanchez, S.; Dos Santos, P.; Franconi, J.M.; Claverol, S.; Bonetto, S.; et al. In vivo phage display to identify new human antibody fragments homing to atherosclerotic endothelial and subendothelial tissues [corrected]. *Am. J. Pathol.* **2012**, *180*, 2576–2589. [CrossRef]
71. Fang, R.H.; Kroll, A.V.; Gao, W.; Zhang, L. Cell Membrane Coating Nanotechnology. *Adv. Mater.* **2018**, *30*, e1706759. [CrossRef]
72. Rao, L.; Meng, Q.F.; Bu, L.L.; Cai, B.; Huang, Q.; Sun, Z.J.; Zhang, W.F.; Li, A.; Guo, S.S.; Liu, W.; et al. Erythrocyte Membrane-Coated Upconversion Nanoparticles with Minimal Protein Adsorption for Enhanced Tumor Imaging. *ACS Appl. Mater. Interfaces* **2017**, *9*, 2159–2168. [CrossRef]
73. Rao, L.; Yu, G.T.; Meng, Q.F.; Bu, L.L.; Tian, R.; Lin, L.S.; Deng, H.Z.; Yang, W.J.; Zan, M.H.; Ding, J.X.; et al. Cancer Cell Membrane-Coated Nanoparticles for Personalized Therapy in Patient-Derived Xenograft Models. *Adv. Funct. Mater.* **2019**, *29*, 1905671. [CrossRef]
74. Wang, D.; Dong, H.; Li, M.; Cao, Y.; Yang, F.; Zhang, K.; Dai, W.; Wang, C.; Zhang, X. Erythrocyte-Cancer Hybrid Membrane Camouflaged Hollow Copper Sulfide Nanoparticles for Prolonged Circulation Life and Homotypic-Targeting Photothermal/Chemotherapy of Melanoma. *ACS Nano* **2018**, *12*, 5241–5252. [CrossRef]
75. Wang, S.; Duan, Y.; Zhang, Q.; Komarla, A.; Gong, H.; Gao, W.; Zhang, L. Drug Targeting via Platelet Membrane-Coated Nanoparticles. *Small Struct.* **2020**, *1*, 2000018. [CrossRef]
76. Chen, M.; Chen, M.; He, J. Cancer cell membrane cloaking nanoparticles for targeted co-delivery of doxorubicin and PD-L1 siRNA. *Artif. Cells Nanomed. Biotechnol.* **2019**, *47*, 1635–1641. [CrossRef]
77. Wang, Y.; Ji, X.; Ruan, M.; Liu, W.; Song, R.; Dai, J.; Xue, W. Worm-Like Biomimetic Nanoerythrocyte Carrying siRNA for Melanoma Gene Therapy. *Small* **2018**, *14*, e1803002. [CrossRef] [PubMed]
78. Park, J.H.; Mohapatra, A.; Zhou, J.; Holay, M.; Krishnan, N.; Gao, W.; Fang, R.H.; Zhang, L. Virus-Mimicking Cell Membrane-Coated Nanoparticles for Cytosolic Delivery of mRNA. *Angew. Chem. Int. Ed. Engl.* **2022**, *61*, e202113671. [CrossRef] [PubMed]
79. Zhuang, J.; Gong, H.; Zhou, J.; Zhang, Q.; Gao, W.; Fang, R.H.; Zhang, L. Targeted gene silencing in vivo by platelet membrane-coated metal-organic framework nanoparticles. *Sci. Adv.* **2020**, *6*, eaaz6108. [CrossRef]
80. Mahmoud, K.; Swidan, S.; El-Nabarawi, M.; Teaima, M. Lipid based nanoparticles as a novel treatment modality for hepatocellular carcinoma: A comprehensive review on targeting and recent advances. *J. Nanobiotech.* **2022**, *20*, 109. [CrossRef] [PubMed]
81. Shinn, J.; Kwon, N.; Lee, S.A.; Lee, Y. Smart pH-responsive nanomedicines for disease therapy. *J. Pharm. Investig.* **2022**, *52*, 427–441. [CrossRef]
82. Heshmati Aghda, N.; Dabbaghianamiri, M.; Tunnell, J.W.; Betancourt, T. Design of smart nanomedicines for effective cancer treatment. *Int. J. Pharm.* **2022**, *621*, 121791. [CrossRef]
83. Krishnan, N.; Fang, R.H.; Zhang, L. Engineering of stimuli-responsive self-assembled biomimetic nanoparticles. *Adv. Drug Deliv. Rev.* **2021**, *179*, 114006. [CrossRef]
84. Salzano, G.; Costa, D.F.; Torchilin, V.P. siRNA Delivery by Stimuli-Sensitive Nanocarriers. *Curr. Pharm. Des.* **2015**, *21*, 4566–4573. [CrossRef]
85. De Maar, J.S.; Suelmann, B.B.M.; Braat, M.; van Diest, P.J.; Vaessen, H.H.B.; Witkamp, A.J.; Linn, S.C.; Moonen, C.T.W.; van der Wall, E.; Deckers, R. Phase I feasibility study of Magnetic Resonance guided High Intensity Focused Ultrasound-induced hyperthermia, Lyso-Thermosensitive Liposomal Doxorubicin and cyclophosphamide in de novo stage IV breast cancer patients: Study protocol of the i-GO study. *BMJ Open* **2020**, *10*, e040162. [CrossRef]
86. Tak, W.Y.; Lin, S.M.; Wang, Y.; Zheng, J.; Vecchione, A.; Park, S.Y.; Chen, M.H.; Wong, S.; Xu, R.; Peng, C.Y.; et al. Phase III HEAT Study Adding Lyso-Thermosensitive Liposomal Doxorubicin to Radiofrequency Ablation in Patients with Unresectable Hepatocellular Carcinoma Lesions. *Clin. Cancer Res.* **2018**, *24*, 73–83. [CrossRef] [PubMed]
87. Yang, W.; Lee, J.C.; Chen, M.H.; Zhang, Z.Y.; Bai, X.M.; Yin, S.S.; Cao, K.; Wang, S.; Wu, W.; Yan, K. Thermosensitive liposomal doxorubicin plus radiofrequency ablation increased tumor destruction and improved survival in patients with medium and large hepatocellular carcinoma: A randomized, double-blinded, dummy-controlled clinical trial in a single center. *J. Cancer Res. Therapeutics* **2019**, *15*, 773–783. [CrossRef]
88. Yingyuad, P.; Mevel, M.; Prata, C.; Kontogiorgis, C.; Thanou, M.; Miller, A.D. Enzyme-triggered PEGylated siRNA-nanoparticles for controlled release of siRNA. *J. RNAi Gene Silencing* **2014**, *10*, 490–499. [PubMed]
89. Zhang, J.; Shrivastava, S.; Cleveland, R.O.; Rabbitts, T.H. Lipid-mRNA Nanoparticle Designed to Enhance Intracellular Delivery Mediated by Shock Waves. *ACS Appl. Mater. Interfaces* **2019**, *11*, 10481–10491. [CrossRef] [PubMed]

pharmaceuticals

Article

Scolicidal and Apoptotic Activities of 5-hydroxy-1, 4-naphthoquinone as a Potent Agent against *Echinococcus granulosus* Protoscoleces

Masoud Moghadaszadeh [1,2,†], Mehdi Khayyati [2,†], Adel Spotin [3,4], Roghayeh Norouzi [5], Abdol Sattar Pagheh [6], Sonia M. R. Oliveira [7,8], Maria de Lourdes Pereira [7,9,*] and Ehsan Ahmadpour [2,3,4,*]

1 Biotechnology Research Center, Tabriz University of Medical Sciences, Tabriz, Iran; masoud.moghadaszadeh@gmail.com
2 Immunology Research Center, Tabriz University of Medical Sciences, Tabriz, Iran; mehdi.khayyati@yahoo.com
3 Infectious and Tropical Diseases Research Center, Tabriz University of Medical Sciences, Tabriz, Iran; adelespotin@gmail.com
4 Department of Parasitology and Mycology, School of Medicine, Tabriz University of Medical Sciences, Tabriz, Iran
5 Department of Pathobiology, Faculty of Veterinary Medicine, University of Tabriz, Tabriz, Iran; roghayehnorouzi123@gmail.com
6 Infectious Diseases Research Center, Birjand University of Medical Sciences, Birjand, Iran; satar2011@googlemail.com
7 CICECO-Aveiro Institute of Materials, University of Aveiro, 3810-193 Aveiro, Portugal; sonia.oliveira@ua.pt
8 Hunter Medical Research Institute, New Lambton, NSW 2305, Australia
9 Department of Medical Sciences, University of Aveiro, 3810-193 Aveiro, Portugal
* Correspondence: mlourdespereira@ua.pt (M.d.L.P.); ehsanahmadpour@gmail.com or ahmadpoure@tbzmed.ac.ir (E.A.); Tel.: +351-234-378141 (M.d.L.P.); +98-413-5428595 (E.A.); Fax: +98-413-3373745 (E.A.)
† These authors contributed equally in this study.

Citation: Moghadaszadeh, M.; Khayyati, M.; Spotin, A.; Norouzi, R.; Pagheh, A.S.; Oliveira, S.M.R.; Pereira, M.d.L.; Ahmadpour, E. Scolicidal and Apoptotic Activities of 5-hydroxy-1, 4-naphthoquinone as a Potent Agent against *Echinococcus granulosus* Protoscoleces. *Pharmaceuticals* **2021**, *14*, 623. https://doi.org/10.3390/ph14070623

Academic Editors: Ana Catarina Silva, Joao Nuno Moreira and Jose Manuel Sousa Lobo

Received: 24 May 2021
Accepted: 22 June 2021
Published: 28 June 2021

Abstract: Cystic hydatid disease (CHD) is a zoonotic disease with different clinical stages caused by the larval stage of the cestode *Echinococcus granulosus*. It is important to highlight as a public health problem in various regions of the world. In the current study, the efficacy and apoptotic activity of the liposomal system containing juglone (5-hydroxy-1,4-naphthoquinone) were assessed against protoscoleces (PSCs) in vitro. To this aim, firstly, liposomal vesicles were prepared by the thin-film method. Their physico-chemical features were assessed using Zeta-Sizer and Scanning Electron Microscope (SEM). Subsequently, various concentrations (50, 100, 200, 400, and 800 μg/mL) of juglone nanoliposomes at different exposure times (15, 30, 60, and 120 min) were used against PSCs. Results showed that juglone nanoliposomes at all tested concentrations induced scolicidal effect, however, 800 μg/mL and 400 μg/mL of juglone nanoliposomes could reach 100% mortality in 60 and 120 min, respectively. Additionally, we found that caspase-3 mRNA expression was higher in PSCs treated with juglone nanoliposomes compared to control groups ($p < 0.001$). Therefore, juglone nanoliposomes are suggested to have a more potent apoptotic effect on PSCs. Generally, optimized doses of juglone nanoliposomes could display significant scolicidal effects. Moreover, further in vivo studies are required to evaluate the efficacy of this nanoliposome.

Keywords: *Echinococcus granulosus*; scolicidal; nanoliposome; juglone; apoptotic activity

1. Introduction

Cystic hydatid disease (CHD) is one of the main neglected helminth diseases, with different clinical complications caused by the larval stage of the cestode *Echinococcus granulosus* in many countries of the world [1]. The metacestode grows as a unilocular cyst that contains an inner germinal layer with totipotent cells that generate capsules with multiple protoscoleces (PSCs) via asexual division, and it is surrounded by a laminated acellular membrane, called the laminar layer [2]. The annual incidence rate of CHD can differ from 1 to 200 per 100,000 populations in numerous endemic areas. The prevalence of CHD in Iran is considered an endemic and hyperendemic area, especially in the southern and northern parts, respectively [3]. CHD has medical and veterinary importance due to broad economic damages and losses of animals [4]. Moreover, the decrease in the quality of meat, milk production, fiber, and the number of surviving offspring are problems of this disease [5]. Humans, sheep, and other mammalian species are intermediate hosts, whereas canids are the definitive hosts for *E. granulosus*. Normally, humans and herbivores get the infection by occasional ingestion of eggs of *E. granulosus* in contaminated food, water, or soil. Oncospheres of eggs are able to penetrate the intestinal mucosa and disseminate through the portal system of the liver and lungs [6]. Vaccination is not a highly effective method for the control of CHD. Although in silico and in vivo studies are being conducted to design vaccines against this parasite [7], to date, there is no appropriate human vaccine against the disease [8,9]. The animal EG95 recombinant vaccine was used for vaccination of sheep against hydatid cyst. Surgery is a routine method for treating the disease, but there are some unexpected side effects, such as anaphylactic shock, disease recurrence, and mortality. Moreover, when cysts are found in the brain and spinal tissues, surgery is not recommended [10,11]. In these cases, chemotherapy and/or puncture-aspiration-injection-respiration (PAIR) technique are alternative resources for the treatment of CHD. Surgery, PAIR technique, and chemotherapy are the most common CHD treatments used today. Removal of the cysts together with chemotherapy, either using albendazole and/or mebendazole before and after surgery, are the best approaches. Nevertheless, some drugs have side effects, such as hepatotoxicity, leucopenia, and thrombocytopenia [12,13].

So far, many natural scolicidal agents have been used to inactivate hydatid cyst PSCs. Among the antiparasite compounds, 5-Hydroxy-1,4-naphthoquinone, also called juglone, is an organic compound with the molecular formula $C_{10}H_6O_3$ that is produced both naturally and industrially from different parts of the fruit, bark, leaves, and roots of some species of walnut from *Juglandaceae* family. The scientific name for juglone is *Juglans regia* [14,15]. Nowadays, walnut is widely cultivated across eastern Asia, northern Africa, southern Europe, and western South America. On the other hand, juglone is a phenolic compound with allopathic activity belonging to the class of naphthoquinones. It also has antibacterial, antiviral, anti-fungal, and anti-tumoral activities [16]. Juglone and its derivatives have a broad potent spectrum of antiparasite activity [17,18]. Nanostructured lipid carriers produced containing the drug enhance the penetration of the incorporated compounds and resolve concerns such as side effects, low drug solubility in water, and lack of adequate drug delivery to the parasite [19]. Here, we evaluated the scolicidal and apoptotic activity of nanoliposomed lipid carriers of juglone against *E. granulosus* PSCs in vitro by the qRT-PCR expression of *caspase-3* gene.

2. Results

2.1. Morphology and Zeta Potential Characterization of Liposomal Systems Containing Juglone

The morphology of nanoliposome systems containing juglone was investigated by SEM. SEM image shows that the morphology of the constituent particles in liposome systems containing essential oil, are spherical displaying a smooth surface and particles are in the range of 10–90 nm (Figure 1). In addition, the surface charge (zeta potential) of the liposome systems containing the juglone was calculated to be −16.7 mV (Figure 1).

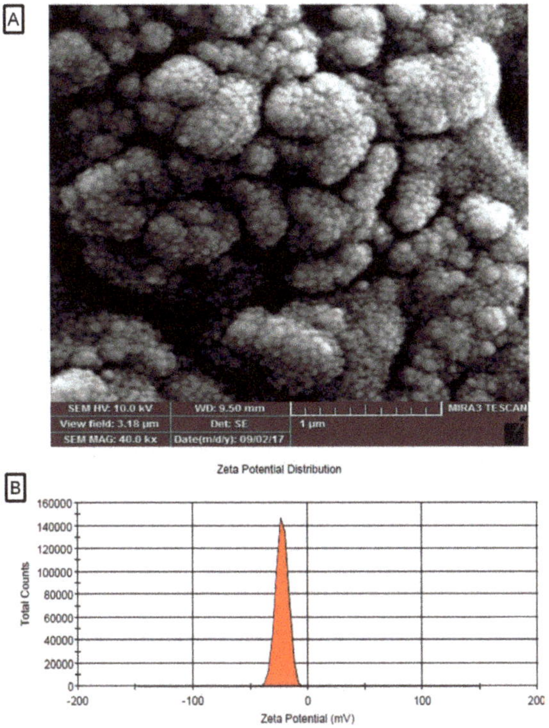

Figure 1. SEM photograph (**A**), zeta potential of the liposomal system containing juglone (**B**).

2.2. Genotyping of E. granulosus PSCs

To identify the *E. granulosus* PSCs genotype, PCR amplification by targeting the *cox1* gene was performed. Based on sequencing analysis (PouyaGostar Gene, Tehran, Iran) the G1 genotype (sheep strain) was confirmed (data not shown) [20].

2.3. Scolicidal Effects of Juglone and Juglone Nanoliposomes

Juglone as an effective agent with various concentrations (50, 100, 200, 400, and 800 µg/mL) was tested at different exposure times (15, 30, 60, and 120 min) against *E. granulosus* PSCs. The results showed that the juglone had a scolicidal effect at all concentrations. Statistically significant differences were observed between 800 µg/mL juglone at exposure times of 120 min (mortality rates of 94%) and the other concentrations and control group (PBS) (Figure 2A). However, the induced scolicidal effect of 50 µg/mL was less than that of other concentrations after 120 min (71%) (Figure 2A).

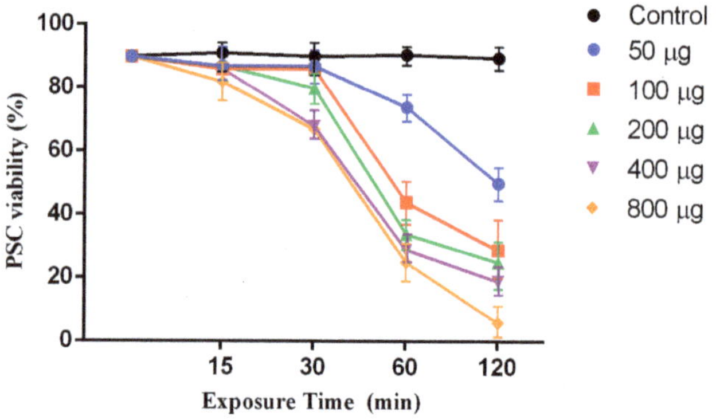

(A)

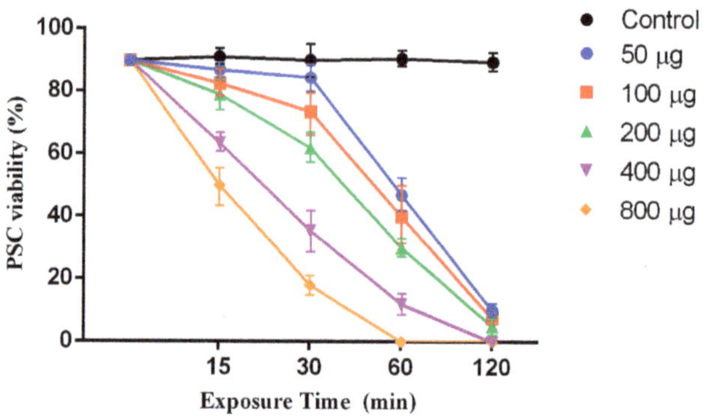

(B)

Figure 2. (**A**) Scolicidal effects of different concentrations of juglone at various times of exposure against PSCs of *E. granulosus*. Each test was performed in triplicate. (**B**) Scolicidal effects of different concentrations of the juglone nanoliposomesat various times of exposure against PSCs of *E. granulosus*. Each test was performed in triplicate.

Remarkably, 800 μg/mL and 400 μg/mL of juglonenanoliposomes could reach 100% mortality at 60 and 120 min, respectively. The scolicidal effect of juglonenanoliposomes at concentrations of 200 μg/mL, 100 μg/mL and 50 μg/mL at exposure times of 120 min were 95%, 92.5%, and 90% mortality rate, respectively (Figure 2B).

2.4. Expression of *caspase-3* Gene

Apoptotic activity was evaluated using the *caspase-3* mRNA expressions assay. The expression of *caspase-3* mRNA was assessed by the qRT-PCR after 15 h of exposure (Figure 3). As a result, *caspase-3* mRNA expression was higher in PSCs treated with juglone nanoliposomes compared to control groups. However, the rate of apoptosis was significantly different between the PSCs treated with juglone nanoliposomes.

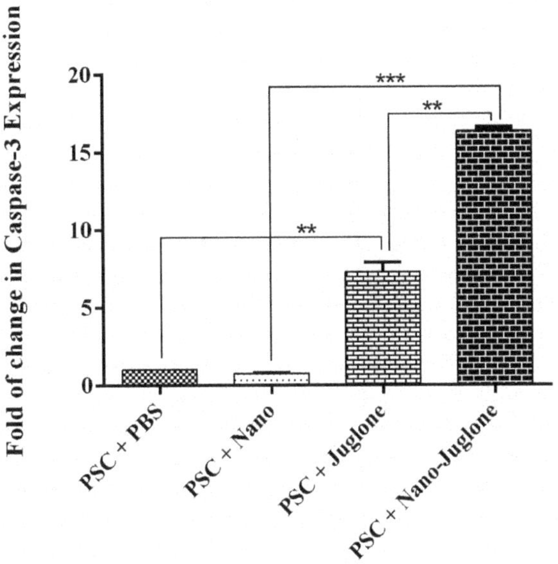

Figure 3. *Caspase-3* gene expression determined by real-time PCR in PSCs treated with PBS (negative control), PSCs treated with nanoliposomes (negative control), PSCs treated with juglone, and PSCs treated with juglone nanoliposomes. The bar graph indicates the mean ± standard deviation. *Caspase-3* mRNA expression was higher in both PSCs treated with juglone nanoliposomes than in control groups (** $p < 0.01$, *** $p < 0.001$).

3. Discussion

In the present study, the scolicidal and apoptotic activity of juglone and juglone nanoliposomes as a novel agent were successfully established against *E. granulosus* PSCs. The survey showed that 800 µg/mL and 400 µg/mL of juglonenanoliposomes have a more effective scolicidal rate (100% mortality at 60 to 120 min of exposure times), respectively, than the rest of concentrations, while 200 µg/mL, 100 µg/mL, and 50 µg/mL at exposure times of 120 min showed 95%, 92.5%, and 90% mortality rate, respectively. Today, surgery is a nominated method for complicated cases of CHD. However, the success of this method depends on the formation of new cysts, relapse, or secondary dissemination of CHD after surgery, which can cause death due to the leakage of the cyst content [10]. In fact, the inactivation and infertilization of PSCs by scolicidal agents accompanied by minimal side effects and high efficacy instead of opening or removing the cyst are highly recommended [21]. So far, several protoscolicidal agents, such as hypertonic saline, mannitol, chlorhexidine gluconate, huaier aqueous, *Allium sativum*, *Sambucus ebulus*, fungal chitosan, and *Berberis vulgaris* have been used to inactivate the content of hydatid cysts [21–24]. Unfortunately, the consumption of these agents has been limited because of their low efficacy, toxicity, and undesirable side effects [25].

Hypertonic saline solution (20%) was considered 100% effective in PSCs of hydatid cyst, but acute hypernatremia can cause severe symptoms in the nervous system, such as necrosis, myelinolysis, convulsions, and intracranial bleeding. Silver nitrate and cetrimide have been shown to be 100% effective against PSCs of the hydatid cyst. However, toxic reactions may also be caused by the absorption of these ingredients [26].

It is accepted that apoptosis played a binary role in the association between host and cystic echinococcosis (CE) in the mechanisms of survival and/or suppression [27,28]. Generally, caspase enzymes play a significant role in apoptotic progression. Among them, caspase-3 proteinase is essential for DNA fragmentation and morphological changes associated with cell death. The apoptotic process of praziquantel and dexamethasone was shown in *E. granulosus* PSCs via terminal deoxynucleotidyl transferase dUTP nick end labeling (TUNEL) assay and *caspase-3* enzymatic activity [29–31]. Importantly, we found that caspase-3 mRNA expression was higher in PSCs treated with juglone nanoliposomes compared to control groups. Our data are complementary to other observations since it has been found that nano compounds have effective apoptotic activity against *E. granulosus* PSCs. A study has shown that silver nanoparticles as a scolicidal agent can affect *E. granulosus* PSCs [32]. A similar study indicated that sulfoxide-loaded PLGA-PEG and albendazole sulfoxide could act as a novel nanopolymeric particle against *E. granulosus* PSCsvb [32]. There are different causes for the effectiveness of nanoliposomes containing juglone, such as increased penetration of the incorporated compounds, high solubility in water, and adequate drug release. On the other hand, juglone as a natural compound has potential therapeutic effects as well as minor side effects against *E. granulosus* PSCs.

Indeed, albendazole sulfoxide is the main choice for the treatment of Echinococcosis, however, persuasive evidence indicates that this drug comes with minor side effects, such as alopecia, leukopenia, musculoskeletal pain, pancytopenia, gastric irritation, headache, and elevation in levels of the liver enzymes [33–35]. Overall, our findings revealed that the optimized doses of nanoliposomes of juglone can induce significant scolicidal effects. In the future, it would be interesting to discover the apoptotic pathways in CE that affect humans that can assist as targets for the development of new scolicidal drugs. Lastly, the side effects of candidate agents must be studied in cells and also in animal models.

4. Materials and Methods

4.1. Preparation of Juglone

Juglone was purchased from Sigma-Aldrich (CAS Number: 481-39-0), and kept as a 100 mM stock solution in dimethyl sulfoxide at 20 °C for in vitro assays. The solution was centrifuged at 1000 rpm for 5 min. The solution was also filtered through a 0.22 mm millipore syringe filter to remove any impurity before use. Then, different concentrations of juglone (50, 100, 200, 400, and 800 μg/mL) were prepared.

4.2. Preparation of Liposomal Systems Containing of Juglone

DL-lactide and glycolide were purchased from Sigma-Aldrich (St. Louis, MO, USA) and recrystallized with ethyl acetate. Stannous octoate (Sn (Oct) 2: stannous 2-ethylhexanoate), nano lipid carriers (molecular weight of 2000, 3000, and 4000), dimethyl sulfoxide, polyethylene glycol (PEGs) and poloxamer 407 were purchased from Sigma-Aldrich. Glyceryl palmitostearate (Precirol® ATO 5) was purchased from Gattefossé (Lyon, France). The nanoliposomes of juglone were prepared using the hot homogenization technique [36]. In this method, the juglone was dissolved in ethanol and added to molten lipidic phase (precirol + myglyol) and mixed completely. Then, the aqueous phase containing the emulsifier was added dropwise to the lipidic phase at the same temperature under homogenization at 20,000 rpm for 20 min. The nanoliposomes of juglone were then produced by solidifying the hot nanoemulsion by cooling to room temperature.

4.3. Size and Zeta Potential Characterizationof Juglonein Liposomal Systems

The particle size and polydispersity of the solution were determined using Zetasizer Nano Particle Analyzer (model 3600, Malvern Instruments, Malvern, UK). The nanoliposomes were measured at an angle of 90° and laser light irradiation at 657 nm at 25 °C was used.

4.4. Morphology of Liposomal Systems Containing Juglone

The surface morphology of the nanocarriers (roughness, shape, smoothing, and mass) was investigated using a Scanning Electron Microscope (SEM: EM3200, KYKY Technology Development Ltd., Beijing, China).

4.5. Collection of *E. granulosus* PSCs

Hydatid cysts of *E. granulosus* were obtained from apparently infected sheep livers in an industrial slaughterhouse in East Azerbaijan, northwest of Iran. The hydatid fluid was removed aseptically and transferred to a container and left to set for 30 min. The PSCs were placed at the bottom of the container and then centrifuged at 800 rpm for 5 min. The supernatant was removed, and the yielded PSCs were washed three times with PBS and tested with 0.1% eosin to assess the viability of protoscoleces. Samples of PSCs with viability greater than 90% were selected for further testing. The protoscoleces were left and the live PSCs were stored at 4 °C for further use.

4.6. Genotyping the PSCs

To identify the *E. granulosus* genotype, genomic DNA from the PSCs was extracted using the commercial kit (DNG-plus™ solution; CinnaGen, Tehran, Iran) according to the manufacturer's instructions. The polymerase chain reaction (PCR) was conducted to amplify the *cox1* (cytochrome *c* oxidase subunit I, accession number: KT154000) in a volume of 25 µL of reaction mixture contained 1 µL of template DNA, 12.5 µL Premix Taq® mix (CinnaGen, Tehran, Iran), 1 µL of 10 µM of each primer, and 9.5 µL nuclease-free water. Details of the primer sequences used for PCR were described previously [32]. The procedure of PCR amplification consisted of 94 °C for 1 min, 30 cycles of 94 °C for 30 s, 56 °C for 30 s, and 72 °C for 1 min, followed by 72 °C for 10 min, with a final holding step at 4 °C. To identify the PSCs genotype, the amplicons (444 bp) were directly sequenced (PouyaGostar Gene, Tehran, Iran).

4.7. Scolicidal Assay

In this study, different concentrations of 5-hydroxy-1,4-naphthoquinone containing 50, 100, 200, 400, and 800 µg/mL were used for different exposure times, including 15, 30, 60, and 120 min. To prepare the mentioned dilutions 50, 100, 200, 400, and 800 µg/mL of agent were dissolved in 1 mL of normal saline in a test tube. Then, the obtained solution was gently mixed. Subsequently, in each experiment, 100 µL of sediment containing 1000 PSCs were added to 100 µL of the solution. After mixing the contents, the test tube was incubated at 37 °C for 15, 30, 60, and 120 min. At the end of incubation periods, in order to assess the viability of PSCs, 10 mL of 0.1% eosin were added to the remaining 20 µL of the PSCs pellet and mixed gently. The stained PSCs were smeared on a manually scaled glass slide, which was covered with a coverslip (24 × 50 mm) and examined under an Olympus BX41TF (Tokyo, Japan) light microscope. Five minutes after the exposure times to the eosin staining, protoscoleces that did not absorb the dye with the movement of the flame cells were verified as potentially viable, otherwise, they were considered as dead PSCs. The percentages of dead PSCs were estimated by counting a minimum of 200 PSCs. The hydatid cyst fluid was considered a negative control group. Besides, 5% NaCl (5 g/100 mL) was used as a positive control group [31]. The experiments were performed in triplicate.

4.8. Quantitative Real-Time Polymerase Chain Reaction (qRT-PCR)

The total RNA of the untreated and treated PSCs after 15 h of exposure time was extracted using the RNX Plus Kit (CinnaGen, Tehran, Iran). The amount and purity of the RNA were assessed using NanoDrop 2000c spectrophotometer (Thermo Fisher Scientific, Waltham, MA, USA). Complementary DNA (cDNA) was synthesized using 1 µg of total RNA, random hexamer primer (Thermo Fisher Scientific, USA). In order to evaluate the apoptotic effects of juglone nanoliposomes on PSCs, the specific primers of *E. granulosuscaspase-3* gene were designed by the Oligo Analyzer v.3.1 tool based on reference accession numbers of AB306934 (EF-1α) and LK028577 (*caspase-3*). Primer sequences and cycling conditions were described previously [20,32]. The real-time PCR amplification of the target gene was performed in a 20µL reaction volume containing 10µLof super SYBR green qPCR mastermix (YTA, Iran), 10 pmol of primer and 1µLof cDNA template (0.05–5 ng/µL) by an initial denaturation step at 95 °C for 5 min followed by 35 cycles at

95 °C for 30 s, 58 °C for 40 s, and 72 °C for 45 s (Roche RealTime PCR system, Applied Biosystems). PCR amplification was performed in triplicate to decrease the experimental error. Relative mRNA expression was measured by the $2^{-\Delta\Delta Ct}$ method, and results were evaluated based on thecycle threshold (Ct) value. The beta-actin gene was used as a house keeping gene (internal control) to normalize the expression of the target gene.

4.9. Statistical Analysis of Data

All statistical analyses were performed using the GraphPad PRISM software version 6 (GraphPad Software, La Jolla, CA, USA; http://www.graphpad.com, accessed on 11 June 2019). Data for each treatment group were analyzed using the chi-square test. The normality of data was assessed using the Kolmogorov–Smirnov test, and the transformation of data was performed where needed. The one-way and two-way analysis of variance (ANOVA) and Tukey HSD post hoc test were used to assess the statistically significant differences between the means. The p values < 0.05 were considered significant.

5. Conclusions

Our results suggest that juglone nanoliposomes have a potent scolicidal effect, and a significant difference in the rate of apoptosis was observed between PSCs treated with juglone and PSCs treated with juglone nanoliposomes. However, further studies are required to evaluate the efficacy of these nanoliposomes in vivo and their clinical applications.

Author Contributions: Conceptualization, E.A., M.M., A.S. and M.d.L.P.; methodology, M.M., M.K., R.N. and A.S.P.; validation, E.A., A.S.P., S.M.R.O. and M.d.L.P.; investigation, M.K., M.M. and A.S.; data curation, E.A. and M.d.L.P.; writing—original draft preparation, M.M., M.K., R.N., A.S.P. and S.M.R.O.; writing—review and editing, E.A., A.S. and M.d.L.P. All authors have read and agreed to the published version of the manuscript.

Funding: This study was part of the M.Sc. thesis of Mehdi Khayyati and financially supported by Immunology Research Center and School of Medicine, Tabriz University of Medical Sciences, Tabriz, Iran (Grant number 59192). M.d.L.P. thanks to project CICECO-Aveiro Institute of Materials, UIDB/50011/2020 and UIDP/50011/2020, national funds by FCT/MCTES.

Institutional Review Board Statement: All experiments were approved by the local Ethics Committee of Tabriz University of Medical Sciences, Tabriz, Iran (No. IR.TBZMED.REC.1397.104, Approval date: 11 June 2018).

Informed Consent Statement: Not applicable.

Data Availability Statement: Data is contained within the article.

Conflicts of Interest: The authors declare no conflict of interest.

References

1. Eckert, J.; Deplazes, P. Biological, Epidemiological, and Clinical Aspects of Echinococcosis, a Zoonosis of Increasing Concern. *Clin. Microbiol. Rev.* **2004**, *17*, 107–135. [CrossRef]
2. Vuitton, D.A. Benzimidazoles for the treatment of cystic and alveolar echinococcosis: What is the consensus? *Expert Rev. Anti-Infect. Ther.* **2009**, *7*, 145–149. [CrossRef]
3. Rokni, M.B. PP-170 Echinococcosis/hydatidosis in Iran. *Int. J. Infect. Dis.* **2009**, *13*, S94–S95. [CrossRef]
4. Eckert, J.; Deplazes, P.; Craig, P.; Gemmell, M.; Gottstein, B.; Heath, D.; Jenkins, D.; Kamiya, M.; Lightowlers, M. Echinococcosis in animals: Clinical aspects, diagnosis, and treatment. In *WHO/OIE Manual on Echinococcosis in Humans and Animals: A Public Health Problem of Global Concern*; World Organization for Animal Health: Paris, France, 2001; pp. 72–99.
5. Battelli, G. Evaluation of the economic costs of Echinococcosis. *Int. Arch. Hidatid.* **1997**, *32*, 33–37.
6. da Silva, A.M. Human echinococcosis: A neglected disease. *Gastroenterol. Res. Pract.* **2010**, *35*, 283–292. [CrossRef] [PubMed]
7. Pourseif, M.M.; Yousefpour, M.; Aminianfar, M.; Moghaddam, G.; Nematollahi, A. A multi-method and structure-based in silico vaccine designing against *Echinococcus granulosus* through investigating enolase protein. *BioImpacts* **2019**, *9*, 131–144. [CrossRef] [PubMed]
8. Šarkūnas, M.; Vienažindienė, Ž.; Rojas, C.A.; Radziulis, K.; Deplazes, P. Praziquantel treatment of dogs for four consecutive years decreased the transmission of *Echinococcus intermedius* G7 to pigs in villages in Lithuania. *Food Waterborne Parasitol.* **2019**, *15*, e00043. [CrossRef] [PubMed]

9. Anvari, D.; Rezaei, F.; Ashouri, A.; Rezaei, S.; Majidiani, H.; Pagheh, A.S.; Shariatzadeh, S.A.; Fotovati, A.; Siyadatpanah, A.; Gholami, S.; et al. Current situation and future prospects of *Echinococcus granulosus* vaccine candidates: A systematic review. *Transbound. Emerg. Dis.* **2021**, *68*, 1080–1096. [CrossRef]
10. Rouhani, S.; Parvizi, P.; Spotin, A. Using specific synthetic peptide (p176) derived AgB 8/1-kDa accompanied by modified patient's sera: A novel hypothesis to follow-up of Cystic echinococcosis after surgery. *Med. Hypotheses* **2013**, *81*, 557–560. [CrossRef] [PubMed]
11. Stamatakos, M.; Sargedi, C.; Stefanaki, C.; Safioleas, C.; Matthaiopoulou, I. Anthelminthic treatment: An adjuvant therapeutic strategy against *Echinococcus granulosus*. *Parasitol. Int.* **2009**, *58*, 115–120. [CrossRef]
12. Adas, G.; Arikan, S.; Kemik, O.; Oner, A.; Sahip, N.; Karatepe, O. Use of albendazole sulfoxide, albendazole sulfone, and combined solutions as scolicidal agents on hydatid cysts (in vitro study). *World J. Gastroenterol.* **2009**, *15*, 112–116. [CrossRef] [PubMed]
13. Smego, R.A., Jr.; Sebanego, P. Treatment options for hepatic cystic echinococcosis. *Int. J. Infect. Dis.* **2005**, *9*, 69–76. [CrossRef] [PubMed]
14. Torres-Giner, S.; Ocio, M.J.; Lagaron, J.M. Development of Active Antimicrobial Fiber-Based Chitosan Polysaccharide Nanostructures using Electrospinning. *Eng. Life Sci.* **2008**, *8*, 303–314. [CrossRef]
15. Kurtyka, R.; Pokora, W.; Tukaj, Z.; Karcz, W. Effects of juglone and lawsone on oxidative stress in maize coleoptile cells treated with IAA. *AoB Plants* **2016**, *8*, plw073. [CrossRef] [PubMed]
16. Blauenburg, B.; Metsä-Ketelä, M.; Klika, K.D. Formation of 5-Hydroxy-3-methoxy-1,4-naphthoquinone and 8-Hydroxy-4-methoxy-1,2-naphthoquinone from Juglone. *ISRN Org. Chem.* **2012**, *2012*, 274980. [CrossRef] [PubMed]
17. Klotz, L.-O.; Hou, X.; Jacob, C. 1,4-Naphthoquinones: From Oxidative Damage to Cellular and Inter-Cellular Signaling. *Molecules* **2014**, *19*, 14902–14918. [CrossRef]
18. Kot, M.; Karcz, W.; Zaborska, W. 5-Hydroxy-1,4-naphthoquinone (juglone) and 2-hydroxy-1,4-naphthoquinone (lawsone) influence on jack bean urease activity: Elucidation of the difference in inhibition activity. *Bioorg. Chem.* **2010**, *38*, 132–137. [CrossRef]
19. Schwendener, R.A. Liposomes as vaccine delivery systems: A review of the recent advances. *Ther. Adv. Vaccines* **2014**, *2*, 159–182. [CrossRef]
20. Ahmadpour, E.; Godrati-Azar, Z.; Spotin, A.; Norouzi, R.; Hamishehkar, H.; Nami, S.; Heydarian, P.; Rajabi, S.; Mohammadi, M.; Perez-Cordon, G. Nanostructured lipid carriers of ivermectin as a novel drug delivery system in hydatidosis. *Parasites Vectors* **2019**, *12*, 1–9. [CrossRef] [PubMed]
21. Fakhar, M.; Chabra, A.; Rahimi-Esboei, B.; Rezaei, F. In vitro protoscolicidal effects of fungal chitosan isolated from *Penicilliumwaksmanii* and *Penicillium citrinum*. *J. Parasit. Dis.* **2013**, *39*, 162–167. [CrossRef]
22. Gholami, S.H.; Rahimi-Esboei, B.; Ebrahimzadeh, M.A.; Pourhajibagher, M. In vitro effect of *Sambucus ebulus* on scolices of Hydatid cysts. *Eur. Rev. Med. Pharmacol. Sci.* **2013**, *17*, 1760–1765. [PubMed]
23. Lv, H.; Jiang, Y.; Liao, M.; Sun, H.; Zhang, S.; Peng, X. In vitro and in vivo treatments of *Echinococcus granulosus* with Huaier aqueous extract and albendazole liposome. *Parasitol. Res.* **2012**, *112*, 193–198. [CrossRef]
24. Kohansal, M.H.; Nourian, A.; Rahimi, M.T.; Daryani, A.; Spotin, A.; Ahmadpour, E. Natural products applied against hydatid cyst protoscolices: A review of past to present. *Acta Trop.* **2017**, *176*, 385–394. [CrossRef] [PubMed]
25. Tappeh, K.H.; Einshaei, A.; Mahmudloo, R.; Mohammadzadeh, H.; Tahermaram, M.; Mousavi, S.J. Effect of Different Concentrations of Hypertonic Saline at Different Times on Protoscoleces of Hydatid Cyst Isolated From Liver and Lung. *Turk. J. Parasitol.* **2011**, *35*, 148–150. [CrossRef]
26. Zhang, J.; Ye, B.; Kong, J.; Cai, H.; Zhao, Y.; Han, X.; Li, F. In vitro protoscolicidal effects of high-intensity focused ultrasound enhanced by a superabsorbent polymer. *Parasitol. Res.* **2012**, *112*, 385–391. [CrossRef] [PubMed]
27. Bakhtiar, N.M.; Spotin, A.; Mahami-Oskouei, M.; Ahmadpour, E.; Rostami, A. Recent advances on innate immune pathways related to host–parasite cross-talk in cystic and alveolar echinococcosis. *Parasites Vectors* **2020**, *13*, 1–8. [CrossRef]
28. Moghaddam, S.M.; Picot, S.; Ahmadpour, E. Interactions between hydatid cyst and regulated cell death may provide new therapeutic opportunities. *Parasite* **2019**, *26*, 70. [CrossRef]
29. De, S.; Pan, D.; Bera, A.; Sreevatsava, V.; Bandyopadhyay, S.; Chaudhuri, D.; Kumar, S.; Rana, T.; Das, S.; Suryanaryana, V.; et al. In vitro assessment of praziquantel and a novel nanomaterial against protoscoleces of *Echinococcus granulosus*. *J. Helminthol.* **2011**, *86*, 26–29. [CrossRef]
30. Hu, H.; Kang, J.; Chen, R.; Mamuti, W.; Wu, G.; Yuan, W. Drug-induced apoptosis of *Echinococcus granulosus*protoscoleces. *Parasitol. Res.* **2011**, *109*, 453–459. [CrossRef] [PubMed]
31. Rahimi, M.T.; Ahmadpour, E.; Esboei, B.R.; Spotin, A.; Koshki, M.H.K.; Alizadeh, A.; Honary, S.; Barabadi, H.; Mohammadi, M.A. Scolicidal activity of biosynthesized silver nanoparticles against *Echinococcus granulosus*protoscolices. *Int. J. Surg.* **2015**, *19*, 128–133. [CrossRef] [PubMed]
32. Naseri, M.; Akbarzadeh, A.; Spotin, A.; Akbari, N.A.R.; Mahami-Oskouei, M.; Ahmadpour, E. Scolicidal and apoptotic activities of albendazole sulfoxide and albendazole sulfoxide-loaded PLGA-PEG as a novel nanopolymeric particle against *Echinococcus-granulosus* protoscoleces. *Parasitol. Res.* **2016**, *115*, 4595–4603. [CrossRef]

33. Yetim, I.; Erzurumlu, K.; Hökelek, M.; Baris, S.; Dervisoglu, A.; Polat, C.; Belet, Ü.; Buyukkarabacak, Y.; Güvenli, A. Results of alcohol and albendazole injections in hepatic hydatidosis: Experimental study. *J. Gastroenterol. Hepatol.* **2005**, *20*, 1442–1447. [CrossRef]
34. Ramírez, T.; Benítez-Bribiesca, L.; Ostrosky-Wegman, P.; Herrera, L.A. In Vitro Effects of Albendazole and Its Metabolites on the Cell Proliferation Kinetics and Micronuclei Frequency of Stimulated Human Lymphocytes. *Arch. Med. Res.* **2001**, *32*, 119–122. [CrossRef]
35. Delatour, P.; Parish, R.C.; Gyurik, R.J. Albendazole: A comparison of relay embryotoxicity with embryotoxicity of individual metabolites. *Ann. Rech. Veter Ann. Veter Res.* **1981**, *12*, 159–167.
36. Mohammadi, M.; Pezeshki, A.; Abbasi, M.M.; Ghanbarzadeh, B.; Hamishehkar, H. Vitamin D3-Loaded Nanostructured Lipid Carriers as a Potential Approach for Fortifying Food Beverages; in Vitro and in Vivo Evaluation. *Adv. Pharm. Bull.* **2017**, *7*, 61–71. [CrossRef] [PubMed]

pharmaceuticals

Article

Development and Characterization of *n*-Propyl Gallate Encapsulated Solid Lipid Nanoparticles-Loaded Hydrogel for Intranasal Delivery

Fakhara Sabir [1], Gábor Katona [1], Ruba Ismail [1,2], Bence Sipos [1], Rita Ambrus [1] and Ildikó Csóka [1,*]

[1] Institute of Pharmaceutical Technology and Regulatory Affairs, Faculty of Pharmacy, University of Szeged, Eötvös Str. 6, H-6720 Szeged, Hungary; fakhra.sabir@gmail.com (F.S.); katona.gabor@szte.hu (G.K.); ruba.ismail@szte.hu (R.I.); sipos.bence@szte.hu (B.S.); ambrus.rita@szte.hu (R.A.)

[2] Department of Applied & Environmental Chemistry, Faculty of Science and Informatics, University of Szeged, Rerrich Béla sqr. 1, H-6720 Szeged, Hungary

* Correspondence: csoka.ildiko@szte.hu; Tel.: +36-62-546-116

Abstract: The objective of the present study was to develop *n*-propyl gallate-loaded solid lipid nanoparticles (PG-SLNs) in a hydrogel (HG) formulation using Transcutol-P (TC-P) as a permeation enhancer. Modified solvent injection technique was applied to produce optimized PG-SLNs via the Quality by Design approach and central composite design. The in vitro mucoadhesion, scavenging activity, drug release, permeation studies of PG from PG-SLNs-loaded HG were evaluated under simulated nasal conditions. Compared with in vitro release behavior of PG from SLNs, the drug release from the PG-SLNs-loaded HG showed a lower burst effect and sustained release profile. The cumulative permeation of PG from PG-SLNs-loaded HG with TC-P was 600 μg/cm^2 within 60 min, which is 3–60-fold higher than PG-SLNs and native PG, respectively. Raman mapping showed that the distribution of PG-SLNs was more concentrated in HG having lower concentrations of hyaluronic acid. The scavenging assay demonstrated increased antioxidant activity at higher concentrations of HG. Due to enhanced stability and mucoadhesive properties, the developed HG-based SLNs can improve nasal absorption by increasing residence time on nasal mucosa. This study provides in vitro proof of the potential of combining the advantages of SLNs and HG for the intranasal delivery of antioxidants.

Keywords: hydrogel; SLNs; nose-to-brain delivery; mucoadhesion; quality by design; antioxidant activity

Citation: Sabir, F.; Katona, G.; Ismail, R.; Sipos, B.; Ambrus, R.; Csóka, I. Development and Characterization of *n*-Propyl Gallate Encapsulated Solid Lipid Nanoparticles-Loaded Hydrogel for Intranasal Delivery. *Pharmaceuticals* **2021**, *14*, 696. https://doi.org/10.3390/ph14070696

Academic Editors: Ana Catarina Silva, João Nuno Moreira and José Manuel Sousa Lobo

Received: 1 June 2021
Accepted: 15 July 2021
Published: 19 July 2021

1. Introduction

In the past few years, the intranasal administration route has gained considerable interest since it provides a non-invasive method to bypass the blood–brain barrier (BBB). Most regions in the central nervous system (CNS) can be directly reached along the olfactory and trigeminal nerves by intranasal administration of drugs. This intranasal administration route is broadly innervated by the olfactory nerve, which is localized in the epithelial tissue of the nasal olfactory mucosa and respiratory mucosa [1]. Various studies provide promising data for the potential of nose-to-brain delivery pathway in the treatment of CNS diseases such as brain tumors, Parkinson's disease and Alzheimer's disease [2,3].

Nose-to-brain delivery is considered very effective for many CNS active drugs that have limited administration because of low bioavailability through other delivery routes including paclitaxel, levetiracetam, cephalexin, dopamine, estrogen or even nerve growth factor-1 [4]. Limited brain uptake can be achieved in numerous intranasally applied compounds from conventional formulations, including chemotherapeutics and antineoplastic agents, due to their low permeability, enzymatic degradation and rapid elimination by mucociliary clearance from the nasal cavity [5–7]. To hurdle these obstacles, the application of nano drug delivery systems can be a suitable tool.

Lipid nanoparticles, including liposomes, niosomes, nanoemulsions and solid lipid nanoparticles (SLNs), are among the most promising drug delivery systems because of their biocompatible nature [8–10]. Moreover, these nanosystems can provide protection of the embedded active pharmaceutical ingredient (API) against efflux transporters (P-glycoprotein), enzymatic degradation or chemical destabilization at nasal conditions [11]. Compared with conventional lipid nanoparticulate drug delivery systems, active targeting has attracted significant attention due to enhanced therapeutic benefits and reduced undesirable side effects.

Hyaluronic acid (HA), a glycosaminoglycan, is a linear polysaccharide that is composed of β-1,4-D-glucoronic acid and 1,3-*N*-acetyl-D-glucosamine disaccharides via alternating glycosidic bonds [12–14]. Hydrogels (HG) containing HA have been successfully developed and evaluated for several promising biomedical applications as carrier systems in nasal, pulmonary, parenteral, topical and ophthalmic delivery [15,16]. Loading nanoparticles into low molecular weight HA-HG can improve nasal absorption by increasing residence time on nasal mucosa through enhanced viscosity and mucoadhesive properties. Improved mechanical stability against degradation and enhanced biochemical functionality of HA can be easily reached using cross-linkers such as glutaraldehyde (GA), divinyl sulfone, carbodiimide or bisepoxide [17,18]. In addition to the gel-forming properties, HA can also be applied in targeted drug delivery [19]. In our experiments, GA was applied due to having high potency to function as a proper cross-linker and because the nasal lining is fairly resistant to aldehyde toxicity below millimolar concentrations [20].

Propyl gallate (PG) (propyl 3,4,5-tri-hydroxybenzoate) is an ester form of gallic acid, and propanol functions as a synthetic antioxidant. Previous studies showed that PG has a high antioxidant capacity, which may contribute to decreasing mitochondrial impairment and to inhibiting cellular respiration. PG has demonstrated anticancer effects on various normal and tumor cells that may lead to DNA genotoxicity, cytotoxicity and fragmentation [21,22]. It has been revealed that PG used along with other anti-tumor agents such as probiotics was effective in mice for tumor treatment [23]. The PG anticancer activity can stop cell proliferation, reduce reactive oxygen species production and stimulate the autophagy of malignant cells [24].

This study aimed to optimize PG containing solid lipid nanoparticles (PG-SLNs) embedded into chemically linked HA-HG as a suitable delivery system for the intranasal route. Intranasal administration of PG can be a promising approach for targeted treatment of brain tumors, e.g., glioblastoma multiforme [25] bypassing the BBB; moreover, this non-invasive way of administration can be more favorable for patients. A further aim was to investigate the effect of excipients as a permeation enhancer for Transcutol-P (TC-P) due to its nontoxicity and biocompatibility and GA as cross-linker for intranasal route. For the formulation optimization, the Quality by Design (QbD) methodology was applied as a quality improvement principle that is able to take into account all critical parameters that have an impact on final product quality, safety and efficacy using a response surface quadratic model.

2. Results

2.1. *Quality by Design Approach and Risk Assessment (RA)*

Screening of the quality target product profile (QTPP) was based on previous experimental data and according to the relevant International Conference on Harmonization (ICH) guidelines (Q8,Q9,Q10,Q11) [26,27]. The QTPP elements in this study were the route of administration, indication, dissolution and permeability profiles, stability and brain distribution [28,29]. QTPPs contain the information required by the mentioned ICH guidelines on the one hand, and the basic assumptions that our product must meet on the other. Based on the QTPPs, the defined aim was to develop a monodisperse PG-containing SLN embedded in a HG formulation that is able to enter the central nervous system via the nose-to-brain pathway as a patient adherence improving drug delivery pathway offering direct transport to the CNS. Figure S1 shows the relations established between the QTPP-

CQA (QTPP-critical quality attribute) and the critical process parameters/critical materials attributes (CPPs/CMA-CQA) elements on a 3-grade scale. During the RA process, the particle characteristics of the nanoformulation were placed under thorough evaluation as they are the key elements during the incorporation to an HG formulation.

Based on the interdependence rating and using the software, quantification of these relations was performed, and severity scores were assigned for each CQA and CPP/CMA element, as presented in Figure 1.

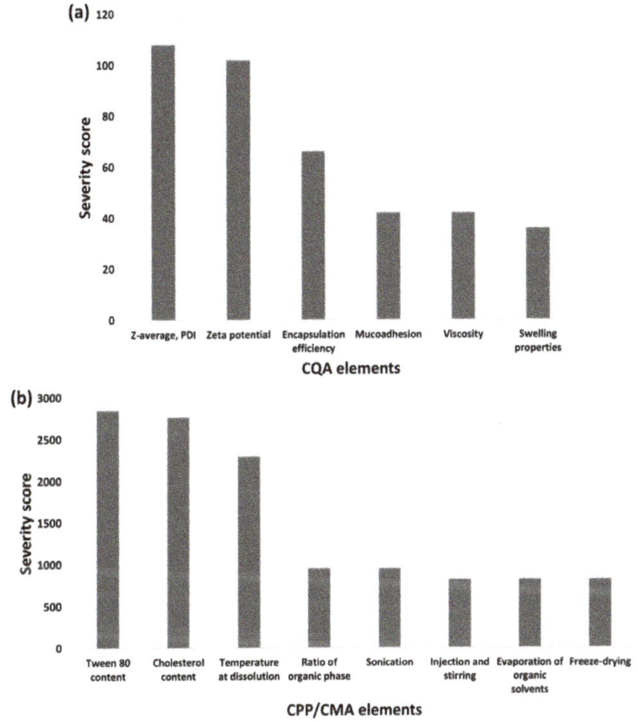

Figure 1. Probability rating of CQA (**a**) and CPP/CMA (**b**) elements. The Pareto charts are presented as the calculated severity scores assigned to the elements.

The interdependence rating (Figure S1) assigned mostly high-grade scores concerning the relations of particle characteristics (Z-average, PDI and zeta potential) which is supported by the higher severity scores in Figure 1a compared with the applicability affecting risk factors such as muco-adhesivity, viscosity and swelling properties. The key element in QbD-driven nanoparticle formulation is to establish the basis for proper particle size and distribution, as these are the main elements influencing the dissolution and permeability profile, which are the first crucial steps in the nasal administration in the nasal cavity and through the nasal mucosa. Based on the calculations, it can be claimed that material attributes such as the concentration of Tween 80 and cholesterol hold the highest risk severity, followed by the temperature at dissolution phase compared with the subprocesses, as seen on Figure 1b. The subprocesses might hold low severity due to the fact that these are either easily controllable processes or because their main function is to achieve the final dosage form, whilst without the appropriate ratios and proportions of the material attributes, the nanosystem cannot be formed.

2.2. Central Composite Design (CCD)

2.2.1. Optimization and Impact of Critical Parameters on Z-Average, Polydispersity Index (PDI), Zeta Potential

Based on the QbD methodology-based RA process, the design of the experiment was conducted according to severity scores. The effect of the characteristics with the highest severity score, i.e., the cholesterol content (A), the Tween 80 content (B) and temperature (°C), were investigated on the independent factors: Z-average, PDI and zeta potential in a 15-formulation experiment series presented in Table 1. We incorporated the results into the software, and as a result, a design expert selected a run (7) depending upon the smallest size, PDI and the characteristic with more negative zeta potential. The software screened the optimized trial with the desirability of 0.99 depending on the lowest Z-average, PDI and more negative zeta potential. The optimized PG-SLNs consisted of 1:6 of Tween 80 and cholesterol. The effects of each individual factor and the combined effect of factors on studied factors are shown in Figure S2a. It was revealed that at a low amount of cholesterol (20 mg), the Z-average was slightly higher than set trials where the maximum amount of it (60 mg) was used. With surfactant addition, the Z-average was less at low concentration of cholesterol due to lower lipid aggregation because of Tween 80 incorporation.

Table 1. Effect of independent variables (temperature, surfactant, cholesterol) on Z-average, PDI and Zeta potential of 15 runs on design of expert. * Data are presented as average ± SD (n = 3 independent measurements).

Number of Runs	Temperature (°C)	Amount of Surfactant (mg)	Amount of Cholesterol (mg)	Z-Average (nm)	PDI	Zeta Potential (mV)
1	45	25	40	150 ± 10	0.30 ± 0.01	−30 ± 8.4
2	20	25	40	220 ± 5.5	0.22 ± 0.02	−29 ± 6.5
3	45	25	40	140 ± 4.5	0.23 ± 0.02	−31 ± 8.4
4	80	10	40	155 ± 5.5	0.25 ± 0.05	−29 ± 8.4
5	45	40	40	500 ± 6.6	0.44 ± 0.07	−5 ± 7.5
6	70	40	20	400 ± 7.8	0.55 ± 0.01	−6 ± 8.5
7 *	70	10	60	120 ± 8.8	0.12 ± 0.08	−38 ± 10.2
8	45	25	40	155 ± 22	0.26 ± 0.09	−29 ± 12
9	45	10	40	200 ± 2.3	0.21 ± 0.08	−29 ± 5.5
10	20	10	20	230 ± 2.4	0.22 ± 0.06	−19 ± 6.5
11	45	25	40	160 ± 40	0.25 ± 0.08	−28 ± 10
12	45	25	40	145 ± 20	0.18 ± 0.05	−28 ± 10.2
13	20	40	60	600 ± 12	0.46 ± 0.01	−4 ± 3.3
14	45	25	20	222 ± 10	0.23 ± 0.02	−20 ± 5.5
15	45	25	60	190 ± 14	0.22 ± 0.02	−19 ± 6.2

* Parameters of optimized formulation.

Even though smaller particle size was obtained at a higher temperature, the temperature effect was not statistically significant. The interaction of individual factors, i.e., cholesterol, on particle size, PDI and zeta potential, are also presented in Figure S2b.

The significance of the applied model was evaluated by F-value and p-value. In the case of particle size analysis, the model F-value of 56.89 implies that the model is significant. The following equations describe the linear and quadratic relations of the individual parameters influencing the dependent factors:

$$\text{Particle size} = 160.57 - 23.74A + 144.53B - 60.62C + 16.88AB - 17.97AC - 50.11BC + 26.74A^2 + 176.21B^2 - 16.67C^2 \quad (1)$$

In the case of zeta potential, the model *F*-value of 10.31 implies that the model is significant. There is only a 0.97% chance that a "model *F*-value" this large could occur due to noise. Values of "Prob > *F*" less than 0.0500 indicate that model terms are significant.

$$\text{Zeta Potential} = -27.42 - 0.8A + 11.08B + 3.45C + 8.7AB - 0.67AC + 2.8BC + 4.78A^2 + 8.2B^2 - 0.73C^2 \quad (2)$$

In the case of PDI, the model *F*-value of 9.41 implies that the model is significant.

$$\text{PDI} = 0.24 - 0.01A + 0.0988B + 0.028C + 0.042AB - 0.057AC + 0.026BC - 0.012A^2 + 0.075B^2 + 0.019C^2 \quad (3)$$

Regarding the particle size, B, C, B^2 are significant model terms, while in the case of the Zeta potential and PDI, B, B^2 are significant models. In all three cases, the values were less than 0.1000, indicating the significance of the applied model. The optimized PG-SLNs were further evaluated for encapsulation efficiency (EE), percentage yield and loading capacity (LC). Optimized PG-SLNs resulted in 84 ± 0.47% EE and 60 ± 0.03% LC. The yield of the PG-SLNs was up to 80 ± 0.1%. Z-average, PDI and zeta potential were also measured for optimized PG-SLNs. The Z-average of PG-SLNs was reported as 103 ± 46 nm with PDI of 0.16 ± 0.001 and zeta potential of −36 ± 4.78 mV.

2.2.2. XRPD and FTIR Analysis

X-ray powder diffractograms (XRPD) of PG show sharp, characteristic peaks confirming its crystalline nature (Figure 2a). The results show that the characteristic peaks of PG (4.1°, 6.2°, 25.8° and 26.4° 2θ) could not be observed in the diffractogram of PG-SLNs, which shows that the crystalline structure of PG is converted into amorphous form and also supports the EE measurement data according to the high amount of PG that was successfully encapsulated into SLNs. In the diffractogram of PG-SLNs, only one peak can be detected at 5.2° 2θ, which corresponds to cholesterol as a carrier base material. These results of PG-SLNs are in agreement with similar experiments reported in the literature [30]. The FTIR spectra (Fourier-transformed infrared spectroscopy) of the components and the formulation are presented in Figure 2b. The characteristic peaks of PG including O–H stretching vibration at 3331 cm^{-1}, C=O stretching of ester at 1539 cm^{-1}, phenol O–H bending at 1246 cm^{-1} as well as C–O–C stretching of aromatic ester at 770 cm^{-1} and 745 cm^{-1} become unobvious in the spectrum of PG-SLNs, which also indicates the encapsulation of PG into SLNs. No other remarkable shift was observed in the other spectral regions, which supports that there is no interaction between SLNs and components.

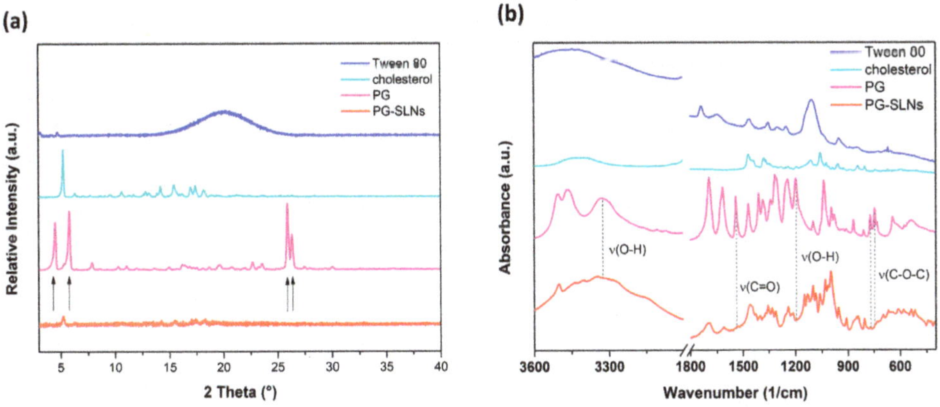

Figure 2. XRPD diffractogram (**a**) and FTIR spectra (**b**) of PG-SLNs and their components.

2.3. *Characterization of Hydrogels*

2.3.1. Evaluation of pH and Drug Contents of Hydrogels

It has been reported in several previous studies that lysozyme as a physiological nasal mucosa enzyme could inhibit specific types of microbes under slightly acidic conditions [31]. Therefore, the pH of an ideal nasal formulation should be in the range of 5.0 to 6.0 to preserve the physiological microbiological defense [32,33]. The pH of the HA-HGs was between 5.2 and 5.9, which is suitable for nasal administration. Drug content of HA-HGs was 78–82% *w*/*v* measured by HPLC, as shown in Table 2.

Table 2. Main physicochemical characteristics of hydrogels at various hyaluronic acid concentrations.

HA Content (% *w*/*v*)	pH Value	Drug Contents (%)	Spreadability (mm^2)	Mucoadhesion Displacement (mm) after 7 h	Viscosity Cross-Linked (Pas)	Viscosity Non-Cross-Linked (Pas)
0.5	5.3 ± 0.2	78 ± 2.5	222.45 ± 0.22	20 *	0.112	0.181
1	5.2 ± 0.3	82 ± 3.3	360 ± 0.33	20	1.88	2.11
2	5.5 ± 0.4	80 ± 1.4	320 ± 0.44	10	14.29	15.45
3	5.9 ± 0.6	79 ± 4.2	340 ± 0.012	1	66.34	157

* After 2 h maximum displacement on agar-mucin plate was already reached.

2.3.2. Raman Chemical Mapping

Raman mapping was carried out in order to examine the distribution of PG-SLNs in non-cross-linked HA-HGs (SLNs-HGnCL) of different concentrations. For localization of nanoparticles, the Raman spectrum of PG-SLNs were set as profile, whose frequency of occurrence is shown in the chemical maps (Figure 3). The different colors of the chemical map show the relative intensity change of PG-SLNs in the gel structure. Red color indicates strong existence of PG-SLNs, whereas blue color marks those regions of the map whose spectral resolution contains different spectra, characteristic for another component. The results reveal that the distribution of PG-SLNs is more concentrated in HGs containing HA in lower concentration (0.5% and 1% *w*/*v*), as shown by high relative intensity values of the Raman map, whereas in the case of higher HA concentration (2% and 3% *w*/*v*), PG-SLNs can be found in well-defined packages.

2.3.3. Spreadability and Swelling Studies of Hydrogel

The spreadability values of both cross-linked (SLNs-HGCL) and non-cross linked (SLNs-HGnCL) SLNs-HGs was investigated. No significant effect of cross-linking was observed in case of spreadability; SLNs-HGs with different concentrations of HA (0.5, 1, 2 and 3% *w*/*v*) showed 222.45 ± 0.22, 360.10 ± 0.33, 320.12 ± 0.44 and 340 ± 0.01 mm^2 spreading surface, respectively (Table 2). Values in this range ensure proper spreading of the hydrogel. The spreadability study showed that the optimized SLNs-HG (1% *w*/*v* HA) resulted in the highest spreading surface [34,35]. Swelling studies were performed both with cross-linked and non-cross-linked hydrogels. The results show that all the non-cross-linked formulations show a higher swelling index than the chemically cross-linked HG, which can be claimed with the hindered diffusion of water into the cross-linked HG network (Figure 4). The formulation's property to spread uniformly and easily on an applied surface is important to deliver a uniform dose of the active compound.

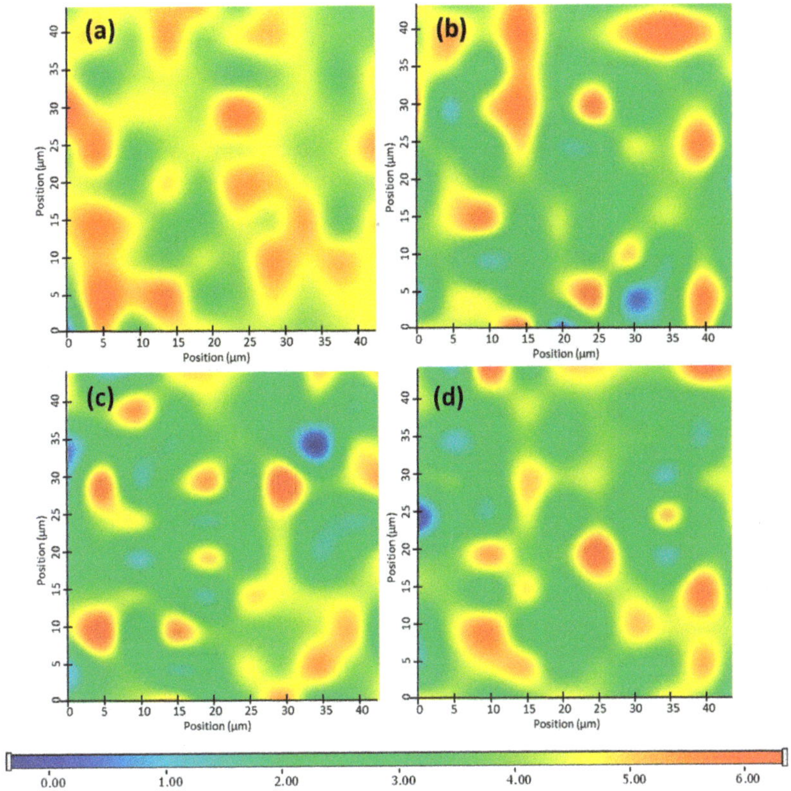

Figure 3. Raman chemical mapping of PG-SLNs in HGs with different concentration of HA: 0.5 (**a**), 1 (**b**), 2 (**c**) and 3% *w*/*v* (**d**).

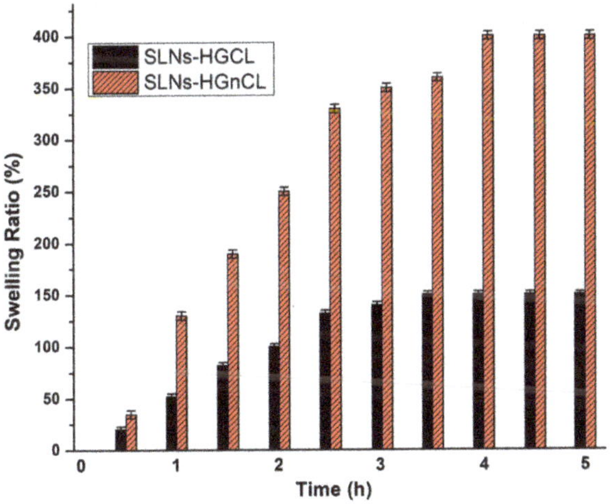

Figure 4. Swelling study of optimized cross-linked (SLNs-HGCL) and non-cross-linked (SLNs-HGnCL) HG (1% *w*/*v* HA). Data are means ± SD (n = 3 independent measurements).

2.3.4. Viscosity Measurement

Viscosity is of paramount importance in the case of the applicability of hydrogels to the intranasal administration route, which influences the mucoadhesive properties of the formulation and can prolong the residence in the nasal cavity. Proper polymer concentration must be set in order to achieve the desired high viscosity value, allowing increased residence time and making it possible to enhance the absorption through the nasal mucosa. However, too high viscosity can also be disadvantageous, resulting in hindered drug release of the formulation in the nasal cavity. The viscosity of both cross-linked and non-cross-linked HGs was measured (Table 2). The viscosity measurement of all formulations showed that there was an inverse relation between shear rate and viscosity of HG, which proves the thixotropic nature of HGs (Figure 5). No significant differences among viscosities of cross-linked and non-cross-linked HGs was observed. Furthermore, the non-cross linked SLNs-HGs were characterized due to the spreadability investigation, where SLNs-HGnCL formulations showed higher swelling ratio and spreadability, along with the non-significant difference experienced in the viscosity compared with cross-linked SLNs-HGs.

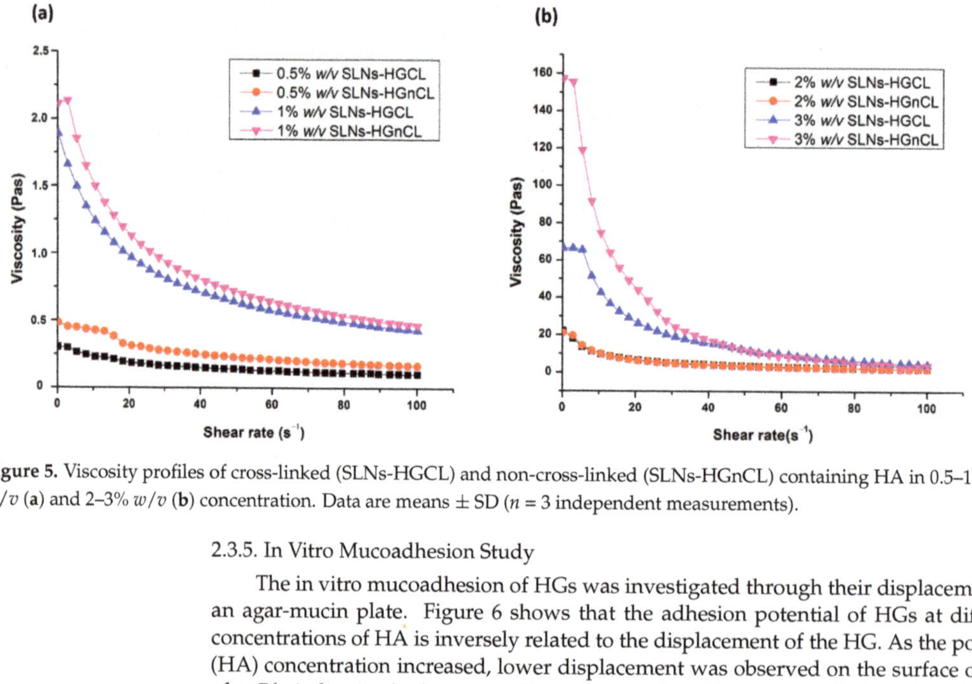

Figure 5. Viscosity profiles of cross-linked (SLNs-HGCL) and non-cross-linked (SLNs-HGnCL) containing HA in 0.5–1% *w*/*v* (**a**) and 2–3% *w*/*v* (**b**) concentration. Data are means ± SD (n = 3 independent measurements).

2.3.5. In Vitro Mucoadhesion Study

The in vitro mucoadhesion of HGs was investigated through their displacement on an agar-mucin plate. Figure 6 shows that the adhesion potential of HGs at different concentrations of HA is inversely related to the displacement of the HG. As the polymer (HA) concentration increased, lower displacement was observed on the surface of agar after 7 h, indicating higher mucoadhesive properties of formulation. This can be related to the increasing strength of chemical interactions (secondary bonding) between mucin and HA. At the highest concentration (3% *w*/*v*) of HA, hardly any displacement was observed during the studied time, indicating remarkable mucoadhesion of formulation. At a lower concentration (0.5% *w*/*v*) of HA, displacement was not adequate for nasal administration, and after 2 h it was totally displaced from the agar-mucin plate. Based on these results, the optimized concentration of HG (1% *w*/*v*) was screened out, as displacement measured at this concentration was adequate and also in accordance with the results of viscosity, spreadability and swelling ratio measured at this specific concentration, as shown in Table 2.

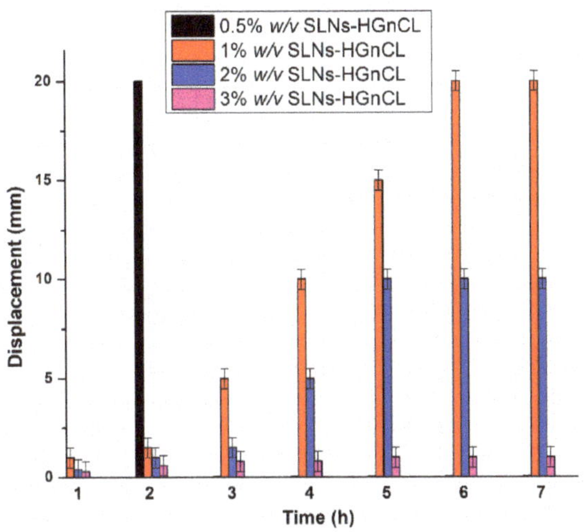

Figure 6. In vitro mucoadhesive studies of SLNs-HGs on agar-mucin gel. Data are means ± SD (n = 5 independent measurements).

2.3.6. Morphological Study of PG-SLNs and PG-SLNs-Loaded HG

SEM images of lyophilized PG-SLNs, shown in Figure 7, also proves that the nanoparticles have spherical morphology and are homogenously distributed in the gel structure. The SEM image of optimized freeze-dried 1% w/v SLNs-HGnCL shows porous structure with a dense cross-linking network.

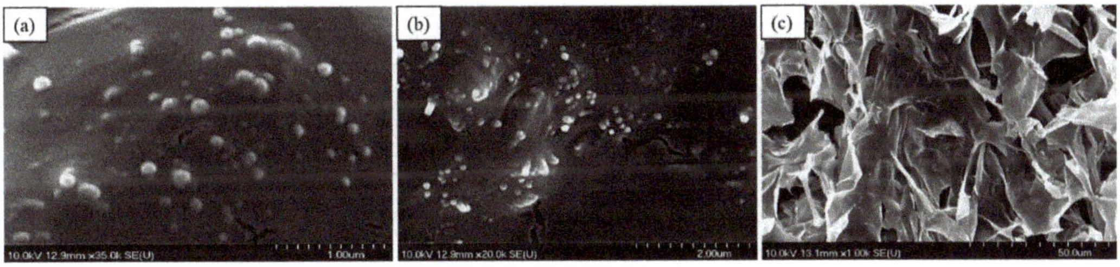

Figure 7. SEM images of optimized lyophilized PG-SLNs (**a**,**b**) and 1% w/v SLNs-HGnCL (**c**) at various resolution.

2.3.7. In Vitro Permeation

Modified Side-Bi-Side® apparatus was used for the in vitro nasal permeation study, whereas the diffusion of PG solution, PG-SLNs, as well as TC-P containing and TC-P-free 1% w/v SLNs-HGnCL was compared. The TC-P was used as permeation enhancer due to its nontoxic and biocompatible nature. Several studies reported its permeation-enhancing effect through a synthetic membrane and on excised skin, reported in previous studies with different drugs [31,36–38]. Figure 8a shows the cumulative PG permeation from donor to acceptor phase through a synthetic cellulose membrane impregnated with isopropyl myristate. The cumulative permeation of PG from PG-SLNs was ~190 μg/cm^2 after 60 min. The TC-P-free 1% w/v SLNs-HGnCL showed a lower permeation of about 180 μg/cm^2, which supports the advantage of application of permeation enhancer. In the case of pure PG dispersion, the permeation was lower than 10 μg/cm^2. The significantly highest permeability was achieved with the HG containing TC-P reaching, with a value around 600 μg/cm^2.

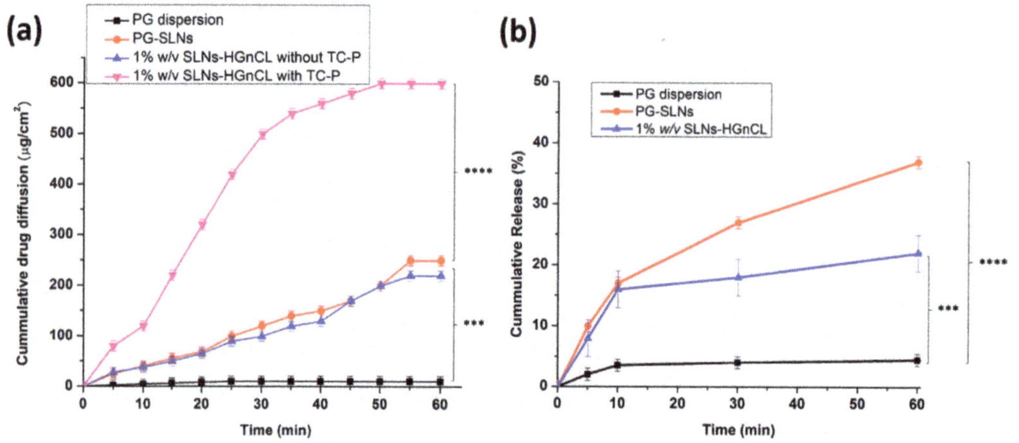

Figure 8. In vitro permeation of pure PG dispersion, PG-SLNs, 1% *w*/*v* SLNs-HGnCL with and without TC-P (**a**). In vitro release study of PG dispersion, PG-SLNs, 1% *w*/*v* SLNs-HGnCL (**b**). Data are means ± SD ($n = 3$ independent measurements). *** $p < 0.001$, **** $p < 0.0001$.

2.3.8. In Vitro Release Study

In vitro release studies of PG-SLNs showed burst release of drug in the first 60 min (~40% of drug) at pH 5.6. After that, the drug release rate decreased following a sustained release tendency, as shown in Figure 8b. In the case of the HG formulation, the initial burst effect was lower, which can be claimed with the controlled release effect of the gel matrix. After 60 min only 15% of PG was released from the HG. To determine the release kinetic of PG from SLNs as well as HG, various dissolution kinetic models including zero-order, first-order, Higuchi, Korsmeyer–Peppas and Hixon–Crowel were fitted to the release data, and kinetic parameters were calculated (Table S1). The drug release both from SLNs and HG followed Higuchi kinetics ($R^2 = 0.96$ and 0.9783 respectively), which can be claimed with the drug release controlling mechanism of lipid matrix and swelling ability of HA-PG matrix in the simulated nasal medium [39]. Fitting the Korsmeyer-Peppas model, the "*n*" value was lower than 0.5, which indicates that both formulations follow Fickian drug diffusion. The significant difference between SLNs and HG can be claimed with the presence of gel network surrounding the SLNs, which decreases the velocity of Fickian diffusion, resulting in sustained release of PG.

2.3.9. In Vitro Antioxidant Activity Evaluation with Hydrogen Peroxide Scavenging Assay

The antioxidant activity of PG was investigated, aiming to confirm that PG-SLNs embedded in HA-HG can preserve antioxidant activity, which is essential in their pharmacological effect. It has been demonstrated that free radicals have a pivotal role in the pathogenesis of different diseases, as well as in several types of cancer [40]. The in vitro scavenging activity of PG-SLN-loaded HA-HGs was investigated containing PG in different concentrations utilizing hydrogen peroxide (H_2O_2) as oxidative medium (Figure 9). It has been revealed that by increasing the polymer concentration in the HG, the antioxidant activity of PG against H_2O_2 was improved, which can be explained by the protective effect of the hydrogel network. The results also support that a strong correlation could be found between the concentration of PG and the rate of inhibition of scavenging activity of H_2O_2. By increasing the concentration of PG, the inhibition was enhanced. At 10 and 30 μg/mL PG containing HGs (containing 2% and 3% *w*/*v* HA), the antioxidant activity was significantly higher in comparison with low HA concentration HGs and PG-SLNs or PG control, which also supports the stabilizing effect of the polymer matrix. In the case of 20 μg/mL, the same tendency of difference was also demonstrated, but it was not significant.

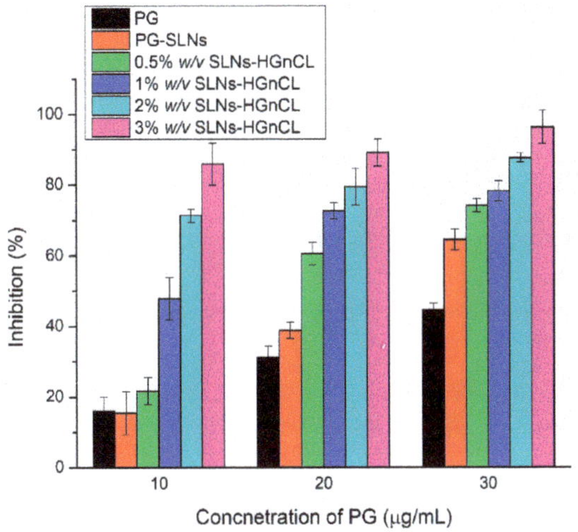

Figure 9. Percentage inhibition of the hydrogen-peroxide-scavenging activity of different concentrations of PG-containing SLNs and PG-SLNs-loaded HA-HG in comparison with the initial PG solution. Data are means ± SD (n = 3 independent measurements). Statistical analysis: t-Test.

3. Discussion

In our previous work we had already investigated the formulation possibilities of PG-loaded liposomes coated with HA [41], as PG has advantageous effects (anti-inflammatory, antioxidant and anticancer activity) in the treatment of brain tumors, e.g., glioblastoma multiforme. As PG is a water-insoluble compound, loading it into a nanocarrier can enhance its water solubility and drug release profile in different administration routes. The present study focused on the formulation of PG-SLNs and loading into HA-HG for brain targeting through intranasal administration. The novelty of our work lies in the fact that our research team explored the first-time application of the PG-SLNs-loaded HA-HG for intranasal delivery route.

SLNs were developed in our study due to their advantageous properties (biocompatibility, increased solubility, protection of drug and permeability enhancement) and loaded into HA-HG as a secondary carrier for facilitating drug transport via the intranasal route. Due to its mucoadhesive property, the role of HA is vital for intranasal drug delivery systems because the nasal cavity is subjected to mucociliary clearance [42,43]. TC-P was utilized as a permeation enhancer as it was previously successfully used as a surfactant or co-surfactant for intranasal application. TC-P has adequate solubilizing property, and it has the ability to enhance the drug's solubility by orders of magnitude compared with other penetration enhancers.

Aiming to develop novel PG-SLNs-loaded into the HA-HG system, the QbD approach was applied. After the determination of the QTPP elements, the relations between CQA and CMA/CPP elements were evaluated, and a risk order was set up based on the software-calculated severity scores. By optimizing the factors having the highest severity via central composite design, the optimized SLNs had a Z-average of 120 ± 8.8 nm, with a PDI of 0.12 ± 0.08 and a zeta potential that was a more negative −38 ± 10.2 mV. The indirect and direct co-effect of cholesterol and Tween 80 on Z-average can be clearly seen in both the single factor and 3D plot (Figure S2a,b). The results show weak repulsion forces between lipid nanoparticles and the surfactant at lower concentration of cholesterol. However, at higher lipid concentrations, prominent repulsion forces can be observed, which can be explained by the presence of the surfactant phase between lipid nanoparticles and the decrease in van der Waals forces, all reducing the aggregation tendency of lipid droplets [44]. The surfactant concentration showed higher impact on the reduction of Z-average and PDI as compared with cholesterol. These results are in accordance with those reported by Azhar Shekoufeh Bahari et al. and Severino et al. [39,45]. The low Z-average and narrow PDI indicate improved nasal absorption, while the highly negative zeta potential due to surface properties of cholesterol supports high stability of formulation. The absolute value of zeta potential was higher than 30 mV, which ensures sufficient repulsive forces to attain better physical and colloidal stability of the nanosystem [46,47]. The morphological studies by SEM showed spherical shaped SLNs with homogenous distribution and nano-range particle size.

Raman mapping showed that the increasing concentration of polymer forms well-designed hydrogel matrix embedding PG-SLNs homogenously, indicating higher stability of nanoparticles avoiding aggregation [48–50]. The swelling study revealed that the polymeric chains were more flexible in cross-linker-free HG, ensuring water diffusion into the gel matrix.

In the case of chemically cross-linked HG, the free association of the polymer chain is hindered, resulting in a decreased swelling ratio. From these results, it can be concluded that by adding a cross-linker, the mechanical strength of the HG was enhanced. More precise controlled release of the nano-carrier from the gel matrix was reached as compared with simple HG, which is mechanically fragile; thus, larger pores may be created through which nano-carriers can easily liberate the active substance initiating a burst release. Previous studies already reported the similar effect of GA with chitosan HG [51–53]. Safety application of GA is based on previous studies, which showed the nose is very resistant to the aldehydes requiring the application of millimolar concentrations before toxic responses [30].

Our results indicate the significant potential of TC-P in enhancing the permeation of PG-SLNs across the artificial cellulose membrane from the HG matrix. TC-P has a greater influence on the thermodynamic driving force. The maximum thermodynamic driving force occurring at saturation is based on Fickian diffusion, according to which the concentration gradient is formed from a high concentration region to a region of lower concentration phase [36]. TC-P was previously used as a surfactant, co-surfactant and permeation enhancer for intranasal delivery in different micro- and nanoemulsions. Several studies demonstrated the influence of TC-P alone or in combination with propylene glycol on clonazepam permeation both in vitro and ex vivo via application of carbomer HGs. Mura et al. revealed that applying TC-P in the concentration range of 10–50% *w*/*w* increased skin penetration of the drug [42].

The anticancer activity of PG is based on its antioxidant property of removing free radicals [54]. The most important mechanism to achieve this goal is to donate hydrogen to free radicals and convert them into nonreactive species. PG can inhibit cellular damage mainly through their free radical scavenging property [40]. Therefore, we aimed to evaluate the antioxidant activity; the hydrogen peroxide (H_2O_2)-scavenging assay results showed enhanced antioxidant activity in case of applying PG as well as HA in higher concentrations. The developed PG-SLNs-loaded HA-HG with the TC-P system, by controlling the drug release, increasing the physical stability and enhancing the drug permeability via nasal mucosa while protecting its antioxidant activity, imparts a promising carrier system for the brain targeting of antioxidant drugs.

4. Materials and Methods

4.1. Materials

PG, the model antioxidant compound, HA (Mw = 14 kDa) and Tween 80 were purchased from Sigma-Aldrich (Budapest, Hungary). Cholesterol, acetone, ethanol (96% *v*/*v*), glutaraldehyde (25% *w*/*v*) and sodium chloride for physiological salt solution were purchased from Molar Chemicals Ltd. (Budapest, Hungary). Transcutol-P (diethyl glycol monoethyl ether) was supplied by Gattefossé (saint-Priest, France).

4.2. Optimization of SLNs by Quality by Design (QbD) Approach and Risk Assessment Strategy

First, the quality target product profile (QTPP) was defined, followed by selecting the critical quality attributes (CQAs) and critical process parameters (CPPs). The next step was to perform the risk assessment (RA) [55–57]. At first, an interdependence rating was established between the QTPP and CQA elements as well as between CPPs and CQAs. The RA was conducted using Lean QbD®® software (QbDworks.com, QbD works LLc., Fremont. CA, USA). Each factor was thoroughly evaluated on a 3-grade scale using low ("L"), medium ("M") and high ("H") attributives reflecting the relations between the elements. Based on the interdependence rating, the next step was to quantify the severity of the risk factors via a probability rating. As a result of the RA, the severity scores of CQAs and CPPs were plotted on Pareto diagrams generated by the software.

4.3. Response Surface Quadratic Model

Stat-Ease Design Expert® version 10 (stat-Ease, INC.2021 East Hennepin Ave., Suite 480 software) was used to optimize the formulation process and product quality of PG encapsulated SLNs. The amount of cholesterol (20–60 mg), Tween 80 (10–40 mg) and temperature (20–70 °C) where chosen as independent factors based on the RA process, while the ratio of aqueous to organic phases (acetone:ethanol) was kept constant (1:4). Central composite design was applied where SLNs were prepared for each trial, and three responses were evaluated—namely, average hydrodynamic diameter (Z-average), polydispersity index (PDI) and zeta potential.

4.4. Development of PG-SLNs by Modified Injection Method

PG-SLNs were prepared through the modified injection method, where 10 mL of 0.2% *w*/*v* Tween 80 aqueous solution and 5 mL of the organic phase (ethanol:acetone 4:1) were added in different ratios. The PG (10 mg) and cholesterol (60 mg) was dissolved in a mixture of the organic phase and injected dropwise into surfactant solution under constant stirring at 700 rpm at 70 °C. After complete evaporation of the organic phase, the formulation was purified using a Hermle Z323K high performance refrigerated centrifuge (Hermle AG, Gossheim, Germany) for 2 h at 13,500 rpm to separate pellets from supernatant and residual solvent. The collected pellets were redispersed in 5 mL purified water and freeze-dried using a Scanvac CoolSafe laboratory freeze-dryer (Labogene, Lynge, Denmark) at −40 °C for 12 h under a 0.013 mbar pressure with additional 3 h secondary drying at 25 °C in presence of 5% *w*/*v* trehalose as cryoprotectant to obtain lyophilized powders. The lyophilized powder was stored at 5 ± 3 °C until further investigation.

4.5. Preparation of Mucoadhesive HA-Based Hydrogel Formulations with PG-SLNs

Different concentrations (0.5, 1, 2 and 3 *w/v*) of HA were used to prepare colloidal HA-HGs, dissolving them in water for half an hour at 400 rpm. After complete swelling of the HA, the freeze-dried SLNs and 0.1% *w*/*v* glutaraldehyde as cross-linker were added into the HA to form an acetal bond among the aldehyde and hydroxyl group by maintaining acidic conditions. After the reaction, 1 mL of TC-P, as permeation enhancer, was added to the HGs.

4.6. Characterization of PG-SLNs

4.6.1. X-ray Powder Diffraction (XRPD)

Structural characterization of PG-SLNs was performed using a BRUKER D8 Advance X-ray powder diffractometer (Bruker AXS GmbH, Karlsruhe, Germany). All the components and formulations were analyzed in a quartz sample holder and were scanned at 40 kV and 40 mA with Cu K λI radiation (λ = 1.5406 Å) using a VANTEC-1 slit detector in the angular range of 3° to 40° 2θ, at a step time of 0.1 s and an increment of 0.007°. Each measurement was carried out at ambient humidity and temperature.

4.6.2. Fourier-Transformed Infrared Spectroscopy (FTIR)

The compatibility and interactions between PG and the components of the formulation were investigated using a Thermo Nicolet AVATAR FTIR instrument (Thermo-Fisher, Waltham, MA, USA). For the investigation, pellets were prepared by co-grinding 10 mg compound with 150 mg potassium bromide (KBr) and compressed with 10 tons using a hydraulic press. The FTIR spectra were measured over the range of 4000–400 cm^{-1} with a resolution of 4 cm^{-1} for 128 scans. The recorded spectra were reported as absorbance as a function of wavenumber.

4.6.3. Measurement of Z-Average, Surface Charge and Polydispersity Index

The measured amount (6 mg) of lyophilized SLNs was reconstituted in 6 mL of purified water and sonicated for 4 min to minimize the inter-particle aggregation. The Z-average, PDI and surface charge (zeta potential) of PG-SLNs were measured in folded capillary cells using a Malvern Zetasizer nano ZS instrument (Malvern Instrument, Worcestershire, UK) at 25 °C, with the refractive index 1.445. All the measurements were conducted in triplicate, and data are presented as average ± SD.

4.6.4. Encapsulation Efficiency (EE), Loading Capacity (LC) and Percentage Yield Determination

EE and LC of PG-SLNs were determined using an indirect method. PG-SLNs were first centrifuged for 1 h at 16,500 rpm at 4 °C in a Hermle laboratory centrifuge (Hermle AG, Gosheim, Germany). The supernatant was collected and diluted 10-fold with purified water. The concentration of PG was determined using HPLC. The EE, as the actual PG content in the optimized formulation, was measured according to the following equation:

$$\text{Encapsulation Efficiency } (\%) = \frac{w_1 - w_2}{w_1} \times 100 \tag{4}$$

where w_1 is the total amount of added PG, and w_2 is the amount of free PG in the supernatant.

The LC was calculated via the following equation:

$$\text{Loading capacity } (\%) = \frac{w_1 - w_2}{w_3} \times 100 \tag{5}$$

where w_1 is the total amount of added PG, and w_2 is the amount of free PG in the supernatant, while w_3 is the total amount of lipid added to the formulation.

The percentage yield was calculated by weighing the dried PG-SLNs and determined by using the following formula [58]:

$$\text{Percentage yield } (\%) = \frac{\text{weight of dried NPs}}{\text{theoretical weight of drug and components}} \times 100 \tag{6}$$

4.6.5. HPLC Method

The PG quantification was carried via HPLC (Agilent 1260, agent technologies, Santa Clara, CA, USA). The stationary phase was C18 column (Gemini-NX® 150 mm × 4.6 mm, 5 μm (Phenomenex, Torrance, CA, USA). Purified water and acetonitrile in 80:20 ratio adjusted pH = 3.0, with phosphoric acid used as mobile phase. A set of 20 μL samples were injected, whereas separation was performed by 10 min isocratic elution at 25 °C temperature with 1 mL/min eluent flow. The UV-Vis diode array detector was applied for the detection of chromatograms at 254 nm. ChemStation B.04.03 Software (Santa Clara, CA, USA) was used for evaluation of data. PG retention time was detected at 4 min. For the calibration line, the linear regression was 0.998. The quantification limit (LOQ) and detection (LOD) of PG were 63 ppm and 21 ppm, respectively [41,59].

4.7. Characterization of PG-SLNs Loaded Hydrogels

4.7.1. Physical Appearance, pH and Drug Contents of Hydrogels

PG-SLN HGs containing HA in different concentrations (0.5, 1, 2 and 3% *w*/*v*) were evaluated apparently for grittiness and uniformity. The pH of HGs was measured directly by dipping pH meter (WTW® inoLab® pH 7110 laboratory pH tester, Thermo Fisher Scientific, Budapest, Hungary). To determine the drug contents in the formulation, 1 g of HG was dispersed in 10 mL of phosphate buffer (pH 7.4). This diluted gel was filtered with a membrane filter (0.45 μm, polypropylene) and analyzed by HPLC. All measurements were carried out in triplicate. Drug content was evaluated by the following formula:

$$\text{Percent Drug contents} = \frac{\text{Actual amount of drug in the formulation}}{\text{Theoretical amount of drug in thr formualtion}} \times 100 \quad (7)$$

4.7.2. Raman Spectroscopy

A Thermo Fisher DXR Dispersive Raman instrument (Thermo Fisher Scientific Inc., Waltham, MA, USA) was used for investigation of SLNs. This instrument was equipped with a 780 nm wavelength diode laser and a CCD camera. The laser power of 12 mW at 50 μm slit aperture size was used for Raman measurements with 2 and 6 s of exposure and acquisition time, for a total of 32 scans per spectrum in the spectral range 3500–200 cm^{-1} with fluorescence and cosmic ray corrections. The PG-SLNs distribution in HGs was determined via Raman chemical mapping in the formulation. For the total of 16 scans, a 45 μm × 45 μm size surface was evaluated with a 10 μm step size. To eliminate the intensity deviation between the measured areas, the normalization of Raman spectra was ensured [60].

4.7.3. Swelling Index

To measure the swelling index of the HGs, the gravimetric method was applied. Lyophilized gel of both cross-linked and non-cross-linked HGs was soaked in phosphate buffer saline (PBS) (pH = 7.4). After swelling, HGs were taken out from the medium and weighed at different time intervals (after every 30 min) until the weight of the swelled HG became constant. Percentage swelling was calculated using the formula [58]:

$$\text{Swelling } (\%) = \frac{w_2 - w_1}{w_1} \times 100 \quad (8)$$

where w_1 is the initial weight of hydrogel, and w_2 is the weight of swollen HG after each sampling point.

4.7.4. Spreadability Test

Spreadability of HGs was measured using the glass slide method. The center of the glass slide was marked with a 1 cm diameter circle upon which 0.5 g of gel was placed. Another glass slide was placed over the HG, forming a sandwich arrangement. The load of the 500 g was placed on the upper plate and weighted for 5 min. After 5 min, the load was removed, and the increment in HG diameter was measured [61]. All the results were evaluated with respect to the spreading area and applied weight by using the following equation:

$$S_i = d^2 \times \frac{\pi}{4} \quad (9)$$

where S_i is the swelling index, d the diameter of the glass slide and π the shear stress.

4.7.5. Viscosity Measurement

Viscosity measurement was performed at 37 °C with a Haake Rheostress 1 instrument (Thermo Scientific, Karlsruhe, Germany). A cone-plate device was used where the cone diameter was 6 cm with an angle of 1° and a 0.052 mm gap size. The apparent viscosity curves of the samples were plotted under the shear rate range of 0.01–100 s^{-1}.

4.8. In Vitro Characterization of Nanoparticles and Hydrogel

4.8.1. In Vitro Mucoadhesion Testing

In vitro mucoadhesion was performed using the displacement method. A specified weighted amount (5 mg) of HG for each respective HA concentration (0.5, 1, 2 and 3% *w/v*) was placed on the top of 1% *w/v* agar and 2% *w/v* mucin aqueous solution casted on a glass plate of 9 cm and was inclined at 60° in an incubator at 37 °C. The downward movement of the HG mass was measured in millimeters hourly up to 7 h. All the measurements were conducted in triplicate [61,62].

4.8.2. Surface Morphology

Scanning electron microscopy (SEM) (Hitachi S4700, Hitachi Scientific Ltd., Tokyo, Japan) was used to characterize the morphology and surface properties of both PG-SLNs-lyophilized formulation and PG-SLNs-loaded HG. A voltage of 10 kV and 10 mA amperage was applied at 1.3–13.1 mPa pressure. A greater vacuum evaporator and argon atmosphere were used to make the sputter-coated samples conductive with gold–palladium (Bio-Rad SC 502, VG Microtech, Uckfield, UK). The gold–palladium coating thickness was approximately 10 nm.

4.8.3. In Vitro Permeation Study

A modified horizontal side-by-side type diffusion apparatus was used for in vitro permeation studies at 37 °C and with 100 rpm constant stirring (Thermo Haake C10-P5, Sigma-Aldrich Co. LLC, St. Louis, MO, USA). The donor and receptor compartments were isolated with an isopropyl myristate impregnated artificial membrane (0.45 µm pore size, Pall Metri-cel cellulose membrane) with a 0.69 cm^2 diffusion surface. The donor compartment consisted of 9 mL simulated nasal electrolyte solution (SNES) with a pH of 5.6, which contained 0.59 g $CaCl_2$, 8.77 g NaCl, 2.98 g KCl anhydrous in 1000 mL of deionized water, where the acceptor compartment consisted of pH 7.4 PBS. The measured amount (5 mg) of formulation was placed in the donor phase 1 mL of each sample (PG, PG-SLNs, PG-SLNs-loaded HG with and without TC-P) and was withdrawn from the acceptor phase every 5 min and replaced with the same volume of fresh medium. The amount of the drug diffused through the membrane was quantified by using HPLC. Each formulation was analyzed in triplicate.

4.8.4. In Vitro Release Study

The in vitro dissolution study was performed under the nasal conditions at 37 °C by using the modified paddle method with a Hanson SR8 Plus apparatus (Teledyne Hanson Research, Chatsworth, CA, USA) at 50 rpm constant stirring. The PG (10 mg) containing formulation was placed into 50 mL SNES (pH 5.60) as dissolution medium, and samples were withdrawn in predetermined time intervals of 5, 15, 30, 60, 180, 360 and 720 min. After filtration (0.45 µm membrane filter), the PG concentration of the aliquots was analyzed using HPLC. All the measurements were performed in triplicate. The in vitro drug release kinetics of each sample were also evaluated, fitting various mathematical models—namely, zero-order, first-order, Higuchi, Korsmeyer–Peppas and Hixon–Crowel models.

4.8.5. Hydrogen Peroxide Scavenging (H_2O_2) Assay

A solution of hydrogen peroxide (40 mM) was prepared in 0.05 M phosphate buffer (pH 7.4). PG SLNs with different drug concentrations (10, 20 and 30 µg/mL) were incorporated in a 0.6 mL and 40 mM hydrogen peroxide solution. After 10 min of addition of hydrogen peroxide, the absorbance at wavelength of 230 nm was determined spectrophotometrically using phosphate buffer as reference [40,61,63]. The hydrogen peroxide percentage scavenging activity was then measured using the following formula:

$$H_2O_2 \text{ scavenging effect } (\%) = A_0 - \frac{A}{A_0} \times 100 \quad (10)$$

where A_o is the absorbance of the control reaction, and A is the absorbance in the presence of initial PG containing sample.

4.9. Statistical Analysis

The statistical analysis was applied to all the results using Microsoft® 13 software (SAS Institute, Cary, NC, USA). All the results were repeated in triplicate, and the means of data are expressed with standard deviation. In vitro permeation and release data were compared using the one-way analysis of variance (ANOVA); differences were considered significant when $p < 0.05$.

5. Conclusions

PG-SLNs were successfully prepared using a modified injection method. For the optimization of formulation and process parameters affecting the quality of the nanosystem, the initial risk assessment study and the design of experiment were applied following the QbD approach. The addition of PG endowed the HG with the ability to facilitate anticancer activity and with significant potential to be co-encapsulated with other anti-glioblastoma drugs. Our optimized platform provided in vitro proof of the potential of combining the advantages of lipid-based NPs with HG as a promising intranasal delivery system.

Supplementary Materials: The following are available online at https://www.mdpi.com/article/10.3390/ph14070696/s1, Figure S1: Interdependence rating amongst QTPP—CQA (a) and CPP/CMA—CQA (b) elements, Figure S2: 3D surface plot (a) and one-factor interaction (b) graph showing the effects of surfactant and cholesterol on Particle Size, PDI and Zeta potential, Table S1: Kinetic parameters of in vitro drug release.

Author Contributions: Conceptualization, F.S., G.K. and I.C.; methodology, F.S., G.K., B.S. and I.C.; software, F.S., G.K. and B.S.; validation, G.K. and I.C.; formal analysis, G.K., R.I. and I.C.; investigation, F.S., G.K. and R.A.; resources, I.C.; data curation, F.S., G.K. and B.S.; writing—original draft preparation, F.S.; writing—review and editing, G.K., R.I. and I.C.; visualization, F.S. and G.K.; supervision, I.C.; project administration, I.C.; funding acquisition, I.C. All authors have read and agreed to the published version of the manuscript.

Funding: The publication was funded by The University of Szeged Open Access Fund (FundRef, Grant No. 5349).

Institutional Review Board Statement: Not applicable.

Informed Consent Statement: Not applicable.

Data Availability Statement: Data is contained within the article and supplementary material.

Acknowledgments: The authors want to express their acknowledgment to the supporters. This study was supported by the Ministry of Human Capacities, Hungary (Grant TKP-2020), and by the National Research, Development and Innovation Office, Hungary (GINOP 2.3.2-15-2016-00060).

Conflicts of Interest: The authors declare no conflict of interest.

Abbreviations

ANOVA	one-way analysis of variance
BBB	blood–brain barrier
CNS	central nervous system

CPPs	critical process parameters
CMA	critical materials attributes
CQA	critical quality attributes
CCD	central composite design
°C	centigrade
EE	encapsulation efficiency
FTIR	Fourier-transformed infrared spectroscopy
GA	glutaraldehyde
HA	hyaluronic acid
HG	hydrogel
HA-HG	hyaluronic acid—hydrogel
HPLC	high proficiency liquid chromatography
H_2O_2	hydrogen peroxide
ICH	International Conference on Harmonization
KBr	potassium bromide
kDa	kilo Dalton
LC	loading capacity
LOQ	limit of quantification
LOD	limit of detection
mV	millivolt
mm	millimol
mA	milliampere
mPa	millipascal
mg	milligram
mm^2	square millimeter
Mw	molecular weight
nm	nanometer
ppm	parts per million
PBS	phosphate buffer saline
PG	propyl gallate
PG-SLNs	PG-solid lipid nanoparticles
PDI	polydispersity index
Pas	pascal
QbD	Quality by Design
QTPP	quality target product profile
RA	risk assessment
SLNs	solid lipid nanoparticles
SEM	scanning electron microscopy
SLNs-HGnCL	SLNs non-cross-linked HG
SLNs-HGCL	SLNs cross-linked HG
TC-P	Transcutol-P
μm	micrometer
w/v	weight/volume
XRPD	X-ray powder diffractograms

References

1. Chung, E.P.; Cotter, J.D.; Prakapenka, A.V.; Cook, R.L.; Diperna, D.M.; Sirianni, R.W. Targeting small molecule delivery to the brain and spinal cord via intranasal administration of rabies virus glycoprotein (RVG29)-modified PLGA nanoparticles. *Pharmaceutics* **2020**, *12*, 93. [CrossRef]
2. Gonçalves, J.; Bicker, J.; Gouveia, F.; Liberal, J.; Oliveira, R.C.; Alves, G.; Falcão, A.; Fortuna, A. Nose-to-brain delivery of levetiracetam after intranasal administration to mice. *Int. J. Pharm.* **2019**, *564*, 329–339. [CrossRef] [PubMed]
3. Kanazawa, T.; Kaneko, M.; Niide, T.; Akiyama, F.; Kakizaki, S.; Ibaraki, H.; Shiraishi, S.; Takashima, Y.; Suzuki, T.; Seta, Y. Enhancement of nose-to-brain delivery of hydrophilic macromolecules with stearate- or polyethylene glycol-modified arginine-rich peptide. *Int. J. Pharm.* **2017**, *530*, 195–200. [CrossRef] [PubMed]
4. Ullah, I.; Chung, K.; Bae, S.; Li, Y.; Kim, C.; Choi, B.; Nam, H.Y.; Kim, S.H.; Yun, C.O.; Lee, K.Y.; et al. Nose-to-Brain Delivery of Cancer-Targeting Paclitaxel-Loaded Nanoparticles Potentiates Antitumor Effects in Malignant Glioblastoma. *Mol. Pharm.* **2020**, *17*, 1193–1204. [CrossRef] [PubMed]

5. Ul Islam, S.; Shehzad, A.; Bilal Ahmed, M.; Lee, Y.S. Intranasal delivery of nanoformulations: A potential way of treatment for neurological disorders. *Molecules* **2020**, *25*, 1929. [CrossRef] [PubMed]
6. Sintov, A.C. AmyloLipid Nanovesicles: A self-assembled lipid-modified starch hybrid system constructed for direct nose-to-brain delivery of curcumin. *Int. J. Pharm.* **2020**, *588*, 119725. [CrossRef] [PubMed]
7. Sabir, F.; Ismail, R.; Csoka, I. Nose-to-brain delivery of antiglioblastoma drugs embedded into lipid nanocarrier systems: Status quo and outlook. *Drug Discov. Today* **2020**, *25*, 185–194. [CrossRef]
8. Agrawal, M.; Konwar, A.N.; Alexander, A.; Borse, V. Nose-to-brain delivery of biologics and stem cells. In *Direct Nose-To-brain Drug Delivery*; Elsevier: Amsterdam, The Netherlands, 2021; pp. 305–328. [CrossRef]
9. Madav, Y.; Wairkar, S. Strategies for enhanced direct nose-to-brain drug delivery. In *Direct Nose-to-Brain Drug Delivery*; Elsevier: Amsterdam, The Netherlands, 2021; pp. 169–184. [CrossRef]
10. Pardeshi, C.V.; Souto, E.B. Surface modification of nanocarriers as a strategy to enhance the direct nose-to-brain drug delivery. In *Direct Nose-to-Brain Drug Delivery*; Elsevier: Amsterdam, The Netherlands, 2021; pp. 93–114. [CrossRef]
11. Battaglia, L.; Panciani, P.P.; Muntoni, E.; Capucchio, M.T.; Biasibetti, E.; De Bonis, P.; Mioletti, S.; Fontanella, M.; Swaminathan, S. Lipid nanoparticles for intranasal administration: Application to nose-to-brain delivery. *Expert Opin. Drug Deliv.* **2018**, *15*, 369–378. [CrossRef]
12. Kadam, T.S.; Agrawal, A. Short Review on the Important Aspects Involved in Preparation, Characterization and Application of Nanostructured Lipid Carriers for Drug Delivery. *Curr. Nanomed.* **2020**, *10*, 188–207. [CrossRef]
13. Mahmood, H.S.; Alaayedi, M.; Ashoor, J.A.; Alghurabi, H. The enhancement effect of olive and almond oils on permeability of nimesulide as transdermal gel. *Int. J. Pharm. Res.* **2019**, *11*, 1200–1206.
14. Fytianos, G.; Rahdar, A.; Kyzas, G.Z. Nanomaterials in cosmetics: Recent updates. *Nanomaterials* **2020**, *10*, 979. [CrossRef]
15. Yasir, M.; Sara, U.V.S.; Chauhan, I.; Gaur, P.K.; Singh, A.P.; Puri, D.; Ameeduzzafar, A. Solid lipid nanoparticles for nose to brain delivery of donepezil: Formulation, optimization by Box–Behnken design, in vitro and in vivo evaluation. *Artif. Cells, Nanomed. Biotechnol.* **2018**, *46*, 1838–1851. [CrossRef]
16. Vasvani, S.; Kulkarni, P.; Rawtani, D. Hyaluronic acid: A review on its biology, aspects of drug delivery, route of administrations and a special emphasis on its approved marketed products and recent clinical studies. *Int. J. Biol. Macromol.* **2020**, *151*, 1012–1029. [CrossRef] [PubMed]
17. Taymouri, S.; Shahnamnia, S.; Mesripour, A.; Varshosaz, J. In vitro and in vivo evaluation of an ionic sensitive in situ gel containing nanotransfersomes for aripiprazole nasal delivery. *Pharm. Dev. and Tech.* **2021**. just-accepted. [CrossRef]
18. Zhang, H.; Fan, T.; Chen, W.; Li, Y.; Wang, B. Recent advances of two-dimensional materials in smart drug delivery nano-systems. *Bioact. Mater.* **2020**, *5*, 1071–1086. [CrossRef]
19. Thompson, C.M.; Gentry, R.; Fitch, S.; Lu, K.; Clewell, H.J. An updated mode of action and human relevance framework evaluation for Formaldehyde-Related nasal tumors. *Crit. Rev. Toxicol.* **2020**, *50*, 919–952. [CrossRef] [PubMed]
20. Huang, H.M.; Wu, P.H.; Chou, P.C.; Hsiao, W.T.; Wang, H.T.; Chiang, H.P.; Lee, C.M.; Wang, S.H.; Hsiao, Y.C. Enhancement of T2* weighted MRI imaging sensitivity of U87MG glioblastoma cells using γ-ray irradiated low molecular weight hyaluronic acid-conjugated iron nanoparticles. *Int. J. Nanomed.* **2021**, *16*, 3789–3802. [CrossRef] [PubMed]
21. Khorsandi, L.; Mansouri, E.; Rashno, M.; Karami, M.A.; Ashtari, A. Myricetin Loaded Solid Lipid Nanoparticles Upregulate MLKL and RIPK3 in Human Lung Adenocarcinoma. *Int. J. Pept. Res. Ther.* **2020**, *26*, 899–910. [CrossRef]
22. Hadavi, R.; Jafari, S.M.; Katouzian, I. Nanoliposomal encapsulation of saffron bioactive compounds; characterization and optimization. *Int. J. Biol. Macromol.* **2020**, *164*, 4046–4053. [CrossRef]
23. Salmanzadeh, R.; Eskandani, M.; Mokhtarzadeh, A.; Vandghanooni, S.; Ilghami, R.; Maleki, H.; Saeeidi, N.; Omidi, Y. Propyl gallate (PG) and tert-butylhydroquinone (TBHQ) may alter the potential anti-cancer behavior of probiotics. *Food Biosci.* **2018**, *24*, 37–45. [CrossRef]
24. Detsi, A.; Kavetsou, E.; Kostopoulou, I.; Pitterou, I.; Pontillo, A.R.N.; Tzani, A.; Christodoulou, P.; Siliachli, A.; Zoumpoulakis, P. Nanosystems for the encapsulation of natural products: The case of chitosan biopolymer as a matrix. *Pharmaceutics* **2020**, *12*, 669. [CrossRef]
25. Yang, J.T.; Lee, I.N.; Lu, F.J.; Chung, C.Y.; Lee, M.H.; Cheng, Y.C.; Chen, K.T.; Chen, C.H. Propyl Gallate Exerts an Antimigration Effect on Temozolomide-Treated Malignant Glioma Cells through Inhibition of ROS and the NF- κ B Pathway. *J. Immunol. Res.* **2017**, *2017*. [CrossRef]
26. Stocker, E.; Becker, K.; Hate, S.; Hohl, R.; Schiemenz, W.; Sacher, S.; Zimmer, A.; Salar-Behzadi, S. Application of ICH Q9 Quality Risk Management Tools for Advanced Development of Hot Melt Coated Multiparticulate Systems. *J. Pharm. Sci.* **2017**, *106*, 278–290. [CrossRef]
27. ICH. *Pharmaceutical Development Q8*; ICH Harmonised Tripartite Guideline; ICH: Geneva, Switzerland, 2009; pp. 1–28.
28. Németh, Z.; Pallagi, E.; Dobó, D.G.; Csóka, I. A proposed methodology for a risk assessment-based liposome development process. *Pharmaceutics* **2020**, *12*, 1164. [CrossRef]
29. Pallagi, E.; Jójárt-Laczkovich, O.; Németh, Z.; Szabó-Révész, P.; Csóka, I. Application of the QbD-based approach in the early development of liposomes for nasal administration. *Int. J. Pharm.* **2019**, *562*, 11–22. [CrossRef]
30. McGregor, D.; Bolt, H.; Cogliano, V.; Richter-Reichhelm, H.B. Formaldehyde and glutaraldehyde and nasal cytotoxicity: Case study within the context of the 2006 IPCS human framework for the analysis of a cancer mode of action for humans. *Crit. Rev. Toxicol.* **2006**, *36*, 821–835. [CrossRef]

31. Pillai, A.M.; Sivasankarapillai, V.S.; Rahdar, A.; Joseph, J.; Sadeghfar, F.; Anuf, A.R.; Rajesh, K.; Kyzas, G.Z. Green synthesis and characterization of zinc oxide nanoparticles with antibacterial and antifungal activity. *J. Mol. Struct.* **2020**, *1211*, 128107. [CrossRef]
32. Mertins, O.; Mathews, P.D.; Angelova, A. Advances in the design of ph-sensitive cubosome liquid crystalline nanocarriers for drug delivery applications. *Nanomaterials* **2020**, *10*, 963. [CrossRef] [PubMed]
33. Rajesh, S.; Zhai, J.; Drummond, C.J.; Tran, N. Synthetic ionizable aminolipids induce a pH dependent inverse hexagonal to bicontinuous cubic lyotropic liquid crystalline phase transition in monoolein nanoparticles. *J. Colloid Interface Sci.* **2021**, *589*, 85–95. [CrossRef]
34. Hao, J.; Zhao, J.; Zhang, S.; Tong, T.; Zhuang, Q.; Jin, K.; Chen, W.; Tang, H. Fabrication of an ionic-sensitive in situ gel loaded with resveratrol nanosuspensions intended for direct nose-to-brain delivery. *Colloids Surfaces B Biointerfaces* **2016**, *147*, 376–386. [CrossRef] [PubMed]
35. Khatoon, M.; Sohail, M.F.; Shahnaz, G.; ur Rehman, F.; Fakhar-ud-Din; ur Rehman, A.; Ullah, N.; Amin, U.; Khan, G.M.; Shah, K.U. Development and Evaluation of Optimized Thiolated Chitosan Proniosomal Gel Containing Duloxetine for Intranasal Delivery. *AAPS PharmSciTech* **2019**, *20*. [CrossRef] [PubMed]
36. Osborne, D.W.; Musakhanian, J. Skin Penetration and Permeation Properties of Transcutol®—Neat or Diluted Mixtures. *AAPS PharmSciTech* **2018**, *19*, 3512–3533. [CrossRef] [PubMed]
37. Chin, L.Y.; Tan, J.Y.P.; Choudhury, H.; Pandey, M.; Sisinthy, S.P.; Gorain, B. Development and optimization of chitosan coated nanoemulgel of telmisartan for intranasal delivery: A comparative study. *J. Drug Deliv. Sci. Technol.* **2021**, *62*, 102341. [CrossRef]
38. Sivasankarapillai, V.S.; Das, S.S.; Sabir, F.; Sundaramahalingam, M.A.; Colmenares, J.C.; Prasannakumar, S.; Rajan, M.; Rahdar, A.; Kyzas, G.Z. Progress in natural polymer engineered biomaterials for transdermal drug delivery systems. *Mater. Today Chem.* **2021**, *19*, 100382. [CrossRef]
39. Varma, L.T.; Singh, N.; Gorain, B.; Choudhury, H.; Tambuwala, M.M.; Kesharwani, P.; Shukla, R. Recent Advances in Self-Assembled Nanoparticles for Drug Delivery. *Curr. Drug Deliv.* **2020**, *17*, 279–291. [CrossRef]
40. Al-Amiery, A.A.; Al-Majedy, Y.K.; Kadhum, A.A.H.; Mohamad, A.B. Hydrogen peroxide scavenging activity of novel coumarins synthesized using different approaches. *PLoS ONE* **2015**, *10*, e0132175. [CrossRef]
41. Sabir, F.; Katona, G.; Pallagi, E.; Dobó, D.G.; Akel, H.; Berkesi, D.; Kónya, Z.; Csóka, I. Quality-by-Design-Based Development of n-Propyl-Gallate-Loaded Hyaluronic-Acid-Coated Liposomes for Intranasal Administration. *Molecules* **2021**, *26*, 1429. [CrossRef]
42. Javadzadeh, Y.; Adibkia, K.; Hamishekar, H. Transcutol® (Diethylene Glycol). In *Percutaneous Penetration Enhancers Chemical Methods in Penetration Enhancement: Modification of the Stratum Corneum*; Springer: Berlin/Heidelberg, Germany, 2015; pp. 195–205. [CrossRef]
43. Khan, A.; Aqil, M.; Imam, S.S.; Ahad, A.; Sultana, Y.; Ali, A.; Khan, K. Temozolomide loaded nano lipid based chitosan hydrogel for nose to brain delivery: Characterization, nasal absorption, histopathology and cell line study. *Int. J. Biol. Macromol.* **2018**, *116*, 1260–1267. [CrossRef] [PubMed]
44. Tapeinos, C.; Battaglini, M.; Ciofani, G. Advances in the design of solid lipid nanoparticles and nanostructured lipid carriers for targeting brain diseases. *J. Control. Release* **2017**, *264*, 306–332. [CrossRef]
45. Bahari, L.A.S.; Hamishehkar, H. The impact of variables on particle size of solid lipid nanoparticles and nanostructured lipid carriers; A comparative literature review. *Adv. Pharm. Bull.* **2016**, *6*, 143–151. [CrossRef]
46. Sarhadi, S.; Gholizadeh, M.; Moghadasian, T.; Golmohammadzadeh, S. Moisturizing effects of solid lipid nanoparticles (SLN) and nanostructured lipid carriers (NLC) using deionized and magnetized water by in vivo and in vitro methods. *Iran. J. Basic Med. Sci.* **2020**, *23*, 337–343. [CrossRef]
47. Naseri, M.; Golmohamadzadeh, S.; Arouiee, H.; Jaafari, M.R.; Nemati, S.H. Preparation and comparison of various formulations of solid lipid nanoparticles (SLNs) containing essential oil of Zataria multiflora. *J. Hortic. Postharvest Res.* **2020**, *3*, 73–84.
48. Zdaniauskienė, A.; Charkova, T.; Ignatjev, I.; Melvydas, V.; Garjonytė, R.; Matulaitienė, I.; Talaikis, M.; Niaura, G. Shell-isolated nanoparticle-enhanced Raman spectroscopy for characterization of living yeast cells. *Spectrochim. Acta Part A Mol. Biomol. Spectrosc.* **2020**, *240*, 118560. [CrossRef]
49. Shringarpure, M.; Gharat, S.; Momin, M.; Omri, A. Management of epileptic disorders using nanotechnology-based strategies for nose-to-brain drug delivery. *Expert Opin. Drug Deliv.* **2021**, *18*, 169–185. [CrossRef]
50. Affes, S.; Aranaz, I.; Acosta, N.; Heras, Á.; Nasri, M.; Maalej, H. Chitosan derivatives-based films as pH-sensitive drug delivery systems with enhanced antioxidant and antibacterial properties. *Int. J. Biol. Macromol.* **2021**, *182*, 730–742. [CrossRef]
51. Lee, H.; Song, C.; Baik, S.; Kim, D.; Hyeon, T.; Kim, D.H. Device-assisted transdermal drug delivery. *Adv. Drug Deliv. Rev.* **2018**, *127*, 35–45. [CrossRef]
52. Abhaihaidelmonem, R.; El Nabarawi, M.; Attia, A. Development of novel bioadhesive granisetron hydrochloride spanlastic gel and insert for brain targeting and study their effects on rats. *Drug Deliv.* **2018**, *25*, 70–77. [CrossRef] [PubMed]
53. Iglesias, N.; Galbis, E.; Valencia, C.; Díaz-Blanco, M.J.; Lacroix, B.; de-Paz, M.V. Biodegradable double cross-linked chitosan hydrogels for drug delivery: Impact of chemistry on rheological and pharmacological performance. *Int. J. Biol. Macromol.* **2020**, *165*, 2205–2218. [CrossRef]
54. Wei, P.L.; Huang, C.Y.; Chang, Y.J. Propyl gallate inhibits hepatocellular carcinoma cell growth through the induction of ROS and the activation of autophagy. *PLoS ONE* **2019**, *14*, e0210513. [CrossRef] [PubMed]

55. Bhise, K.; Kashaw, S.K.; Sau, S.; Iyer, A.K. Nanostructured lipid carriers employing polyphenols as promising anticancer agents: Quality by design (QbD) approach. *Int. J. Pharm.* **2017**, *526*, 506–515. [CrossRef] [PubMed]
56. Pallagi, E.; Ambrus, R.; Szabó-Révész, P.; Csóka, I. Adaptation of the quality by design concept in early pharmaceutical development of an intranasal nanosized formulation. *Int. J. Pharm.* **2015**, *491*, 384–392. [CrossRef] [PubMed]
57. Pallagi, E.; Ismail, R.; Paál, T.L.; Csóka, I. Initial Risk Assessment as part of the Quality by Design in peptide drug containing formulation development. *Eur. J. Pharm. Sci.* **2018**, *122*, 160–169. [CrossRef] [PubMed]
58. Qindeel, M.; Ahmed, N.; Sabir, F.; Khan, S.; Ur-Rehman, A. Development of novel pH-sensitive nanoparticles loaded hydrogel for transdermal drug delivery. *Drug Dev. Ind. Pharm.* **2019**, *45*, 629–641. [CrossRef] [PubMed]
59. Katona, G.; Balogh, G.T.; Dargó, G.; Gáspár, R.; Márki, Á.; Ducza, E.; Sztojkov-Ivanov, A.; Tömösi, F.; Kecskeméti, G.; Janáky, T.; et al. Development of meloxicam-human serum albumin nanoparticles for nose-to-brain delivery via application of a quality by design approach. *Pharmaceutics* **2020**, *12*, 97. [CrossRef]
60. Sipos, B.; Szabó-Révész, P.; Csóka, I.; Pallagi, E.; Dobó, D.G.; Bélteky, P.; Kónya, Z.; Deák, Á.; Janovák, L.; Katona, G. Quality by design based formulation study of meloxicam-loaded polymeric micelles for intranasal administration. *Pharmaceutics* **2020**, *12*, 697. [CrossRef] [PubMed]
61. Rajinikanth, P.S.; Chellian, J. Development and evaluation of nanostructured lipid carrier-based hydrogel for topical delivery of 5-fluorouracil. *Int. J. Nanomedicine* **2016**, *11*, 5067. [CrossRef]
62. Youssef, N.A.H.A.; Kassem, A.A.; Farid, R.M.; Ismail, F.A.; EL-Massik, M.A.E.; Boraie, N.A. A novel nasal almotriptan loaded solid lipid nanoparticles in mucoadhesive in situ gel formulation for brain targeting: Preparation, characterization and in vivo evaluation. *Int. J. Pharm.* **2018**, *548*, 609–624. [CrossRef] [PubMed]
63. Porfiryeva, N.N.; Semina, I.I.; Salakhov, I.A.; Moustafine, R.I.; Khutoryanskiy, V.V. Mucoadhesive and mucus-penetrating Interpolyelectrolyte complexes for nose-to-brain drug delivery. *Nanomed. Nanotechnol. Biol. Med.* **2021**, 102432. [CrossRef]

pharmaceuticals

Article

Transfer Investigations of Lipophilic Drugs from Lipid Nanoemulsions to Lipophilic Acceptors: Contributing Effects of Cholesteryl Esters and Albumin as Acceptor Structures

Sabrina Knoke [1] and Heike Bunjes [1,2,*]

1 Technische Universität Braunschweig, Institut für Pharmazeutische Technologie und Biopharmazie, Mendelssohnstraße 1, 38106 Braunschweig, Germany; sabrina.knoke@tu-braunschweig.de
2 Technische Universität Braunschweig, Zentrum für Pharmaverfahrenstechnik (PVZ), Franz-Liszt-Straße 35a, 38106 Braunschweig, Germany
* Correspondence: heike.bunjes@tu-braunschweig.de; Tel.: +49-531-391-5652

Abstract: When studying the release of poorly water-soluble drugs from colloidal drug delivery systems designed for intravenous administration, the release media should preferentially contain lipophilic components that represent the physiological acceptors present in vivo. In this study, the effect of different acceptor structures was investigated by comparing the transfer of fenofibrate, retinyl acetate, and orlistat from trimyristin nanoemulsion droplets into lipid-containing hydrogel particles, as well as to bovine serum albumin (BSA). A nanodispersion based on trimyristin and cholesteryl nonanoate was incorporated into the hydrogel particles (mean diameter ~40 μm) in order to mimic the composition of lipoproteins. The course of transfer observed utilizing the lipid-containing hydrogel particles as an acceptor was in relation to the lipophilicity of the drugs: the higher the logP value, the slower the transfer. There was no detectable amount of the drugs transferred to BSA in liquid solution, demonstrating clearly that albumin alone does not contribute substantially as acceptor for the lipophilic drugs under investigation in this study. In contrast, cholesteryl nonanoate contributes to a much greater extent. However, in all cases, the partition equilibrium of the drugs under investigation was in favor of the trimyristin emulsion droplets.

Keywords: drug transfer; in vitro release; colloidal drug carriers; lipid nanoparticles; hydrogel beads; cholesteryl nonanoate; bovine serum albumin

Citation: Knoke, S.; Bunjes, H. Transfer Investigations of Lipophilic Drugs from Lipid Nanoemulsions to Lipophilic Acceptors: Contributing Effects of Cholesteryl Esters and Albumin as Acceptor Structures. *Pharmaceuticals* **2021**, *14*, 865. https://doi.org/10.3390/ph14090865

Academic Editors: Ana Catarina Silva, João Nuno Moreira and José Manuel Sousa Lobo

Received: 3 August 2021
Accepted: 26 August 2021
Published: 28 August 2021

1. Introduction

To overcome issues arising from the poor water solubility of many newly discovered drugs, lipid-based colloidal dispersions are under investigation as a promising formulation approach for the parenteral administration of these substances [1]. Such dispersions may, e.g., be liposomes, nanoemulsions, or may contain solid or liquid crystalline nanoparticles [2–4]. Information on the release behavior (or drug retention properties, respectively) of the lipid carrier particles is crucial for quality control, as well as to predict in vivo behavior. Since there is no officially approved test, efforts are being made to design appropriate setups for release testing of nanoparticulate drug carriers [5].

Challenges to face are, for example, related to the small size of the carrier particles. Only drugs with special properties, such as fluorescence, acidic/basic moieties, or electrochemically active groups, enable the detection of released drug with analytical methods that do not interfere with the dispersed phase particles [6–8]. Hence, many methods described in the literature require a separation step, such as filtration or centrifugation, in order to perform quantitative analysis of the released drug [9,10]. Other approaches are based on membrane barrier techniques [11–13] or continuous flow setups [14,15]. Depending on the method, the drug release behavior may be affected by the experimental conditions, e.g., due to high shear stress or long high-speed circulation times, insufficient time resolution, fluctuations in flow rates, or filter clogging [12,16–19].

For dosage forms that are designed to deliver lipophilic drugs via the intravenous (i.v.) route, release testing should be performed in an appropriate medium that reflects the physiological environment. Lipophilic compounds display poor aqueous solubility, and their distribution into mainly aqueous release media, for instance, simple buffer solutions, is limited. As an example, (lipo)proteins or cell compartments represent lipophilic acceptors in the blood that may be available for drug binding. Studies addressing this issue, e.g., investigated the transfer of lipophilic fluorescent dyes or temoporfin as model drugs into the oily droplets of o/w emulsions as acceptor using a flow cytometric approach [20], or focused on liposomes as acceptor, applying asymmetrical flow field-flow fractionation [21].

As an even closer approach to physiological conditions, Roese and Bunjes investigated drug transfer into porcine serum and blood using a method based on differential scanning calorimetry (DSC) for detection [22]. This method circumvents the necessity of separating the donor from the acceptor compartment, but may be limited in applicability to supercooled trimyristin donor nanoparticles and similar systems.

The highest proportion of proteins in human plasma can be attributed to albumin (~55%) [23]. Upon entering the bloodstream after parenteral administration, many drugs do not only associate with albumin, but also with lipoproteins [24]. Studies that analyzed the transfer properties of temoporfin from liposomes to some of the individual lipoprotein fractions and albumin in human plasma found significant differences regarding the distribution profiles of the drug [25,26]. After i.v. administration of liposomal amphotericin B, a large fraction of the drug was transferred to high density lipoproteins (HDL) [27]. For α-tocopherol, in contrast, low density lipoproteins (LDL) seem to be the predominant transport vehicle, as this substance was found to considerably associate with LDL after incubation in human plasma [28].

In order to predict the release performance in vivo, it is most desirable to investigate drug transfer into the original media relevant for administration. Unfortunately, the small size of the carrier particles on the one hand, as well as the complexity of the physiological environment present in vivo on the other hand, entails complications. During in vitro method development, it may thus be preferable to replace the very complex physiological media with simple and robust in vitro media that only contain the ingredients essential for the drug release process.

In a recent study, the transfer of lipophilic drugs from drug-loaded trimyristin emulsions was investigated using an unloaded trimyristin nanoemulsion incorporated into small calcium alginate hydrogel microbeads as a lipophilic acceptor [29]. This setup combined the advantages of small acceptor particles (with a large corresponding interfacial area) with a simple, filtration-based separation procedure from the donor particles. However, trimyristin emulsion droplets alone may not be sufficiently representative as components of "model-blood", since other lipophilic substances, such as albumin and lipoproteins, might also have an impact on the drug distribution process. For example, LDL, which represent a large proportion of the plasma lipoprotein fraction, consist, for the most part, of cholesteryl esters [30,31].

To achieve an even closer approximation to the lipophilic acceptors in the blood, the trimyristin emulsion employed in the previous study was supplemented in the present study by the additional incorporation of a cholesteryl nonanoate dispersion into the hydrogel particles. Cholesteryl nonanoate was chosen as model cholesteryl ester as it forms nanodispersions in which it remains physically stable in a supercooled liquid crystalline state over a long period of time [3]. As another advantage, the saturated fatty acid chain of the cholesteryl nonanoate molecule is more resistant to chemical degradation, such as oxidation, in comparison to unsaturated derivates. It was an aim of this study to comprehensively characterize the trimyristin and cholesteryl nonanoate-containing hydrogel particles in order to perform transfer studies in a more advanced transfer medium. Using this approach, the contribution of the "model lipoprotein" acceptor hydrogel particles to the transfer of fenofibrate, retinyl acetate, and orlistat was investigated from trimyristin donor emulsions. Additionally, the transfer performance of these drugs was investigated from the same donor emulsions into albumin solution as acceptor by applying the DSC method for drug detection [22].

2. Results and Discussion

2.1. Characteristics of Donor and Acceptor Particles

2.1.1. Particle Sizes

According to photon correlation spectroscopy (PCS) measurements, all intensity-weighted mean diameters (z-Averages) of the loaded and unloaded trimyristin (TM) nanoemulsions were between 113 and 126 nm, with polydispersity indices (PdIs) ≤0.10, indicating a monomodal size distribution. The z-Average diameters of the cholesteryl nonanoate (CN) dispersions and the mixed trimyristin–cholesteryl nonanoate (CNTM) dispersions were about 130 nm, and the PdIs were <0.11 (Table 1).

Table 1. Particle sizes, lipid content, and drug load of the different nanodispersions used as donors in transfer studies or as acceptor particles to be incorporated into the hydrogel microbeads.

Nanodispersion	Z-Average (nm)	PdI	Lipid Content (%) DSC	Lipid Content (%) HPLC	Drug Load Related to Trimyristin (%)
Trimyristin donor emulsions					
FFB donor	126	0.09	9.66	-	2.89
RA donor	113	0.10	9.97	-	2.94
ORL donor	115	0.09	9.36	-	3
Acceptor dispersions (n = 3 batches ± SD)					
Trimyristin (TM)	118 ± 4	<0.10	9.60 ± 1.01	9.53 ± 1.07	-
Cholesteryl nonanoate (CN)	133 ± 0.8	<0.11	-	9.08 ± 0.16	-
Mixed trimyristin–cholesteryl nonanoate (CNTM)	132 ± 0.2	<0.10	8.91 ± 0.30	9.03 ± 0.16	-

The particle sizes in each batch of the hydrogel particles containing the CNTM dispersion were determined via laser diffraction. In order to compare the drug transfer results obtained from this study with the results obtained from a previous study, hydrogel particles with a mean diameter between 35 and 42 µm were produced and utilized in transfer experiments (Figure 1). The D10 diameter was not below 8 µm so that the acceptor gel particles could be separated from the nanosized donor via filtration. The particle diameters, as well as the particle size distributions, were reproducible and very similar to those of the particles obtained in an earlier study [29].

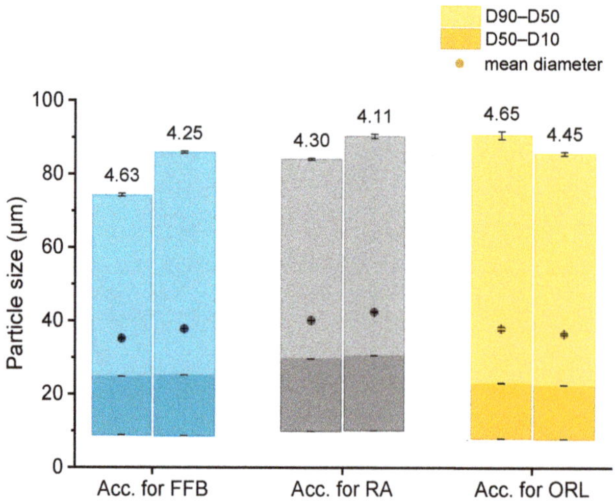

Figure 1. Particle size (represented as bars, all values n = 3 measurements ± SD) and lipid concentration (%) as determined by DSC (respective values above bars) of the different lipid-containing hydrogel bead dispersions utilized as acceptors (Acc.) in the respective transfer experiments. Further abbreviations: FFB—fenofibrate, RA—retinyl acetate, ORL—orlistat.

2.1.2. Drug Load of Donor Emulsions

Drug loading into the nanoemulsions was performed by dissolving the drug in the melted trimyristin prior to homogenization. All drugs were loaded in a concentration of ~3% in relation to the trimyristin matrix (based on lipid determination via DSC), leading to the final concentrations as shown in Table 1.

Please note that the given concentration of orlistat is the weighed-in amount, since it was not possible to determine orlistat with UV spectroscopy. This does not affect the accuracy of the calculated amount of transferred orlistat, as explained in Section 3.9. None of the drugs displayed significant adsorption on the PES filter membrane used during the transfer experiments, since recovery after filtration was close to 100% for all drugs (data not shown).

2.1.3. Determination of Lipid Content

Knowledge of the lipid content in the nanodispersions, as well as in the lipid-containing hydrogel bead dispersions, was of essential importance for the adjustment of the lipid–mass ratio between donor and acceptor in the transfer studies. Differential scanning calorimetry (DSC) measurements were employed to evaluate the trimyristin content in the hydrogel particle dispersions, loaded and unloaded trimyristin-containing dispersions, whereas high performance liquid chromatography (HPLC) measurements were performed for the same unloaded emulsions, as well as the cholesteryl nonanoate dispersions. This procedure enabled a precise and verified lipid determination in the hydrogel bead dispersions and was necessary for two reasons. First, dispersed triglycerides are prone to forming different polymorphs that exhibit different crystallization enthalpies that may falsify the lipid quantification via DSC [32]. Second, it was not possible to completely dissolve the hydrogel beads in an appropriate solvent, such as tetrahydrofurane or acetonitrile, to extract the lipid in order to perform HPLC measurements. Thus, the lipid content in the acceptor dispersions had to be evaluated based on the DSC measurements and was calculated by multiplying the evaluated trimyristin content by 10, provided that the amount of cholesteryl nonanoate and trimyristin was accurately adjusted to 9 + 1. Comparing these two methods, the lipid determination of the TM and CNTM dispersions revealed very similar results in both cases (Table 1). Thus, applying the DSC method for the determination of the overall lipid content in the hydrogel bead dispersions seemed appropriate (please refer to the Supplementary Material for further detail). In general, the lipid content of the hydrogel bead dispersions was adjusted to ~4.4% by adding water (corresponding to approximately 44 mg/mL). A certain fraction of water surrounding the hydrogel particles was required to ensure thorough mixing of the donor and acceptor on the one hand, and to be able to draw a sufficient volume of sample out of the transfer vial for drug quantification on the other hand [29,33]. The lipid concentration of the hydrogel particle dispersions used for the transfer studies, as determined via DSC, are indicated in Figure 1.

2.1.4. Structure Investigations

The different liquid crystalline phases of cholesteryl nonanoate can clearly be characterized by the combination of, e.g., thermal analysis and small-angle X-ray scattering (SAXS). As demonstrated in Figure 2a for the bulk material, the liquid crystalline phase transitions of cholesteryl nonanoate cause very small but distinct signals. Upon heating using DSC, the crystalline bulk material melted into the smectic mesophase and transformed immediately into the cholesteric mesophase at around 80 °C (Figure 2a) [3]. Upon further heating, the isotropic melt was formed at ~92 °C. Whilst cooling, the isotropic melt transformed back into the cholesteric phase which was present until transition into the smectic mesophase at around 76 °C. During heating of the dispersions (also inside the hydrogel beads), no melting peak was observed, demonstrating that all lipids were in a liquid (TM) or liquid crystalline (CN) state after production via hot melt homogenization (Figure 2b). The minor endothermic event occurring in all samples upon heating at about 72 °C corresponds to the transformation of CN from the smectic into the cholesteric mesophase. The main transition at about 87 °C is attributed to the melting of the cholesteric phase. The respective phase transitions upon cooling occurred in the same temperature range as upon heating. In comparison to the bulk material, a small temperature shift of the phase transitions was observed that is most likely related to the presence of the nanodispersed particles, as this was observed in another study as well [3]. However, the presence of trimyristin in the CNTM dispersion did not influence the formation of the liquid crystalline phases. No crystallization event was observed for CN within cooling to −10 °C, confirming the presence of the smectic mesophase of cholesteryl nonanoate. The exothermic event at <10 °C corresponds to the crystallization signal of the supercooled trimyristin droplets that was used for quantification (cf. Section 3.6).

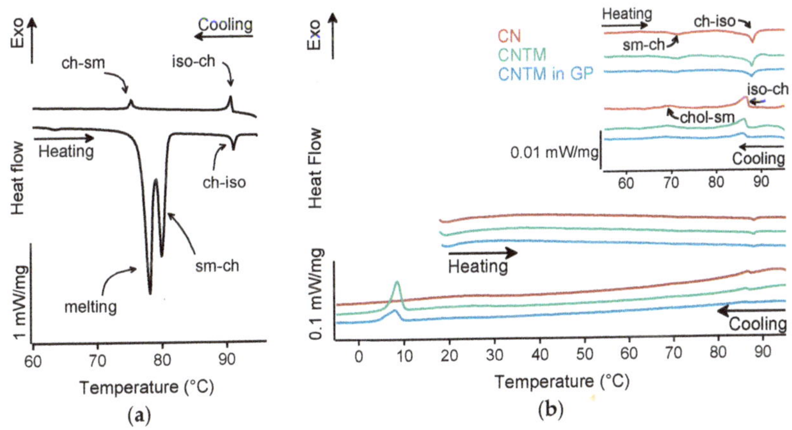

Figure 2. DSC curves of (**a**) cholesteryl nonanoate bulk material, (**b**) nanodispersions of pure cholesteryl nonanoate (CN), mixed cholesteryl nonanoate and trimyristin (CNTM), and the CNTM dispersion incorporated in hydrogel particles (CNTM in GP). The insert shows the transitions in the upper temperature range at a higher magnification. Further abbreviations: sm—smectic, ch—cholesteric, iso—isotropic melt. Scan rate: 5 K/min.

The smectic mesophase of cholesteryl nonanoate can be clearly identified by its very sharp and characteristic SAXS reflection [34]. The d-spacing of the CN dispersion was calculated to be 28.0 Å at about 20 °C (Figure 3), which is within the same range as literature data [3]. Neither the addition of trimyristin, nor encapsulation into the hydrogel matrix led to a prominent shift of the reflection (calculated to be 28.0 Å for the CNTM dispersion and 28.1 Å when incorporated into the hydrogel particles). These findings are in accordance with the phase transition events observed by DSC and confirm the presence of the smectic mesophase of CN in all dispersions, also, when incorporated in the hydrogel beads. The strong increase in scattering intensity at lower angles observed for the sample containing the CNTM dispersion in the hydrogel beads seemed to be caused by the hydrogel network, since the same phenomenon was observed by measuring the lipid-free hydrogel particles as control.

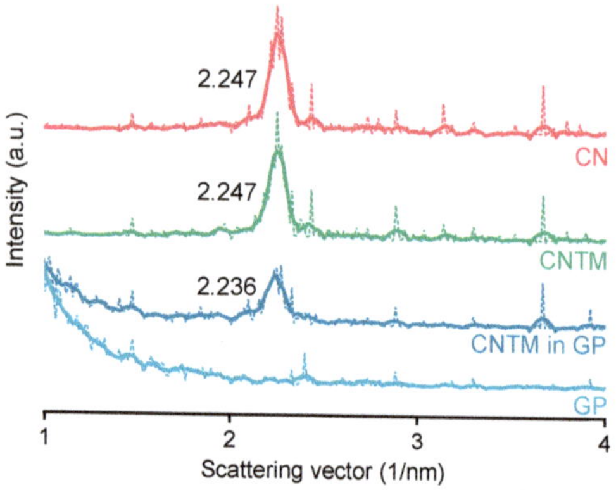

Figure 3. SAXS patterns of different nanodispersions and hydrogel beads at 20 °C. The values state the peak positions (q) upon which the calculation of the d-spacings was based. Abbreviations: CN—cholesteryl nonanoate, CNTM—cholesteryl nonanoate–trimyristin, GP—gel particle.

Preserving the properties of the incorporated lipid nanoparticles was an important aim for the use of lipid-containing hydrogel microspheres as acceptor in the transfer experiments. During spraying upon hydrogel bead production, the lipid-containing alginate dispersion was exposed to high shear forces, which may have a negative effect on the integrity or state of the dispersed particles. Cryo-scanning electron microscopy (cryo-SEM) measurements were performed to depict the inner structure of the plain placebo and the lipid-containing hydrogel beads. The cryo-SEM images illustrate that the nanoparticles were associated with the hydrogel network and that their individuality seemed to be preserved in most cases (Figure 4). This is in accordance with the results obtained in earlier studies, in which the melting pattern of incorporated trimyristin particles was analyzed, and which indicated the presence of small nanoparticles inside the hydrogel beads [29].

The shape of the particles in the images implied that the incorporated lipids were no longer in their initial state (supercooled liquid in the case of trimyristin or smectic state in the case of cholesteryl nonanoate, as verified via DSC and SAXS), but seemed to be solidified due to the sample preparation procedure. In spite of that, the formation of the characteristic platelet-like shape of the crystalline lipid nanoparticles [32,35] seems to have been prevented, e.g., by the extremely rapid high-pressure freezing process or due to limited available space inside the hydrogel pores.

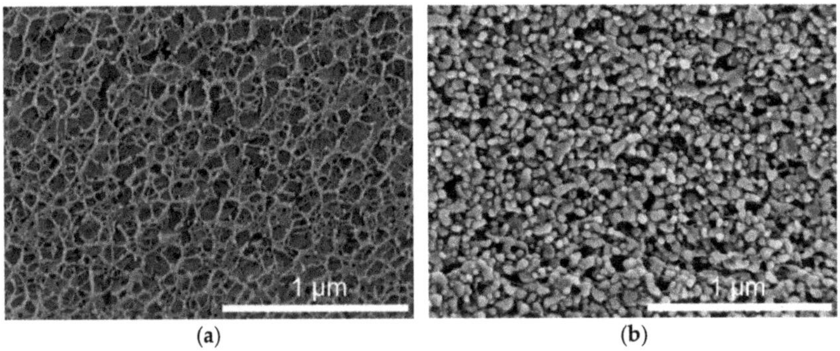

Figure 4. Cryo-SEM cross-sections of hydrogel particles. (**a**) Pure crosslinked alginate matrix. (**b**) Hydrogel particle containing mixed cholesteryl nonanoate–trimyristin dispersion.

2.2. Investigation of Drug Transfer

2.2.1. Transfer into CNTM-Containing Hydrogel Beads as Acceptor

Drug transfer from trimyristin emulsions (donor; d) into CNTM-containing alginate microspheres (acceptor; a) was investigated for three different drugs loaded at a concentration of ~3% (drug related to matrix lipid). After mixing of donor and acceptor, fenofibrate (logP 4.86) transfer was completed within a few minutes, whereas retinyl acetate (logP 6.56) transferred more slowly and reached equilibrium at >40 h. Orlistat (logP 7.61) transfer seemed to be completed after about 70 h (Figure 5). The transfer course of all drugs was very similar to that obtained in earlier studies using trimyristin-nanodroplet-containing hydrogel microbeads as acceptor; however, the extent of drug transfer was distinctly smaller in the present case [29]. Assuming an equal distribution between the donor and acceptor lipids, a maximum fraction of 90% transferred drug would have been expected based on the adjusted lipid–mass ratio of 1 + 9 (d + a). In this case, however, the maximum fraction of transferred drug was ~74% for fenofibrate and retinyl acetate, whereas orlistat transferred to an extent of about 62%. The observed concentration equilibrium of the drugs was clearly shifted in favor of the donor. Thus, the affinity of all drugs seemed to be higher to trimyristin droplets instead of to the cholesteryl nonanoate particles. Bearing in mind that the hydrogel particles contained CN and TM in a mixture of 9 + 1, the contribution of the cholesteryl nonanoate as acceptor seemed very small in comparison to the trimyristin. Partition of the drugs can be assumed to be equal between the trimyristin of the donor emulsion and the trimyristin acceptor droplets that were incorporated in the hydrogel particles. In the case of fenofibrate and retinyl acetate, about 26% of the drugs were not transferred to the acceptor compartment but remained in the trimyristin donor emulsion. As a consequence, only approximately 50% of fenofibrate or retinyl acetate are presumably located in the cholesteryl nonanoate acceptor particles, considering that one tenth of the acceptor lipid is also composed of trimyristin. For orlistat, only ~62% of drug transfer to the acceptor particles was observed, corresponding to about 30% of the drug that is located in the cholesteryl nonanoate particles.

Reasons for this observation may be related to the lower lipophilicity of CN (CN eluted prior to TM from an RP column in the HPLC measurements). It may also be attributed to the presence of the liquid crystalline state. In the more ordered state of the liquid crystalline mesophase, the cholesteryl ester molecules are motionally restricted, which possibly made it more difficult for the drugs to associate with them [34]. Cholesteryl nonanoate was chosen as a model compound to mimic the cholesteryl ester fraction in lipoproteins present in the blood. At body temperature, LDL undergoes a phase transition, which is predominantly related to the phase transition of the cholesteryl esters into a more disordered, liquid-like state [30,36]. It might be conceivable that the drug transfer will be affected by the phase transition of LDL present in vivo. This remains to be investigated.

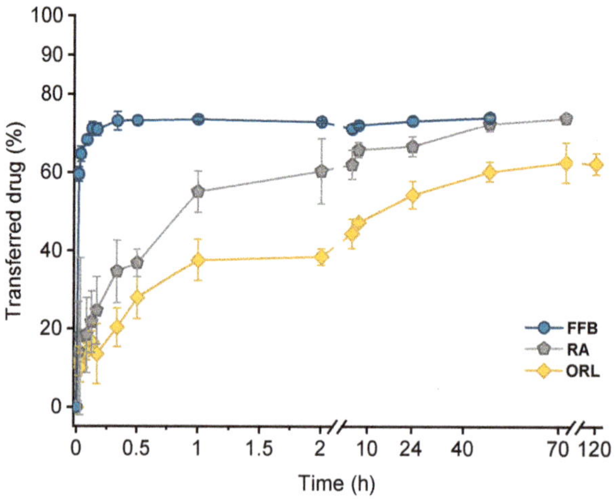

Figure 5. Drug transfer into CNTM-containing hydrogel beads. Each value represents mean ± SD ($n = 3$). Abbreviations: FFB—fenofibrate, RA—retinyl acetate, ORL—orlistat.

Lipophilicity, estimated based on the calculated logP values of the drugs, was a major factor determining the course of the drug transfer, which indicates that the transfer observed in these experiments is a partition driven process and that the characteristics of the drug (and not those of the carrier system) dominate the release performance. These findings are in accordance with the literature since drug release from lipid nanoemulsions has previously been reported to occur very rapidly [9,17,20,22]. A diffusion barrier due to the presence of the hydrogel matrix appeared not to be experimentally relevant for fenofibrate but seemed to be more critical for rather slowly transferring drugs, as already described in an earlier study in more detail [29].

2.2.2. Bovine Serum Albumin (BSA) as Acceptor

In order to investigate albumin as acceptor for the lipophilic drugs under investigation, all drug-containing donor emulsions were incubated in BSA solution over 24 h. Directly after sampling at different time points, the samples were cooled from 25 °C to 0 °C via DSC, and the crystallization temperature of trimyristin ($T_{cryst.}$) was evaluated. Using this procedure, no filtration step was required, but control experiments were performed by incubating drug-free nanoemulsion in the BSA solution, as well as in pure PBS buffer.

Crystallization temperatures of control samples, as well as of a drug-loaded donor emulsion (exemplarily for fenofibrate), are plotted in Figure 6a. The presence of BSA solution did not influence the crystallization temperature of the unloaded trimyristin emulsion, which remained constant at about the same value as when incubated in pure PBS buffer (after 24 h, 10.63 ± 0.01 °C in BSA and 10.65 ± 0.02 °C in PBS, respectively). Consequently, obvious changes in $T_{cryst.}$ of the drug-loaded samples should only result from drug transfer from the nanoemulsion to BSA. Within the time frame of the experiment, the crystallization temperature of the FFB donor emulsion remained unchanged, but within the standard fluctuations of the measurement device. Consequently, the change of the crystallization temperature ($\Delta T_{cryst.}$) of the fenofibrate-containing trimyristin emulsion in comparison to the unloaded nanoemulsion used as control remained very similar, indicating no transfer to BSA (Figure 6a,b).

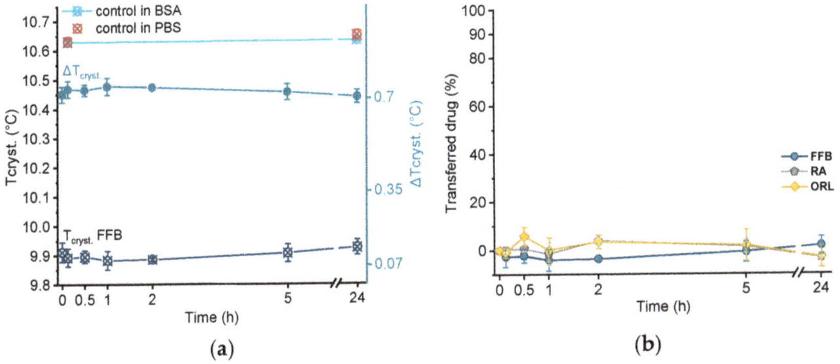

Figure 6. (**a**) Crystallization temperatures ($T_{cryst.}$) of unloaded trimyristin emulsion (control) and fenofibrate-containing emulsion (FFB), as well as the change of $T_{cryst.}$ ($\Delta T_{cryst.}$) within 24 h. (**b**) Transferred percentage of fenofibrate (FFB), retinyl acetate (RA), and orlistat (ORL) to the BSA fraction.

Moreover, for retinyl acetate and orlistat no clear change in crystallization temperature was detected beyond the deviations of the measurement device, indicating that virtually no drug transferred to BSA (Figure 6b).

In previous studies, albumin was added to the aqueous release media as a solubilizing agent to enhance drug release from lipid nanocarriers. For example, Magenheim et al. and Levy and Benita investigated the release of miconazole and diazepam from triglyceride nanoemulsions applying sink conditions and found an increased amount of released drug in comparison to pure Hepes buffer [9,11].

In contrast, Reshetov et al. found no significant proportion of temoporfin bound to albumin in the presence of other lipophilic components [37]. Studies investigating the transfer of orlistat through oil–water interfaces revealed no effect on the transfer of orlistat by adding albumin, and found the partitioning of orlistat to be in favor of the oil phase, regardless of the composition of the aqueous phase [38]. These findings are in accordance with the results presented in this study.

In the case of fenofibrate, Pas et al. reported an increased solubility by a multiple in comparison to pure water. However, the absolute concentration did not exceed ~0.006 mg/mL [39]. The lack of transfer of fenofibrate to BSA in the present study is, thus, not particularly surprising, considering that the fenofibrate concentration applied in the present experiments was ~0.3 mg/mL. It might be conceivable that a very small amount of fenofibrate (and, consequently, retinyl acetate and orlistat) did transfer to BSA (up to their respective solubility limit), but was not detectable using the DSC method in this case. Dilution by many orders would seem to be required in this case to attain appropriate conditions that allow an adequate amount of drug to partition into the release medium.

In spite of that, it was clearly demonstrated that BSA, used here to mimic HSA, alone does not contribute substantially as an acceptor for the lipophilic drugs under investigation in this study. In contrast, cholesteryl nonanoate, utilized as a model compound to mimic the cholesteryl ester portion in lipoproteins, does contribute to a much greater extent. Yet, the partitioning of the drugs was in favor of the trimyristin in all cases. With regard to intravenous administration in humans, a significantly greater dilution, e.g., 1 + 1000, would be necessary to attain an even more realistic approach. For drugs under partition control, an increased transfer may be expected in vivo, if sufficient acceptor is provided. This remains to be investigated in further detail.

3. Materials and Methods

3.1. Materials

The triglyceride trimyristin (Dynasan® 114) was donated by IOI Oleo, Witten, Germany, and the surfactant poloxamer 407 (Kolliphor® P127) by BASF AG, Ludwigshafen,

Germany. Sodium alginate (Manugel® GMB) was a kind gift from FMC International, Wallingstown, Ireland. As estimated by the supplier, the molecular weight was ~124 kDa, the content of guluronic acid was 60–70%, and that of mannuronic acid was 30–40%. Cholesteryl nonanoate was purchased from TCI, Zwijndrecht, Belgium. Tetrahydrofuran (HPLC grade), acetonitrile (HPLC grade), bovine serum albumin (BSA, heat shock fraction, pH 7, ≥98%), and the drugs fenofibrate and retinyl acetate were obtained from Sigma-Aldrich, Steinheim, Germany. Orlistat was donated by Formosa Laboratories Inc., Taoyuan, Taiwan. Sodium azide, anhydrous glycerol, calcium chloride, acetonitrile (LC MS grade), and tetrahydrofuran (ultra LC MS grade) were obtained from Carl Roth, Karlsruhe, Germany. All materials were used as received. Water was purified by deionization and filtration (EASYpureTM LF, Barnstead, Dubuque, IA, USA) or was of bidistilled quality. The logP values of the drugs were obtained from DrugBank (calculated by ALOGPS).

3.2. *Preparation of Donor and Acceptor Lipid Nanodispersions*

The nanoemulsions consisted of 10% trimyristin (TM) as lipid phase, which was dispersed in an aqueous phase containing 5% poloxamer 407 as a stabilizer. The aqueous phase was isotonized with 2.25% anhydrous glycerol. Additionally, nanodispersions were prepared that contained 10% cholesteryl nonanoate (CN) as lipid phase. These dispersions were stabilized with 8% poloxamer 407. All lipid nanodispersions were preserved with 0.05% sodium azide. The concentrations are given related to the total weight of the dispersions (*w/w*).

The aqueous and lipid phases were preheated separately to 75 °C (TM nanoemulsions) or 95 °C (CN dispersions). After mixing, a pre-emulsion was formed using an Ultra-Turrax (T25 digital, IKA, Staufen, Germany) for four minutes at 11,000 rpm. Subsequently, the mixture was processed in the heat by high-pressure homogenization in 10 cycles at 700 bar (TM emulsions) or 900 bar (CN dispersions) using a Microfluidizer (M110-PS, interaction chamber type F12Y DIXC, Microfluidics, Newton, MA, USA).

After homogenization, all dispersions were filtered through a polyvinylidene fluoride (PVDF) filter with 0.45 µm pore size (Rotilabo®, Karlsruhe, Germany) and stored in glass vials at 20 °C. Under these conditions, TM remained in a liquid state due to supercooling [22], whereas the CN transformed into a liquid crystalline state [3]. The trimyristin nanoemulsion and the cholesteryl nonanoate dispersion were mixed in a ratio of 9 CN + 1 TM (CNTM dispersion; lipid ratio based on quantification via HPLC), and served as the acceptor system to be incorporated in alginate beads (cf. Section 3.4).

For the preparation of donor emulsions to be studied in transfer experiments, fenofibrate, retinyl acetate, or orlistat were dissolved in the melted trimyristin prior to emulsification. In order to exclude any possible influence of the drug loading on the transfer kinetics, all emulsions were loaded at the same concentration of ~3% related to trimyristin.

3.3. *Lipid Quantification via High Performance Liquid Chromatography*

A slight reduction in the lipid concentration may occur during dispersion production by dilution with process water remaining in the homogenization device. In order to achieve the lipid mixing ratio of 9 CN + 1 TM accurately, the lipid content of the unloaded dispersions was determined by HPLC after preparation. A Dionex UltiMate 3000 HPLC system (Thermo Fisher Scientific, Waltham, MA, USA) equipped with an LPG-3400SD pump, a WPS-3000TSL autosampler, and a Corona Veo Charged Aerosol detector was used to perform the analysis. The column (Thermo Fisher Scientific Hypersil Gold C18, 2.1 × 150 mm, 1.9 µm) was kept at 25 °C and the flow rate was set to 0.3 mL/min. The mobile phase consisted of acetonitrile/tetrahydrofuran 70/30 (*v/v*). Under these conditions, the retention time of both lipids was between 3 and 5 min, with cholesteryl nonanoate eluting from the column prior to trimyristin.

For sample preparation, dispersions were dissolved in tetrahydrofuran/acetonitrile 50/50 (*v/v*) and diluted to an appropriate detector response; 1 µL was injected and detected at a nebulizer temperature of 50 °C. Every sample was diluted twice and every dilution measured two times (n = 4). Lipid concentrations were calculated with the Chromeleon 7.2 software (Thermo Fisher Scientific, Waltham, MA, USA) using a calibration curve for trimyristin or cholesteryl nonanoate in different concentrations.

3.4. Preparation of Lipid-Containing Alginate Beads

Calcium alginate beads were produced with a spraying method as described earlier, with minor modifications [29]. The lipid nanodispersion that was incorporated into the hydrogel beads was composed of cholesteryl nonanoate and trimyristin (lipid mixing ratio 9 + 1 as determined by HPLC). The drug-free lipid nanodispersion was mixed with the same volume of bidistilled water (final volume approximately 20–25 mL each per batch) and 2% (*w/w*) sodium alginate was added to the dispersion. Under stirring at 200 rpm, the mixture was left to swell overnight. With the aid of a syringe pump (Fusion 200, Chemyx, Stafford, TX, USA), the resulting alginate-containing dispersion was fed (1 mL/min) into the two-fluid spray nozzle (diameter: 0.7 mm) of a BÜCHI Mini Spray Dryer B-191 (BÜCHI Labortechnik AG, Flawil, Switzerland) and sprayed under compressed air (650 L/h) into a continuously stirred 5% (*w/w*) $CaCl_2$ solution (approximately 500 mL). The hydrogel particles were stored in the $CaCl_2$ solution overnight to ensure thorough cross-linking. After hardening, excess $CaCl_2$ was washed off with purified water via centrifugation (SIGMA® 3–15, Sigma Laborzentrifugen GmbH, Osterode am Harz, Germany) three times at 3200 rpm. The microbeads were stored in water and used as acceptor particles. The resulting volume of each batch of dispersion was about 40–50 mL in total. The overall lipid concentration encapsulated in each batch of hydrogel bead dispersion was evaluated via DSC (cf. Section 3.6). Plain microbeads used for the cryo-SEM and SAXS analysis were produced in the same way but without lipid dispersion.

3.5. Particle Size Analysis

The particle size of the lipid nanodispersions was measured by PCS using a Zetasizer Nano ZS (Malvern Instruments, Worcestershire, UK). Prior to the measurement, samples were diluted with purified water to an appropriate scattering intensity (attenuator 5–7). After an equilibration time of 300 s, three consecutive measurements of 5 min each were performed at 25 °C using a laser wavelength of 633 nm at an angle of 173°. As an average of three runs, the z-Average and the PdI were calculated.

The particle sizes of the hydrogel beads were determined via laser diffraction (LD; Beckman Coulter LS 13 320, Beckman Coulter GmbH, Krefeld, Germany). The samples were diluted with water to an appropriate optical density in the measuring chamber. Three consecutive measurements of 90 s each were averaged and the volume distribution, mean particle size, and D10, D50, and D90 values were calculated using Fraunhofer approximation.

3.6. Differential Scanning Calorimetry

Differential scanning calorimetry (DSC) measurements were carried out using a DSC 1 calorimeter (Mettler Toledo, Gießen, Germany) equipped with an FRS 5+ sensor that was calibrated with indium. The calibration was checked by measuring indium before a series of measurements. About 20 mg of the samples were accurately weighed into 40 µL aluminum pans (Mettler Toledo, Gießen, Germany), which were hermetically sealed by cold welding. An empty pan was used as reference and all measurements were performed under nitrogen purge.

To examine the trimyristin concentration in the hydrogel bead dispersion, as well as in the drug-loaded and unloaded trimyristin-containing dispersions, samples were heated from 20 °C to 70 °C (20 K/min) and subsequently cooled to −5 °C with a scan rate of 10 K/min. The crystallization enthalpies from the cooling curves were evaluated and the trimyristin content was calculated using a calibration curve obtained from measuring different amounts of bulk trimyristin under the same conditions. The overall lipid content in mixed CNTM dispersions (composed of 9 CN + 1 TM), as well as the lipid amount in the hydrogel particle dispersions, was calculated by multiplying the determined trimyristin amount by 10.

The onset value of the crystallization signal of trimyristin was determined as an indicator for the crystallization temperature ($T_{cryst.}$). Samples from transfer experiments were cooled from 25 °C to 0 °C with a scan rate of 2.5 K/min. The changes in $T_{cryst.}$ of drug-loaded nanoemulsions were used to quantify the transferred amount of drug, as described in earlier studies; cf. Section 3.9.

In order to obtain information on the liquid crystalline structure, the cholesteryl no-nanoate dispersion and the CNTM-containing nanodispersion (also enclosed in the hydrogel beads) were heated from 15 °C to 100 °C (5 K/min), and subsequently cooled to −10 °C (5 K/min). The phase transitions indicated in the resulting curves were examined to characterize the structure of the incorporated lipid particles in comparison to those of unencapsulated counterparts.

If necessary, baseline correction was performed using OriginLab 2018.

3.7. *Cryo-SEM*

To evaluate the inner appearance of the placebo and the lipid-containing hydrogel beads, cryo-scanning electron microscopy (cryo-SEM) was performed using a Helios G4 CX DualBeam system and a Through the Lens Detector (FEI, Hillsboro, OR, USA). For sample preparation, the hydrogel microbeads were frozen in a high-pressure freezer (Leica EM ICE, Leica Microsystems GmbH, Wetzlar, Germany) using liquid nitrogen, subsequently fractured in the cryo-chamber at −150 °C, and sputtered with a 4 nm platinum layer in a high-vacuum coater (Leica EM ACE600, Leica Microsystems GmbH, Wetzlar, Germany). Imaging was performed at a voltage of 3 kV at different magnifications. The samples were kept under cryo conditions throughout the entire workflow.

3.8. *X-ray Scattering*

Small-angle X-ray scattering (SAXS) was performed to investigate the liquid crystalline structure of the cholesteryl-nonanoate-containing dispersions. The measurements were conducted with a SAXSess mc2 system (Anton Paar GmbH, Graz, Austria) using Cu Kα radiation ($\lambda = 0.154$) and a CCD detector (measurement range: $q = 0 - 6\ nm^{-1}$). The nanodispersions, as well as hydrogel beads (lipid-containing and placebo), were measured at room temperature in a 1 mm capillary, which was positioned in the beam path at a distance of 309 mm to the CCD detector.

Background and dark current subtraction, as well as desmearing, were performed using the SAXSquant software (Anton Paar GmbH, Graz, Austria). The raw data (dotted lines in Figure 3) were appropriately smoothed (solid lines; Figure 3), and the scattering vector q (nm^{-1}) was determined using OriginLab 2018. The position of the reflections was used to calculate the layer spacing (d) according to Bragg's law: $d = 2\pi/q$.

3.9. *Investigation of Drug Transfer*

3.9.1. CNTM-Containing Hydrogel Beads as Acceptor

The procedure for drug transfer investigations using lipid-containing hydrogel beads as an acceptor was described earlier [29,33]. Briefly, drug-loaded nanoemulsions were mixed with the microsphere dispersion in 3 mL glass vials in a donor (d) to acceptor (a) lipid mass ratio of 1 + 9 (based on the results of lipid determination by DSC). This lipid ratio was chosen to ensure comparability of the present transfer results with those of a previous study [29]. The transfer started when the donor emulsion (~70 µL) was added to the required amount of acceptor particle dispersion (resulting in a total volume of approximately 1.5 mL in each transfer vial). For each time point of sampling, a separate transfer vial was used. During transfer, the samples were placed on a horizontal shaker (Vibrax VXR Basic, IKA-Werke GmbH & Co. KG, Staufen, Germany) and agitated with 300 rpm at ~23 °C. Samples were withdrawn using a 2 mL plastic syringe via filtration at predetermined time points. For this purpose, a polyethersulfone (PES) membrane with

1.2 µm pore size (Pieper Filter GmbH, Bad Zwischenahn, Germany) was mounted into a custom-built screw cap that was attached to the transfer vial shortly before sampling.

For fenofibrate and retinyl acetate, the drug load of the donor nanoemulsions, as well as the remaining amount of drug in the nanoemulsions during transfer experiments, was quantified via UV spectroscopy (Specord 40, Analytik Jena AG, Jena, Germany). Samples were dissolved in tetrahydrofuran/water 9/1 (*v/v*) and measured at wavelengths of 287 nm (fenofibrate) or 360 nm (retinyl acetate) three times. Where required, the measured absorptions were corrected for the blank absorptions of the dissolved unloaded nanoemulsion that had been treated in the same way as the respective drug-containing nanoemulsion. Calibration curves for each drug were obtained by preparing at least six different dilutions containing varying amounts of the respective drug. The amount of transferred drug was calculated by subtracting the amount in the sampled aqueous donor system from the originally applied one.

Orlistat could not be quantified via UV spectroscopy in the presence of trimyristin because of overlapping absorption signals. Thus, orlistat transfer from the trimyristin nanoemulsion into the lipophilic acceptor was investigated by DSC. The change in crystallization temperature ($\Delta T_{cryst.}$, determined upon cooling) is in a linear relation to the decrease in drug content [22]. The respective donor emulsion, diluted with water in the same volume as that of the acceptor system (which corresponded to 0% drug transfer), and an unloaded trimyristin nanoemulsion with comparable characteristics (corresponding to 100% drug transfer; measured as control) were used to calculate the transferred amount of orlistat by applying the rule of three. Control experiments were performed by incubating unloaded trimyristin emulsion with the lipid-containing microsphere dispersion under the same conditions. Fluctuations in the crystallization temperature of the donor emulsion that were not caused by drug transfer could thus be identified and included into the calculations of the transferred amount of drug [22].

3.9.2. Albumin Solution as Acceptor

The overall amino acid sequence identity of BSA in comparison to human serum albumin (HSA) is ~76%, leading to a similar tertiary structure of these molecules, with similar binding sites [40,41]. In order to evaluate the contribution of albumin as a potential acceptor for lipophilic drugs in blood, BSA was used for screening purposes in this study.

BSA solution was freshly prepared before use by dissolving 43 mg/mL BSA in PBS buffer under continuous stirring at 200 rpm. This concentration was chosen for two reasons. First, the concentration of albumin in human plasma is 35–50 mg/mL [23] and, second, the concentration of lipid acceptor in the studies performed here with CNTM-containing dispersion that was incorporated in microspheres was in the same range (cf. Section 2.1.3). Thus, the chosen BSA concentration offered the possibility to compare the contribution of (different) available acceptor structures used in this study on the one hand, and also provided a realistic approach to the albumin concentration in vivo.

A total of 70 µL of the drug-loaded donor emulsions were mixed in a ratio of 1 + 9 (ratio adjusted based on the lipid quantification in the donor emulsion, as determined using DSC) with the acceptor solution in a 3 mL vial and incubated for 24 h in the same way as described above (total volume ~1.5 mL/vial). At various time points, samples were withdrawn using an Eppendorf pipette and directly measured by DSC. In contrast to the hydrogel-bead-based setup, no filtration step was necessary using this method. The change in crystallization temperature ($\Delta T_{cryst.}$) determined upon cooling was used to calculate the transferred amount of each drug under investigation, as described in Section 3.9.1 for orlistat. For the control experiments, an unloaded trimyristin emulsion with comparable characteristics was incubated in the acceptor solution and in PBS buffer, and measured by DSC as well.

All transfer results are presented by plotting the fraction of transferred drug (%) against the time (hours, h). All transfer studies were performed in triplicate.

4. Conclusions

The liquid (trimyristin) and liquid crystalline (cholesteryl nonanoate) state, as well as the integrity of the nanoparticles, could be preserved during hydrogel bead production, and the resulting system was successfully applied as lipophilic acceptor in transfer studies. The course of transfer observed using the lipid-containing hydrogel particles as the acceptor was in relation to the lipophilicity of the drugs: the higher the logP value, the slower the transfer. In all cases, the partition equilibrium of the drugs under investigation was found to be in favor of the trimyristin emulsion droplets. Given that there is no officially approved method to investigate the release of lipophilic drugs from nanosized carriers, the hydrogel-bead-based setup can be helpful in order to compare the contribution of different lipophilic acceptors to the release performance of colloidal drug delivery systems. The nature of the lipophilic acceptor in release studies is essential, as it strongly affects the release behavior. No detectable fraction of the drugs was transferred to BSA, demonstrating clearly that albumin seemed to be of minor importance as lipophilic acceptor for the drugs under investigation in the present study. Albumin as solubilizing agent to be used in transfer experiments should thus be evaluated thoughtfully, especially for drugs with high lipophilicities. The lipophilic substances used in the present study as an acceptor were selected as model compounds in order to mimic different lipophilic acceptors present in the blood. Thus, a closer approach to the physiological environment was provided than with many other release media currently applied. However, many other aspects, e.g., the physical state of the acceptor particles and, with special regard to the intravenous route of administration, a realistic dilution of the donor system, should be taken into consideration for future investigations, as they may also affect the drug release performance.

Supplementary Materials: The following are available online at https://www.mdpi.com/article/10.3390/ph14090865/s1, Figure S1: Lipid determination of an exemplary batch of different lipid nanodispersions used as acceptor particles to be incorporated into the hydrogel beads.

Author Contributions: Conceptualization, S.K. and H.B.; investigation, S.K.; writing—original draft preparation, S.K.; writing—review and editing, S.K. and H.B.; visualization, S.K.; supervision, H.B. All authors have read and agreed to the published version of the manuscript.

Funding: This work has been carried out within the framework of the SMART BIOTECS alliance between the Technische Universität Braunschweig and the Leibniz Universität Hannover, an initiative supported by the Ministry of Science and Culture (MWK) of Lower Saxony, Germany. We also acknowledge support by the Open Access Publication Funds of Technische Universität Braunschweig.

Institutional Review Board Statement: Not applicable.

Informed Consent Statement: Not applicable.

Data Availability Statement: Data is contained within the article and supplementary material.

Acknowledgments: Bogdan Semenenko is kindly acknowledged for his contributions to the electron microscopic investigations. The authors thank Britta Meier for the support in the SAXS measurements.

Conflicts of Interest: The authors declare no conflict of interest.

References

1. Bunjes, H. Lipid nanoparticles for the delivery of poorly water-soluble drugs. *J. Pharm. Pharmacol.* **2010**, *62*, 1637–1645. [CrossRef]
2. Fahr, A.; Liu, X. Drug delivery strategies for poorly water-soluble drugs. *Expert Opin. Drug Deliv.* **2007**, *4*, 403–416. [CrossRef]
3. Kuntsche, J.; Koch, M.H.J.; Fahr, A.; Bunjes, H. Supercooled smectic nanoparticles: Influence of the matrix composition and in vitro cytotoxicity. *Eur. J. Pharm. Sci.* **2009**, *38*, 238–248. [CrossRef] [PubMed]
4. Angelova, A.; Garamus, V.M.; Angelov, B.; Tian, Z.; Li, Y.; Zou, A. Advances in structural design of lipid-based nanoparticle carriers for delivery of macromolecular drugs, phytochemicals and anti-tumor agents. *Adv. Colloid Interface Sci.* **2017**, *249*, 331–345. [CrossRef]
5. Shen, J.; Burgess, D.J. In vitro dissolution testing strategies for nanoparticulate drug delivery systems: Recent developments and challenges. *Drug. Deliv. Transl. Res.* **2013**, *3*, 409–415. [CrossRef]

6. Landry, F.B.; Bazile, D.V.; Spenlehauer, G.; Veillard, M.; Kreuter, J. Release of the fluorescent marker Prodan® from poly(D,L-lactic acid) nanoparticles coated with albumin or polyvinyl alcohol in model digestive fluids (USP XXII). *J. Control. Release* **1997**, *44*, 227–236. [CrossRef]
7. Washington, C.; Evans, K. Release rate measurements of model hydrophobic solutes hydrophobic solutes from submicron triglyceride emulsions. *J. Control. Release* **1994**, *33*, 383–390. [CrossRef]
8. Kontoyannis, C.G.; Douroumis, D. Release study of drugs from liposomic dispersions using differential pulse polarography. *Anal. Chim. Acta* **2001**, *449*, 135–141. [CrossRef]
9. Magenheim, B.; Levy, M.Y.; Benita, S. A new in vitro technique for the evaluation of drug release profile from colloidal carriers-ultrafiltration technique at low pressure. *Int. J. Pharm.* **1993**, *94*, 115–123. [CrossRef]
10. Danhier, F.; Lecouturier, N.; Vroman, B.; Jérôme, C.; Marchand-Brynaert, J.; Feron, O.; Préat, V. Paclitaxel-loaded PEGylated PLGA-based nanoparticles: In vitro and in vivo evaluation. *J. Control. Release* **2009**, *133*, 11–17. [CrossRef]
11. Levy, M.Y.; Benita, S. Drug release from submicronized o/w emulsion: A new in vitro kinetic evaluation model. *Int. J. Pharm.* **1990**, *66*, 29–37. [CrossRef]
12. Chidambaram, N.; Burgess, D.J. A novel in vitro release method for submicron-sized dispersed systems. *AAPS PharmSci* **1999**, *1*, 32–40. [CrossRef] [PubMed]
13. Henriksen, I.; Sande, S.A.; Smistad, G.; Ågren, T.; Karlsen, J. In vitro evaluation of drug release kinetics from liposomes by fractional dialysis. *Int. J. Pharm.* **1995**, *119*, 231–238. [CrossRef]
14. Bhardwaj, U.; Burgess, D.J. A novel USP apparatus 4 based release testing method for dispersed systems. *Int. J. Pharm.* **2010**, *388*, 287–294. [CrossRef] [PubMed]
15. Salmela, L.; Washington, C. A continuous flow method for estimation of drug release rates from emulsion formulations. *Int. J. Pharm.* **2014**, *472*, 276–281. [CrossRef] [PubMed]
16. Wallace, S.J.; Li, J.; Nation, R.L.; Boyd, B.J. Drug release from nanomedicines: Selection of appropriate encapsulation and release methodology. *Drug. Deliv. Transl. Res.* **2012**, *2*, 284–292. [CrossRef] [PubMed]
17. Washington, C. Drug release from microdisperse systems: A critical review. *Int. J. Pharm.* **1990**, *58*, 1–12. [CrossRef]
18. Washington, C.; Koosha, F. Drug release from microparticulates; deconvolution of measurement errors. *Int. J. Pharm.* **1990**, *59*, 79–82. [CrossRef]
19. D'Souza, S.S.; DeLuca, P.P. Methods to assess in vitro drug release from injectable polymeric particulate systems. *Pharm. Res.* **2006**, *23*, 460–474. [CrossRef]
20. Petersen, S.; Fahr, A.; Bunjes, H. Flow cytometry as a new approach to investigate drug transfer between lipid particles. *Mol. Pharm.* **2010**, *7*, 350–363. [CrossRef]
21. Hinna, A.; Steiniger, F.; Hupfeld, S.; Brandl, M.; Kuntsche, J. Asymmetrical flow field-flow fractionation with on-line detection for drug transfer studies: A feasibility study. *Anal. Bioanal. Chem.* **2014**, *406*, 7827–7839. [CrossRef] [PubMed]
22. Roese, E.; Bunjes, H. Drug release studies from lipid nanoparticles in physiological media by a new DSC method. *J. Control. Release* **2017**, *256*, 92–100. [CrossRef]
23. Anderson, N.L.; Anderson, N.G. The human plasma proteome: History, character, and diagnostic prospects. *Mol. Cell. Proteom.* **2002**, *1*, 845–867. [CrossRef] [PubMed]
24. Wasan, K.M.; Cassidy, G.M. Role of plasma lipoproteins in modifying the biological activity of hydrophobic drugs. *J. Pharm. Sci.* **1998**, *87*, 411–424. [CrossRef] [PubMed]
25. Decker, C.; Steiniger, F.; Fahr, A. Transfer of a lipophilic drug (temoporfin) between small unilamellar liposomes and human plasma proteins: Influence of membrane composition on vesicle integrity and release characteristics. *J. Liposome Res.* **2013**, *23*, 154–165. [CrossRef]
26. Holzschuh, S.; Kaeß, K.; Bossa, G.V.; Decker, C.; Fahr, A.; May, S. Investigations of the influence of liposome composition on vesicle stability and drug transfer in human plasma: A transfer study. *J. Liposome Res.* **2018**, *28*, 22–34. [CrossRef]
27. Wasan, K.M.; Brazeau, G.A.; Keyhani, A.; Hayman, A.C.; Lopez-Berestein, G. Roles of liposome composition and temperature in distribution of amphotericin B in serum lipoproteins. *Antimicrob. Agents Chemother.* **1993**, *37*, 246–250. [CrossRef]
28. Gurusinghe, A.; de Niese, M.; Renaud, J.F.; Austin, L. The binding of lipoproteins to human muscle cells: Binding and uptake of LDL, HDL, and alpha-tocopherol. *Muscle Nerve* **1988**, *11*, 1231–1239. [CrossRef]
29. Knoke, S.; Bunjes, H. Transfer of lipophilic drugs from nanoemulsions into lipid-containing alginate microspheres. *Pharmaceutics* **2021**, *13*, 173. [CrossRef]
30. Deckelbaum, R.J.; Shipley, G.G.; Small, D.M. Structure and interactions of lipids in human plasma low density lipoproteins. *J. Biol. Chem.* **1977**, *252*, 744–754. [CrossRef]
31. Friedewald, W.T.; Levy, R.I.; Fredrickson, D.S. Estimation of the concentration of low-density lipoprotein cholesterol in plasma, without use of the preparative ultracentrifuge. *Clin. Chem.* **1972**, *18*, 499–502. [CrossRef]
32. Bunjes, H.; Unruh, T. Characterization of lipid nanoparticles by differential scanning calorimetry, X-ray and neutron scattering. *Adv. Drug Delivery Rev.* **2007**, *59*, 379–402. [CrossRef]
33. Strasdat, B.; Bunjes, H. Development of a new approach to investigating the drug transfer from colloidal carrier systems applying lipid nanosuspension-containing alginate microbeads as acceptor. *Int. J. Pharm.* **2015**, *489*, 203–209. [CrossRef] [PubMed]
34. Ginsburg, G.S.; Atkinson, D.; Small, D.M. Physical properties of cholesteryl esters. *Prog. Lipid Res.* **1984**, *23*, 135–167. [CrossRef]

35. Kuntsche, J.; Koch, M.H.J.; Steiniger, F.; Bunjes, H. Influence of stabilizer systems on the properties and phase behavior of supercooled smectic nanoparticles. *J. Colloid Interface Sci.* **2010**, *350*, 229–239. [CrossRef]
36. Kumar, V.; Butcher, S.J.; Öörni, K.; Engelhardt, P.; Heikkonen, J.; Kaski, K.; Ala-Korpela, M.; Kovanen, P.T. Three-dimensional cryoEM reconstruction of native LDL particles to 16Å resolution at physiological body temperature. *PLoS ONE* **2011**, *6*, e18841. [CrossRef] [PubMed]
37. Reshetov, V.; Zorin, V.; Siupa, A.; D'Hallewin, M.-A.; Guillemin, F.; Bezdetnaya, L. Interaction of liposomal formulations of meta-tetra(hydroxyphenyl)chlorin (temoporfin) with serum proteins: Protein binding and liposome destruction. *Photochem. Photobiol.* **2012**, *88*, 1256–1264. [CrossRef] [PubMed]
38. Tiss, A.; Lengsfeld, H.; Hadváry, P.; Cagna, A.; Verger, R. Transfer of orlistat through oil-water interfaces. *Chem. Phys. Lipids* **2002**, *19*, 41–49. [CrossRef]
39. Pas, T.; Struyf, A.; Vergauwen, B.; van den Mooter, G. Ability of gelatin and BSA to stabilize the supersaturated state of poorly soluble drugs. *Eur. J. Pharm. Biopharm.* **2018**, *131*, 211–223. [CrossRef] [PubMed]
40. Nakamura, K.; Era, S.; Ozaki, Y.; Sogami, M.; Hayashi, T.; Murakami, M. Conformational changes in seventeen cystine disulfide bridges of bovine serum albumin proved by Raman spectroscopy. *FEBS Lett.* **1997**, *417*, 375–378. [CrossRef]
41. Majorek, K.A.; Porebski, P.J.; Dayal, A.; Zimmerman, M.D.; Jablonska, K.; Stewart, A.J.; Chruszcz, M.; Minor, W. Structural and immunologic characterization of bovine, horse, and rabbit serum albumins. *Mol. Immunol.* **2012**, *52*, 174–182. [CrossRef] [PubMed]

pharmaceuticals

MDPI

Article

Imidazole-Based pH-Sensitive Convertible Liposomes for Anticancer Drug Delivery

Ruiqi Huang †, Vijay Gyanani †, Shen Zhao, Yifan Lu and Xin Guo *

Thomas J. Long School of Pharmacy, University of the Pacific, Stockton, CA 95211, USA; r_huang9@u.pacific.edu (R.H.); v_gyanani@u.pacific.edu (V.G.); s_zhao5@u.pacific.edu (S.Z.); y_lu5@u.pacific.edu (Y.L.)
* Correspondence: xguo@pacific.edu
† These authors contributed equally to this work.

Abstract: In efforts to enhance the activity of liposomal drugs against solid tumors, three novel lipids that carry imidazole-based headgroups of incremental basicity were prepared and incorporated into the membrane of PEGylated liposomes containing doxorubicin (DOX) to render pH-sensitive convertible liposomes (ICL). The imidazole lipids were designed to protonate and cluster with negatively charged phosphatidylethanolamine-polyethylene glycol when pH drops from 7.4 to 6.0, thereby triggering ICL in acidic tumor interstitium. Upon the drop of pH, ICL gained more positive surface charges, displayed lipid phase separation in TEM and DSC, and aggregated with cell membrane-mimetic model liposomes. The drop of pH also enhanced DOX release from ICL consisting of one of the imidazole lipids, *sn*-2-((2,3-dihexadecyloxypropyl)thio)-5-methyl-1H-imidazole. ICL demonstrated superior activities against monolayer cells and several 3D MCS than the analogous PEGylated, pH-insensitive liposomes containing DOX, which serves as a control and clinical benchmark. The presence of cholesterol in ICL enhanced their colloidal stability but diminished their pH-sensitivity. ICL with the most basic imidazole lipid showed the highest activity in monolayer Hela cells; ICL with the imidazole lipid of medium basicity showed the highest anticancer activity in 3D MCS. ICL that balances the needs of tissue penetration, cell-binding, and drug release would yield optimal activity against solid tumors.

Keywords: pH-sensitive; liposome; imidazole; anticancer; drug delivery; multicellular spheroids

Citation: Huang, R.; Gyanani, V.; Zhao, S.; Lu, Y.; Guo, X. Imidazole-Based pH-Sensitive Convertible Liposomes for Anticancer Drug Delivery. *Pharmaceuticals* **2022**, *15*, 306. https://doi.org/10.3390/ph15030306

Academic Editors: Ana Catarina Silva, João Nuno Moreira and José Manuel Sousa Lobo

Received: 8 February 2022
Accepted: 25 February 2022
Published: 3 March 2022

1. Introduction

The past two decades have seen a surge in the medical use of nanotechnology. Tens of nanomedicines, mostly liposomes, have been approved by Food and Drug Administration (FDA) or European Medicines Agency (EMA) to treat or diagnose many serious diseases, especially various types of cancer [1–4]. Liposomal formulations of doxorubicin (DOX) [4–6] represent an important group of nanomedicines, which are indicated for a wide range of cancers. Many studies have demonstrated that, compared with free DOX, DOX-loaded nanomedicines offer substantially lower cardiotoxicity and higher efficacy, both owing to their preferred accumulation at tumor sites [7,8].

One abnormal feature in many solid tumors is a fenestrated vasculature [9], which allows nano-formulations of anticancer drugs to permeate selectively from the blood circulation to the tumor interstitium. The nano-formulations can then accumulate in solid tumors due to their lack of lymphatic drainage, a phenomenon known as the enhanced permeability and retention (EPR) effect. Many long-circulating nano-formulations have been developed to take advantage of the EPR effect, including PEGylated liposomes, hydrophilic polymers, and solid lipid nanoparticles [10,11]. However, the fenestrated vasculature distributes mainly in the peripheral of solid tumors, which could limit the distribution of nano-drug formulations to the tumor core, and hence limit their ability to eradicate the entire tumor cell population [12].

Another abnormality of tumor tissue is its acidic microenvironment. Whereas normal cells in healthy tissues have an intracellular pH (pH_i) of 7.2 and a slightly higher extracellular pH (pH_e) of 7.4, cancer cells in tumors are characterized by a pH_i of 7.2 but a significantly lower pH_e of 6.2–7.0 [13,14]. The lower pH_e in the tumor interstitium results from the accumulation of lactate, an acidic by-product of the elevated anaerobic metabolism by the cancer cells in the hypoxic tumor microenvironment [15]. In response, many pH-sensitive drug delivery systems have been developed, including pH-sensitive liposomes, antibody-drug conjugates with acid-labile linkers, and pH-sensitive polymeric nanoparticles [16–18]. A number of pH-sensitive drug delivery systems have shown enhanced anticancer activity compared to their pH-insensitive counterparts in preclinical research [19,20]. However, pH-sensitive nano-drug delivery systems have not yet been approved to treat cancer patients.

Imidazole represents an important pH-sensitive functional group in pharmaceutical sciences. Imidazoles carry pKa values around 5.0–6.5 and thus can protonate to assume a positive charge in response to weakly acidic pH in pathophysiological settings [21]. The incorporation of imidazole-based lipids into nano-formulations has enhanced their intracellular delivery of proteins and nucleic acids [22,23]. However, very few studies [24] have been reported on imidazole-based nano-formulations for anticancer drug delivery.

Herein, we report a novel type of imidazole lipids and their pH-sensitive liposomes. Our goal is to develop imidazole lipids that trigger the liposomes in cooperation with phosphatidylethanolamine-polyethylene glycol conjugates (PE-PEG), which is a key component to stabilize liposomes in blood circulation for anticancer drug delivery. At pH 7.4, the imidazole lipids are mostly uncharged, while at acidic pH, they would protonate and cluster with negatively charged PE-PEG to induce lipid phase conversions. Such liposomes are thus called imidazole-based convertible liposomes (ICL) (Figure 1). ICL was loaded with the anticancer drug doxorubicin (DOX) and subjected to physicochemical and morphological characterizations. The pH-sensitivity of ICL was assessed by Differential Scanning Calorimetry (DSC), change of ζ-potential, interaction with negatively charged model lipid membranes, and pH-dependent drug release. The anticancer activities of ICL were assessed against both 2D monolayer cancer cells and 3D multicellular tumor spheroids (MCS), which mimic more features of solid tumors than 2D cell cultures, including the acidic microenvironment, the dense ECM, and the hypoxic core [9,25]. PEGylated liposomes containing DOX but not the pH-sensitive, imidazole-based lipids were also studied, both as a pH-insensitive control and as a benchmark of clinically used liposomal formulations. The effects of cholesterol on the physicochemical properties, pH-sensitivity and anticancer activities of ICL were also investigated. We report the physicochemical properties and the superior anticancer activities of ICL in both monolayer cancer cells and MCS of multiple cancer cell lines in correlation to their pH-sensitivity.

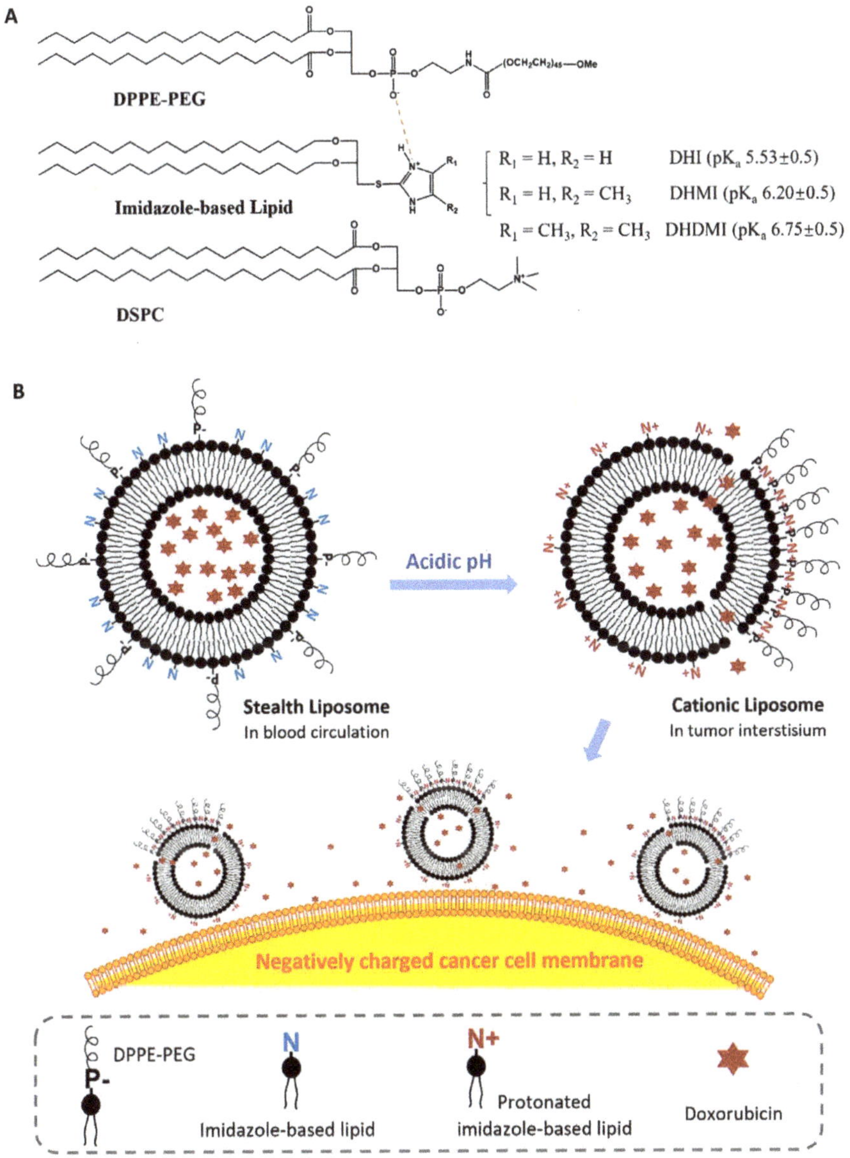

Figure 1. Imidazole-based convertible liposome (ICL). (**A**) Chemical structures of lipids that constitute ICL. (**B**) Schematic of ICL turning from stealth liposomes into cationic liposomes in acidic tumor interstitium. P−, negatively charged phosphate group in DPPE-PEG; N/N+, basic amine in imidazole-based lipids.

2. Results

2.1. Imidazole-Based pH-Sensitive Lipids

Three novel lipids (Figure 2), namely *sn*-2-((2,3-dihexadecyloxypropyl)thio)-1H-imida -zole (DHI), *sn*-2-((2,3-dihexadecyloxypropyl)thio)-5-methyl-1H-imidazole (DHMI), and *sn*-2-((2,3-dihexadecyloxypropyl)thio)-4,5-dimethyl-1H-imidazole (DHDMI) were designed as a critical component of ICL. Each of the lipids contains two saturated hexadecyl (C16) hydrocarbon chains as the tail and an imidazole-based headgroup. In a typical anticancer liposome formulation, the C16 chains would make the novel lipids more compatible with other lipids, which would also carry long, saturated hydrocarbon chains to enhance the physicochemical stability of the formulation. All the imidazole-based headgroups of the three lipids are expected to interact with the negatively charged DPPE-PEG at lowered pH, but they would each have slightly different pH-sensitivity due to their different substituents. Specifically, the imidazole headgroup of DHI, DHMI, and DHDMI carries zero, one, and two electron-donating methyl groups, respectively, which would yield incrementally higher pKa of the lipids (Figure 2). ICL containing such lipids would therefore be triggered at incrementally higher pH. The three lipids were all synthesized from dihexadecyl glycerol (DHG) in two steps: first, its activation into DHG-tosylate, and then conjugation with the appropriately methylated mercaptoimidazole (Figure 3).

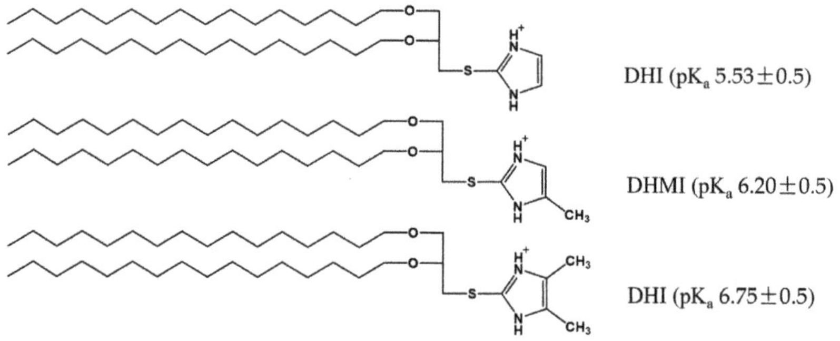

Figure 2. Imidazole-based, pH-sensitive lipids under study: chemical structures and calculated pKa by the ACD/pKa DB software.

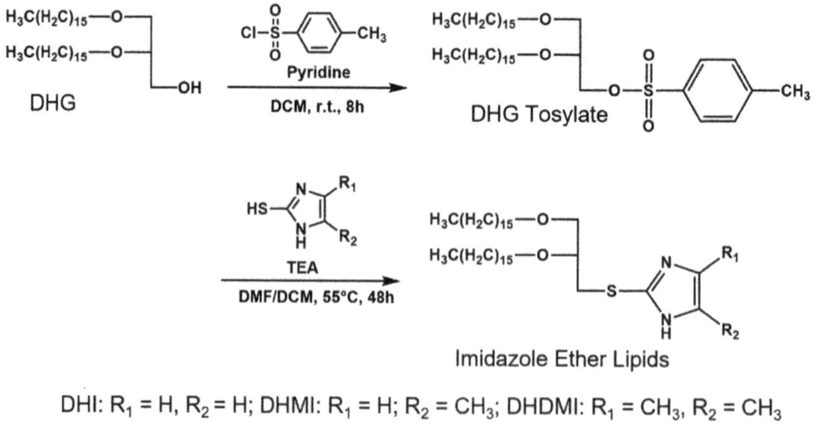

Figure 3. Synthesis of imidazole-based, pH-sensitive lipids.

2.2. Composition of Imidazole-Based Convertible Liposomes (ICL)

The imidazole-based lipids (DHI, DHMI, and DHDMI) were each mixed with 1,2-distearoyl-*sn*-glycero-3-phosphocholine (DSPC) and 1,2-dipalmitoyl-*sn*-glycero-3-phosphoe -thanolamine-*N*-[azido(polyethylene glycol)-2000 (DPPE-PEG (2000)) at 25/70/5 molar ratio to construct their corresponding ICL. DSPC is a phospholipid with a neutrally charged choline headgroup and a tail of two long (C18), saturated hydrocarbon chains; DPPE-PEG is a conjugate of PEG2000 and phosphoethanolamine with a negative charge from the phosphate, and a tail of two long (C16) saturated hydrocarbon chains. At pH 7.4, the lipids would assemble into a stable lipid membrane of ICL that is evenly coated by PEG as in sterically hindered, long-circulating liposomes [6,8]. In response to lowered pH, the imidazole-based lipids in ICL would be protonated to assume positive charges and cluster with negatively charged DPPE-PEG (2000) by electrostatic interactions (Figure 1B). Such pH-triggered clustering of lipids would expose part of the ICL surface that is no longer sterically hindered by PEG, which would then enhance the interaction between ICL and cancer cells in the acidic tumor interstitium [26]. The ICL-cancer cell interactions could also be enhanced by the excess positive charges on the ICL surface [26]. Furthermore, the pH-triggered lipid clustering could enhance the release of the liposome contents through the edges between the DPPE-PEG-rich and DPPE-PEG-poor regions of the liposome membrane based on our prior studies on liposomes consisting of pH-sensitive conformational switches of lipid tails [27,28]. As a common lipid component to improve the stability of liposomes, cholesterol [29,30] was included in some of the formulations under investigation. Cholesterol was incorporated at 25 mol%, a level that tends to improve the liposome stability both on the shelf and in blood circulation. Analogous liposomes without imidazole-based lipids were also prepared and characterized as pH-insensitive controls.

2.3. Physicochemical Characteristics of ICL

After lipidic film hydration, freeze-anneal-thawing and sequential extrusion through 400 nm, 200 nm and 100 nm polycarbonate membranes, ICL consisting of 25 mol% DHI, DHMI or DHMI were successfully prepared with mean hydrodynamic diameters smaller than 130 nm (Table 1). The Polydispersity Index (PDI), a measure of the heterogeneity of the size of particles in a mixture, was lower than 0.3 for all the liposome formulations. The liposomes with 25 mol% cholesterol showed generally smaller PDI than the cholesterol-free formulations. After being loaded with DOX, all the formulations were characterized with larger sizes and PDI. Nevertheless, the sizes of all the DOX-loaded formulations were below or around 200 nm in diameter. The DOX-loaded ICL with 25% cholesterol showed smaller sizes and PDI than the DOX-loaded ICL without cholesterol. The encapsulation efficiency (EE) of all the formulations was 50% or higher, and ICL with cholesterol were characterized with considerably higher EE than cholesterol-free ICL.

Table 1. Physicochemical characteristics of DOX-free and DOX-loaded ICL in comparison with pH-insensitive stealth liposomes.

		Before DOX-Loading		After DOX-Loading		
Lipid Compositions	**Molar Ratio**	**Size (nm)**	**PDI**	**Size (nm)**	**PDI**	**EE (%)**
DHI/DSPC/DPPE-PEG	25/70/5	114.9 ± 10.9	0.205 ± 0.008	200.8 ± 14.6	0.522 ± 0.047	56.62 ± 2.06
DHMI/DSPC/DPPE-PEG	25/70/5	117.9 ± 3.6	0.220 ± 0.033	189.3 ± 22.3	0.546 ± 0.055	53.18 ± 1.12
DHDMI/DSPC/DPPE-PEG	25/70/5	104.8 ± 3.5	0.176 ± 0.035	194.9 ± 7.0	0.253 ± 0.130	59.54 ± 0.59
DSPC/DPPE-PEG	95/5	101.8 ± 3.0	0.125 ± 0.067	136.9 ± 13.7	0.364 ± 0.085	57.74 ± 0.98
DHI/DSPC/DPPE-PEG/Chol	25/45/5/25	122.7 ± 8.19	0.081 ± 0.020	142.2 ± 9.5	0.113 ± 0.035	71.38 ± 0.61
DHMI/DSPC/DPPE-PEG/Chol	25/45/5/25	116.5 ± 11.9	0.075 ± 0.030	128.1 ± 8.3	0.078 ± 0.021	89.86 ± 1.27
DHDMI/DSPC/DPPE-PEG/Chol	25/45/5/25	114.0 ± 5.6	0.074 ± 0.008	128.6 ± 14.2	0.104 ± 0.020	92.97 ± 1.10
DSPC/DPPE-PEG/Chol	70/5/25	119.9 ± 5.4	0.066 ± 0.037	138.4 ± 5.6	0.165 ± 0.092	60.98 ± 1.66

Size values are hydrodynamic diameters based on cumulative intensity. Data are presented as mean ± SD, $N = 3$.

2.4. pH-Triggered Acquisition of Positive Charges on ICL Surface

The ζ-potentials of ICL and pH-insensitive liposomes at pH 6.0, 6.5, 7.0, and 7.4, 37 °C were measured to assess the surface charge of ICL in relationship to pH. As shown in Figure 4A, all three ICL consisting of DHI, DHMI, or DHDMI but no cholesterol showed a significant increase of ζ-potential when pH was lowered from 7.4 to 6.0. Particularly, the ζ-potential of ICL containing DHMI or DHDMI was elevated from below to above zero, indicating the conversion of such ICL to assume positive surface charges in response to the pH drop. Furthermore, the higher the pK_a of the imidazole-based lipid (DHDMI > DHMI > DHI), the larger was the increase of the ζ-potential of its ICL. This result indicated that the pH-triggered acquisition of positive charges on the ICL surface was rendered by the protonation of the imidazole-based lipids DHI, DHMI and DHDMI. By contrast, the pH-insensitive liposomes (DSPC/DPPE-PEG) displayed negative ζ-potentials below −10 mV at both physiological and acidic pH. However, as can be seen in Figure 4B, ICL containing 25 mol% cholesterol didn't show incremental elevation of ζ-potentials at pH 6.0–7.4 but fluctuated between −5 mV and −20 mV, indicating that the pH-sensitivity of ICL, as shown by the pH-triggered acquisition of positive surface charges, was prohibited by the addition of 25 mol% cholesterol.

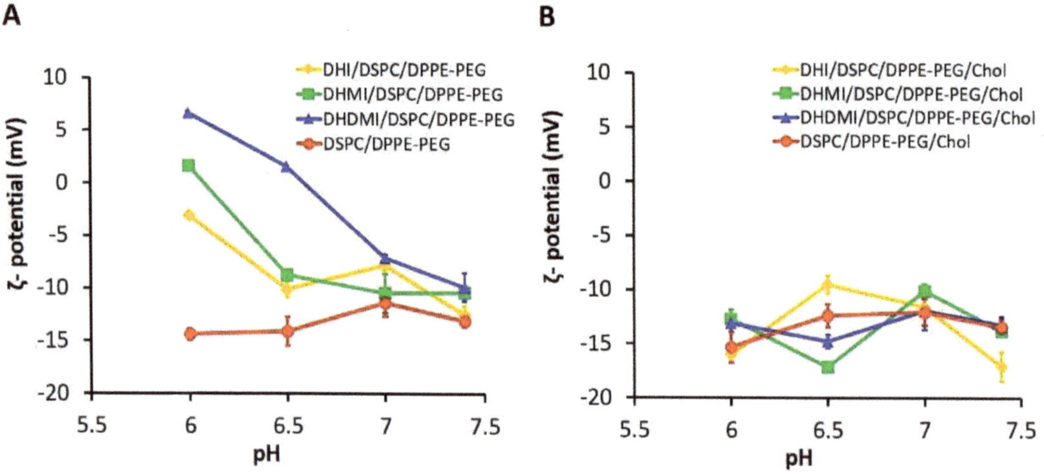

Figure 4. pH-triggered acquisition of positive surface charges by ICL. ζ-potential of ICL without (**A**) or with (**B**) 25% cholesterol were measured at 37 °C, pH 6.0, 6.5, 7.0, and 7.4. Data are presented as mean ± SD, $N = 3$.

2.5. pH-Triggered Interaction between ICL and Model Liposome

To test if lowered pH can enhance ICL's interaction with cell membrane, model liposomes (negatively charged, ~200 nm in diameter) that mimicked the composition of the plasma membrane [31] were prepared and mixed with ICL at a 1:1 lipid molar ratio. The mixture was then exposed to pH 7.4, 7.0, 6.5, and 6.0 and characterized by dynamic light scattering (Figure 5). ICL consisting of DHI, DHMI, or DHDMI but no cholesterol (Figure 5A) showed a remarkable increase of diameter from ~200 nm up to ~1300 nm as the pH decreased from 7.4 to 6.0, indicating the aggregation of ICL with the model liposomes in response to the drop of pH. It is worth noting that ICL aggregated with the cell membrane-mimetic liposomes even at near-zero ζ-potentials (DHMI and DHDMI at pH 6.5), indicating that acquisition of excessive positive charge is not necessary for ICL to adsorb onto the model liposomes. Instead, the aggregation may be attributed to the loss of negative charges on the ICL surface when the positively charged imidazole lipids cluster with negatively charged DPPE-PEG. As shown in Figure 5B, the mixture of model liposomes and liposomes consisting of both imidazole-based lipids and cholesterol did not show any size increase, which indicated that the incorporation of 25 mol% cholesterol hindered the interaction between ICL and the model liposomes at the acidic pHs under this investigation.

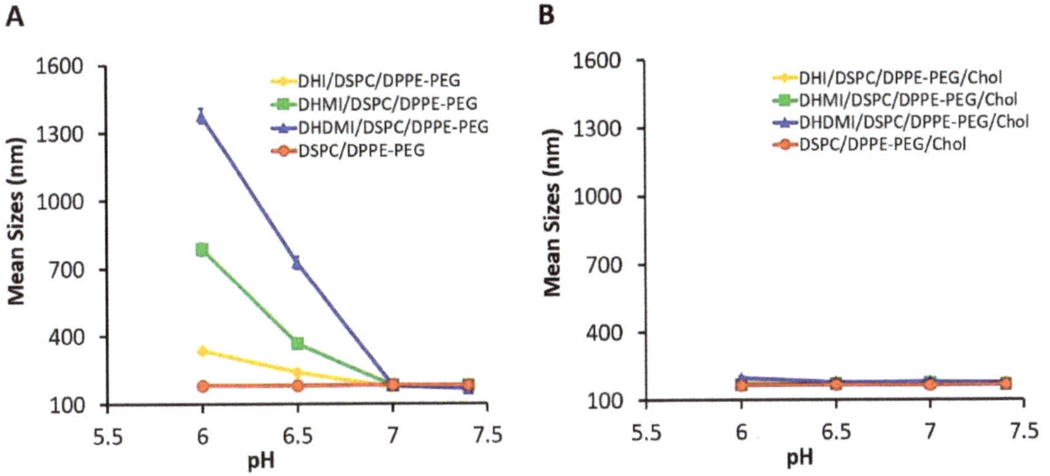

Figure 5. pH-triggered interaction between ICL and model liposomes. Mean sizes of equimolar mixture of model liposome and ICL without (**A**) or with (**B**) 25% cholesterol were measured at 37 °C, pH 6.0, 6.5, 7.0, and 7.4. Data are presented as mean ± SD, $N = 3$.

2.6. pH-Triggered Drug Release from ICL

Drug release from ICL and the pH-insensitive control liposomes were monitored at various pHs over 12 h to further characterize the stability and pH-sensitivity of ICL. As shown in Figure 6A–D, the ICL formulations consisting of DHI, DHMI, DHDMI but no cholesterol and the pH-insensitive control liposomes without cholesterol released 64.53 ± 1.74%, 53.65 ± 2.27%, 20.36 ± 0.83% and 29.56 ± 0.70% of the encapsulated DOX, respectively, after incubation at pH 7.4 for 12 h, which indicated that the stability of DHDMI/DSPC/DPPE-PEG and of the pH-insensitive DSPC/DPPE-PEG liposomes was higher than DHI/DSPC/DPPE-PEG and DHMI/DSPC/DPPE-PEG liposomes at the physiological pH 7.4. More importantly, the DHMI/DSPC/DPPE-PEG showed remarkably higher drug release at pH 6.0 than pH 7.4 (~50% vs. ~25%), but the DHI/DSPC/DPPE-PEG, DHMI/DSPC/DPPE-PEG and the pH-insensitive liposomes showed no noticeable enhancement of drug release under the same condition. In the presence of 25 mol% cholesterol, the ICL consisting of DHI, DHMI, DHDMI and the pH-insensitive liposomes released 56.19 ± 0.78%, 47.11 ± 0.60%, 40.32 ± 0.99% and 57.70 ± 3.03% DOX, respectively after incubation at pH 7.4 for 12 h. Compared to their cholesterol-free counterparts, the DHI and the DHMI liposomes with cholesterol (Figure 6E,F) released a similar percentage of DOX at pH 7.4, while the DHDMI (Figure 6G) and the pH-insensitive control liposomes (Figure 6H) released a higher percentage of DOX at pH 7.4. None of the formulations with cholesterol showed enhanced drug release at lowered pH, which indicates that the addition of cholesterol prevented any acidic pH-triggered drug release from ICL.

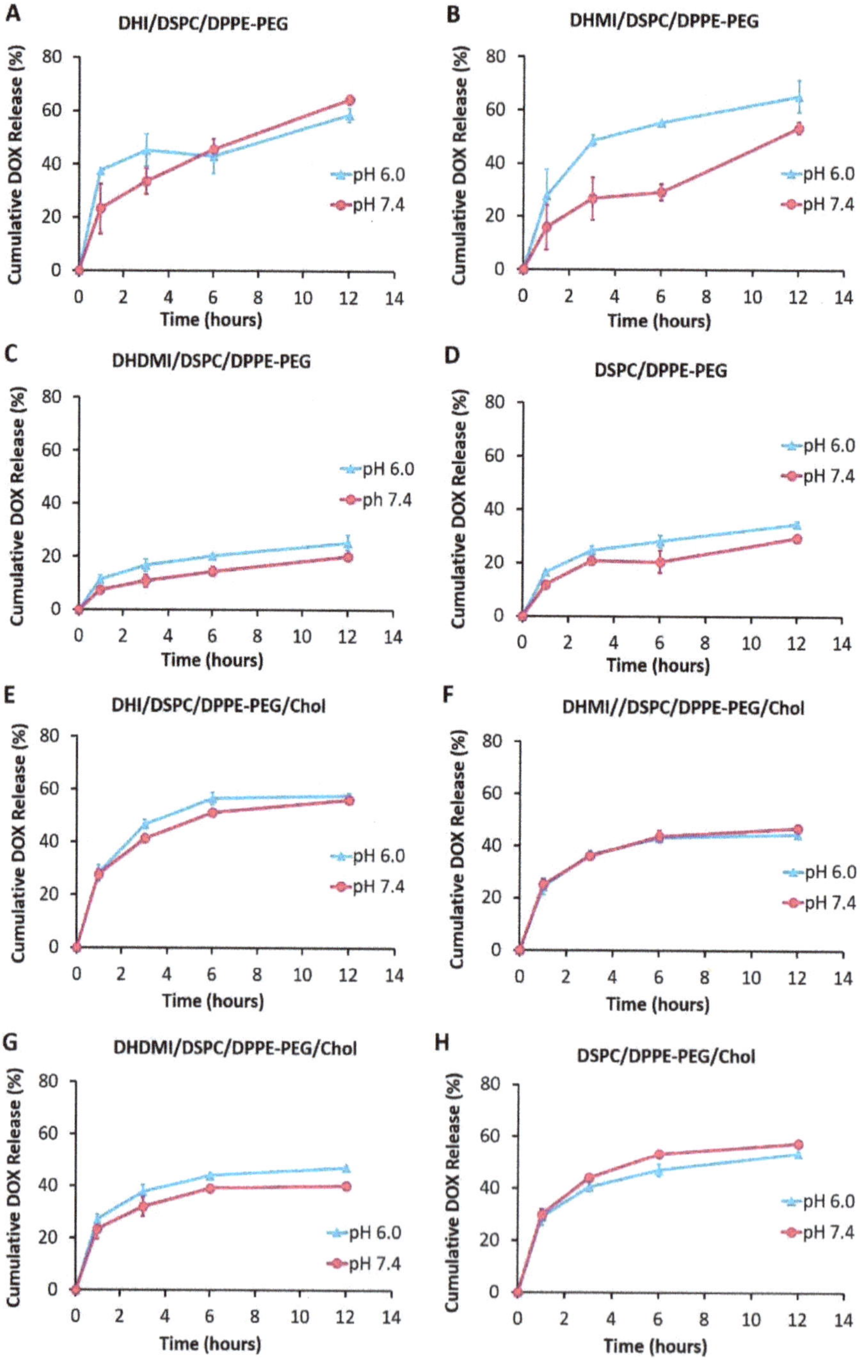

Figure 6. Release of DOX from liposomes without cholesterol (**A–D**) and with 25% cholesterol (**E–H**) over 12 h of incubation at 37 °C, pH 6.0 and 7.4. Data are presented as mean ± SD, $N = 3$.

2.7. Morphological Studies on ICL under TEM

Based on the aforementioned three pH-sensitivity studies, the ICL formulations consisting of DHI, DHMI, or DHDMI but no cholesterol were further characterized by TEM (Figure 7). Such ICL formulations showed spherical vesicle structures at pH 7.4, thus confirming the formation of liposomes. While DHI/DSPC/DPPE-PEG and DHMI/DSPC/DPPE-PEG formulations showed vesicles of smooth staining, those of DHDMI/DSPC/DPPE-PEG showed bright patches of light staining at pH 7.4. Upon exposure to lower pH 6.0, all the three ICL formulations showed more bright patches, especially the DHDMI/DSPC/DPPE-PEG formulation, which showed vesicles predominantly with clearly distinguishable bright and dark areas, which most probably represent separated lipid phases that are differentially stained by uranyl acetate. DHMI/DSPC/DPPE-PEG and DHDMI/DSPC/DPPE-PEG ICL also showed larger and brighter vesicles at the lower pH 6.4. Because the positively charged uranyl ions ($UO^{2+}{}_2$) of the TEM stain preferably bind to the phosphate groups in lipid bilayers [32], the bright patches probably represent areas of ICL surface where the protonated imidazole-based lipids cluster with phosphate groups of DPPE-PEG and thus hinder their binding with the uranyl ions. At pH 6.0, the DHMI/DSPC/DPPE-PEG formulation also showed some collapsed, non-vesicle structures, which would explain its acidic pH-enhanced release of DOX (Figure 6B).

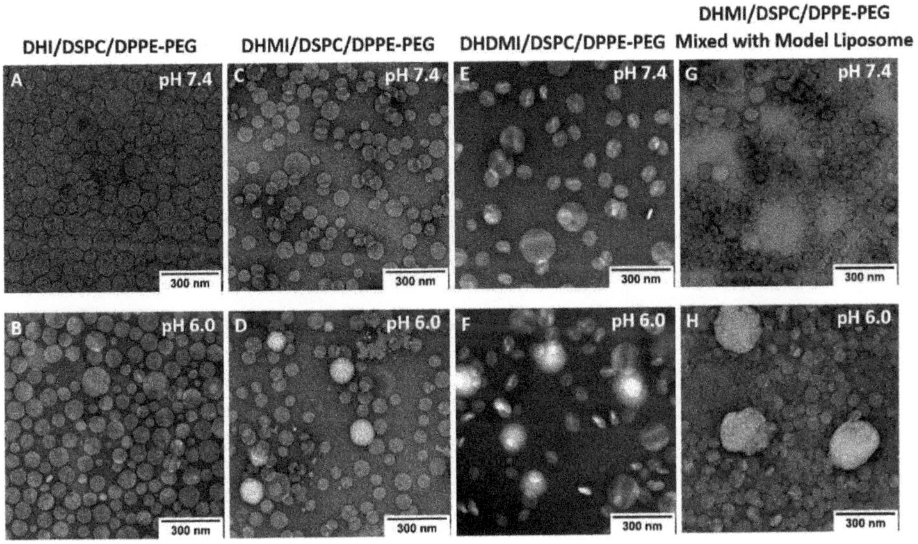

Figure 7. TEM images of DOX-loaded ICL formulations (**A–F**) and mixture of DHMI liposomes with model liposomes (**G**,**H**) at pH 7.4 (**A**,**C**,**E**,**G**) and pH 6.0 (**B**,**D**,**F**,**H**).

The mixture of DHMI/DSPC/DPPE-PEG and model liposomes also showed different morphology at pH 7.4 and 6.0. At pH 7.4, the mixture consisted mainly of smoothly stained vesicles; at pH 6.0, the mixture showed both vesicles with bright patches and substantially larger and brighter structures that appear to be aggregates of multiple ICL and model liposomes.

2.8. Differential Scanning Calorimetry of ICL

In order to further elucidate the phase behavior of ICL, DHI/DSPC/DPPE-PEG liposomes were characterized by differential scanning calorimetry. As the temperature was gradually increased from 40 °C to 75 °C at pH 7.4, the DSC thermogram of DHI/DSPC/DPPE-PEG liposomes (Figure 8A) showed one broad and tilted peak between 56 °C and 65 °C, which indicated that the liposomes went through mainly one phase transition and therefore started with mainly one lipid phase of a mixture of DHI, DSPC, and DPPE-PEG. At pH 6.0, the DSC thermogram showed two distinct peaks, one at a similar range between 60 °C and 64 °C, and another new peak at around 52 °C (Figure 8A), which indicated the formation of at least two lipid phases in the liposome membrane. The new peak most probably represents a lipid phase that is rich in DSPC because liposomes of only DSPC have a very similar gel-to-liquid phase transition temperature at 54 °C [33]. The DSC thermogram of the pH-insensitive control liposome DSPC/DPPE-PEG (Figure 8B) showed one phase-transition peak around 53 °C at pH 7.4 and 6.0, indicating that the control liposomes had homogenous mixing of lipids at both pHs.

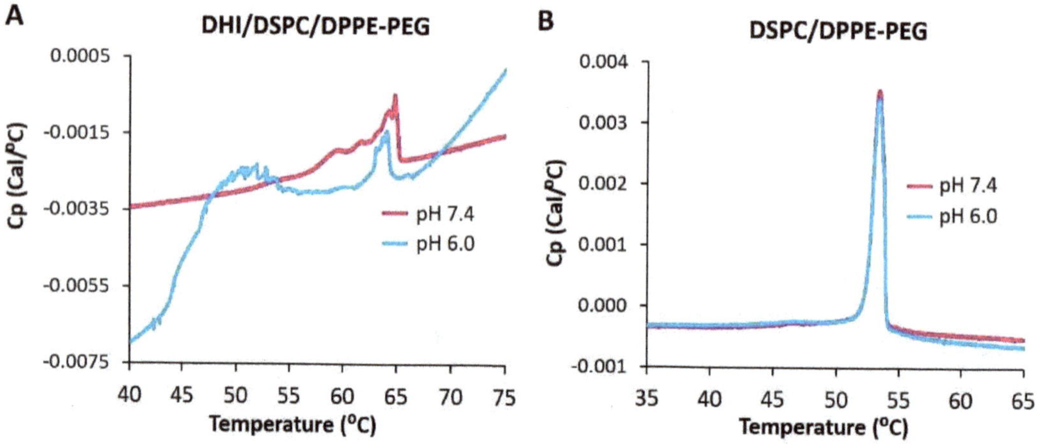

Figure 8. DSC thermograms of pH-sensitive ICL (DHI/DSPC/DPPE-PEG) (**A**) and pH-insensitive stealth liposome DSPC/DPPE-PEG (**B**) at pH 7.4 and 6.0.

As DSPC carries the longest hydrophobic tail (two C18 chains) among all the lipids of the DHI/DSPC/DPPE-PEG formulation, the phase transition peak in the high-temperature region of 56 °C to 65 °C indicates strong interactions between different types of lipid molecules, most probably DHI and DPPE-PEG, rather than interactions between the same type of lipid molecules in the liposome membrane.

2.9. Anticancer Activity of ICL on 2D Monolayer Cells

The anticancer activity of ICL formulations was tested by the decrease of the viability of 2D monolayer cancer cells (HeLa) at both neutral and mildly acidic pH 6.0–6.5 as seen in tumor interstitium. As the culture media pH was adjusted from 7.4 to 6.0, the ICL formulations that consisted of an imidazole-based pH-sensitive lipid but no cholesterol showed higher anticancer activity (Figure 9), especially at 10 μg/mL DOX concentration, where all the ICL formulations under study showed significantly higher anticancer activity (see * in Figure 9) at pH 6.0 than pH 7.4 ($p < 0.05$). Among the three ICL formulations, the DHDMI/DSPC/DPPE-PEG liposomes that contained the imidazole lipid (DHDMI) of the highest pKa showed the best anticancer activity on the monolayer HeLa cells. By contrast, no difference in the anticancer activity of the pH-insensitive control liposomes (DSPC/DPPE-PEG) was detected between pH 7.4 and 6.0. As the positive control, free DOX showed the highest anticancer activity (~50% cell viability at 10 μg/mL), but such activity was the same at both pH 7.4 and pH 6.0.

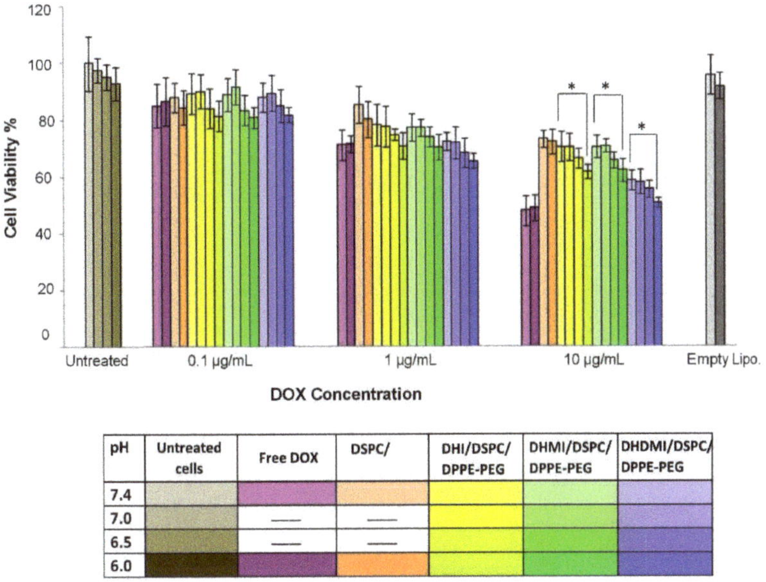

Figure 9. Cell viability of 2D HeLa cells treated with free DOX, cholesterol-free ICL and pH-insensitive liposomes at pH 7.4, 7.0, 6.5, and 6.0 for 12 h. Data are presented as mean ± SD, N = 4. * $p < 0.05$. pH was adjusted in the growth media.

2.10. Anticancer Activity of ICL on 3D Multicellular Spheroids

The ICL formulations were also tested against 3D multicellular spheroids (MCS) of a number of cancer cell lines, including HeLa (cervical cancer), MDA-MB-231 (breast cancer), MDA-MB-468 (breast cancer), and A549 (lung cancer). Compared to monolayer cells, MCS better mimic many features of solid tumors, including a cell cluster structure that hinders drug penetration, a hypoxic microenvironment, and an acidic interstitium. Similar to prior reports [34,35], confocal imaging of MCS in our studies confirmed the presence of pH-gradient from 7–8 at the peripheral to 5.5–6.4 at the core (Supplementary Materials, Figure S4 and Table S2 [36]).

After growth to about 500 µm in diameter to ensure the development of a necrotic core and an acid microenvironment, MCS were exposed to incremental concentrations of cholesterol-free ICL, pH-insensitive control liposomes and free DOX for 72 h followed by assessment of the dose-dependent decrease of cancer cell viability. Against HeLa MCS (Figure 10A), the DHI/DSPC/DPPE-PEG and DHMI/DSPC/DPPE-PEG ICL formulations showed significantly better anticancer activity (IC_{50} = 3.82 ± 1.13 and 2.07 ± 1.13 µM, respectively, Table 2) than the pH-insensitive control liposomes (IC_{50} = 11.41 ± 1.28 µM, $p < 0.001$). However, such improvement in anticancer activity was not observed in the DHDMI/DSPC/DPPE-PEG formulation (IC_{50} = 9.51 ± 1.15 µM, $p = 0.0693$, Table 2). Against MDA-MB-468 MCS (Figure 10D), all the three ICL formulations consisting of DHI, DHMI or DHDMI showed better anticancer activity (IC_{50} = 0.38 ± 0.21, 0.31 ± 0.15, and 0.63 ± 0.10 µM, respectively, Table 2) than the pH-insensitive control liposomes (IC_{50} = 1.24 ± 0.13 µM; $p < 0.001$ for DHI and DHMI, $p < 0.01$ for DHDMI) but the improvement was not as large as on HeLa MCS. Against both HeLa and MDA-MB-468 MCS, the DHMI/DSPC/DPPE-PEG ICL showed the best anticancer activity, which was comparable to that of the positive control, free DOX. However, ICL did not show noticeable improvement in activity against A549 (Figure 10B) or MDA-MB-231 (Figure 10C) MCS, compared with pH-insensitive control liposomes. When 25 mol% cholesterol was included in the lipid composition

(Figure 10E–G), all the ICL formulations showed similar but not better anticancer activity compared with pH-insensitive liposomes against HeLa, A549, or MDA-MB-231 MCS.

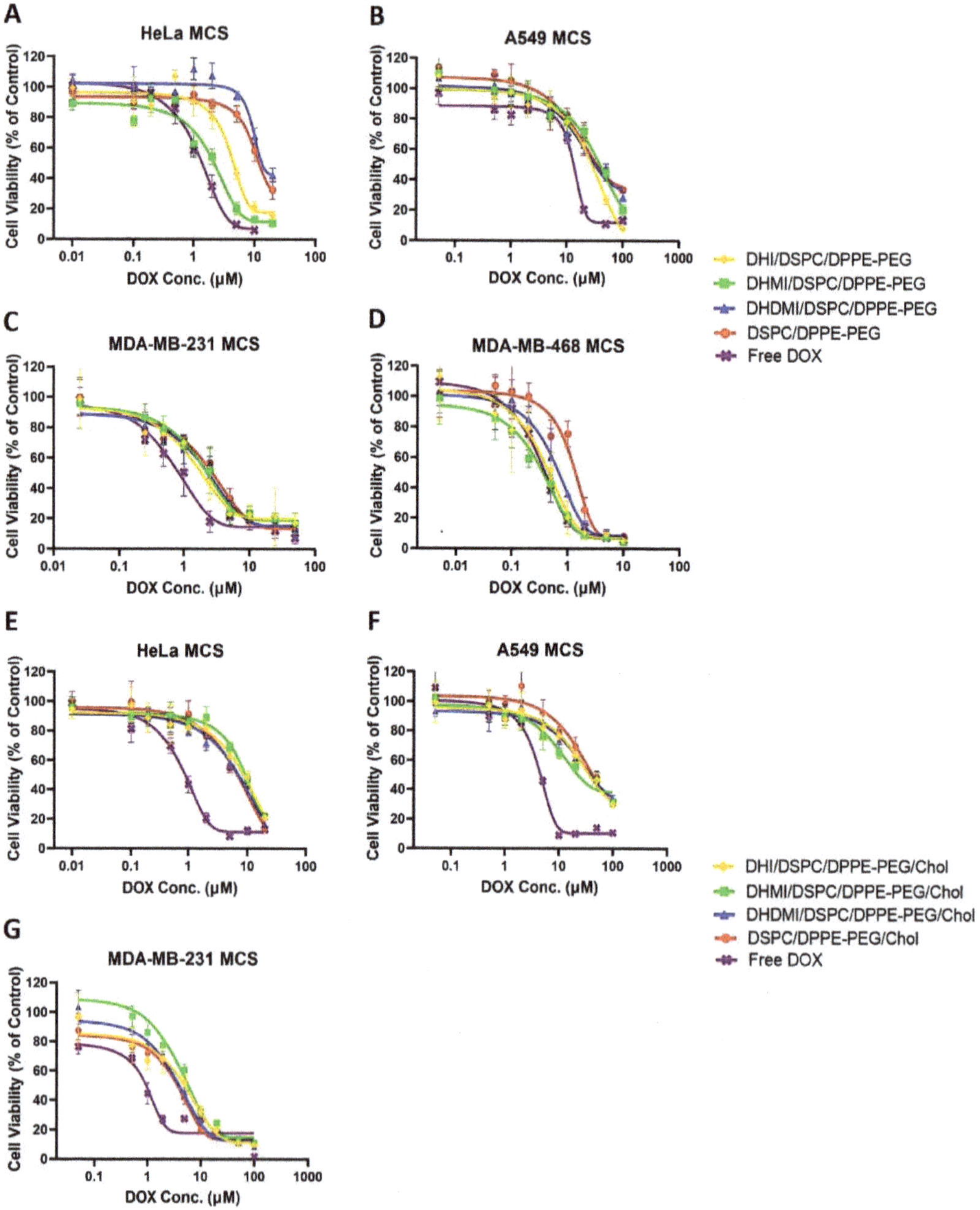

Figure 10. Cell viability of Hela, A549, MDA-MB-231, and MDA-MB-468 MCS after treatment with incremental concentrations of ICL formulations, pH-insensitive liposome, or free DOX. ICL consisted of either no cholesterol (**A–D**) or 25 mol% cholesterol (**E–G**). Data are presented as mean ± SD, $N = 4$.

Table 2. IC50 values of DOX-loaded liposomes and free DOX on HeLa, A549, MDA-MB-231, and MDA-MB-468 3D MCS.

Liposome Membrane Composition	Lipid Molar Ratio	IC_{50} $ (μM)			
		Hela	A549	MDA-MB-231	MDA-MB-468
DHI/DSPC/DPPE-PEG	25/70/5	3.82 ± 1.13 ***	~30 #	1.38 ± 1.31	0.38 ± 0.21 **
DHMI/DSPC/DPPE-PEG	25/70/5	2.07 ± 1.13 ***	~40 #	1.77 ± 1.21	0.31 ± 0.15 ***
DHDMI/DSPC/DPPE-PEG	25/70/5	9.51 ± 1.15	~35 #	1.86 ± 1.24	0.63 ± 0.10 **
DSPC/DPPE-PEG	95/5	11.41 ± 1.28	~35 #	2.37 ± 1.29	1.24 ± 0.13
DHI/DSPC/DPPE-PEG/Chol	25/45/5/25	~10 #	~30 #	5.13 ± 1.46	-
DHMI/DSPC/DPPE-PEG/Chol	25/45/5/25	10.38 ± 1.33	29.07 ± 2.73	3.62 ± 1.17	-
DHDMI/DSPC/DPPE-PEG/Chol	25/45/5/25	~10 #	24.06 ± 1.40	3.26 ± 1.18	-
DSPC/DPPE-PEG/Chol	70/5/25	~10 #	33.88 ± 1.62	3.98 ± 1.10	-
Free DOX	-	1.26 ± 0.04	12.59 ± 1.05	1.18 ± 0.29	0.32 ± 0.12

$ Calculated from dose-response data using GraphPad software. Data are presented as mean ± SD, $N = 4$. ** $p < 0.01$, *** $p < 0.001$ compared to the IC_{50} of DSPC/DPPE-PEG. # Visual estimation from dose-response curve.

3. Discussion

Two decades of investigations on nano-drug delivery systems have established the importance of their physicochemical properties in targeting the payload drug to cancer cells (also known as physical targeting) [37]. Such physicochemical properties include size, shape, surface charge, surface hydrophilicity, drug-loading, and drug release [37]. The introduction of new characteristics such as active targeting or pH-sensitivity needs to be accomplished in coordination with such properties, which poses a considerable challenge to formulation development.

In this study on ICL, the three imidazole-based lipids triggered PEGylated liposomes by efficiently clustering with phospholipid-PEG conjugates. Such a feature differentiates them from the imidazole lipid reported by Ju et al. [24] and represents a novel approach to construct stealth liposomes with pH-sensitivity. The clustering action is most probably achieved by the three lipids' unique structure, in which the imidazole headgroup is linked to the lipid tail at the C2 position through a carbon-sulfur bond so that both nitrogen atoms of the imidazole group can serve as H-bond donors upon protonation at acidic pH (Figure 2). The protonated imidazole groups can then each bind with negatively charged phosphate groups from two different DPPE-PEG molecules, which in turn crosslink DPPE-PEG molecules into clusters on the ICL surface. As PEGylation serves as a key method to construct long-circulating liposomes for anticancer drug delivery by the EPR effect, the imidazole-based lipids under this study have the potential for wide applications in vivo.

Compared to the doxorubicin-loaded PEG liposomes (Doxil®) that are in current clinical use, ICL carries the advantage of pH-sensitivity while preserving the physicochemical properties that favor passive targeting to solid tumors. The drug-free ICL carried sizes under 130 nm in diameter while the DOX-loaded ICL formulations carried sizes under or around 200 nm, both of which were within the size range for the EPR effect [9]. The increase of size and PDI of ICL upon DOX-loading was probably due to the aggregation of DOX molecules with the liposomes because our attempts to load higher concentrations of DOX led to precipitation and because DOX had been reported to aggregate with negatively charged liposomes [38]. DOX can be loaded into ICL at >50% encapsulation efficiency (EE) and at sufficiently high concentrations (Table 1) for anticancer studies in cell culture [39]. The payload DOX concentration of ICL could be further elevated by concentrating DOX-loaded ICL using Tangential Flow Filtration [40]. Although DOX is elected as the cargo drug in this study for better comparison between ICL and clinically established liposomal formulations, we anticipate that the imidazole lipids under this study can be used to trigger PEGylated liposomes containing various water-soluble anticancer drugs.

In response to the drop of pH, ICL without cholesterol demonstrated a number of substantial changes in their physicochemical properties, including acquisition of positive surface charges (ζ-potential elevation in Figure 4A), lipid phase separation (DSC studies in Figure 8A and TEM images in Figure 7), binding with the bio-mimetic membrane (aggregation with model liposomes in Figure 5A), and enhanced release of the payload drug DOX (Figure 6). The extent of most of the changes, namely the positive surface charge acquisition, lipid phase separation, and binding with bio-mimetic membrane, are correlated with higher basicity of the imidazole lipid (DHDMI > DHMI >DHI). This correlation can be explained by our proposed mechanism of ICL's pH-sensitivity, where the more basic imidazole lipid would be protonated more at the same mildly acidic pH, which would yield more positive charges on liposome surface and more electrostatic interaction between the imidazole lipid and DPPE-PEG, which would, in turn, promote phase separation of ICL membranes and binding between ICL and bio-mimetic membranes. Interestingly, DOX release from ICL did not follow such correlation in that only ICL consisting of DHMI showed substantially enhanced DOX release when the pH dropped from 7.4 to 6.0. TEM images of DHMI/DSPC/DPPE-PEG in comparison to DHI/DSPC/DPPE-PEG and DHDMI/DSPC/DPPE-PEG suggest that this pH-triggered release may be caused by DHMI/DSPC/DPPE-PEG's unique tendency to collapse into non-lamellar structures at pH 6.0. Alternatively, DHMI/DSPC/DPPE-PEG's membrane might also have more structural defects at the edge between the separated lipid phases at pH 6.0 to enhance the DOX release.

The incorporation of 25 mol% cholesterol prevented the size increase of ICL during DOX-loading; it also elevated the EE and the payload DOX concentration in ICL. This was probably because cholesterol can improve the stability of the lipid bilayer structure in the ICL formulations. During drug-loading, when the temperature is above the lipid bilayer transition temperature ($T > T_m$), the liposome membrane was in the fluid phase, in which the lipid molecules were free to move laterally. The addition of cholesterol was found to help suppress the mobility of lipid bilayers in the fluid phase and reduce their permeability to water, thus improving the membrane stability and drug retention during drug loading [41]. The introduction of cholesterol also diminished the pH-sensitivity of ICL (Figures 4–7), probably because the incorporation of cholesterol obstructed the lateral movements of lipids in bilayers at $T < T_m$. The nonpolar cholesterol molecules were found to tie up the neighboring lipid's hydrocarbon chains to minimize cholesterol molecules' thermodynamically unfavorable exposure to water at the membrane-water interface [42]. In ICL, such cholesterol-lipid interaction would substantially limit the movement of the imidazole-based lipids and DPPE-PEG, thus hindering their clustering at acidic pH. Furthermore, ICL with cholesterol maintained negative ζ-potentials at acidic pH, indicating that the protonation of the imidazole-based lipids was also suppressed by cholesterol (Figure 4B). This is probably because the addition of cholesterol increases the hydrophobicity of the liposome membrane, which in turn reduces its affinity with cations [43].

The targeting of cytotoxic chemotherapy drugs to enhance their efficacy and safety is a complicated process with multiple challenges that all need to be addressed by the drug delivery system, including preferred distribution of the drug molecules from blood circulation to the tumor interstitium, sufficient permeation of the drug molecules to all areas of the solid tumor, and uptake of the drug molecules by virtually all the cancer cells in the tumor. It is therefore critical that anticancer drug delivery systems are evaluated by biological models that simulate these multiple challenges. ICL formulations under this study were evaluated by both monolayer cancer cells and 3D MCS in culture in order to test the potential of their pH-sensitivity to enhance the anticancer activity [34].

In monolayer Hela cells, ICL's higher ability to suppress cell viability is strongly correlated with lower pH and higher pKa, which are both correlated with the acquisition of positive charges on the ICL surface, ICL's phase separation, and ICL's interaction with negatively charged bio-mimetic membranes. Such strong correlations suggest that ICL's activities to suppress monolayer cell viabilities can be attributed to ICL's enhanced binding to the cancer cells at lowered pH. More specifically, the drop of pH protonates the imidazole lipids, which cluster DPPE-PEG lipids to expose a de-PEGylated and positively charged ICL surface, which in turn binds to the cancer cell surface to induce the endocytosis of the DOX-loaded ICL and consequently the cell death.

The ICL's pattern of suppressing the cell viability in 3D multicellular spheroids was quite different from that in 2D monolayer cells. Overall, ICL consisting of DHMI, the imidazole lipid of the second-highest calculated pKa (6.20 $\pm$ 0.5), yielded the highest activity to suppress MCS viability, rather than DHDMI of the highest calculated pKa (6.75 $\pm$ 0.5). This is probably due to the dynamic balance between the binding of ICL to the cancer cells in MCS and the penetration of ICL to reach the most cancer cells in MCS. On the one hand, DHI may carry too low a pKa (5.53 $\pm$ 0.5) to sufficiently trigger its ICL in the mildly acidic microenvironment of MCS; on the other hand, DHDMI may carry too high a pKa, which would trigger most of its ICL to bind to only the cancer cells in the peripheral region of MCS. Paradoxically, DHMI may carry the optimal basicity (pKa 6.20 $\pm$ 0.5, closest to the measured interstitial pH of MCS) to facilitate both the penetration and the cellular binding of its ICL. Furthermore, among all the ICL under this study, DHMI/DSPC/DPPE-PEG showed the unique property of pH-enhanced drug release, which would allow such ICL to selectively release DOX in the MCS interstitium to kill multiple adjacent cancer cells, also known as the bystander effect [44].

4. Materials and Methods

4.1. Materials

1,2-Di-O-hexadecyl-*rac*-glycerol (DHG), 2-mercaptoimidazole, 4-methyl-1H-imidazole-2-thiol, and 4,5-dimethyl-1H-imidazole-2-thiol were purchased from Santa Cruz Biotechnology (Dallas, TX, USA). *p*-Toluenesulfonyl chloride, 2-[4-(2-hydroxyethyl)piperazin-1-yl]-ethanesulfonic acid (HEPES), and 2-(N-morpholino)ethanesulfonic acid (MES) were purchased from Fisher Scientific (Hampton, NH, USA). Triethylamine (TEA) was purchased from Alfa Aesar (Haverhill, MA, USA). The lipids 1,2-distearoyl-*sn*-glycero-3-phosphocholine (DSPC), 1,2-dipalmitoyl-*sn*-glycero-3-phosphoethanolamine-*N*-[azido(poly -ethylene glycol)-2000 (DPPE-PEG (2000)), 1-palmitoyl-2-oleoyl-*sn*-glycero-3-phosphocholine (POPC), 1-palmitoyl-2-oleoyl-*sn*-glycero-3-phosphoethanolamine (POPE), 1-palmitoyl-2-oleoyl-*sn*-glycero-3-phospho-L-serine (sodium salt) (POPS) and L-α-phosphatidylinositol (Soy) (L-R-PI) were purchased from Avanti Polar Lipids, Inc. (Alabaster, AL, USA). Cholesterol, Dowex® 50WX-4 (50–100 mesh), Sephadex G-25, and Uranyl acetate (UA) were purchased from Sigma-Aldrich (St. Louis, MO, USA). Doxorubicin hydrochloride was purchased from Biotang (Waltham, MA, USA). Carbon-coated copper grids (200 mesh) for electron microscopy were purchased from Polysciences (Warrington, PA, USA). The HeLa, A549, MDA-MB-231 and MDA-MB-468 cell lines were purchased from ATCC (Manassas, VA, USA). The Dulbecco's Modified Eagle's Medium (DMEM), Advanced DMEM/F12 medium, Trypsin-EDTA, L-glutamine, fetal bovine serum, and collagen were purchased from Thermo-Fisher Scientific (Waltham, MA, USA). The RPMI 1640 medium, penicillin-streptomycin, 96-well Ultra-low Attachment round-button microplates, 96-well solid white microplates, CellTiter-Glo 3D cell viability assay kits and MTS CellTiter 96® AQueous One Solution cell proliferation assay kits (Promega Corp., WI, USA) were purchased from VWR (Radnor, PA, USA). All other organic solvents and chemicals were purchased from Sigma-Aldrich (St. Louis, MO, USA), Fisher Scientific (Hampton, NH, USA) or VWR (Radnor, PA, USA).

4.2. Synthesis of 2,3-di-O-Hexadecyl-1-rac-glyceryl-tosylate (DHG-Tosylate)

1,2-Di-O-hexadecyl-*rac*-glycerol (DHG) (2.30 g, 4.25 mmol) was mixed with anhydrous dichloromethane (20 mL) and pyridine (18.6 mL, 225 mmol). *p*-Toluenesulfonyl chloride (1.90 g, 9.97 mmol) was dissolved in ~0.5 mL anhydrous dichloromethane and transferred into the mixture. The reaction mixture was stirred under argon at room temperature for 8 to 12 h. The reaction mixture was then mixed well with 10 mL anhydrous dichloromethane and washed with saturated Na_2CO_2 solution 3 times. The organic phase was separated from the aqueous phase, dried with $MgSO_4$, filtered, and then evaporated into dryness under vacuum. The resultant residue was separated by silica gel chromatography with dichloromethane as the mobile phase to yield 2.53 g solid (86%). DART Mass Spectrum: 695.5; calculated, 695.6 $(MH)^+$. 1H-NMR (600 MHz, $CDCl_3$, δ ppm): 0.87 (t, 6H, 2 $CH_3(CH_2)_{15}$-), 1.18–1.31 (m, 52H, 2 $OCH_2CH_2(CH_2)_{13}CH_3$), 1.46 (m, 4H, 2 $OCH_2CH_2(CH_2)_{13}CH_3$), 2.44 (s, 3H, -$(C_6H_4)CH_3$), 3.31–3.62 (m, 7H, glyceryl/hexadecyl -CH_2O and -CHO-), δ 4.14 (m, 2H, -CH_2OSO_2-), δ 7.33 (d, 2H, aromatic protons ortho to -CH_3), and δ 7.78 (d, 2H, aromatic protons ortho to -SO_2-).

4.3. Synthesis of sn-2-((2,3-Dihexadecyloxypropyl)thio)-1H-imidazole (DHI)

2-Mercaptoimidazole (0.91 g, 9.06 mmol) was dissolved in 8–9 mL of anhydrous N, N-dimethylformamide (DMF). DHG-tosylate (1.265 g, 1.82 mmol) was dissolved in 7–8 mL of anhydrous dichloromethane and transferred into the above-mentioned solution, followed by the addition of triethylamine (TEA, 1.27 mL, 9.08 mmol). The reaction mixture was stirred under argon at 55 °C for 48 h. The solvent was evaporated under a vacuum, and the resultant residue was dissolved in dichloromethane. The solution was washed with saturated sodium bicarbonate solution 3 times, dried with sodium carbonate, filtered, and then evaporated into dryness under vacuum. The resultant residue was then separated by silica gel chromatography with 1–5 vol% methanol in dichloromethane as the mobile gradient phase to yield DHI (25–30%). DART Mass Spectrum: 623.48 (Figure S1); calculated, 623.55 $(MH)^+$. 1H-NMR (Figure S2, 600 MHz, $CDCl_3$): δ 0.87 (t, 6H, 2 $CH_3(CH_2)_{15}$-), δ 1.19–1.32 (m, 54H, 2 -$OCH_2CH_2(CH_2)_{13}CH_3$ and -H_2CSCNH-), δ 1.55 (m, 4H, 2 $OCH_2CH_2(CH_2)_{13}CH_3$, δ 3.2–3.7 (m, 7H, glyceryl/hexadecyl -CH_2O and -CHO-), δ 7.02 (d, 1H, H_2CSC-NHC*H*=CH-N=), δ 7.21 (d, 1H, H_2CSC-NHCH=C*H*-N=). Elemental analysis: C 73.27%, H 12.25%, N 4.56%; calculated: C 73.25%, H 11.97%, N 4.50%. Calculated pK_a using ACD/pKa DB software: 5.53 ± 0.5.

4.4. Synthesis of sn-2-((2,3-Dihexadecyloxypropyl)thio)-5-methyl-1H-imidazole (DHMI)

4-Methyl-1H-imidazole-2-thiol (1.03 g, 9.03 mmol) was used to prepare DHMI, using the same synthesis method as DHI. Yield: 25–30%. DART Mass Spectrum: 637.55 (Figure S1); calculated, 637.57 $(MH)^+$. 1H-NMR (Figure S2, 600 MHz, $CDCl_3$): δ 0.87 (t, 6H, 2 $CH_3(CH_2)_{15}$-), δ 1.19–1.34 (m, 54H, 2 -$OCH_2CH_2(CH_2)_{13}CH_3$ and -H_2CSCNH-), δ 1.53 (m, 4H, 2 $OCH_2CH_2(CH_2)_{13}CH_3$), δ 2.41 (s, 3H, -H_2CSC-NH-C(CH_3)-), δ 3.2–3.7 (m, 7H, glyceryl/hexadecyl -CH_2O and -CHO-), δ 6.81 (s, 1H, -H_2CSC=N-C*H*=). Elemental analysis: C 73.63%, H 12.08%, N 4.35%; calculated: C 73.52%, H 12.02%, N 4.40%. Calculated pK_a using ACD/pKa DB software: 6.20 ± 0.5.

4.5. Synthesis of sn-2-((2,3-Dihexadecyloxypropyl)thio)-4,5-dimethyl-1H-imidazole (DHDMI)

4,5-Dimethyl-1H-imidazole-2-thiol (1.15 g, 9.03 mmol) was used to prepare DHDMI, using the same synthesis method as DHI. Yield: 25–30%. DART Mass Spectrum: 651.56 (Figure S1); calculated, 651.59 $(MH)^+$. 1H-NMR (Figure S2, 600 MHz, $CDCl_3$): δ 0.87 (t, 6H, 2 $CH_3(CH_2)_{15}$–), δ 1.19–1.34 (m, 54H, 2 -$OCH_2CH_2(CH_2)_{13}CH_3$ and -H_2CSCNH-), δ 1.53 (m, 4H, 2 $OCH_2CH_2(CH_2)_{13}CH_3$), δ2.22 (s, 3H, -H_2CSC-NHC(CH_3)=), δ2.24 (s, 3H, -H_2CSC=N-C(CH_3)=), δ 3.3–3.7 (m, 7H, glyceryl/hexadecyl -CH_2O and -CHO-). Elemental analysis: C 73.78%, H 12.24%, N 4.16%; calculated: C 73.78%, H 12.07%, N 4.30%. Calculated pK_a using ACD/pKa DB software: 6.72 ± 0.5.

4.6. Preparation of ICL Formulations

A dichloromethane solution of an imidazole-based lipid and a chloroform solution of other lipids were mixed in a round-bottom flask. The organic solvents were evaporated under reduced pressure to form a lipidic film at 70 °C. The lipidic film was further dried in a high vacuum for over 4 h at room temperature to remove the residual solvent. The lipidic film was then hydrated with HEPES buffer (pH 7.4, 30 mM HEPES) containing 300 mM $MnSO_4$ by intermittent agitation in a 70 °C water bath under argon to obtain a liposome suspension containing 20 mM total lipids. The liposome suspension was freeze-anneal-thawed by rapidly freezing in liquid nitrogen, immerging in the ice-water mixture for 2 min and incubating in a 70 °C water bath for 4 min. The freeze-anneal-thawing was repeated 11 times. The liposome suspension was sequentially extruded 21 times each through 400 nm, 200 nm and 100 nm polycarbonate membranes (Nucleopore Corp., Pleasanton, CA, USA) using a hand-held Mini-extruder (Avanti Polar Lipids Inc., Alabaster, AL, USA) at 70 °C to reduce and homogenize the size of liposomes. DOX was then loaded into the liposomes as follows, using a transmembrane $MnSO_4$ gradient [45]. The extruded liposomes were separated from the unencapsulated MnSO4 by size exclusion chromatography using a Sephadex G-75 column pre-equilibrated with isotonic HEPES buffer (pH 7.4, 5 mM HEPES, 140 mM NaCl). DOX (0.75 mg/mL) dissolved in the same isotonic HEPES buffer was then mixed with the liposome suspension in a 1:2 (v/v) ratio, and the mixture was incubated in a 70 °C water bath for 90 min. The cation-exchange resin Dowex® 50WX-4, 50–100 mesh was pre-treated with NaOH and NaCl [46], mixed with the DOX-liposome mixture at DOX: resin = 1:60 (w/w), and then shaken gently for 25 min to remove the unencapsulated DOX from the DOX-loaded liposomes. The resin was separated from the DOX-loaded liposomes by filtration. A tangential flow filtration column (MicroKros®, Spectrum, Stamford, CT, USA) was used to concentrate the liposome suspension by partially removing the extra-liposomal buffer. Typically, a 2 mL liposome suspension was extruded 14 times through the tangential flow filtration column to yield a ~0.5 mL concentrated formulation. The lipid composition of the liposomes under study is listed in Table 3.

Table 3. Lipid composition of liposomes under study.

	Mol %					
Formulations	**DHI**	**DHMI**	**DHDMI**	**DSPC**	**DPPE-PEG**	**Chol**
I	25	-	-	70	5	-
II	-	25		70	5	-
III	-	-	25	70	5	-
IV	-	-	-	95	5	-
V	25	-	-	45	5	25
VI	-	25	-	45	5	25
VII	-	-	25	45	5	25
VIII	-	-	-	70	5	25

I–III and V–VII are ICL; IV and VIII are PEGylated, pH-insensitive liposomes as controls; V–VIII contain cholesterol, and I–IV does not contain cholesterol.

4.7. Size Measurement

An aliquot (2.5–5 μL) of a liposome suspension was diluted in 150 μL isotonic buffer, and the size was measured at room temperature by dynamic light scattering (Zetasizer ZS90, Malvern Instruments Ltd., Malvern, UK). The data were analyzed based on light intensity distribution to give hydrodynamic diameters.

4.8. Quantification of Encapsulation Efficiency (EE)

An aliquot (10 μL) of DOX-loaded liposome suspension was lysed with 90 μL lysis buffer (90% (v/v) isopropanol, 0.075 M HCl) [46] in a 96-well Black Clear Bottom Polystyrene microplate (Corning®, NY, USA), together with 10 μL DOX standard solutions diluted in the same lysing buffer (90 μL). The microplate was covered with foil, and the fluorescence of the samples (λ_{ex} = 486 nm, λ_{em} = 590 nm) was recorded on a Synergy HT microplate reader (Biotek, Winooski, VT, USA). The concentration of the payload DOX of liposomes was estimated using a standard calibration curve from the fluorescence of the DOX standard solutions. The encapsulation efficiency (EE) of the liposomes was then calculated by the following formula.

$$EE = \frac{\text{Encapsulated DOX Conc.}}{\text{Input DOX Conc. for drug loading}} \times 100\%$$

4.9. Differential Scanning Calorimetry

A VP-DSC Instrument (MicroCal, LLC, Northampton, MA, USA) was used for the differential scanning calorimetry (DSC) studies. DSC scans were performed on 0.5 mL liposome suspensions containing 2.5 mM total lipids at pH 7.4 and pH 6.0. The thermograms of liposome suspensions were acquired from 40 °C to 75 °C at a scan rate of 5 °C/h. Each excess heat capacity curve of a liposome sample was normalized by subtraction of the thermogram of the buffer acquired simultaneously under identical conditions.

4.10. pH-Triggered Change of ζ-Potential

In order to enhance the detection of changes in liposome surface charge, the liposomes were prepared by hydration in an isotonic buffer of low ionic strength (pH 7.4, 5 mM HEPES, 5% (*w*/*v*) Glucose) [47]. Aliquots (50–100 μL) of the resultant liposome suspensions were diluted in 900 μL isotonic MES buffer (final pH 6.0 and 6.5, 10 mM MES, 5% (*w*/*v*) Glucose) and 900 μL isotonic HEPES buffer (final pH 7.0 and 7.4, 10 mM HEPES, 5% (*w*/*v*) Glucose). The ζ-potential was then measured at 37 °C based on electrophoresis mobility under applied voltage (Zetasizer ZS90, Malvern Instruments Ltd., Malvern, UK).

4.11. pH-Dependent Interaction with Model Liposomes

The model liposomes (POPC:POPE:POPS:L-R-PI:cholesterol = 50:20:5:10:15 (mol%)) mimicking the lipid composition and surface charge of biomembranes were prepared based on a previous report [31]. As measured by Zetasizer ZS90, the mean size of the model liposomes was 192.7 nm in diameter, and the ζ-potential was −51.77 ± 1.18 mV. Suspensions of ICL and pH-insensitive control liposomes were each mixed with the model liposomes at a 1:1 total lipid molar ratio. An aliquot (5 μL) of each mixture was diluted in 150 μL isotonic MES buffer (final pH 6.0 and 6.5, 10 mM MES, 140 mM NaCl) and isotonic HEPES buffer (final pH 7.0 and 7.4, 10 mM HEPES, 140 mM NaCl), and incubated at 37 °C for 5 min. The particle size of the diluted mixtures was measured at 37 °C by dynamic light scattering (Zetasizer ZS90, Malvern Instruments Ltd., Malvern, UK).

4.12. pH-Dependent Drug Release

Each liposome formulation was severally diluted (100 μL aliquots) with 500 μL MES buffer (final pH 6.0 and 6.5, 100 mM MES, 1.7% (*w*/*v*) Glucose) and HEPES buffer (final pH 7.0 and 7.4, 100 mM HEPES, 1.7% (*w*/*v*) Glucose). An aliquot (10 μL) of each diluted liposome formulation was immediately lysed with 90 μL lysis buffer (90% (*v*/*v*) isopropanol, 0.075 M HCl) in a 96-well Black Clear Bottom Polystyrene microplate and the initial DOX concentration C_i (as at the 0-h time point) was qualified with standard DOX solutions. The liposome samples diluted by buffers at various pH (6.0, 6.5, 7.0, 7.4) were then mixed with cation-exchange resin Dowex® 50WX-4 (50–100 mesh) at DOX:resin = 1:200 (*w*/*w*) ratio. The mixtures were incubated and gently shaken at 37 °C. At different time points (1, 3, 6, 12 h), each mixture was allowed to settle briefly, and an aliquot (10 μL) of the resultant supernatant was harvested, lysed, and its DOX concentration measured as mentioned before. The percentage of DOX release was determined by the following equation,

$$\%\ \text{Release} = \left(1 - \frac{C_s}{C_i}\right) \times 100\%$$

where C_s is the concentration of DOX in the supernatant of the liposome-resin mixture at different time points, C_i is the initial liposomal DOX concentration.

4.13. Transmission Electron Microscopy

The morphology of ICL formulations was observed on a JEOL-JEM 1230 Electron Microscope (JEOL, Tokyo, Japan). Carbon-coated copper TEM grids (200 mesh) were subjected to glow discharge before usage to increase their hydrophilicity. An aliquot (5 μL) of diluted ICL suspension (approximately 1 mM total lipids) at pH 7.4 or 6.0 was dripped onto the grid to wet its surface for 1 min and then blotted with filter paper to generate a thin film. The sample film was then wetted five times with 5 μL of the negative stain 2% uranyl acetate (UA) between blotting. The grid was dried at room temperature and then transferred into the electron microscope for imaging at an accelerating voltage of 100 kV. The samples of ICL mixed with model liposomes were prepared and imaged by the same method.

4.14. Cell Culture

Cervical cancer cell line HeLa, lung cancer cell line A549, and breast cancer cell lines MDA-MB-231 and MDA-MB-468 were cultured to construct 3D MCS in order to evaluate the anticancer activities of ICL. Hela cells were also cultured into monolayer cells. HeLa cells were maintained in DMEM media; A549 cells were maintained in RPMI 1640 media; MDA-MB-231 and MDA-MB-468 cells were maintained in advanced DMEM/F12 media. All media were supplemented with 10% fetal bovine serum, 1% Penicillin-Streptomycin, and 1% L-glutamine. All cells were grown in a humidified atmosphere of 5% CO_2 in air at 37 °C and passaged at 85% confluence. In all studies, the cells were sub-cultured every 2–3 days and used for experiments at passages 5–20.

4.15. Cytotoxicity Assays on 2D Monolayer Hela Cells

Monolayer HeLa cells at ~85% confluence were suspended by trypsinization, and the cell density was determined with a Handheld Automated Cell Counter (Millipore, Burlington, MA, USA). The cells were then diluted to ~80,000 cells/mL in complete growth media and seeded into 96-well Clear Microplates (Corning, NY, USA) at ~8000 cells/well by transferring 100 μL of the cell suspension into each well. The cytotoxicity assay was carried out on the cells 8 h after they were seeded. The cells were washed with PBS and treated with DOX-loaded liposomes or free DOX solutions in complete growth media at incremental concentrations. The pH of the media (10 mL) was adjusted to 7.4, 7.0, 6.5, and 6.0 with glacial acetic acid. After 12-h incubation, the media was removed, and the cells were washed with 100 μL PBS buffer and supplemented with 100 μL/well complete growth media and 20 μL/well MTS CellTiter 96® AQueous One Solution. The mixture was incubated for 4 h at 37 °C with 5% CO_2. The cell viability was quantified by UV/visible absorbance at 490 nm on a Synergy HT microplate reader (Biotek, Winooski, VT, USA). The Hela cells treated with growth media at corresponding pHs without free DOX or DOX-loaded liposomes were referred to as 100% cell viability.

4.16. Cytotoxicity Assays on 3D Multicellular Spheroids

Monolayer cells in T75 flasks were trypsinized, and the cell density in the suspensions was determined with a Handheld Automated Cell Counter. The cells were then seeded into 96-well Ultra-low Attachment (ULA) round-bottom microplates (Corning, NY, USA) at ~500 Hela cells/well, ~5000 A549 cells/well, ~3000 MDA-MB-231 cells/well, and ~2000 MDA-MB-468 cells/well by transferring 100 μL properly diluted cell suspensions in complete growth media containing collagen (0% for HeLa, 0.3% for A549, 1% for MDA-MB-231, and 1% for MDA-MB-468 cell lines). If needed, the microplates were centrifuged at 7 °C to promote cell aggregation (Table S1). Complete growth media (100 μL) was added to each well on the second day after seeding. The growth media were then partially exchanged every other day by replacing 100 μL of media in each well with 100 μL fresh media to maintain a 200 μL/well total media volume. The cytotoxicity assays were carried out on selected MCS whose diameter reached or exceeded 500 μm (Figure S3) [48,49]. Part of the growth media (100 μL/well) was replaced with the same volume of DOX-loaded liposomes or free DOX solutions in complete growth media at incremental concentrations. After 72 h incubation, each MCS was transferred into a well of a 96-well Solid White microplate (Corning, NY, USA) together with 100 μL media. Then, 100 μL reagent of the CellTiter-Glo 3D cell viability assay was then added to each well, and the microplate was covered with foil, shaken on an orbital shaker for 5 min, and then incubated for 25 min at room temperature. The viability of MCS was then measured by luminescence intensity on a Synergy HT microplate reader (Biotek, Winooski, VT, USA). The MCS treated by growth media without free DOX or DOX-loaded liposomes was referred to as 100% cell viability.

5. Conclusions

Novel imidazole-based convertible liposomes (ICL) have been designed and constructed. ICL carries a PEG-coating and slight excess of negative surface charges at pH 7.4. As pH decreased to 6.0, the imidazole-based lipids assumed positive charges and clustered with negatively charged PE-PEG conjugates in ICL, which in turn partially de-PEGylated the liposomes to enhance their adsorption to negatively charged, bio-mimetic membranes. The drop of pH to 6.0 also enhanced the release of the anticancer drug DOX from ICL that consisted of the imidazole lipid DHMI (>50% release in 6 h), but not those of the other two imidazole-based lipids. TEM studies suggest that DHMI enhanced the drug release from ICL due to its ability to convert the liposomal membrane into non-lamellar structures. The incorporation of cholesterol improved the colloidal stability of ICL but diminished their pH-sensitivity. ICL demonstrated substantially higher anticancer activities than the analogous PEGylated, pH-insensitive liposomes containing doxorubicin, which is a common type of nano-formulations in clinical use. While the anticancer activities of ICL against monolayer Hela cells are correlated with higher pKa of the imidazole lipid, the anticancer activities against 3D multicellular spheroids are the highest in ICL that consisted of the imidazole lipid DHMI, which possesses the medium pKa and enhances the liposomal drug release at pH 6.0. Our studies on ICL suggest that nano-drug delivery systems that balance the needs of intratumoral penetration, adsorption to cancer cells, and enhanced drug release would yield optimal anticancer activities.

Supplementary Materials: The following supporting information can be downloaded at: https://www.mdpi.com/article/10.3390/ph15030306/s1, Figure S1: DART Mass Spectra of imidazole-based lipids DHI (A), DHMI (B), and DHDMI (C); Figure S2: 1H-NMR Spectra (600 MHz, CDCl3) of imidazole-based lipids DHI (A), DHMI (B), and DHDMI (C); Figure S3: Representative morphology of MCS with a diameter of ~500 μm in the ULA 96-well microplates for anticancer drug treatment; Figure S4: Representative confocal images of 3D MCS for intra-MCS pH measurements; Table S1: Conditions to culture 3D MCS of cancer cells; Table S2: Calculated pH in 3D MCS of Hela, A549, and MDA-MB-468 cancer cells based on fluorescent images of confocal microscopy.

Author Contributions: Conceptualization, X.G.; methodology, R.H., V.G., S.Z., Y.L. and X.G.; validation, X.G., R.H. and Y.L.; formal analysis, R.H., V.G. and Y.L.; investigation, R.H., V.G., S.Z. and Y.L.; resources, X.G.; writing—original draft preparation, R.H. and V.G.; writing—review and editing, X.G.; supervision, X.G.; project administration, X.G.; funding acquisition, X.G. All authors have read and agreed to the published version of the manuscript.

Funding: This research received no external funding.

Institutional Review Board Statement: Not applicable.

Informed Consent Statement: Not applicable.

Data Availability Statement: Data is contained within the article and Supplementary Materials.

Acknowledgments: The fluorescence, UV absorbance and luminescence intensity were quantified with the Synergy HT microplate reader from John C. Livesey (Department of Physiology and Pharmacology, University of the Pacific). The cells for MCS construction were centrifuged in the lab of William K. Chan (Department of Pharmaceutics and Medicinal Chemistry, University of the Pacific). The TEM study was carried with the help from Fei Guo (Technical Director of Department of Molecular and Cellular Biology, UC Davis) at the BioEM Facility, which is supported by discretionary funds from Professor Jodi Nunnari (MCB) and a grant provided by NIH R00-GM080249 (J. Al-Bassam). The DSC experiments were carried out at San Jose State University in Daryl Eggers' lab (instrumental support from the National Science Foundation, CHE-0723278).

Conflicts of Interest: The authors declare no conflict of interest.

References

1. U.S. Food and Drug Administration Resources on Drugs and Devices. Available online: https://clinicaltrials.gov/ct2/info/fdalinks (accessed on 8 February 2022).
2. Anselmo, A.C.; Mitragotri, S. Nanoparticles in the clinic. *Bioeng. Transl. Med.* **2016**, *1*, 10–29. [CrossRef] [PubMed]
3. Anselmo, A.C.; Mitragotri, S. Nanoparticles in the clinic: An update. *Bioeng. Transl. Med.* **2019**, *4*, e10143. [CrossRef] [PubMed]
4. Bulbake, U.; Doppalapudi, S.; Kommineni, N.; Khan, W. Liposomal Formulations in Clinical Use: An Updated Review. *Pharmaceutics* **2017**, *9*, 12. [CrossRef] [PubMed]
5. Beltrán-Gracia, E.; López-Camacho, A.; Higuera-Ciapara, I.; Velázquez-Fernández, J.B.; Vallejo-Cardona, A.A. Nanomedicine review: Clinical developments in liposomal applications. *Cancer Nanotechnol.* **2019**, *10*, 11. [CrossRef]
6. Wang, R.; Billone, P.S.; Mullett, W.M. Nanomedicine in Action: An Overview of Cancer Nanomedicine on the Market and in Clinical Trials. *J. Nanomater.* **2013**, *2013*, 629681. [CrossRef]
7. Gabizon, A.; Shmeeda, H.; Barenholz, Y. Pharmacokinetics of Pegylated Liposomal Doxorubicin. *Clin. Pharmacokinet.* **2003**, *42*, 419–436. [CrossRef]
8. Immordino, M.L.; Dosio, F.; Cattel, L. Stealth liposomes: Review of the basic science, rationale, and clinical applications, existing and potential. *Int. J. Nanomed.* **2006**, *1*, 297–315.
9. Millard, M.; Yakavets, I.; Zorin, V.; Kulmukhamedova, A.; Marchal, S.; Bezdetnaya, L. Drug delivery to solid tumors: The predictive value of the multicellular tumor spheroid model for nanomedicine screening. *Int. J. Nanomed.* **2017**, *12*, 7993–8007. [CrossRef]
10. Vladimir, T. Tumor delivery of macromolecular drugs based on the EPR effect. *Adv. Drug Deliv. Rev.* **2011**, *63*, 131–135. [CrossRef]
11. Kommineni, N.; Mahira, S.; Domb, A.J.; Khan, W. Cabazitaxel-Loaded Nanocarriers for Cancer Therapy with Reduced Side Effects. *Pharmaceutics* **2019**, *11*, 141. [CrossRef]
12. Maeda, H. Toward a full understanding of the EPR effect in primary and metastatic tumors as well as issues related to its heterogeneity. *Adv. Drug Deliv. Rev.* **2015**, *91*, 3–6. [CrossRef] [PubMed]
13. Reshetnyak, Y.K. Imaging tumor acidity: pH-low insertion peptide probe for optoacoustic tomography. *Clin. Cancer Res.* **2015**, *21*, 4502–4504. [CrossRef] [PubMed]
14. Zagaynova, E.V.; Druzhkova, I.N.; Mishina, N.M.; Ignatova, N.I.; Dudenkova, V.V.; Shirmanova, M.V. Imaging of intracellular pH in tumor spheroids using genetically encoded sensor SypHer2. In *Multi-Parametric Live Cell Microscopy of 3D Tissue Models*; Springer: Berlin/Heidelberg, Germany, 2017; pp. 105–119.
15. Warburg, O.; Wind, F.; Negelein, E. The metabolism of tumors in the body. *J. Gen. Physiol.* **1927**, *8*, 519–530. [CrossRef]
16. Drummond, D.C.; Zignani, M.; Leroux, J.-C. Current status of pH-sensitive liposomes in drug delivery. *Prog. Lipid Res.* **2000**, *39*, 409–460. [CrossRef]
17. Fang, Y.; Vadlamudi, M.; Huang, Y.; Guo, X. Lipid-Coated, pH-Sensitive Magnesium Phosphate Particles for Intracellular Protein Delivery. *Pharm. Res.* **2019**, *36*, 81. [CrossRef]
18. Zheng, Y.; Liu, X.; Samoshina, N.M.; Samoshin, V.V.; Franz, A.H.; Guo, X. Fliposomes: Trans-2-aminocyclohexanol-based amphiphiles as pH-sensitive conformational switches of liposome membrane—A structure-activity relationship study. *Chem. Phys. Lipids* **2017**, *210*, 129–141. [CrossRef]
19. He, X.; Li, J.; An, S.; Jiang, C. pH-sensitive drug-delivery systems for tumor targeting. *Ther. Deliv.* **2013**, *4*, 1499–1510. [CrossRef]
20. Liu, J.; Huang, Y.; Kumar, A.; Tan, A.; Jin, S.; Mozhi, A.; Liang, X.J. pH-sensitive nano-systems for drug delivery in cancer therapy. *Biotechnol. Adv.* **2014**, *32*, 693–710. [CrossRef]
21. Oya, T.A.; Ishiyama, A.A.; Nishikawa, N.A. Imidazole Compound and Liposome Containing Same. European Patent EP 3170812A1, 2017. Available online: https://data.epo.org/publication-server/document?iDocId=5335445&iFormat=0 (accessed on 8 February 2022).
22. Chatin, B.; Mével, M.; Devallière, J.; Dallet, L.; Haudebourg, T.; Peuziat, P.; Colombani, T.; Berchel, M.; Lambert, O.; Edelman, A.; et al. Liposome-based Formulation for Intracellular Delivery of Functional Proteins. *Mol. Ther. Nucleic Acids* **2015**, *4*, e244. [CrossRef]
23. He, J.; Xu, S.; Mixson, A.J. The Multifaceted Histidine-Based Carriers for Nucleic Acid Delivery: Advances and Challenges. *Pharmaceutics* **2020**, *12*, 774. [CrossRef]

24. Ju, L.; Cailin, F.; Wenlan, W.; Pinghua, Y.; Jiayu, G.; Junbo, L. Preparation and properties evaluation of a novel pH-sensitive liposomes based on imidazole-modified cholesterol derivatives. *Int. J. Pharm.* **2017**, *518*, 213–219. [CrossRef] [PubMed]
25. Däster, S.; Amatruda, N.; Calabrese, D.; Ivanek, R.; Turrini, E.; Droeser, R.A.; Zajac, P.; Fimognari, C.; Spagnoli, G.C.; Iezzi, G.; et al. Induction of hypoxia and necrosis in multicellular tumor spheroids is associated with resistance to chemotherapy treatment. *Oncotarget* **2017**, *8*, 1725–1736. [CrossRef] [PubMed]
26. Miller, C.R.; Bondurant, B.; McLean, S.D.; McGovern, K.A.; O'Brien, D.F. Liposome−Cell Interactions in Vitro: Effect of Liposome Surface Charge on the Binding and Endocytosis of Conventional and Sterically Stabilized Liposomes. *Biochemistry* **1998**, *37*, 12875–12883. [CrossRef] [PubMed]
27. Brazdova, B.; Zhang, N.; Samoshin, V.V.; Guo, X. trans-2-Aminocyclohexanol as a pH-sensitive conformational switch in lipid amphiphiles. *Chem. Commun.* **2008**, *39*, 4774–4776. [CrossRef]
28. Samoshina, N.M.; Liu, X.; Brazdova, B.; Franz, A.H.; Samoshin, V.V.; Guo, X. Fliposomes: pH-Sensitive Liposomes Containing a trans-2-morpholinocyclohexanol-Based Lipid That Performs a Conformational Flip and Triggers an Instant Cargo Release in Acidic Medium. *Pharmaceutics* **2011**, *3*, 379–405. [CrossRef]
29. Nakhaei, P.; Margiana, R.; Bokov, D.O.; Abdelbasset, W.K.; Kouhbanani, M.A.J.; Varma, R.S.; Marofi, F.; Jarahian, M.; Beheshtkhoo, N. Liposomes: Structure, Biomedical Applications, and Stability Parameters with Emphasis on Cholesterol. *Front. Bioeng. Biotechnol.* **2021**, *9*, 705886. [CrossRef]
30. Briuglia, M.-L.; Rotella, C.M.; McFarlane, A.; Lamprou, D.A. Influence of cholesterol on liposome stability and on in vitro drug release. *Drug Deliv. Transl. Res.* **2015**, *5*, 231–242. [CrossRef]
31. Chen, H.; Zhang, H.; McCallum, C.M.; Szoka, F.C.; Guo, X. Unsaturated Cationic Ortho Esters for Endosome Permeation in Gene Delivery. *J. Med. Chem.* **2007**, *50*, 4269–4278. [CrossRef]
32. Ting-Beall, H.P. Interactions of uranyl ions with lipid bilayer membranes. *J. Microsc.* **1980**, *118*, 221–227. [CrossRef]
33. Koyama, T.M.; Stevens, C.R.; Borda, E.J.; Grobe, K.J.; Cleary, D.A. Characterizing the Gel to Liquid Crystal Transition in Lipid-Bilayer Model Systems. *Chem. Educ.* **1999**, *4*, 12–15. [CrossRef]
34. Anderson, M.; Moshnikova, A.; Engelman, D.M.; Reshetnyak, Y.K.; Andreev, O.A. Probe for the measurement of cell surface pH in vivo and ex vivo. *Proc. Natl. Acad. Sci. USA* **2016**, *113*, 8177–8181. [CrossRef] [PubMed]
35. Cody, S.H.; Dubbin, P.N.; Beischer, A.D.; Duncan, N.D.; Hill, J.S.; Kaye, A.H.; Williams, D.A. Intracellular pH mapping with SNARF-1 and confocal microscopy. I: A quantitative technique for living tissue and isolated cells. *Micron* **1993**, *24*, 573–580. [CrossRef]
36. Sun, B.; Leem, C.H.; Vaughan-Jones, R.D. Novel chloride-dependent acid loader in the guinea-pig ventricular myocyte: Part of a dual acid-loading mechanism. *J. Physiol.* **1996**, *495*, 65–82. [CrossRef] [PubMed]
37. Matsumura, Y.; Maeda, H. A new concept for macromolecular therapeutics in cancer chemotherapy: Mechanism of tumoritropic accumulation of proteins and the antitumor agent smancs. *Cancer Res.* **1986**, *46*, 6387–6392.
38. Fonseca, M.; van Winden, E.; Crommelin, D. Doxorubicin induces aggregation of small negatively charged liposomes. *Eur. J. Pharm. Biopharm.* **1997**, *43*, 9–17. [CrossRef]
39. Anderson, M.; Omri, A. The Effect of Different Lipid Components on the In Vitro Stability and Release Kinetics of Liposome Formulations. *Drug Deliv.* **2004**, *11*, 33–39. [CrossRef]
40. Anders, C.B.; Baker, J.D.; Stahler, A.C.; Williams, A.J.; Sisco, J.N.; Trefry, J.C.; Wooley, D.P.; Sizemore, I.E.P. Tangential Flow Ultrafiltration: A "Green" Method for the Size Selection and Concentration of Colloidal Silver Nanoparticles. *J. Vis. Exp.* **2012**, *68*, e4167. [CrossRef]
41. Corvera, E.; Mouritsen, O.; Singer, M.; Zuckermann, M. The permeability and the effect of acyl-chain length for phospholipid bilayers containing cholesterol: Theory and experiment. *Biochim. Biophys. Acta Biomembr.* **1992**, *1107*, 261–270. [CrossRef]
42. Huang, J. Exploration of Molecular Interactions in Cholesterol Superlattices: Effect of Multibody Interactions. *Biophys. J.* **2002**, *83*, 1014–1025. [CrossRef]
43. Magarkar, A.; Dhawan, V.; Kallinteri, P.; Viitala, T.; Elmowafy, M.; Róg, T.; Bunker, A. Cholesterol level affects surface charge of lipid membranes in saline solution. *Sci. Rep.* **2014**, *4*, 5005. [CrossRef]
44. Yan, Y.; Rubinchik, S.; Wood, A.L.; Gillanders, W.E.; Dong, J.-Y.; Watson, D.K.; Cole, D.J. Bystander Effect Contributes to the Antitumor Efficacy of CaSm Antisense Gene Therapy in a Preclinical Model of Advanced Pancreatic Cancer. *Mol. Ther.* **2006**, *13*, 357–365. [CrossRef] [PubMed]
45. Cheung, B.C.; Sun, T.H.; Leenhouts, J.M.; Cullis, P.R. Loading of doxorubicin into liposomes by forming Mn2+-drug complexes. *Biochim. Biophys. Acta Biomembr.* **1998**, *1414*, 205–216. [CrossRef]
46. Amselem, S.; Barenholz, Y.; Gabizon, A. Optimization and Upscaling of Doxorubicin-Containing Liposomes for Clinical Use. *J. Pharm. Sci.* **1990**, *79*, 1045–1052. [CrossRef] [PubMed]
47. Carneiro-Da-Cunha, M.G.; Cerqueira, M.A.; Souza, B.W.; Teixeira, J.A.; Vicente, A.A. Influence of concentration, ionic strength and pH on zeta potential and mean hydrodynamic diameter of edible polysaccharide solutions envisaged for multinanolayered films production. *Carbohydr. Polym.* **2011**, *85*, 522–528. [CrossRef]

48. Cox, M.C.; Reese, L.M.; Bickford, L.R.; Verbridge, S.S. Toward the Broad Adoption of 3D Tumor Models in the Cancer Drug Pipeline. *ACS Biomater. Sci. Eng.* **2015**, *1*, 877–894. [CrossRef]
49. Huang, Y.; Wang, S.; Guo, Q.; Kessel, S.; Rubinoff, I.; Chan, L.L.-Y.; Li, P.; Liu, Y.; Qiu, J.; Zhou, C. Optical Coherence Tomography Detects Necrotic Regions and Volumetrically Quantifies Multicellular Tumor Spheroids. *Cancer Res.* **2017**, *77*, 6011–6020. [CrossRef]

pharmaceuticals

Article

Development of Dapagliflozin Solid Lipid Nanoparticles as a Novel Carrier for Oral Delivery: Statistical Design, Optimization, In-Vitro and In-Vivo Characterization, and Evaluation

Aziz Unnisa [1,*], Ananda K. Chettupalli [2], Turki Al Hagbani [3], Mohammad Khalid [4], Suresh B. Jandrajupalli [5], Swarnalatha Chandolu [5] and Talib Hussain [6]

1 Department of Pharmaceutical Chemistry, College of Pharmacy, University of Hail, Hail 81442, Saudi Arabia
2 Department of Pharmaceutical Sciences, School of Pharmacy, Anurag University, Hyderabad 500088, India; anandphd88@gmail.com
3 Department of Pharmaceutics, College of Pharmacy, University of Hail, Hail 81442, Saudi Arabia; t.alhagbani@uoh.edu.sa
4 Department of Pharmacognosy, College of Pharmacy, Prince Sattam Bin Abdulaziz University, Al-Kharj 11942, Saudi Arabia; m.khalid@psau.edu.sa
5 Department of Preventive Dental Sciences, College of Dentistry, University of Hail, Hail 81442, Saudi Arabia; s.jandrajupalli@uoh.edu.sa (S.B.J.); s.chandolu@uoh.edu.sa (S.C.)
6 Department of Pharmacology and Toxicology, College of Pharmacy, University of Hail, Hail 81442, Saudi Arabia; mdth_ah@yahoo.com
* Correspondence: khushiazeez@yahoo.co.in; Tel.: +966-537860207

Citation: Unnisa, A.; Chettupalli, A.K.; Al Hagbani, T.; Khalid, M.; Jandrajupalli, S.B.; Chandolu, S.; Hussain, T. Development of Dapagliflozin Solid Lipid Nanoparticles as a Novel Carrier for Oral Delivery: Statistical Design, Optimization, In-Vitro and In-Vivo Characterization, and Evaluation. *Pharmaceuticals* **2022**, *15*, 568. https://doi.org/10.3390/ph15050568

Academic Editors: Ana Catarina Silva, João Nuno Moreira and José Manuel Sousa Lobo

Received: 20 February 2022
Accepted: 21 April 2022
Published: 2 May 2022

Abstract: Controlling hyperglycemia and avoiding glucose reabsorption are significant goals in type 2 diabetes treatments. Among the numerous modes of medication administration, the oral route is the most common. Introduction: Dapagliflozin is an oral hypoglycemic agent and a powerful, competitive, reversible, highly selective, and orally active human SGLT2 inhibitor. Dapagliflozin-loaded solid lipid nanoparticles (SLNs) are the focus of our present investigation. Controlled-release lipid nanocarriers were formulated by integrating them into lipid nanocarriers. The nanoparticle size and lipid utilized for formulation help to regulate the release of pharmaceuticals over some time. Dapagliflozin-loaded nanoparticles were formulated by hot homogenization followed by ultra-sonication. The morphology and physicochemical properties of dapagliflozin-SLNs have been characterized using various techniques. The optimized dapagliflozin-SLNs have a particle size ranging from 100.13 ± 7.2 to 399.08 ± 2.4 nm with 68.26 ± 0.2 to 94.46 ± 0.7% entrapment efficiency (%EE). Dapagliflozin-SLNs were optimized using a three-factor, three-level Box–Behnken design (BBD). Polymer concentration (X1), surfactant concentration (X2), and stirring duration (X3) were chosen as independent factors, whereas %EE, cumulative drug release (%CDR), and particle size were selected as dependent variables. Interactions between drug substances and polymers were studied using Fourier transform infrared spectroscopy (FTIR) and scanning electron microscopy (SEM). Differential scanning calorimetry (DSC), X-ray diffraction (XRD), and atomic force microscopy (AFM) analysis indicated the crystalline change from the drug to the amorphous crystal. Electron microscope studies revealed that the SLNs' structure is nearly perfectly round. It is evident from the findings that dapagliflozin-SLNs could lower elevated blood glucose levels to normal in STZ-induced diabetic rats, demonstrating a better hypoglycemic impact on type 2 diabetic patients. The in vivo pharmacokinetic parameters of SLNs exhibited a significant rise in C_{max} (1258.37 ± 1.21 mcg/mL), AUC (5247.04 mcg/mL), and oral absorption (2-fold) of the drug compared to the marketed formulation in the Sprague Dawley rats.

Keywords: dapagliflozin; solid lipid nanoparticles; Box–Behnken design; FTIR; DSC; XRD; SEM; AFM; in vitro Franz diffusion cells

1. Introduction

The Food and Drug Administration (FDA) approved dapagliflozin in 2014 as a novel oral hypoglycemic medication. In terms of structure, it is a tetrahydro-2H-pyran-3, 4, 5-triol fitting to the gliflozin family of compounds. Type 2 diabetes mellitus (T2DM) is currently treated with this drug. Dapagliflozin's poor oral bioavailability is due to its poor solubility and stability [1]. Dapagliflozin increases urine glucose excretion and lowers blood glucose levels by blocking the transporter protein sodium-glucose co-transporter-2 (SGLT2) in the proximal renal tubule, inhibiting renal glucose reabsorption. Extensive follow-up periods of 1–4 years suggested that the dapagliflozin effects are sustained, and the drug is typically well-tolerated, making it a desirable therapy of choice.

Increased blood sugar levels (>70–110 mg/dL) are connected with the peril of microvascular impairment such as nephropathy, neuropathy, and retinopathy in T2DM [2,3]. About 95% of T2DM cases are found in the elderly, caused by genetics, fat, and lifestyle habits [4]. Anti-diabetic medications are currently used to treat diabetes, and their mechanisms include an increase in insulin production, lowering insulin resistance, and blocking glucose reabsorption from the Henley loop [5].

Researchers have observed various lipid-based nano preparations for improving the solubility, absorption, and dissolution characteristics of poorly soluble substances [6–8]. The SLNs have a nano size, a unique structure, a tall drug loading capacity, are biocompatible [9,10], and improve lipophilic drug absorption while also achieving effective concentration at the receptor location [11]. SLNs can bypass the apical transporter protein and enhance the therapeutic permeability [12]. They protect drugs from acidic breakdown and improve drug absorption into the vascular system [13]. The physicochemical properties of SLNs are greatly affected by several reactions such as particle size, %EE, %CDR, and loading efficiency [14].

SLNs, a possible nanotechnology-based drug delivery method, have been identified [15]. The advantages of conventional colloidal carriers should be combined with SLNs while the disadvantages are avoided. Drug targeting and controlled drug release are two highlighted benefits [16]. With an increased pharmacodynamics profile and improved drug efficacy, the carrier is biodegradable and may be used to incorporate both lipophilic and hydrophilic drugs [17].

Hadgraft et al., 2001 and Patel et al., 2012 suggested incorporating Compritol 888 ATO, a chylomicron-forming chemical, in the formulation of SLNs which enhanced glibenclamide bioavailability [18,19]. The improved bioavailability of the medication was attributed to the SLNs' decreased efflux transport and increased surface area [18].

Dapagliflozin-loaded nanostructured lipid carriers (NLCs) were developed by Ameeduz Zafar et al., 2020 to improve oral administration. Dapagliflozin had a twofold release pattern, with a quick initial release followed by a 24 h steady-state release. In another investigation by Kazi et al., 2021, the self-nano emulsifying drug delivery systems (SNEDDS) were used to produce an oral combination dose for two anti-diabetic drugs. Dapagliflozin oral absorption in the rat model was two times more with SNEDDS than with the commercially available drug, as shown by in-vivo pharmacokinetic parameters C_{max}, AUC, and oral absorption. Anti-diabetic trials demonstrated that SNEDDS significantly reduced glucose levels in diabetic mice [19].

Many researchers have reported using various statistical designs (central composite design (CCD), Box–Behnken design (BBD), D-optimal, Taguchi, 2-level factorial, Placket Burman) for formulation optimization [20–23], as it reduces the number of trials and saves time. BBD design is an innovative method for formulation optimization. The response surfaces methodology aims to understand the influence of fundamental elements on the response and attain optimal formulations that produce the desired results [24].

SLNs were explicitly created for this research to enhance dapagliflozin oral administration. SLNs were formulated using the hot homogenization approach. The dapagliflozin-loaded SLNs were produced by combining heat homogenization with ultrasonic agitation. SLNs properties such as size, distribution, surface charge, and entrapment effectiveness were analyzed. The optimized formulation will be further assessed for solid-state characterization, drug release, in vivo anti-diabetic, and biochemical evaluation.

2. Results

2.1. Design of Dapagliflozin-SLNs

2.1.1. Solubility of Dapagliflozin in Lipids

The highest solubility of dapagliflozin was used to choose solid lipids for the development of SLNs. Figure 1A shows the solubility profile of dapagliflozin in various lipids. The order of dapagliflozin's solubility in different solid lipids was observed as Compritol 888 ATO, Precirol ATO55, glyceryl monostearate, stearic acid, palmitic acid, and myristic acid. Compritol 888 ATO was preferred as the best solid lipid for manufacturing dapagliflozin-SLNs because it had the maximum partitioning of dapagliflozin [25].

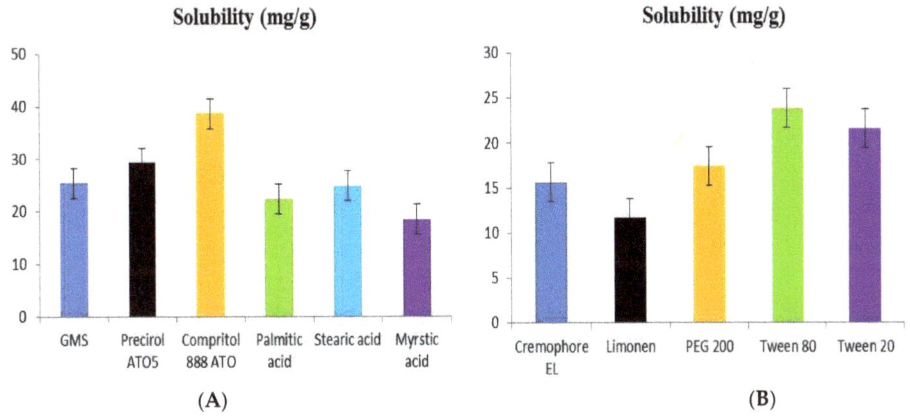

Figure 1. Determination of the solubility of (**A**) solid lipids, (**B**) surfactants.

2.1.2. Selection of Surfactant

The screening of surfactants was done based on dapagliflozin solubility. The solubility profile of dapagliflozin in different surfactants is shown in Figure 1B. The order of solubility of dapagliflozin in surfactant is Tween 80 $\geq$ Tween 20 $\geq$ PEG200 $\geq$ Cremophore EL $\geq$ Limonene. Tween 80 was selected for the formulation of dapagliflozin-SLNs as the drug exhibited the highest solubility in Tween 80 [26].

2.1.3. Selection of Sonication Time and Amplitude

Larger particles were observed at 20% amplitude compared to 40% and 50% amplitude when sonication was done for 5 min. This could be due to a lack of proper sonication time and amplitude. Whereas particle size achieved at 40% amplitude was 200 nm after 2 min of sonication time only, and a larger particle size was seen at 20% and 50% amplitude with a sonication time of 2 min, the accurate amplitude was discovered to be 40%; at an amplitude of 20%, sonication remains incomplete, and above this level (at 50%), the formulation begins to form aggregates. %EE was shown to diminish as the amplitude and sonication duration was increased steadily. As a result, the appropriate amplitude and sonication time were 40% and 2 min, respectively, which were chosen to prepare SLNs [27].

2.2. Preparation and Characterization of Dapagliflozin-SLNs

Dapagliflozin-SLNs were formulated using the modified high shear homogenization and ultrasonication method, after screening different concentrations of solid lipids, surfactants, and sonication time by applying hot a homogenization process with an ultrasonic phase method, as the drug exhibited enhanced solubility in the molten lipid state. It is a pretty straightforward and repeatable procedure. Seventeen batches of dapagliflozin-loaded SLNs were made using a BBD, with three independent variables: lipid content (X1), surfactant concentration (% *w/v*) (X2), and sonication time (X3). Table 1 shows the findings of using %EE, % CDR, and particle size as dependent variables: formulation composition of dapagliflozin SLNs using statistical BBD against independent and dependent variables [28].

Table 1. Experimental runs conducted using BBD and values obtained for various parameters.

	Independent Variables			Dependent Variables				
F. Code	X1 (% *w/v*)	X2 (% *w/v*)	X3 (min)	Y1 (%EE)	Y2 (CDR %)	Y3 (PS) (nm)	Zeta	PDI
F1	+1	0	−1	92.06 ± 1.2	75.13 ± 2.8	280.23 ± 8.9	−27.8 ± 1.01	0.45 ± 0.05
F2	0	0	0	86.08 ± 2.3	86.06 ± 2.4	190.13 ± 4.6	−26.4 ± 0.62	0.56 ± 0.01
F3	0	−1	+1	75.31 ± 0.5	88.08 ± 0.7	189.08 ± 4.2	−22.5 ± 0.72	0.42 ± 0.06
F4	−1	−1	0	79.10 ± 0.7	89.28 ± 0.2	150.37 ± 4.6	−35.8 ± 0.22	0.37 ± 0.01
F5	+1	0	+1	68.26 ± 0.2	83.34 ± 1.1	398.49 ± 2.1	−33.4 ± 0.62	0.41 ± 0.02
F6	+1	+1	0	82.34 ± 1.8	76.29 ± 1.8	199.05 ± 2.8	−31.9 ± 1.64	0.80 ± 0.07
F7	−1	+1	0	84.61 ± 0.4	65.43 ± 2.7	320.11 ± 8.4	−38.7 ± 1.06	0.58 ± 0.01
F8	+1	−1	0	76.81 ± 2.8	77.09 ± 3.5	162.18 ± 6.2	−30.9 ± 0.62	0.41 ± 0.02
F9	0	0	0	87.12 ± 0.6	87.29 ± 4.1	210.12 ± 3.7	−33.5 ± 0.92	0.47 ± 0.01
F10	−1	0	−1	78.84 ± 1.5	73.73 ± 1.9	399.08 ± 2.4	−29.7 ± 1.08	0.80 ± 0.07
F11	0	0	0	86.09 ± 1.1	86.26 ± 3.7	202.23 ± 5.4	−28.7 ± 0.62	0.92 ± 0.10
F12	**0**	**−1**	**0**	**94.46 ± 0.7**	**99.08 ± 0.4**	**100.13 ± 7.2**	**−34.4 ± 1.64**	**0.32 ± 0.02**
F13	0	0	−1	88.21 ± 0.2	84.26 ± 2.4	220.29 ± 5.1	−25.6±1.13	0.58 ± 0.01
F14	0	+1	−1	89.37 ± 1.6	62.83 ± 5.1	278.84 ± 4.9	−31.1 ± 0.72	0.82 ± 0.04
F15	0	0	−1	86.31 ± 0.5	86.13 ± 2.4	198.29 ± 3.4	−30.4 ± 1.44	0.80 ± 0.07
F16	−1	0	+1	87.94 ± 0.2	88.07 ± 1.5	355.71 ± 0.9	−32.3 ± 1.61	0.47 ± 0.01
F17	0	+1	+1	89.29 ± 1.5	87.01 ± 2.8	315.25 ± 3.4	−29.1 ± 0.62	0.41 ± 0.02

2.2.1. Effect of Independent Variables on %EE

The centrifugation technique was used to estimate the %EE of each experimental run of dapagliflozin-SLNs, and the findings are shown in Table 1. The impacts of variables on the %EE were shown using the polynomial equation, 3D plots, and contour plots, and the %EE was found to be in the range of 68.26 ± 0.2–94.46 ± 0.7% (Figure 2). A 2 to 5% increase in lipid concentration causes an increase in EE. The %EE increased due to the increased space for drugs in the lipid matrix. On %EE, Tween 80 showed biphasic character. Dapagliflozin increased solubility and reduced drug partition in the aqueous phase, causing an increase in %EE [29,30]. Further increase in concentration resulted in the development of micelles and an increase in dapagliflozin solubility in the aqueous phase system, and a decrease in %EE. Particle breakdown and medication leaching occur [31,32]. As a result, the %EE decreased.

$$EE = +86.40 - 1.25A + 2.50B - 4.25C + 0.2500AB - 8.25AC + 4.75BC - 5.82A^2 - 0.3250B^2 + 0.6750C^2$$

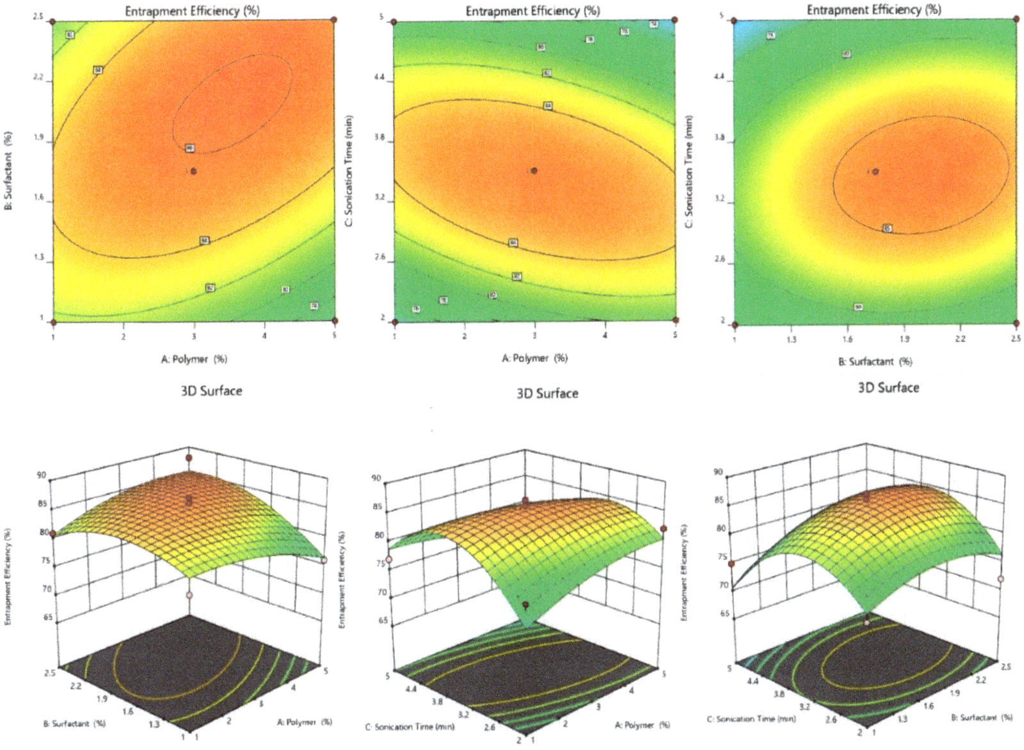

Figure 2. Effect of independent variables on %EE counterplots and 3D response surface plots.

The F-value of 150.25 for the model indicates that it is significant. An F-value of this magnitude has a 0.01% chance of occurring due to noise. A, B, C, AC, BC, and A^2 are important model terms in this situation. The F-value of 50.86 for the Lack of Fit indicates that it is not significant compared to the pure error. Due to noise, a significant Lack of Fit F-value has a 10.18% chance of occurring. It is okay if there is a minor mismatch. The Adjusted R^2 of 0.993 is reasonably close to the Predicted R^2 of 0.916, i.e., the difference is less than 0.2. Adeq Precision measures the signal-to-noise ratio. It is preferable to have a ratio of more than four. The signal-to-noise ratio of 46.18 suggests a good signal. The design space can be navigated using this concept. The lipid concentration variable was slightly negative, indicating that as the drug concentration was increased beyond a certain point, %EE dropped, possibly due to the lipid's inability to load a significant amount of drug. The positive coefficient of B implies that increased %EE leads to increased surfactant concentration. This could be due to the extra scope offered by acylglycerols for medicines to become entrapped. Although the lipid's water solubility increased as the sonication time increased, %EE dropped. However, our research discovered that increasing surfactant content enhanced %EE. The growing effect is due to Tween 80, as previously discussed. It is also possible that stabilizer affects %EE [33].

2.2.2. Effect of Independent Variables on %CDR

Before pharmacological testing, determining %CDR is critical for evaluating drug release from optimized SLN formulations [34]. In all formulations, the %CDR ranged from 62.83 ± 5.1 to 99.08 ± 0.4. (Table 1). For various levels of surfactant concentrations, it was seen that %CDR increased as phospholipid concentrations climbed. This variance in %CDR followed the same pattern as the change in % EE. As a result, the particle size, %EE, and %CDR of dapagliflozin-SLNs are thought to be intensely dependent on the polymer content, surfactant, and stirring speed.

$$\%CDR = +86.40 + 0.500A - 6.75B + 5.75C + 5.75AB - 1.75AC + 6.75BC - 5.83A^2 - 3.83B^2 - 0.8250C^2$$

At 24 h, there was an inverse link between surfactant concentration and %CDR. The decrease in drug release could be caused by an increase in lipid concentration, which causes nanoparticles to grow in size, reducing the effective surface area available to interact with the release medium. Furthermore, as the size of the nanoparticles grows, the length of the drug's diffusion from organic to the aqueous phase grows, lowering drug release. The capacity of surfactant to reduce particle size and enhance surface area and drug release could explain an enhancement in drug release with growing lipid content [29].

The significance of the model is indicated by the Model F-value of 54.26. Model terms with p-values less than 0.05 are significant. B, C, AB, AC, BC, A^2, and B^2 are essential to model terms in this case. The model terms are not necessary if the value is bigger than 0.1. The F-value of 2.78 for the Lack of Fit indicates that it is insignificant to the pure error. Due to noise, a significant Lack of Fit F-value has a 15.64% chance of occurring. It is okay if there is a minor mismatch. The Adjusted R^2 of 0.945 is reasonably close to the Predicted R^2 of 0.920; the difference is less than 0.2. Adeq Precision measures the signal-to-noise ratio. A ratio of more than four is desirable. Your signal-to-noise ratio of 48.870 indicates a good signal. The design space can be navigated using this concept [30].

2.2.3. Effect of Independent Variables on Particle Size

Dapagliflozin-SLNs have particle sizes that vary from 100.13 ± 7.2 to 399.08 ± 2.4 nm. The effect of a variable on particle size was discussed using the polynomial equation, 3D plots, and contour plots (Figure 2). The lipid has an agonistic effect on the size of SLNs. The size of the SLNs increased as the lipid concentration increased from 1 to 5%. The aggregation of particles causes the particles to grow in size. The second factor, Tween 80, negatively influences particle size, i.e., when the concentration is increased from 1 to 2.5%, the SLN size drops. The size reduction could be related to decrease interfacial tension between two phases, slowing particle aggregation [33]. The homogenization speed aids in particle breaking. The size of the SLNs reduced as the homogenization speed increased due to particle breakdown into smaller sizes [29].

$$\text{Particle Size} = +202.00 - 16.88A + 63.88B + 18.75C - 45.75AB + 40.50AC - 0.5000BC + 59.13A2 - 65.88B2 + 96.88C2$$

When the variable value is increased, the positive and negative coefficients of the variable in the coded equation showed an increase and decrease in the response, respectively. The model was significant, with an F-value of 33.59 and a p-value of 0.0001. A, B, C, BC, A^2, B^2, and C^2 were significant model terms with $p > 0.05$ in the analysis of particle size (Y3). To improve the model, unimportant model terms were deleted. The adjusted R^2 was 0.9974, while the standard R^2 was 0.9915, reasonably close to the adjusted R^2. Y1, with a signal-to-noise ratio of 56.9332, has adequate accuracy. The lack of fit was barely noticeable. The particle size ranged from 100.13 ± 7.2 nm to 399.08 ± 0.2.4 nm (Table 1). The equation reveals that as the lipid concentration increased, the particle size grew. The particle size was unaffected by the surfactant concentration, which was 2.5% when employed with a 5% lipid. Despite this, particle size rose considerably after reaching a concentration of >1%, which could be due to a large number of unentrapped drug particles. The positive coefficient of factor B indicated that lipids had a more significant impact on particle size. Increased lipid concentration in the SLNs may cause coalescence and increase viscosity, resulting in increased particle size [31].

Furthermore, as the lipid concentration increases, the overall surface area reduces, allowing more space for drug entrapment, resulting in larger particle size. Large particles are formed at high lipid concentrations because sonication does not perform well in more viscous liquids. On the other hand, raising the concentration of surfactant, as shown by the factor in the equation and the response surface plot, resulted in smaller particles. Because it lowers surface tension and increases surface free energy. It inhibits aggregate formation by breaking down of melting lipid droplets, resulting in smaller particles and a more stable dispersion. However, the declining effect was detected up to a certain point. A positive C^2 result showed that increasing the sonication duration beyond the limit could cause the particle size to surpass the particle size limit by generating micelles. According to the equation, the particle size is reduced by the interaction of lipid and surfactant. This could be due to the surfactant that coats the lipid droplets and aids in reducing size. The positive coefficient of other key model factors (A^2, C^2) implies that a rise in surfactant, like sonication time and lipid concentration, increases particle size after a level [32].

2.2.4. 3D-Response Surface and Contour Plot

As shown in Table 1, 17 experimental runs involving three factors at three levels were obtained. These plots show the effects of independent variables on a single response (Figures 2–4). Table 2 shows the sum of squares, df, mean squares, F-value, *p*-value, R^2, Lack of Fit, and residual of the best fitted quadratic model. Table 3 summarizes the statistical significance of each model (Linear, 2FI, and Quadratic) for both responses. The R^2, Adjusted R^2, and Predicted R^2 values for each response model varied, with the quadratic model having the highest R^2, so the quadratic model was chosen for each response. The optimized dapagliflozin-SLNs have a high %EE and optimal average particle size. The optimum SLNs formula was created using BBD software's point prediction, which included lipid content (Compritol® 888 ATO—1% *w*/*v*), surfactant (tween 80–20% *w*/*v*), and homogenization stirring speed (2 min). The particle size, %EE, and %CDR of optimized dapagliflozin-SLNs were determined to be 100.13 ± 7.2 nm, 94.46 ± 0.7%, and 99.08 ± 0.4%, respectively. The closeness of these expected results and actual values demonstrate the robustness of the optimization process employed for dapagliflozin-SLNs production. The optimized dapagliflozin-SLNs formulation's PDI, zeta-potential, and drug load were 0.32 ± 0.02, −34.4 ± 1.64 mV, and 15.5 ± 0.86%, respectively.

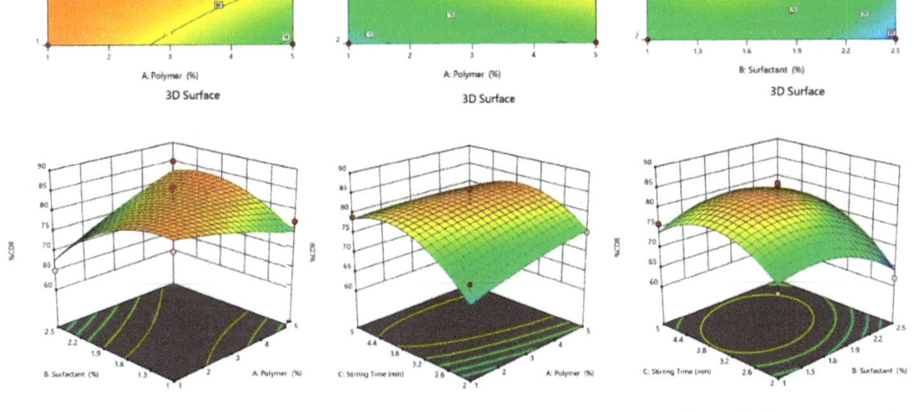

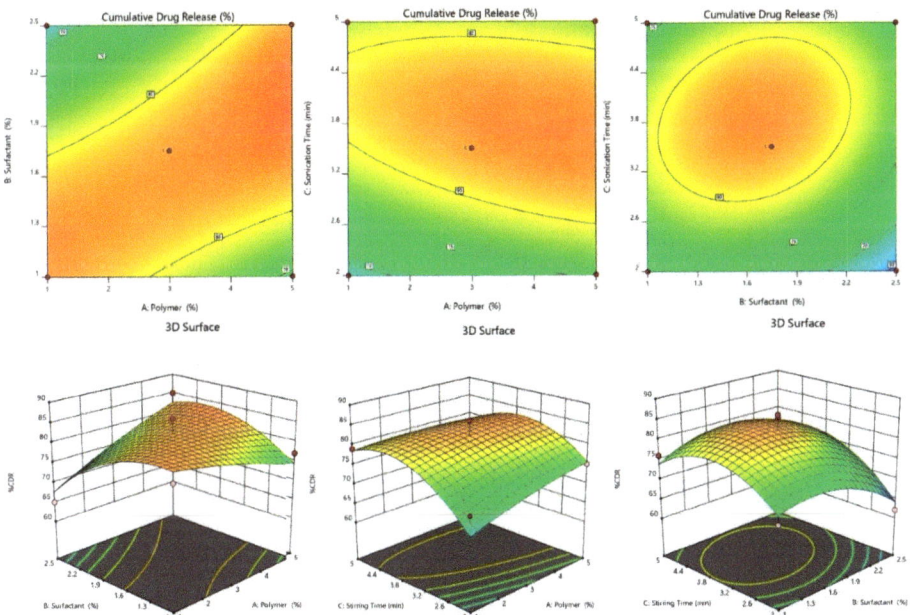

Figure 3. Effect of independent variables on %CDR counterplots and 3D response surface plots.

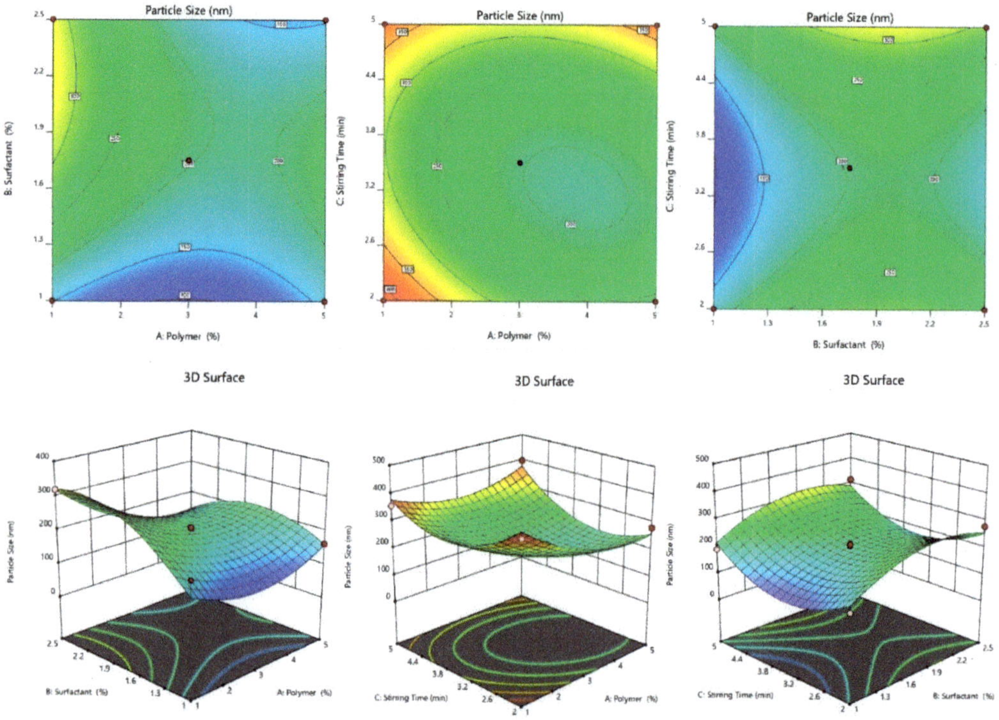

Figure 4. Effect of independent variables on CDR counterplots and 3D response surface plots.

Table 2. Optimized quadratic model for all responses: ANOVA results.

Parameter	Source	Df	Sum of Squares	Mean of Squares	F-Values	*p*-Values
%EE	Model	9	714.83	79.43	50.86	<0.0001
	Residual	7	10.93	1.56		
	Lack of Fit	4	10.18	2.55	10.18	
	Pure Error	3	0.7500	0.2500		
%CDR	Model	9	1143.14	127.02	54.26	<0.0001
	Residual	7	16.39	2.34		
	Lack of Fit	4	15.64	3.91	15.64	
	Pure Error	3	0.7500	0.2500		
Particle size	Model	9	1.204×10^5	13,377.76	33.59	<0.0001
	Residual	7	398.30			
	Lack of Fit	4	645.03	9.30		
	Pure Error	3	69.33			

Table 3. Regression coefficient values of the selected responses during optimization.

	Y_1 (%EE)			Y_2 (CDR %)			Y_3 (PARTICLE SIZE)		
Model	R^2	**Adjusted R^2**	**Predicted R^2**	R^2	**Adjusted R^2**	**Predicted R^2**	R^2	**Adjusted R^2**	**Predicted R^2**
Linear	0.296	0.134	−0.437	0.473	0.352	−0.038	0.299	0.137	−0.383
2FI	0.810	0.697	0.172	0.806	0.691	0.269	0.416	0.067	−1.646
Quadratic	**0.993**	**0.985**	**0.916**	**0.975**	**0.945**	**0.920**	**0.997**	**0.993**	**0.991**
Cubic	0.891	0.645		0.812	0.654		0.726	0.564	
p-value		<0.0001			<0.0001			<0.0001	

2.2.5. Optimization of SLNs Formulation

The formulation was optimized by using the BBD. The independent variables were chosen based on preliminary trial study results. Applying certain constraints, an optimized formula was generated from the software Design Expert Version 12.0.3.0. All 17 formulations with five center points and their responses are presented in Table 1. In the present study, three different responses were used in the three-factor, three-level BBD. The variables used in the study were results of optimization. The optimization results showed that the F12 formulation was 100.13 ± 7.2 nm for particle size, 94.46 ± 0.7 for %EE, and 99.08 ± 0.4 %CDR. Table 2 shows the results of an ANOVA of the fitted regression model (quadratic) for each dependent variable (Y1, Y2, and Y3). A quadratic model of all responses had a $p < 0.0001$ value, indicating that the created model was significant. The lack of fit of the model was found to be insignificant ($p > 0.05$), indicating that there is minor variation in the actual and projected values and that the model is well fitted, with independent factors having a significant effect on responses. All applicable models' R^2 regression values were presented, with quadratic R^2 0.999 being the highest (Table 3). The best-fit model for particle size, %EE, and %CDR was quadratic.

Each of the three components (lipid, surfactant, and stirring speed) is represented by the letters X1, X2, and X3 on a scale from one to three hundred. When a positive sign is used, it indicates a positive effect, and when a negative sign is used, it indicates a negative effect. When tested with 95 percent confidence, all replies revealed a statistically significant lack of match ($p > 0.05$). Other quadratic model parameters, including the remainder of the coefficients, were found to be statistically significant ($p < 0.0001$), with a high F-value and "Adeq Precision" (>4) as well. As a result, the model performed admirably when tested against acceptable data.

2.3. Fourier Transform Infrared (FTIR)

FTIR was used to look at the possibility of drugs interacting with the SLN components. The intensity of the peaks and the shifting of the peaks, were studied. The compatibility of the drug, Compritol ATO888, and optimized dapagliflozin-SLNs was determined using FTIR spectral analysis [34]. The characteristic bands of O–H, C=C, aromatic C–O, O–H, C=O, and C=C groups were visible in pure dapagliflozin. Pure dapagliflozin exhibited absorption peaks at 3367.10 cm^{-1} (OH stretching), 1613.16 cm^{-1} (C=C, aromatic), and 1246.70 cm^{-1} (C–O ester stretching) in the FTIR spectrum. The compounds had a 1018 cm^{-1} peak for the C–Cl bond, a 3375 cm^{-1} peak for the O–H elastic response, and a 1614 cm^{-1} peak for the C–C bond as peaks generated from dapagliflozin in common.

The absorption bands in the FTIR spectrum of the physical mixture of drug, lipid, and poloxamer 188 did not change, showing that there were no chemical interactions between the medication and excipients in the solid form, while lowering the intensity of the lipid's carbonyl C=O group peak may indicate hydrogen bonding or dipole-dipole interaction with the medication due to electrostatic attraction. In the melting lipid, minor lipophilic dapagliflozin interaction was probably acceptable.

It was observed that the aromatic C–H and C–Cl stretchings of the drug were no longer present in the SLNs formulation (F12) as a result of the creation of hydrogen bonds, with a notable expansion of the O–H stretching at 3420 cm^{-1}. When FTIR spectra of optimized dapagliflozin-SLNs were analyzed, the usual O–H stretching peak was identified at 3367.10 cm^{-1}, the C=O stretching peak was found at 1246.70 cm^{-1}, and the aromatic C=C stretching peak was detected at 1613.16 cm^{-1}. Additionally, the C=O peak of lipid (to 1637 cm^{-1}) and the aromatic C=C peak of dapagliflozin (to 1637 cm^{-1}) shifted (to 1615.12 cm^{-1}).

In the optimized dapagliflozin-SLNs spectra, the absolute peak of Compritol ATO888 and dapagliflozin was also present. Dapagliflozin was shown to be compatible with the components of SLNs (no interaction). Figure 5 shows the FTIR spectra of dapagliflozin (pure API), Compritol ATO888, Tween 80, and improved dapagliflozin SLNs [35]. The FTIR spectra of the optimized dapagliflozin formulation contained all of the functional group peaks found in pure drug spectra, with no extra peaks. This implies that the drug and excipients used in manufacturing the dapagliflozin-loaded SLNs had no interaction [23].

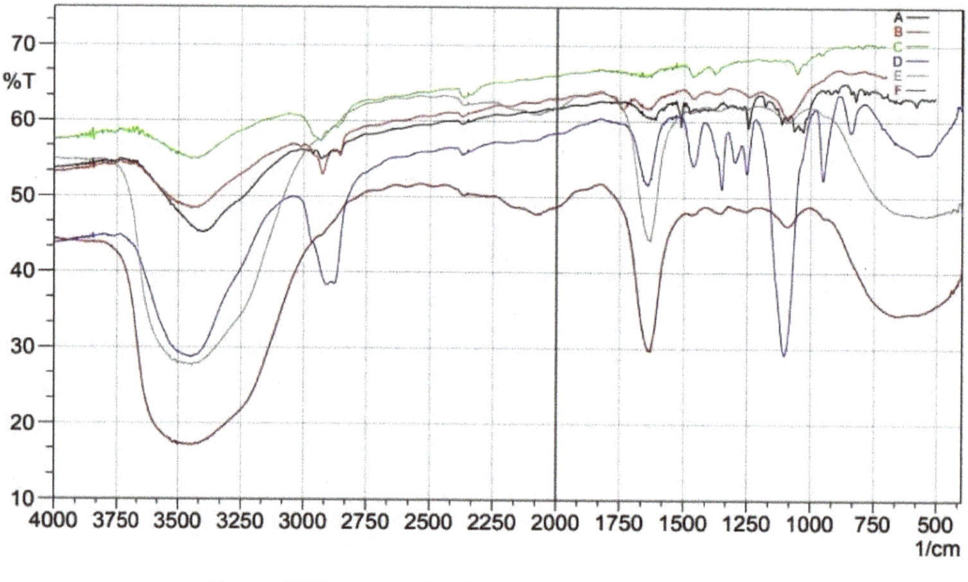

Figure 5. FTIR spectra studies of (**A**) pure drug, (**B**) Compritol 888ATO, (**C**) Tween 80, (**D**) Poloxamer 188, (**E**) control, (**F**) optimized formulation.

2.4. DSC Studies

Differential scanning calorimetry (DSC) is a technique for measuring thermal changes in a material without any mass change. Because the exposure duration to the harsh condition was short in this experimental approach, it was difficult to detect a significant change in dapagliflozin, although the crystal form may be lost over long-term exposure, according to reference literature. Dapagliflozin's surfactant thermogram indicated a pronounced endothermic peak at 76.2 °C and 52.6 °C (Figure 6), revealing its crystalline nature. The shift of the drug from crystalline nature to amorphous is indicated by a change in the thermal behavior of endothermic peaks of optimized formulation.

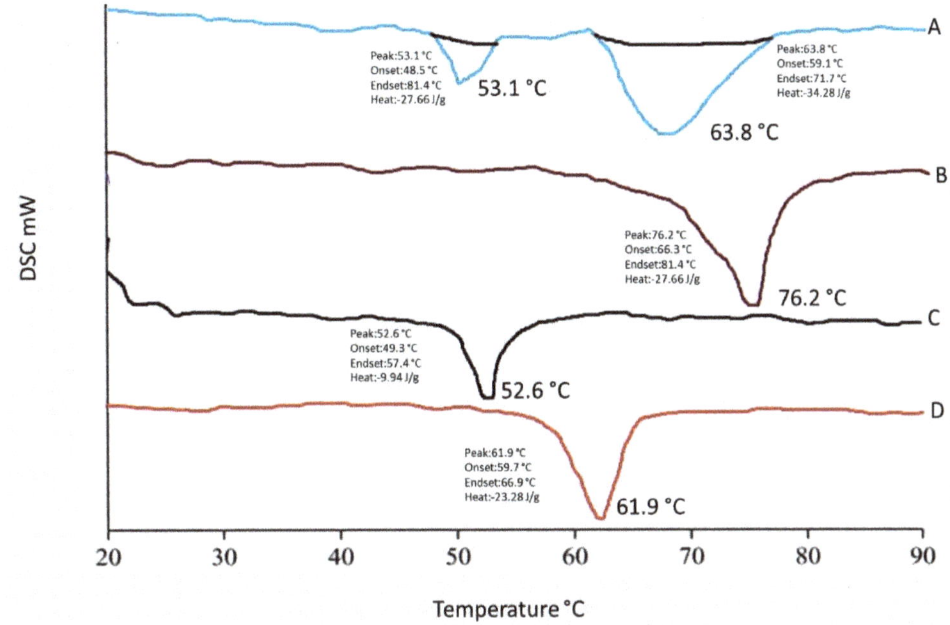

Figure 6. DSC thermogram of (**A**) optimized formulation, (**B**) pure drug, (**C**) Tween 80, (**D**) Compritol 888 ATO.

A Compritol® 888 ATO melting peak at 61.9 °C was observed in improved dapagliflozin-SLNs rather than an endothermic dapagliflozin melting peak. Compritol® 888 ATO endothermic peak shifted towards higher melting temperature in optimized dapagliflozin-SLNs. Compritol® 888 ATO has a lower melting temperature due to nano-sized particles. It has a greater surface area than Compritol® 888 ATO, lowering the melting point because melting a large crystal takes time and energy. This is due to a surfactant (tween 80) and Compritol® 888 ATO's scattered nature. Dapagliflozin did not have a melting endotherm in the thermogram of drug-loaded SLNs, indicating that the drug was entirely encapsulated in its amorphous form inside the lipid matrix of the SLNs. With the lack of the drug melting peak, the thermal profile of the dapagliflozin-loaded SLNs formulation (F12) showed a shift to 53.1 and 63.8 °C for the lipid and surfactant peaks, respectively. This revealed that the lipid's phase transition temperature increased after being loaded with dapagliflozin. These findings revealed a strong interaction with increased amorphous drug entrapment in the SLNs. The lack of drug peaks in SLNs spectra indicates that amorphization completely encapsulated the drug. The results were consistent with those previously published [36]. As shown in Figure 6, the melting temperature, offset temperature, and the area beneath the curve is displayed on the DSC curve.

2.5. *XRD Crystallography*

The powder-XRD analysis confirmed the drug's molecular dispersion state in the established formulation method. Powder-XRD was conducted to investigate the polymorphic behavior and crystallinity of dapagliflozin. Figure 7 shows the diffraction patterns of SLNs (F12) compared to Tween 80, pure dapagliflozin, and Compritol® 888 ATO. The average bulk composition of the studied material after finely powdered and homogenized. Dapagliflozin XRD spectrum shows multiple intense distinct peaks at diffraction angles (2 theta degree), namely 17.2 (d-5.15), 19.0 (d-4.66), 20.2 (d-4.399), 21.9 (d-4.05), 38.0

(d-2.366), and 44.2 (d-2.04). This lattice was observed at 2° theta diffraction angles of 20.6 and 24.8.

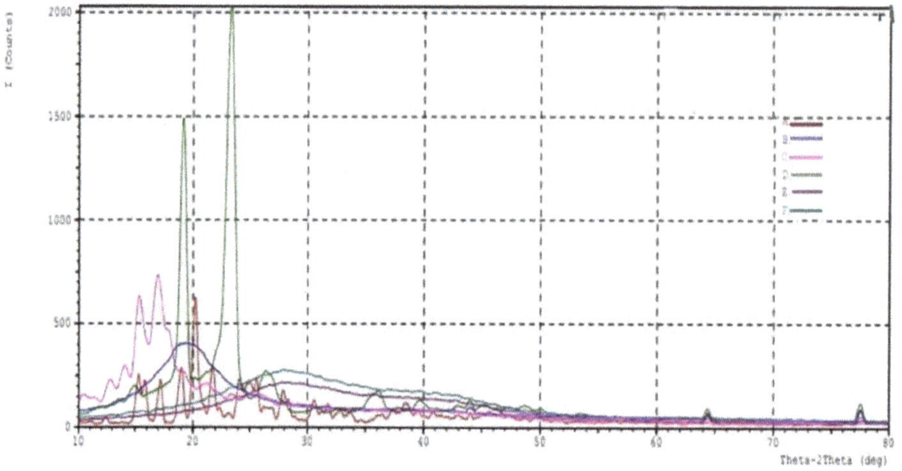

Figure 7. XRD pattern of (**A**) pure drug, (**B**) Compritol 888ATO, (**C**) Tween 80, (**D**) Poloxamer 188, (**E**) formulation (F4), (**F**) optimized formulation (F12).

Because of lipidic polymorphism, Compritol® 888 ATO exhibited a distinctive lattice at 2° theta diffraction angles of 20.6 and 24.8. At the beginning of the diffraction patterns for both formulations, the two minor peaks belong to Compritol® 888 ATO. The diffraction pattern of SLNs (F12) showed peaks intensity similar to the diffraction pattern of the blank formula. Many publications have made similar observations about the diffraction pattern of Compritol® 888 ATO. Dapagliflozin's crystalline nature was severely disturbed and was shifted to the amorphic state in optimized (F12) formulation. An X-ray powder diffraction analysis validated the results of the DSC investigation. ATO peak was identified in the XRD spectra of optimized dapagliflozin-SLNs, but no dapagliflozin peak was identified. The nano-size range of SLNs, encapsulation, and solubilization of dapagliflozin in the lipid matrix and its amorphization in the lipid matrix all contribute to this conclusion [37–39].

2.6. SEM Image Studies

SEM was used to examine the form and surface morphology of optimized dapagliflozin-SLNs, and the image revealed a spherical shape with smooth surfaces and no aggregation. As demonstrated in Figure 8, SEM describes the surface morphology of the medication and excipient [40]. This nanometric size indicates that SLNs can be absorbed by Peyer's patches and delivered to the intestinal lymphatic system without going through the liver, increasing the drug's oral bioavailability. Malvern's particle size measurement is somewhat more significant than that of SEM. This can be explained in the following way: the hydrodynamic size of a nanoparticle is assessed by differential light scattering, which is the size of the nanoparticle plus the liquid layer around it, whereas the size is determined by SEM, which is the actual size of the nanoparticle. For absorption through cells and into lymphatic tissue, round and smooth particles are frequently preferred [41].

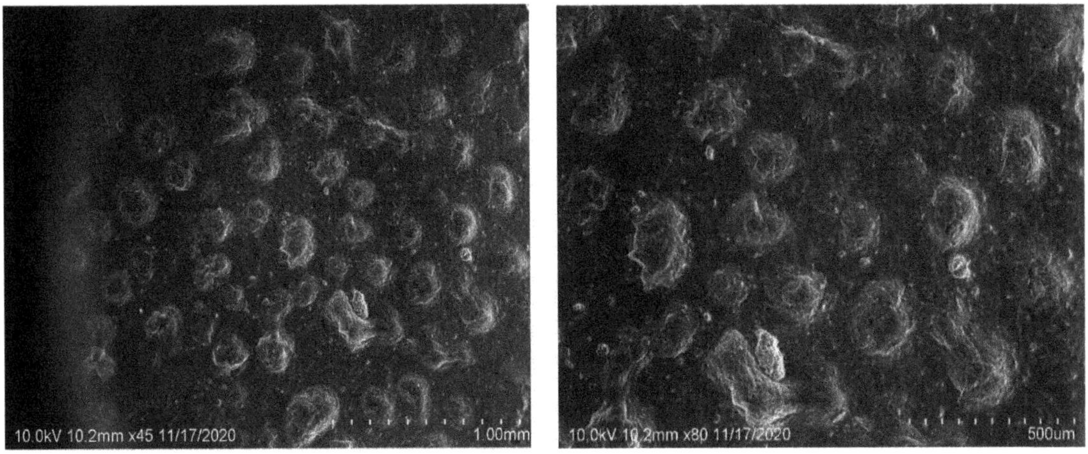

Figure 8. SEM micrographs of dapagliflozin-loaded SLNs of optimized formulation with different scales of measurement (10× magnification).

2.7. Zeta Potential and PDI of the Formulation

The electric potential differential throughout the ionic layer around a positive ion in colloids is zeta potential. The lower the zeta potential value, the less aggregation. Their zeta potentials influence dapagliflozin-SLNs' potential stability. The zeta potential assessment is one of the quick tests for reducing candidate formulation stability investigations, reducing experimental time and testing costs, and boosting shelf-life [42]. F1–F17 are stable if their zeta potential ranges between −22.5–34.4 ± 1.64 mV. The optimized zeta potential is −34.4 ± 1.64 mV (Figure 9).

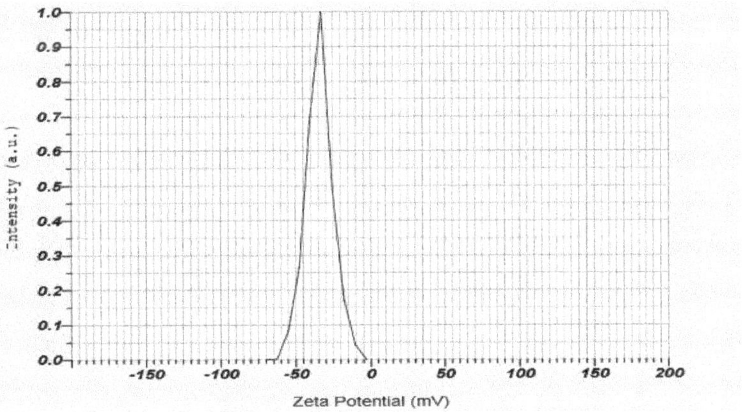

Figure 9. Zeta potential of dapagliflozin-loaded SLNs of optimized formulation.

The zeta potential indicates the electrical voltage difference in surface-charged particles and forecasts the formulation's stability; its optimal range is more than ±30 mV. The formulation's zeta potential (-potential) was determined in the original dispersion media. For very stable suspensions, the absolute value of -potential should be around ±30 mV. This number may be lower in the case of combination electrostatic and steric stabilization (due to the usage of ionic and non-ionic surfactants). A longer homogenization time resulted in nanoparticles with a higher zeta potential. The observed behavior can be explained by better surfactant mixing in dispersion, which results in higher zeta potential values and, as a result, improved formulation stability, as evidenced by the backscattering profiles described below [43].

For a homogenous SLNs distribution, a PDI near 0 is appropriate, and a PDI of up to 0.5 is acceptable for narrow size distribution. Our research discovered that raising the surfactant content reduced PDI (Table 2). The causes for this could be the same as for particle size. The PDI was nearly identical to the surfactant concentration, ranging from 1 to 2.5%. This means that increasing surfactant concentration decreases PDI until a certain point, which may remain unchanged. The PDI was shown to improve when the surfactant and lipid concentrations were increased. However, with the maximum quantity of lipid comprising 2.5% and 1% of the surfactant than 2 min of sonication time, the PDI was lowered, implying that the presence of free drug raises the PDI. The PDI values of 0.32 ± 0.02–0.82 ± 0.04 indicate that the system has a relatively narrow size distribution, which can be called monodisperse. The obtained results are linked with previous data presented in the literature and show that increasing the sonication time reduces the size of nanoparticles and lowers PDI values [44].

2.8. AFM

The topology of nanocarriers was examined using AFM, which is essential when building drug delivery systems. Figure 10 shows the AFM pictures of dapagliflozin-SLNs on mica. The examination of SLNs morphology using AFM tapping and non-contact mode techniques is possible without any sample treatment such as staining, labeling, or fixation. The tip's intermittent contact motion, in particular, reduces later or shears pressures that might otherwise deform or scrape the material. The ability to operate with greater fidelity in air or fluid in real time and on the nanometer scale is the key benefit of this approach. However, once deposited on mica support, SLNs can change shape by employing tapping mode and functioning in an aqueous solution (about 10–15 min) while still moistened and plugged in water. It depends on the vesicle composition, the contact between the sample and the substrate, and the provided sufficient tip, which might cause deformation [45].

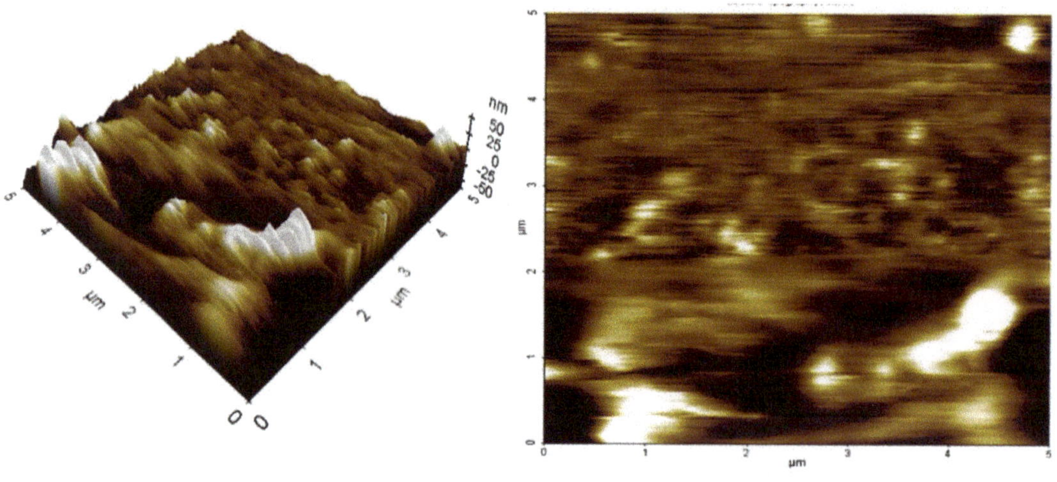

Figure 10. AFM analysis (within 10–15 min) on deposition on mica support.

The SLN was found to be spherical, with particles measuring roughly 200 nm in diameter, according to an AFM analysis (Figure 10). The size range reported by AFM and the size determined by dynamic light scattering is linked. The average roughness of SLN was discovered to be 10.27 nm, indicating its surface smoothness.

The outcomes of our experiments support the ideas proposed in the literature. The flattening of nanoparticles on the support was shown by comparing the diameter and height values of our SLNs just a few minutes after deposition. This revealed that the SLNs on a mica substrate were only moderately stable. Even though the diameters were more significant than the equivalent heights, the SLNs maintained a spherical, well-defined shape (Figure 10, 3D reconstruction). SLNs demonstrated a progressive tendency to change into an asymmetrical and irregular form defined as planar vesicles 20 min after deposition (data not shown). As others have discovered, this behavior can detect dried or partially dried liposomes.

2.9. Studies of In Vitro Drug Release

The release pattern of optimized dapagliflozin-SLNs was compared to pure dapagliflozin under the same conditions. Optimized dapagliflozin-SLNs had a higher and long-lasting release, 69.23 ± 2.35% in 8 h, compared to a pure drug, which had a poor release pattern, 37.85 ± 4.26% (Figure 11). Dapagliflozin released from optimized dapagliflozin-SLNs had a twofold release profile, with an initial burst release within 8 h followed by a continuous release pattern [46]. The rapid release of dapagliflozin adsorbed on the surface of the SLNs resulted in this type of release behavior. Subsequently, solubilized or dispersed dapagliflozin is released slowly from the inside of the lipid core matrix via diffusion processes, resulting in a protracted drug release. The presence of Compritol® 888 ATO as a solid lipid and Tween 80 as a surfactant in the SLNs resulted in much-increased drug release, which aids in the release of weakly soluble medicines. Different release kinetic models were used to suit the data. Because it has the highest R^2, the Korsmeyer–Peppas model was chosen as the best-fit release model. It implies that the release process is controlled by diffusion, which is then followed by lipid matrix erosion [47].

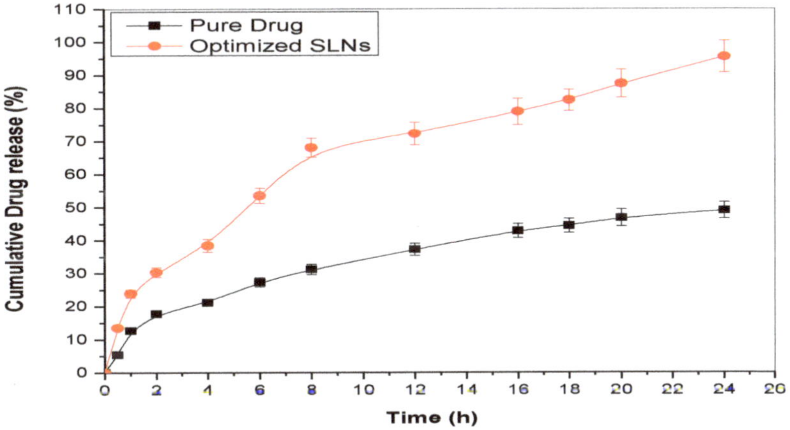

Figure 11. In vitro release studies on optimized SLNs and comparison with pure drug solution-Dapagliflozin.

2.10. Histopathology Studies

In acute toxicity trials, dapagliflozin-SLNs were found to be non-toxic. At any given dosage, no lethality or toxic reaction was observed. As shown in Figure 12, histopathological evidence backed up the non-toxic nature of the substance. The liver, kidneys, stomach, testis, and pancreas tissues are unaffected by dapagliflozin-SLNs.

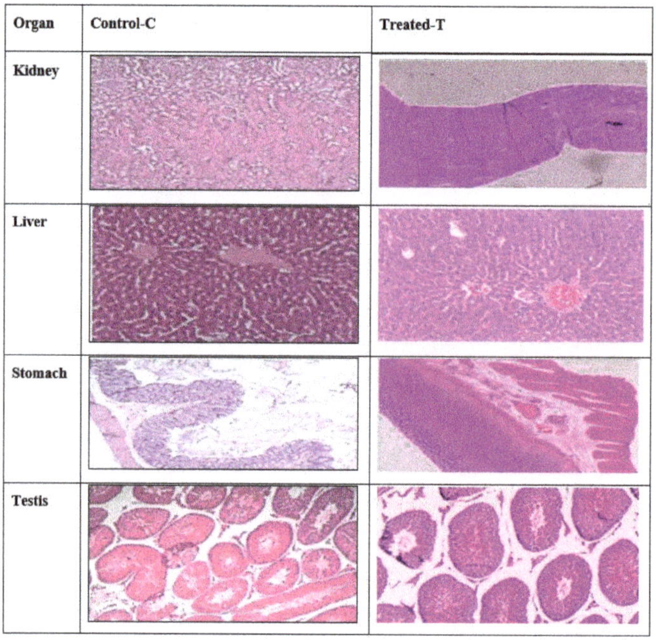

Figure 12. Histopathology of vital organs, namely liver, kidney, stomach, testis, and spleen in the rat during acute toxicity studies. C—Control, T—Treated. Dose, highest dose of 15 mg/kg b.wt of dapagliflozin. All sections were stained with H&E, ×400.

2.11. *In Vivo Study*

Healthy male Wistar rat of either sex weighing 180 to 250 g were employed. They were kept in conventional circumstances, with a temperature of 25 °C and relative humidity of 45 to 55%.

Rats were fed with an essential pellet diet and had free access to water. All animals were carefully monitored and cared for by CPCSEA criteria for experimental animal control and monitoring.

Group I was the vehicle control, Group II was the streptozotocin (STZ) control (STZ 65 mg/kg), Groups III and IV were the testing groups, receiving 5 and 10 dosage mg/kg of dapagliflozin-SLNs, respectively, and Group V was the standard group, receiving dapagliflozin. The treatment was repeated every day for 21 days.

2.12. *Effect of Dapagliflozin-SLNs on Insulin, HbA1c, and Blood Glucose Levels in STZ-Induced Diabetic Rats*

Diabetes mellitus is characterized by high blood sugar levels that disrupt metabolism and glucose recovery over time [47,48]. STZ is commonly used to induce diabetes in laboratory animals by killing beta cells. It degrades into isocyanates and methyl diazo hydroxide before reaching the cell. Alkylation of DNA in beta-pancreatic cells by methyl diazo-hydroxide. After 28 days of treatment, blood glucose levels in groups III, IV, and V were normalized but still higher than in group I (Figure 13A,B).

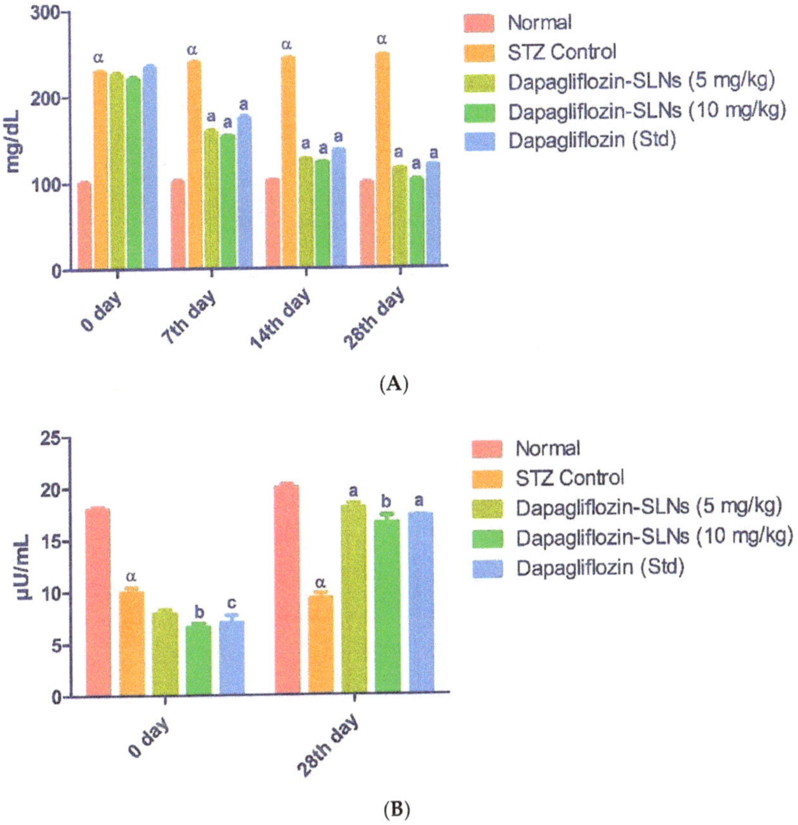

Figure 13. (**A**) Effect of dapagliflozin-SLNs on glucose levels in STZ-induced diabetic rats. Data are presented as the mean, standard error of the mean ($n = 6$), and analyzed using one-way ANOVA followed by Tukey's test to compare means. $p < 0.001$ when compared to the control group; a $p < 0.001$ compared to the STZ group. (**B**) Effect of dapagliflozin-SLNs on serum insulin of STZ treated diabetic rats. Data are expressed as mean ± SEM ($n = 6$) and were analyzed by one-way analysis of variance (ANOVA) followed by Tukey's test to compare means. α $p < 0.001$, when compared to the normal group; a $p < 0.001$, b $p < 0.01$, c $p < 0.05$ compared to STZ control.

Insulin deficiency causes metabolic changes like higher blood glucose and better lipid profile. As shown in Figure 13B, STZ-induced diabetic rats had significantly lower insulin levels. The diabetes control group's HbA1c was higher ($p < 0.01$) than the regular control group's (Figure 14).

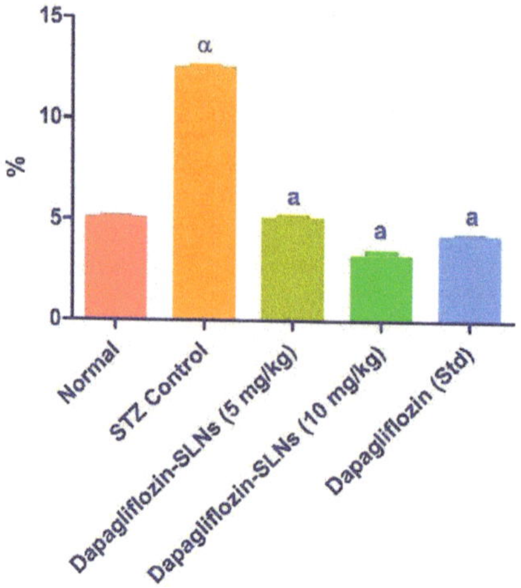

Figure 14. Dapagliflozin-SLNs on glycosylated hemoglobin (HbA1c) of STZ-treated diabetic rats. Data are presented as the mean, standard error of the mean (n = 6), and were analyzed using one-way ANOVA followed by Tukey's test to compare means. $\alpha\ p < 0.001$ when compared to the control group; a $p < 0.001$ when contrasted to the STZ group.

2.13. *Lipid Profiles*

Lipids are critical in the progression of diabetes mellitus. Hypertriglyceridemia and hypercholesterolemia are frequent lipid abnormalities in this illness. In this investigation, diabetic rats had higher plasma cholesterol, triglycerides, and LDL, which are key risk factors for cardiovascular disease [49,50]. In normal rats, STZ therapy increased total cholesterol, plasma triglycerides, LDL-C, and lowered HDL-C levels (Figure 15).

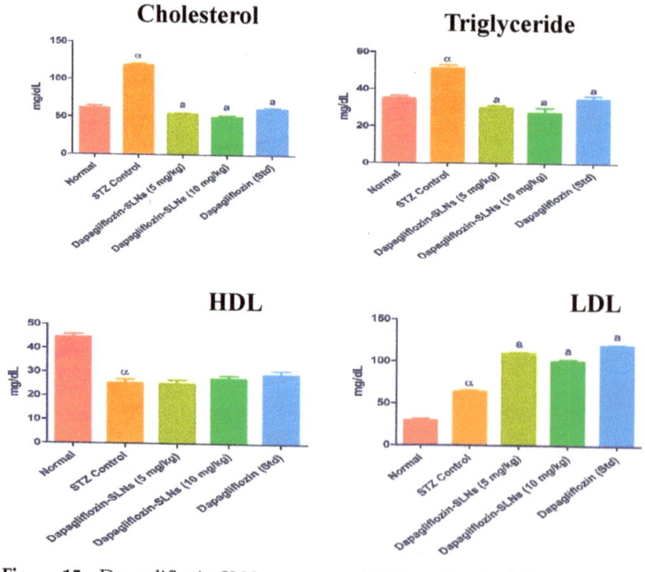

Figure 15. Dapagliflozin-SLNs on serum lipid profiles in STZ-induced diabetic rats. Data are presented as the mean, standard error of the mean (n = 6), and were analyzed using one-way ANOVA followed by Tukey's test to compare means. $\alpha\ p < 0.001$ when compared to the control group; a $p < 0.001$ compared to the STZ group.

2.14. Biochemical Enzymes

The decreased structural integrity of the liver produced by STZ induction and a high-fat diet has been linked to differences in SGOT, SGPT, and ALP. The liver function tests on dapagliflozin-SLNs revealed a reduction in serum ALP, SGOT, and SGPT to normal levels, demonstrating plasma membrane stability and hepatic tissue damage preparation, as shown in Figure 16.

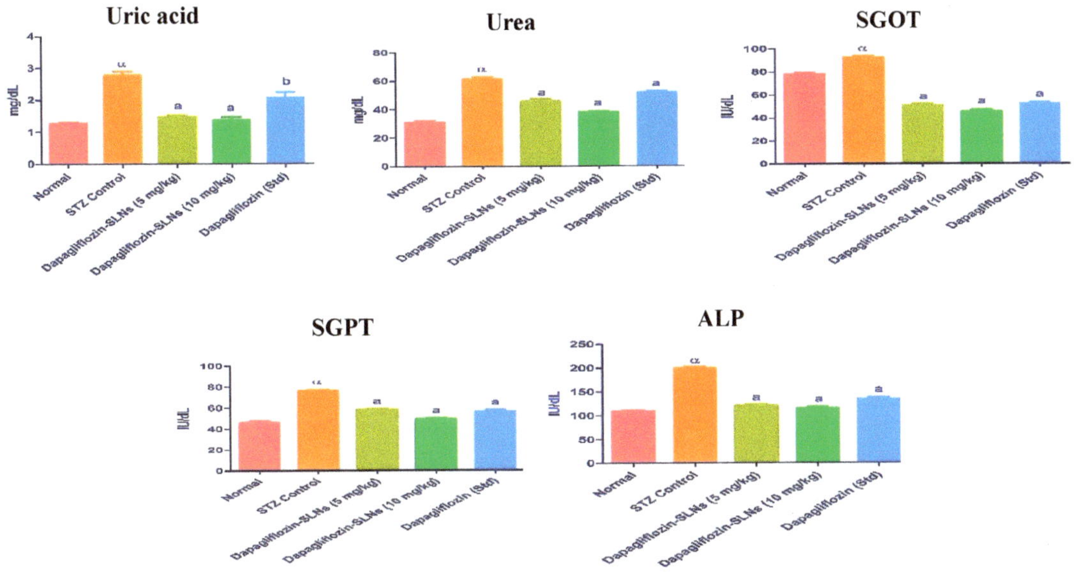

Figure 16. Dapagliflozin-SLNs on serum biomarkers in STZ-induced diabetic rats. Data are presented as the mean, standard error of the mean (n = 6), and were analyzed using one-way ANOVA followed by Tukey's test to compare means. α $p < 0.001$ when compared to the control group; a $p < 0.001$, b $p < 0.01$ compared to the STZ group.

2.15. Oral Bioavailability Studies

The in vivo pharmacokinetic behavior of the typical optimized dapagliflozin-SLNs formulation was investigated to quantify dapagliflozin in rat plasma following oral administration in the current study [51]. The study found that dapagliflozin is well absorbed following oral treatment, with peak plasma levels reaching within 8 h. Figure 17 shows that the C_{max} of dapagliflozin after oral administration of a commercial product was 621.57 ± 0.52 μg/mL. Nonetheless, the C_{max} of dapagliflozin after oral administration of our optimized dapagliflozin-SLNs was 1258.37 ± 1.21 μg/mL. The C_{max} of dapagliflozin from the SLNs formulation was enhanced significantly from 184.67 ± 3.12 to 1258.37 ± 1.21 mcg mL^{-1} ($p < 0.05$) (Figure 16). The AUC of dapagliflozin in the SLNs-treated group increased considerably from 113.03 ± 0.19 to 6310.89 ± 0.04 when compared to the sole marketed product treated group (mcg mL^{-1}). Compared to the commercial development, the oral bioavailability of dapagliflozin from our optimized dapagliflozin SLNs was twofold higher in vivo testing (Table 4) [52].

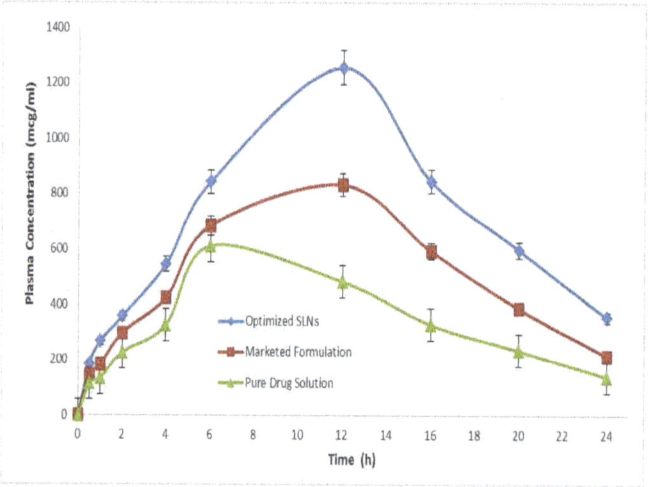

Figure 17. Plasma concentration vs. time profile of dapagliflozin after oral administration of optimized formulation and compared with the marketed and pure drug solution.

Table 4. Pharmacokinetic parameters of optimized SLNs compared with the marketed and pure drug solution.

Pharmacokinetic Parameters	Pure Drug Solution	Marketed Formulation	Optimized SLNs
Intercept	2.378	2.481	2.582
Slope	0.0019	0.0076	0.011
Co (mcg/mL)	238.850	303.024	382.68
K (h^{-1})	0.0044	0.0175	0.027
Dose (mg)	100	100	100
Dose (mcg)	100,000	100,000	100,000
Vd (mL)	41.86	33.00	26.13
Vd (L)	0.041	0.033	0.026
t1/2 (h)	155.26	39.54	25.20
Cl (L/h)	0.0001	0.0005	0.0007
$AUC_{o\text{-}t}$ (mcg.h/mL)	59.83	54.23	95.79
$AUC_{1\text{-}t}$ (mcg.h/mL)	8531.975	12,744.44	18,036.93
$AUC_{1\text{-}inf}$ (mcg.h/mL)	31,425.20	12,349.3	12,885.67
AUC_{total} (mcg.h/mL)	22,833.39	449.326	5247.046
C_{max} (mcg/mL/h)	834.26	621.57	1258.37
Tmax (mL/min)	12.1	5.97	12.06

These findings suggest that the proposed SLNs could improve the oral bioavailability of the anti-diabetic drug dapagliflozin, which could be used in combination with sitagliptin to treat T2DM. The results of diabetic studies show that combining dapagliflozin and sitagliptin has better efficacy and outcomes in lowering blood glucose levels. However, we only studied dapagliflozins in in vivo pharmacokinetics. For product performance, it was essential to correlate drug solubility and % age solubilized with bioavailability. This would allow for proper in vitro and in vivo drug correlation [53]. The increased bioavailability of dapagliflozin may be due to increased solubility and faster uptake of the nanoemulsion by enterocytes at the absorption site (Table 4). These findings for dapagliflozin were previously reported and are expected for sitagliptin.

2.16. Stability Studies

Stability is the main issue for the commercial application of SLNs. A series of stability studies (ICH guideline Q1A (R2) were carried out on the optimized formulation (F12) to determine its stability to the determining factors of vesicle size, polydispersity index, and %EE [54]. The recrystallization of the amorphous form of SLNs takes place on storage for a long time, leading to decreased drug content and release. Table 5 shows the stability results for dapagliflozin-SLNs in drug content and release.

Table 5. Results for stability studies of dapagliflozin-SLNs.

Months	Temperature (°C)	EE (%)	CDR (%)	Drug Content (%)	Vesicle Size (nm)	Zeta Value (mv)
1st Month	Refrigeration	94.46 ± 0.7	99.08 ± 0.4	98.49 ± 2.1	150.37 ± 4.6	−34.4 ± 1.64
2nd Month	temperature	92.34 ± 2.1	96.45 ± 0.1	98.12 ± 1.1	167.42 ± 3.8	−32.1 ± 1.1
3rd Month	(4 ± 2 °C)	89.26 ± 0.5	92.46 ± 0.4	97.89 ± 1.3	180.64 ± 2.4	−30.9 ± 1.4
1st Month	Room	94.46 ± 0.7	99.08 ± 0.4	98.49 ± 2.1	150.37 ± 4.6	−34.4 ± 1.64
2nd Month	temperature	94.13 ± 0.1	99.02 ± 0.2	98.15 ± 1.1	155.26 ± 2.5	−33.1 ± 0.38
3rd Month	(30 ± 2 °C)	93.46 ± 0.4	98.19 ± 0.1	97.89 ± 0.3	160.45 ± 1.4	−32.41 ± 0.26

3. Discussion

First, the solubility of dapagliflozin in various lipids and surfactants was investigated. The lipid Compritol 888 ATO solid lipid has the highest solubility of dapagliflozin, 38.67 ± 2.08 mg/g. Tween 80 contains the surfactant (23.84 ± 2.65 mg/g), which was chosen to produce SLNs. Tween 80 is a non-ionic surfactant that is physiologically non-toxic to humans. It is a hydrophilic surfactant with a high emulsification capability (HLB = 15).

Hot homogenization-ultra-sonication is the most straightforward and practical approach for manufacturing SLNs in laboratories. Poloxamer 188 and Compritol 888 ATO were utilized as lipids, surfactants, and co-surfactants. The homogenization time was set at 10 min at 15,000 pm, while the sonication time was 5 min at 50 W. An optimal formula was developed by applying specific constraints to the software Design Expert Version 12. The quadratic model was the best fit for all of the responses investigated, including mean particle size, %EE, and %CDR.

FTIR spectroscopy, DSC, and XRD crystallography were used to characterize the generated formulations. The pure dapagliflozin is crystalline, according to SEM images. In the improved formulation, the crystalline form of dapagliflozin was converted to an amorphous state. As illustrated in Figure 9, the size of dapagliflozin-SLNs ranges from 10 to 1000 nm.

The zeta potential is the charge that forms at the contact between a solid surface and its surrounding liquid. Stability is created when scattered particles in water have large amounts of either positive or negative zeta potential, which causes them to resist one another. Because of this, the particles become unstable due to the dispersant's shallow zeta potential, which makes it impossible to keep them apart. F1 and F17 are stable if their zeta potential is between –22.5 to 34.4 ± 1.64 mV. The optimized zeta potential is −34.4 mv. The morphology of nanocarriers, which is crucial in designing drug delivery systems, was ascertained from the high-resolution nanoscale AFM images.

Studies on in vitro drug release, as shown in Figure 10, show that slow diffusion (release) of dapagliflozin was responsible for the first phase (burst release) and the second phase (slow release) of dapagliflozin release from the polymeric matrix.

From the results of the stability studies, it can be observed that there were no significant changes in either the release or concentration of the medicine being studied. Dapagliflozin-SLNs produced using the heat homogenization-ultrasonication process were therefore maintained in an amorphous condition throughout storage.

Dapagliflozin-SLNs were tested in STZ-induced diabetic rats in vivo to see how they affected blood glucose, insulin, and HbA1c levels. Dapagliflozin-SLNs might drop high blood glucose levels to normal in STZ-induced diabetic rats, indicating a more significant hypoglycemic effect, according to the findings of this study. In STZ and high-fat diabetic animals, dapagliflozin-SLNs reduced glucose levels. In diabetic rats, STZ significantly reduced insulin levels, as shown in Figure 12. Diabetic rats administered with dapagliflozin exhibited considerably higher insulin levels than diabetic rats in control group II. Increased insulin sensitivity could be one of the active mechanisms by which dapagliflozin-SLNs exert their anti-diabetic effects [14]

The diabetic control group's HbA1c level was slightly higher ($p < 0.01$) than the standard control group's HbA1c level. The dapagliflozin-SLNs and dapagliflozin significantly decreased diabetic rats' blood levels of HbA1c compared to the control diabetic community (Figure 13). The standard glycemic regulation indicator HbA1c demonstrates the decreasing concentration in treated animals.

The lipid profile of STZ diabetic rats was considerably reduced by dapagliflozin-SLNs ($p \leq 0.01$). Triglycerides, total cholesterol, and LDL-C levels were significantly lowered in diabetic rats administered dapagliflozin-SLNs. However, HDL-C levels in all treated diabetic rats were considerably more significant than in diabetic control groups (Figure 14). As a result, the hypolipidemic activity of dapagliflozin-SLNs has been proposed. Dapagliflozin-SLNs affected serum GOT, GPT, and ALP in normal and diabetic rats, as shown in Figure 15. According to the data, the diabetic rats had greater serum GOT, GPT, and ALP levels than the control rats. Compared to diabetic rats in the control group, dapagliflozin-SLNs administration significantly reduced serum GOT, GPT, and ALP high levels ($p \leq 0.01$).

4. Materials and Methods

4.1. Materials

Dapagliflozin was obtained as a gift sample from Hetero Drugs Lab (Hyderabad, India). Poloxamer-188, stearic acid (SA), and cetostearyl alcohol (CSA) phospholipids were procured from Research-lab fine chem industries in Mumbai; glycerol monostearate, Mohini Organics Pvt. Ltd. (Mumbai, India), Bangalore provided Tween 80, methanol, and chloroform. SD fine chemicals Pvt. Ltd., Mumbai, India, provided Precirol® ATO5 and Compritol® 888 ATO.

4.2. Measurement of Dapagliflozin Solubility in Lipids

The solubility studies were not performed due to the solid nature of the lipids; a different method was used to determine the drug's solubility in solid lipids. In brief, 10 mg of dapagliflozin was precisely weighed and placed in a screw-capped glass bottle with an aluminum foil covering. About 200 mg of lipid (stearic acid, cetostearyl alcohol, GMS, Precirol ATO5, and Compritol 888ATO) was added to the bottle and cooked at 80 °C while swirling continuously [8]. Then, more lipid was added in small increments while constantly stirring and heating at 80 °C until a clear solution was created. The mixture was centrifuged for 10 min at 6000 rpm (Remi centrifuge) to separate the aqueous phase. After suitable dilution in triplicate, the concentration of dapagliflozin in the aqueous phase was determined using a UV spectrophotometer (UV-1800, Shimadzu, Japan). The entire amount of lipid added to achieve a clear solution was monitored [55].

4.2.1. Selection of Appropriate Surfactant

First, 1 mL surfactant (Tween 20, Tween 80, PEG200, Limonene, and Cremophore EL) was added to an Eppendorf tube, and the excess dapagliflozin and the tube were shaken for 15 min. The mixture was left to stand for 72 h in an orbital shaker. After centrifuging the mixture at 5000 rpm for 15 min, the supernatant was collected and separated [56]. After proper dilution, the amount of dapagliflozin was determined at 235 nm using a UV–Vis spectrophotometer (Shimadzu, 1800, Tokyo, Japan).

4.2.2. Selection of Sonication Time and Amplitude

Probe sonication was chosen because of its better repeatability ratio and targeted intensity. By raising the ultrasonic strength and sonication time, the particle size decreases. However, if the amplitude and time increase beyond a certain point, particle size rises due to particle aggregation. The optimum amplitude and time for the sonication process were determined through experiments. 2.5% lipid, 1% surfactant, and a stabilizer were used to make SLNs. EE and particle size were measured after formulas were sonicated at 20, 40, and 50% amplitude for 2 to 5 min [57].

4.3. RP-HPLC Conditions for Analysis of Dapagliflozin

RP-HPLC (prominence HPLC, Shimadzu, Kyoto, Japan) with an autosampler and a UV detector (SPD 20A) set at 235 nm was used to measure dapagliflozin. The medication was separated chromatographically at room temperature using a C18 column (Phenomenex, C-18, 5 μm, 150 4.5 mm). The injection volume was set at 20 μL. Acetonitrile and water (50:50) were used as a mobile phase, with a 0.5 mL/min flow rate.

4.4. Preparation of SLNS

The dapagliflozin-loaded SLNs were made using a hot homogenization process with an ultrasonic phase. Dapagliflozin (100 mg) was dissolved in melted lipid (Compritol 888 ATO) and then dissolved in 20 mL chloroform: methanol (1:1) at 75 °C. The aqueous process used a surfactant called Poloxamer-188 and a co-surfactant called Tween 80, which were dissolved in 20 mL of distilled water to make a 2% solution heated to 80 °C. The heated aqueous phase solution was applied to the lipid phase held at 75 °C after the clear homogeneous lipid phase was collected in a beaker. Ultra Turrax T10 (T-10 simple ULTRA-TURRAX-IKA, Germany) was homogenized for 10 min at 15,000 rpm in a high-speed homogenizer. The pre-emulsion was subsequently ultra-sonicated at 50 w for 5 min using a probe sonicator (Frontline Sonicator). After that, the mixture was placed into cold water (between 1 and 40 °C) and mixed with a magnetic agitator. The SLNs were recrystallized at room temperature before being diluted with deionized water to make a dapagliflozin-SLN dispersion of up to 100 mL [58].

4.5. Experimental Design and Statistical Analysis

SLNs for dapagliflozin were optimized using a triadic, three-level BBD. Research into the quadratic solution surface and the second-order polynomial model may be carried out using this tool. Each edge of the multidimensional cube has a central point and a set of characteristics that define the exciting region. To determine the best-fitted model, all of the responses from each run were fitted to linear, 2F1, and quadratic models. The software generated contour and 3D plots, which were used to evaluate the independent factor for each answer. The actual value of each response is quantitatively compared to the software-predicted values [59]. The BBD created the generic polynomial equation for the quadratic model to check the effect of independent variables on the answer. In the synthesis of SLNs, polymer concentration (X1), surfactant concentration (X2), and stirring speed (X3) were three independent variables. Additionally, the % of drug release, EE, and particle size were selected as the dependent variables (Y1, Y2, and Y3, respectively). Runs were then conducted at various levels of each element to determine process parameters. Each run's answers were examined using the Design EXPERT 12.0.3.0 (Table 6).

Table 6. Dependent and independent variables of SLNs.

Parameter	Units	Low (−1)	High (+1)
X1- Polymer concentration	% (*w*/*v*)	1	5
X2- Surfactant	% (*w*/*v*)	2	2.5
X3- Stirring Speed	min	2	5
Dependent Variables		Low	High
Y1- %EE		68.26 ± 0.2	94.46 ± 0.7
Y2- %CDR		62.83 ± 5.1	99.08 ± 0.4
Y3- Particle Size		100.13 ± 7.2	399.08 ± 2.4

The non-linear quadratic model is given by this design as

$$Yi = b0 + b2X2 + b3X3 + b12X1X2 + b13X1X3 + b23X2X3 + b11X21 + b22X22 + b33X23X23$$

Results were analyzed using linear regression with particle size, %EE, and %CDR as response variables, lipid amount and surfactant concentration, organic phase volume, and sonication duration as factors at various levels. ANOVA and the mean effects plot for particle size and zeta potential were utilized to identify the critical variables. Pareto and contour diagrams were also used to demonstrate the effects of different factors on particle size. Design expert was used for all statistical analysis [60].

4.6. Measurement of Particle Size, PDI, and Zeta Potential of SLNs

Size, polydispersity index (PDI), and zeta potential (ZP) of SLNs were determined using a Zeta Sizer (Nano ZS90, Malvern, Worcestershire) (ZP). Dilution with double-distilled water was done to determine the best 50–200 kilo counts per second [61]. The calculation itself is electrophoresis of particles, with the Doppler effect of laser light dispersed by the moving particles determining the particle velocity. Using the Helmholtz–Smouches equation, the field strength was 20 V/cm; electrophoretic mobility was translated into zeta potential (mV) [62].

4.7. Drug Loading

Centrifugation was used to determine the drug load of the improved formulation (dapagliflozin-SLNs). The sample was deposited in a centrifuge tube and centrifuged for 30 min at 18,000 rpm with a cooling centrifuge (Sigma 3-1 KL IVD, Germany). After the supernatant was recovered, the SLNs particle was rinsed with water and dispersed in methanol. The material was then sonicated for 15 min with a probe sonicator and re-centrifuged. Finally, the supernatant was collected, and the dapagliflozin content was measured in triplicate using a UV spectrophotometer set to 235 nm. The drug loading was determined using the formula below [63].

$$\%\ Drug\ loading = \frac{Concentration\ of\ the\ drug\ in\ SLNs}{Total\ weight\ of\ SLNs} \times 100$$

4.8. %EE

Surfactant and co-surfactant aqueous solution-free drug concentrations were separated using a cooling centrifuge to compute the %EE. Centrifuge-controlled (Remi Instruments Ltd., Mumbai, India) decantation of the SLNs dispersion resulted in the free (unentrapped) drug sedimenting at 12,000 rpm, 4 °C for 20 min. A UV spectrophotometric method was utilized for the aqueous phase dapagliflozin concentration, and it was represented as %EE [64].

$$\%EE = (\text{Total Amount} - \text{Entrapped drug})/(\text{Total amount of drug}) \times 100$$

4.9. *Solid-State Characterizations*

4.9.1. FTIR

These experiments are conducted to estimate the chemical reaction between drugs and excipients. The pellet approach is used for potassium bromide (KBr), and the background spectrum is obtained in the same case. Dapagliflozin was prepared using an electrically operated KBr press model, potassium bromide (KBr) discs with the drug. Approximately 2 mg of dapagliflozin was shredded with about 5 mg of dry KBr and then pneumatically pressed into the pellet. The Fourier transform spectrometer (Shimadzu, 8400S) was used to obtain IR spectra from the prepared dapagliflozin pellet. Every spectrum is extracted from single average scans obtained against a background interferogram in the 400–4000 cm^{-1} range [65].

4.9.2. DSC

DSC is conducted to estimate studies of association and polymorphism, thermotropic properties, and thermal behaviors of drugs and excipients used in the formulation. Around 5 mg of the sample was sealed and heated at 10 C/min in the aluminum pans. The temperature range of 4 to 30 °C was covered under a nitrogen atmosphere with a 100 mL/min flow rate [66].

4.9.3. XRD

XRD patterns are determined for the physical mixture of the drug and other excipients to establish crystalline properties of drugs and excipients. A copper-targeted X-ray diffractometer at a voltage of 49 KV and a current of 20 MA was used to understand the crystallinity of the compound. Patterns were performed at 0.3 °C/min [67].

4.9.4. SEM

The form and size of produced particles were examined using SEM. Microscopy was used to investigate dispersion patterns of nanoparticles, which were deposited on a thin carbon sheet and pumped out of the chamber. A high-intensity primary electron beam scans the sample row by row, passing through lenses that focus the electrons to a tiny point. Ionization causes secondary electrons to be generated when the concentrated electron beam reaches the location on the material. Secondary electrons are counted using a detector. A collector collects electrons positioned laterally and sends them to an amplifier [68].

4.9.5. AFM

The SLNs were imaged using a Veeco NanoScope Dimension V AFM (Plainview, NY, USA) and an RT ESP Veeco tube scanner. A silicon cantilever with an ultralow-resonance resonating at 250–331 kHz and a force of 20–80 N/m was used [68]. The scanning frequency was set at 0.5 Hz. Before being seen, lipid nanoparticles were allowed to stick to a new mica surface in the solution for 24 h. After cleaning, the surfaces were washed with double-distilled water and dried in the shade [69]. A drop of dispersion sample was placed on a copper grid and dried at room temperature for one hour to conduct an examination [69].

4.10. *In Vitro Drug Release Studies and In Vivo Anti-Diabetic Studies*

The dialysis bag technique checked the release studies of optimized dapagliflozin-SLNs and pure drug solution. An enhanced open dialysis bag was used to study dapagliflozin in vitro release from improved SLNs. Before being linked to the diffusion cell, the dialysis membrane was kept for 24 h in double-distilled water at room temperature. The dialysis bag was filled with pure drug solution and optimized dapagliflozin-SLNs (equal to 2.0 mg dapagliflozin). It was submerged in 200 mL of 0.1 N HCl as a release medium for 2 h before being transferred to phosphate buffer (200 mL, pH 7.4). Throughout the experiment, the medium was continuously agitated at 60 rpm with 37 ± 0.5 °C. The aliquot (5 mL) was removed at regular intervals and replaced with newly released media in the same volume to maintain the concentration gradients. The amount of Dapagliflozin released was computed using the concentration of dapagliflozin measured using a UV spectrophotometer at each time point. The released data were fitted into multiple kinetic release models to determine the best-fit release model for improved dapagliflozin-SLNs [70].

In the in vivo investigations, SD rats of either sex (weight: 150–200 g; age: 8–10 weeks) were employed. Normal rats' blood glucose levels were in the 80–120 mg/dL range. The rats were obtained from the National Institute of Nutrition's animal house in Hyderabad, India. The rats were acclimated to a 12-h dark/light cycle in typical animal house facilities. Before the investigation, each animal's blood glucose levels (BGL) were measured. For 15 days before diabetic induction, the experimental animals were provided a fat-rich meal (powdered regular pellet food, coconut oil, casein protein, vitamin, cholesterol, sucrose, sodium chloride, DL-methionine, and fructose). Their nutrition was a standard pellet meal provided by Hindustan Lever (Kolkata, India), and they had access to water at all times in clean polypropylene cages [70]. The animals were kept in a typical laboratory environment for a week before the experiment. The ethics committee approved the study protocol-with registered number-I/IAEC/NCP/013/2020-SAM.

4.10.1. High-Fat Diet

With a calorie density of 13.2 kJ/g calories, the average rat diet contains 54% carbohydrates and 4% lipids. The high-fat diet had a calorie content of 22.1 kJ/g and consisted of 40% ordinary diet, 5.1% carbohydrate, 20% edible lard, 34% egg (*w*/*w*), and 0.9% salt chloride. Diabetes was produced in albino rats by feeding them a high-fat diet and administering a single modest dose (35 mg/kg) of STZ intraperitoneally. A digital glucometer was used to test the fasting BGL after 72 h of STZ treatment (Accu Check, Roche, Mannheim, Germany). Fasting BGL levels of less than 220 mg/dL were considered diabetic and were used in an experiment.

4.10.2. Acute Toxicity Studies (Fixed-Dose Procedure)

Acute oral toxicity testing was performed following the 2001 OECD-420 recommendations. We used male albino Wistar rats randomly selected for the acute toxicity study. The animals were grouped into four classes ($n = 6$) and fasted overnight with free access to water. As a control, the first group received normal saline orally. Groups II, III, and IV were given the improved formulation by oral bolus at doses of 5 mg/kg, 10 mg/kg, and 15 mg/kg body weight, respectively, with filtered water. During the first 12 h after treatment, the animals were monitored at 0, 15, 30, and 60 min. They were monitored for 14 days for death and toxic symptoms. After the observation period, the surviving rats were euthanized and autopsied. The kidneys, liver, stomach, testes, and pancreas were examined.

4.10.3. Induction of Diabetes

Wistar rats were placed into five classes of six after acclimatization. The first group of rats received a citrate buffer dose of 65 mg/kg (group I). Groups II, III, IV, and V diabetic rats were fed a high-fat diet for two weeks before receiving a single intraperitoneal injection of STZ (35 mg/kg b.w) (0.1 M, pH 4.5). The enhanced formulation was administered orally (with filtered water) for 28 days, beginning three days after the STZ injection. The fifth group of rats (group V) was given dapagliflozin at a dose of 1 mg/kg per day for 28 days. The rats were administered a 5% glucose solution for 48 h after STZ. Diabetic rats had blood glucose levels of 250 mg/dL or higher in subsequent testing [71].

4.10.4. Biochemical Estimations

Blood samples were taken from the animals' retro-orbital plexus after 28 days of testing. Total cholesterol, triglycerides, LDL, and HDL were determined using serum lipid profiles and blood glucose levels. ALP, SGOT, and SGPT levels were tested to identify abnormalities. A standard kit (Span Diagnostic Limited, Surat, India) was used to measure serum insulin levels, while a glycosylated hemoglobin kit was used to measure HbA1c levels (Stangen Immunodiagnostics, Hyderabad, India). At pH 7.4 and 3000 rpm/min, the livers of the rats were homogenized in a five mM Tris-HCl buffer with two mM EDTA and centrifuged at four °C for 10 min at the same temperature. MDA, CAT, GSH-Px, and SOD were analyzed using commercial kits and the manufacturers' activity manuals in the collected supernatant [72].

4.10.5. Statistical Analysis

All three results (n = 3) were presented as mean, standard deviation (SD). In vivo experiments used one-way ANOVA and Tukey's tests, with results expressed as mean and standard error, mean using GraphPad Prism software. One-way ANOVA and Dunnett's multiple comparison tests with a 95% confidence interval compared stability results to a new sample. The one-way ANOVA significance level was set at 0.05.

4.11. In Vivo Oral Bioavailability Studies

4.11.1. Animals

The Nalgonda Pharmacy College Laboratory Animal Center provided male rats (SD, 200–220 g). A representative optimized dapagliflozin-SLNs (F12) (group A) and marketed drug (group B) were each given to six rats (group B). After a 12-h fast, the rats were given optimized dapagliflozin-SLNs (5 mg/kg). This was conducted by NIH Publications No. 80–23 (1996) and after receiving ethical clearance (No. I/IAEC/NCP/013/2020-SAM). The animals were kept in a temperature-controlled room with a 12-h light/dark cycle, with free access to food and water until 12 h before treatment.

4.11.2. Pharmacokinetic Studies and Experimental Design

In the dapagliflozin investigation, the bioavailability of the enhanced SLNs was compared to that of the commercial product. At various time intervals, 0.5 mL of blood was drawn from the retro-orbital plexus in a heparinized tube (at 0.0, 0.5, 1, 2, 4, 6, 12, 16, 20, and 24 h). Blood samples were stored at 80 °C after being centrifuged for 15 min at 6000 rpm to separate the plasma. Using HPLC, a 775 L sample of plasma was mixed with a 225 L aliquot of methanol to determine the amount of dapagliflozin in plasma. After 1 min of vortex mixing, the product was centrifuged at 6000 rpm for 10 min, and the organic layer was transferred to a clean tube and dried at 45 °C under a mild nitrogen stream. Then, 225 L of mobile phase was used to re-dissolve the residue, and 5 L was injected into an HSS C18 (2.1 × 50 mm, 1.8 m) analytical column. Cmax, Tmax, and AUC (0–1) were calculated using nonlinear pharmacokinetics [73].

4.12. In Vitro UP-HPLC Analysis of Plasma Samples for Pharmacokinetic Assessment

The pharmacokinetic study assessed dapagliflozin concentrations in rat plasma after oral administration. Dapagliflozin, the model drug, was extracted from rat plasma using liquid-liquid extraction. Plasma was collected in 1.5 mL Eppendorf tubes. All plasma samples received 1 μg/mL internal standard solution in addition to methanol. Then, it was centrifuged for 10 min at 5000 rpm. The organic layer supernatant was transferred to a clean centrifuge tube and dried at 45–50 °C under nitrogen gas. It was reconstituted in 225 μL of the mobile phase. This was vortexed and autosampled for UPHPLC analysis. Thermo Scientific's Di-onexVR UPHPLC system (Ultimate 3000, Bedford, MA, USA) separated the DN and plasma samples. Methanol with 0.1% formic acid and 0.2% PhA) aqueous solution (28:72) and ACN (82/18 v/v) was used as a mobile phase at 0.4 mL/min. The analysis took 6 min to complete with a 2 μL sample injection volume. Q2A I (R1), 2005) were used to validate this plasma analysis method. The method's linearity (R^2 = 0.9999) was validated in the 100–10,000 μg/mL range [74].

4.13. Stability Study

The stability study of dapagliflozin-SLNs was done as per the ICH guidelines [54]. The sample was stored in Active-vials® for six months in a humidity-controlled oven (TH90S/G, Thermo lab, India) at intermediate storage conditions (30 °C 2 °C/65% RH 5% RH). The

Active-vial® is used to prevent moisture absorption by the samples during storage because, to avoid moisture absorption, it has a flip-top closed vial with an integrated molecular filter sleeve. The samples were withdrawn at predetermined time intervals (0, 1, 2, 3 months), and drug content and drug release were evaluated at 262 nm using a UV spectrophotometer.

5. Conclusions

Hot homogenization developed the SLNs followed by an ultra-sonication method using Compritol 888 ATO as lipid and Tween 80 as surfactant. The three-level, three-factor Box–Behnken experimental design was influential in optimizing dapagliflozin-SLNs. The optimized formulation showed small particle size and high %EE, optimum PDI, and zeta potential. The effect of selected independent variables on the quantity of drug release and %CDR may be predicted using the polynomial equation. Between the expected and observed values, closeness was observed. The quadratic response surface was studied for the amount of drug release, which helped understand the interaction effects of the selected independent variables and %CDR. Using the architecture of Box–Behnken to optimize the floating drug delivery system with an adequate response, a high degree of prediction was thus obtained. The IR data showed no incompatibility in the formulation between the drug and the excipients used. Optimized formulations of SLNs showed kinetics and drug release of Korsmeyer–Peppas model release. The optimized formulation was more significant ($p < 0.05$) than the pure drug solution. It confirms that the drug has higher therapeutic effectiveness after being encapsulated into SLNs.

Author Contributions: Formal analysis, M.K.; funding acquisition, A.U.; investigation, A.K.C. and T.H.; methodology, A.K.C., T.A.H. and T.H.; project administration, A.U., M.K. and S.C.; software, A.U. and T.A.H.; supervision, S.C.; writing—original draft, S.B.J. All authors have read and agreed to the published version of the manuscript.

Funding: The research was funded by the scientific research deanship at the University of Hail, Hail, Saudi Arabia: RG 20165.

Institutional Review Board Statement: The animal study protocol was approved by the Institutional Animal Ethics Committee (IAEC)—wide registered number I/IAEC/NCP/013/2020-SAM.

Informed Consent Statement: Not applicable.

Data Availability Statement: Data is contained within the article.

Acknowledgments: The authors are thankful to the scientific research deanship at the University of Hail, Hail, Saudi Arabia for funding our research work through the research grant number RG 20165.

Conflicts of Interest: The authors declare no conflict of interest.

References

1. Muzzalupo, R.; Tavano, L.; Cassano, R.; Trombino, S.; Ferrarelli, T.; Picci, N. A new approach for the evaluation of niosomes as effective transdermal drug delivery systems. *Eur. J. Pharm. Biopharm.* **2011**, *79*, 28–35. [CrossRef] [PubMed]
2. Wild, S.; Roglic, G.; Green, A.; Sicree, R.; King, H. Global prevalence of diabetes: Estimates for the year 2000 and projections for 2030. *Diabetes Care* **2004**, *27*, 1047–1053. [CrossRef] [PubMed]
3. Zelniker, T.A.; Wiviott, S.D.; Raz, I.; Im, K.; Goodrich, E.L.; Bonaca, M.P.; Mosenzon, O.; Kato, E.T.; Cahn, A.; Furtado, R.H.M.; et al. SGLT2 inhibitors for primary and secondary prevention of cardiovascular and renal outcomes in type 2 diabetes: A systematic review and meta-analysis of cardiovascular outcome trials. *Lancet* **2019**, *393*, 31–39. [CrossRef]
4. Kolb, H.; Martin, S. Environmental/lifestyle factors in the pathogenesis and prevention of type 2 diabetes. *BMC Med.* **2017**, *15*, 131. [CrossRef]
5. Canivell, S.; Mata-Cases, M.; Real, J.; Franch-Nadal, J.; Vlacho, B.; Khunti, K.; Gratacòs, M.; Mauricio, D. Glycaemic control after treatment intensification in patients with type 2 diabetes uncontrolled on two or more non-insulin antidiabetic drugs in a real-world setting. *Diabetes Obes. Metab.* **2019**, *21*, 1373–1380. [CrossRef]
6. Spinks, C.B.; Zidan, A.S.; Khan, M.A.; Habib, M.J.; Faustino, P.J. Pharmaceutical characterization of novel tenofovir liposomal formulations for enhanced oral drug delivery: In vitro pharmaceutics and Caco-2 permeability investigations. *Clin. Pharmacol. Adv. Appl.* **2017**, *9*, 29. [CrossRef]
7. Alsulays, B.B.; Anwer, M.K.; Soliman, G.A.; Alshehri, S.M.; Khafagy, E.-S. Impact of penetratin stereochemistry on the oral bioavailability of insulin-loaded solid lipid nanoparticles. *Int. J. Nanomed.* **2019**, *14*, 9127. [CrossRef]

8. Mishra, A.; Imam, S.S.; Aqil, M.; Ahad, A.; Sultana, Y.; Ameeduzzafar; Ali, A. Carvedilol nano lipid carriers: Formulation, characterization and in-vivo evaluation. *Drug Deliv.* **2016**, *23*, 1486–1494. [CrossRef]
9. Paudel, A.; Imam, S.S.; Fazil, M.; Khan, S.; Hafeez, A.; Ahmad, F.J.; Ali, A. Formulation and optimization of candesartan cilexetil nano lipid carrier: In vitro and in vivo evaluation. *Curr. Drug Deliv.* **2017**, *14*, 1005–1015. [CrossRef]
10. Mishra, V.; Bansal, K.K.; Verma, A.; Yadav, N.; Thakur, S.; Sudhakar, K.; Rosenholm, J.M. Solid lipid nanoparticles: Emerging colloidal nano drug delivery systems. *Pharmaceutics* **2018**, *10*, 191. [CrossRef]
11. Ganesan, P.; Ramalingam, P.; Karthivashan, G.; Ko, Y.T.; Choi, D.-K. Recent developments in solid lipid nanoparticle and surface-modified solid lipid nanoparticle delivery systems for oral delivery of phyto-bioactive compounds in various chronic diseases. *Int. J. Nanomed.* **2018**, *13*, 1569. [CrossRef] [PubMed]
12. Stella, B.; Peira, E.; Dianzani, C.; Gallarate, M.; Battaglia, L.; Gigliotti, C.L.; Boggio, E.; Dianzani, U.; Dosio, F. Development and characterization of solid lipid nanoparticles loaded with a highly active doxorubicin derivative. *Nanomaterials* **2018**, *8*, 110. [CrossRef] [PubMed]
13. Trevaskis, N.L.; Kaminskas, L.M.; Porter, C.J.H. From sewer to saviour—Targeting the lymphatic system to promote drug exposure and activity. *Nat. Rev. Drug Discov.* **2015**, *14*, 781–803. [CrossRef] [PubMed]
14. Porter, C.J.H.; Trevaskis, N.L.; Charman, W.N. Lipids and lipid-based formulations: Optimizing the oral delivery of lipophilic drugs. *Nat. Rev. Drug Discov.* **2007**, *6*, 231–248. [CrossRef]
15. Cross, S.E.; Roberts, M.S. Physical enhancement of transdermal drug application: Is delivery technology keeping up with pharmaceutical development? *Curr. Drug Deliv.* **2004**, *1*, 81–92. [CrossRef]
16. Jain, N.K. *Advances in Controlled and Novel Drug Delivery*; CBS Publishers & Distributors: New Delhi, India, 2008.
17. Barry, B.W. Novel mechanisms and devices to enable successful transdermal drug delivery. *Eur. J. Pharm. Sci.* **2001**, *14*, 101–114. [CrossRef]
18. Kandavilli, S.; Nair, V.; Panchagnula, R. Polymers in transdermal drug delivery systems. *Pharm. Technol.* **2002**, *26*, 62–81.
19. Sharma, S. Topical preparations are used for the localized effects at the site of their application by virtue of drug penetration into the underlying layers of skin or mucous membranes. *Pharm. Rev.* **2008**, *6*, 1–10.
20. Carbone, C.; Tomasello, B.; Ruozi, B.; Renis, M.; Puglisi, G. Preparation and optimization of PIT solid lipid nanoparticles via statistical factorial design. *Eur. J. Med. Chem.* **2012**, *49*, 110–117. [CrossRef]
21. Ansari, M.D.; Ahmed, S.; Imam, S.S.; Khan, I.; Singhal, S.; Sharma, M.; Sultana, Y. CCD based development and characterization of nano-transethosome to augment the antidepressant effect of agomelatine on Swiss albino mice. *J. Drug Deliv. Sci. Technol.* **2019**, *54*, 101234. [CrossRef]
22. Abedullahh, M.H. Box-behnken design for development and optimization of acetazolamide microspheres. *India* **2014**, *5*, 1228–1239.
23. Abdallah, M.H.; Sabry, S.A.; Hasan, A.A. Enhancing Transdermal Delivery of Glimepiride Via Entrapment in Proniosomal Gel. *J. Young Pharm.* **2016**, *8*, 335–340. [CrossRef]
24. Hosny, K.M.; Khalid, M.; Alkhalidi, H.M. Quality by design approach to screen the formulation and process variables influencing the characteristics of carvedilol solid lipid nanoparticles. *J. Drug Deliv. Sci. Technol.* **2018**, *45*, 168–176. [CrossRef]
25. Nepal, P.R.; Han, H.-K.; Choi, H.-K. Preparation and in vitro–in vivo evaluation of Witepsol®H35 based self-nanoemulsifying drug delivery systems (SNEDDS) of coenzyme Q10. *Eur. J. Pharm. Sci.* **2010**, *39*, 224–232. [CrossRef] [PubMed]
26. Date, A.A.; Nagarsenker, M.S. Design and evaluation of self-nanoemulsifying drug delivery systems (SNEDDS) for cefpodoxime proxetil. *Int. J. Pharm.* **2007**, *329*, 166–172. [CrossRef]
27. Sharma, J.B.; Bhatt, S.; Saini, V.; Kumar, M. Pharmacokinetics and pharmacodynamics of curcumin-loaded solid lipid nanoparticles in the Management of Streptozotocin-Induced Diabetes Mellitus: Application of central composite design. *Assay Drug Dev. Technol.* **2021**, *19*, 262–279. [CrossRef] [PubMed]
28. Wei, L.; Yang, Y.; Shi, K.; Wu, J.; Zhao, W.; Mo, J. Preparation and characterization of loperamide-loaded dynasan 114 solid lipid nanoparticles for increased oral absorption in the treatment of diarrhea. *Front. Pharmacol.* **2016**, *7*, 332. [CrossRef]
29. Manoochehri, S.; Darvishi, B.; Kamalinia, G.; Amini, M.; Fallah, M.; Ostad, S.N.; Atyabi, F.; Dinarvand, R. Surface modification of PLGA nanoparticles via human serum albumin conjugation for controlled delivery of docetaxel. *DARU J. Pharm. Sci.* **2013**, *21*, 58. [CrossRef]
30. Lalani, J.; Patil, S.; Kolate, A.; Lalani, R.; Misra, A. Protein-functionalized PLGA nanoparticles of lamotrigine for neuropathic pain management. *AAPS Pharmscitech* **2015**, *16*, 413–427. [CrossRef]
31. Das, S.; Ng, W.K.; Tan, R.B.H. Are nanostructured lipid carriers (NLCs) better than solid lipid nanoparticles (SLNs): Development, characterizations and comparative evaluations of clotrimazole-loaded SLNs and NLCs? *Eur. J. Pharm. Sci.* **2012**, *47*, 139–151. [CrossRef]
32. Ozturk, A.; Yenilmez, E.; Arslan, R.; Şenel, B.; Yazan, Y. Dexketoprofen trometamol loaded solid lipid nanoparticles (SLNs): Formulation, in vitro and in vivo evaluation. *J. Res. Pharm.* **2020**, *24*, 82–99.
33. Shah, M.; Pathak, K. Development and statistical optimization of solid lipid nanoparticles of simvastatin by using 23 full-factorial design. *AAPS Pharmscitech* **2010**, *11*, 489–496. [CrossRef] [PubMed]
34. Sumana Chompootaweep, M.D. The pharmacokinetics of pioglitazone in Thai healthy subjects. *J. Med. Assoc. Thail.* **2006**, *89*, 2116–2122.

35. Ghasemiyeh, P.; Mohammadi-Samani, S. Solid lipid nanoparticles and nanostructured lipid carriers as novel drug delivery systems: Applications, advantages and disadvantages. *Res. Pharm. Sci.* **2018**, *13*, 288. [PubMed]
36. Kovacevic, A.; Savic, S.; Vuleta, G.; Mueller, R.H.; Keck, C.M. Polyhydroxy surfactants for the formulation of lipid nanoparticles (SLN and NLC): Effects on size, physical stability and particle matrix structure. *Int. J. Pharm.* **2011**, *406*, 163–172. [CrossRef] [PubMed]
37. Thapa, C.; Ahad, A.; Aqil, M.; Imam, S.S.; Sultana, Y. Formulation and optimization of nanostructured lipid carriers to enhance oral bioavailability of telmisartan using Box–Behnken design. *J. Drug Deliv. Sci. Technol.* **2018**, *44*, 431–439. [CrossRef]
38. Venkateswarlu, V.; Manjunath, K. Preparation, characterization and in vitro release kinetics of clozapine solid lipid nanoparticles. *J. Control. Release* **2004**, *95*, 627–638. [CrossRef]
39. Kumar, V.V.; Chandrasekar, D.; Ramakrishna, S.; Kishan, V.; Rao, Y.M.; Diwan, P.V. Development and evaluation of nitrendipine loaded solid lipid nanoparticles: Influence of wax and glyceride lipids on plasma pharmacokinetics. *Int. J. Pharm.* **2007**, *335*, 167–175. [CrossRef]
40. Martin-Garcia, B.; Pimentel-Moral, S.; Gómez-Caravaca, A.M.; Arraez-Roman, D.; Segura-Carretero, A. Box-Behnken experimental design for a green extraction method of phenolic compounds from olive leaves. *Ind. Crops Prod.* **2020**, *154*, 112741. [CrossRef]
41. Kushwaha, A.K.; Vuddanda, P.R.; Karunanidhi, P.; Singh, S.K.; Singh, S. Development and evaluation of solid lipid nanoparticles of raloxifene hydrochloride for enhanced bioavailability. *Biomed Res. Int.* **2013**, *2013*, 584549. [CrossRef]
42. Mohsin, K.; Alamri, R.; Ahmad, A.; Raish, M.; Alanazi, F.K.; Hussain, M.D. Development of self-nanoemulsifying drug delivery systems for the enhancement of solubility and oral bioavailability of fenofibrate, a poorly water-soluble drug. *Int. J. Nanomed.* **2016**, *11*, 2829.
43. Agarwal, S.; Murthy, R.S.R.; Harikumar, S.L.; Garg, R. Quality by design approach for development and characterisation of solid lipid nanoparticles of quetiapine fumarate. *Curr. Comput. Aided. Drug Des.* **2020**, *16*, 73–91. [CrossRef] [PubMed]
44. Gade, S.; Patel, K.K.; Gupta, C.; Anjum, M.M.; Deepika, D.; Agrawal, A.K.; Singh, S. An ex vivo evaluation of moxifloxacin nanostructured lipid carrier enriched in situ gel for transcorneal permeation on goat cornea. *J. Pharm. Sci.* **2019**, *108*, 2905–2916. [CrossRef]
45. Pandey, S.; Patel, P.; Gupta, A. Novel solid lipid nanocarrier of glibenclamide: A factorial design approach with response surface methodology. *Curr. Pharm. Des.* **2018**, *24*, 1811–1820. [CrossRef]
46. Gonçalves, L.M.D.; Maestrelli, F.; Mannelli, L.D.C.; Ghelardini, C.; Almeida, A.J.; Mura, P. Development of solid lipid nanoparticles as carriers for improving oral bioavailability of glibenclamide. *Eur. J. Pharm. Biopharm.* **2016**, *102*, 41–50. [CrossRef]
47. Sefidgar, S.M.; Ahmadi-Hamedani, M.; Javan, A.J.; Sani, R.N.; Vayghan, A.J. Effect of crocin on biochemical parameters, oxidative/antioxidative profiles, sperm characteristics and testicular histopathology in streptozotocin-induced diabetic rats. *Avicenna J. Phytomed.* **2019**, *9*, 347.
48. Nabi, S.A.; Kasetti, R.B.; Sirasanagandla, S.; Tilak, T.K.; Kumar, M.V.J.; Rao, C.A. Antidiabetic and antihyperlipidemic activity of Piper longum root aqueous extract in STZ induced diabetic rats. *BMC Complement. Altern. Med.* **2013**, *13*, 37. [CrossRef]
49. Pandey, R.; Sharma, S.; Khuller, G.K. Oral solid lipid nanoparticle-based antitubercular chemotherapy. *Tuberculosis* **2005**, *85*, 415–420. [CrossRef] [PubMed]
50. Heiati, H.; Tawashi, R.; Phillips, N.C. Drug retention and stability of solid lipid nanoparticles containing azidothymidine palmitate after autoclaving, storage and lyophilization. *J. Microencapsul.* **1998**, *15*, 173–184. [CrossRef]
51. Kazi, M.; Al-Swairi, M.; Ahmad, A.; Raish, M.; Alanazi, F.K.; Badran, M.M.; Khan, A.A.; Alanazi, A.M.; Hussain, M.D. Evaluation of self-nanoemulsifying drug delivery systems (SNEDDS) for poorly water-soluble talinolol: Preparation, in vitro and in vivo assessment. *Front. Pharmacol.* **2019**, *10*, 459. [CrossRef]
52. Kazi, M.; Shahba, A.A.; Alrashoud, S.; Alwadei, M.; Sherif, A.Y.; Alanazi, F.K. Bioactive self-nanoemulsifying drug delivery systems (Bio-SNEDDS) for combined oral delivery of curcumin and piperine. *Molecules* **2020**, *25*, 1703. [CrossRef]
53. Zhang, X.; Chen, G.; Zhang, T.; Ma, Z.; Wu, B. Effects of PEGylated lipid nanoparticles on the oral absorption of one BCS II drug: A mechanistic investigation. *Int. J. Nanomed.* **2014**, *9*, 5503.
54. Agency, E.M. ICH Topic Q 1 A (R2) Stability Testing of New Drug Substances and Products. 2003. Available online: https://www.ema.europa.eu/en/ich-q1a-r2-stability-testing-new-drug-substances-drug-products (accessed on 17 January 2022).
55. Ahmad, J.; Mir, S.R.; Kohli, K.; Amin, S. Effect of oil and co-surfactant on the formation of Solutol HS 15 based colloidal drug carrier by Box–Behnken statistical design. *Colloids Surf. A Physicochem. Eng. Asp.* **2014**, *453*, 68–77. [CrossRef]
56. Ahmad, J.; Kohli, K.; Mir, S.R.; Amin, S. Formulation of self-nanoemulsifying drug delivery system for telmisartan with improved dissolution and oral bioavailability. *J. Dispers. Sci. Technol.* **2011**, *32*, 958–968. [CrossRef]
57. Behbahani, E.S.; Ghaedi, M.; Abbaspour, M.; Rostamizadeh, K. Optimization and characterization of ultrasound assisted preparation of curcumin-loaded solid lipid nanoparticles: Application of central composite design, thermal analysis and X-ray diffraction techniques. *Ultrason. Sonochem.* **2017**, *38*, 271–280. [CrossRef] [PubMed]
58. Amasya, G.; Aksu, B.; Badilli, U.; Onay-Besikci, A.; Tarimci, N. QbD guided early pharmaceutical development study: Production of lipid nanoparticles by high pressure homogenization for skin cancer treatment. *Int. J. Pharm.* **2019**, *563*, 110–121. [CrossRef] [PubMed]
59. Ali, J.; Bhatnagar, A.; Kumar, N.; Ali, A. Others Chitosan nanoparticles amplify the ocular hypotensive effect of cateolol in rabbits. *Int. J. Biol. Macromol.* **2014**, *65*, 479–491.

60. Imam, S.S.; Bukhari, S.N.A.; Ahmad, J.; Ali, A. Others Formulation and optimization of levofloxacin loaded chitosan nanoparticle for ocular delivery: In-vitro characterization, ocular tolerance and antibacterial activity. *Int. J. Biol. Macromol.* **2018**, *108*, 650–659.
61. Agarwal, V.; Siddiqui, A.; Ali, H.; Nazzal, S. Dissolution and powder flow characterization of solid self-emulsified drug delivery system (SEDDS). *Int. J. Pharm.* **2009**, *366*, 44–52. [CrossRef]
62. Atef, E.; Belmonte, A.A. Formulation and in vitro and in vivo characterization of a phenytoin self-emulsifying drug delivery system (SEDDS). *Eur. J. Pharm. Sci.* **2008**, *35*, 257–263. [CrossRef]
63. Shaveta, S.; Singh, J.; Afzal, M.; Kaur, R.; Imam, S.S.; Alruwaili, N.K.; Alharbi, K.S.; Alotaibi, N.H.; Alshammari, M.S.; Kazmi, I.; et al. Development of solid lipid nanoparticle as carrier of pioglitazone for amplification of oral efficacy: Formulation design optimization, in-vitro characterization and in-vivo biological evaluation. *J. Drug Deliv. Sci. Technol.* **2020**, *57*, 101674. [CrossRef]
64. Ekambaram, P.; Sathali, A.A.H. Formulation and evaluation of solid lipid nanoparticles of ramipril. *J. Young Pharm.* **2011**, *3*, 216–220. [CrossRef] [PubMed]
65. Ahmad, I.; Pandit, J.; Sultana, Y.; Mishra, A.K.; Hazari, P.P.; Aqil, M. Optimization by design of etoposide loaded solid lipid nanoparticles for ocular delivery: Characterization, pharmacokinetic and deposition study. *Mater. Sci. Eng. C* **2019**, *100*, 959–970. [CrossRef]
66. Chadha, R.; Bhandari, S. Drug–excipient compatibility screening—Role of thermoanalytical and spectroscopic techniques. *J. Pharm. Biomed. Anal.* **2014**, *87*, 82–97. [CrossRef] [PubMed]
67. Tamjidi, F.; Shahedi, M.; Varshosaz, J.; Nasirpour, A. Design and characterization of astaxanthin-loaded nanostructured lipid carriers. *Innov. Food Sci. Emerg. Technol.* **2014**, *26*, 366–374. [CrossRef]
68. Montenegro, L.; Sinico, C.; Castangia, I.; Carbone, C.; Puglisi, G. Idebenone-loaded solid lipid nanoparticles for drug delivery to the skin: In vitro evaluation. *Int. J. Pharm.* **2012**, *434*, 169–174. [CrossRef]
69. Colas, J.-C.; Shi, W.; Rao, V.S.N.M.; Omri, A.; Mozafari, M.R.; Singh, H. Microscopical investigations of nisin-loaded nanoliposomes prepared by Mozafari method and their bacterial targeting. *Micron* **2007**, *38*, 841–847. [CrossRef]
70. Aljaeid, B.M.; Hosny, K.M. Miconazole-loaded solid lipid nanoparticles: Formulation and evaluation of a novel formula with high bioavailability and antifungal activity. *Int. J. Nanomed.* **2016**, *11*, 441. [CrossRef]
71. Guo, X.; Wang, Y.; Wang, K.; Ji, B.; Zhou, F. Stability of a type 2 diabetes rat model induced by high-fat diet feeding with low-dose streptozotocin injection. *J. Zhejiang Univ. B* **2018**, *19*, 559–569. [CrossRef]
72. Trinder, P. Determination of glucose in blood using glucose oxidase with an alternative oxygen acceptor. *Ann. Clin. Biochem.* **1969**, *6*, 24–27. [CrossRef]
73. Pappa, H.; Farru, R.; Vilanova, P.O.; Palacios, M.; Pizzorno, M.T. A new HPLC method to determine Donepezil hydrochloride in tablets. *J. Pharm. Biomed. Anal.* **2002**, *27*, 177–182. [CrossRef]
74. Abdelbary, G.A.; Tadros, M.I. Brain targeting of olanzapine via intranasal delivery of core–shell difunctional block copolymer mixed nanomicellar carriers: In vitro characterization, ex vivo estimation of nasal toxicity and in vivo biodistribution studies. *Int. J. Pharm.* **2013**, *452*, 300–310. [CrossRef] [PubMed]

pharmaceuticals

MDPI

Article

Multi-Dose Intravenous Administration of Neutral and Cationic Liposomes in Mice: An Extensive Toxicity Study

Stéphanie Andrade [1,2,†], Joana A. Loureiro [1,2,†], Santiago Ramirez [3], Celso S. G. Catumbela [3], Claudio Soto [3], Rodrigo Morales [3,4,*] and Maria Carmo Pereira [1,2,*]

1 LEPABE, Department of Chemical Engineering, Faculty of Engineering, University of Porto, 4200-465 Porto, Portugal; stephanie@fe.up.pt (S.A.); jasl@fe.up.pt (J.A.L.)
2 ALiCE—Associate Laboratory in Chemical Engineering, Faculty of Engineering, University of Porto, Rua Dr. Roberto Frias, 4200-465 Porto, Portugal
3 Department of Neurology, The University of Texas Health Science Center at Houston, 6431 Fannin St., Houston, TX 77030, USA; santiago.d.ramirez@uth.tmc.edu (S.R.); celso.catumbela@uth.tmc.edu (C.S.G.C.); claudio.soto@uth.tmc.edu (C.S.)
4 Centro Integrativo de Biologia y Quimica Aplicada (CIBQA), Universidad Bernardo O'Higgins, Santiago 1497, Chile
* Correspondence: rodrigo.moralesloyola@uth.tmc.edu (R.M.); mcsp@fe.up.pt (M.C.P.)
† These authors contributed equally to this work.

Abstract: Liposomes are widely used as delivery systems for therapeutic purposes. However, the toxicity associated with the multi-dose administration of these nanoparticles is not fully elucidated. Here, we evaluated the toxicity of the prolonged administration of liposomes composed of neutral or cationic phospholipids often used in drug and gene delivery. For that purpose, adult wild-type mice (C57Bl6) were randomly distributed into three groups receiving either vehicle (PBS), neutral, or cationic liposomes and subjected to repeated intravenous injections for a total of 10 doses administered over 3 weeks. Several parameters, including mortality, body weight, and glucose levels, were monitored throughout the trial. While these variables did not change in the group treated with neutral liposomes, the group treated with the positively charged liposomes displayed a mortality rate of 45% after 10 doses of administration. Additional urinalysis, blood tests, and behavioral assays to evaluate impairments of motor functions or lesions in major organs were also performed. The cationic group showed less forelimb peak force than the control group, alterations at the hematological level, and inflammatory components, unlike the neutral group. Overall, the results demonstrate that cationic liposomes are toxic for multi-dose administration, while the neutral liposomes did not induce changes associated with toxicity. Therefore, our results support the use of the well-known neutral liposomes as safe drug shuttles, even when repetitive administrations are needed.

Keywords: lipid-based nanoparticles; nanocarrier; surface charge; delivery systems; chronic treatment; mice

Citation: Andrade, S.; Loureiro, J.A.; Ramirez, S.; Catumbela, C.S.G.; Soto, C.; Morales, R.; Pereira, M.C. Multi-Dose Intravenous Administration of Neutral and Cationic Liposomes in Mice: An Extensive Toxicity Study. *Pharmaceuticals* **2022**, *15*, 761. https://doi.org/10.3390/ph15060761

Academic Editor: Jianping Qi

Received: 16 May 2022
Accepted: 17 June 2022
Published: 18 June 2022

1. Introduction

The poor pharmacokinetics, reduced bioavailability, and high toxicity of most therapeutic molecules are some of the aspects that decrease their therapeutic efficacy. Such limitations can be overcome using delivery systems to protect molecules from degradation and direct them to the desired target site [1].

Liposomes are spherical vesicles composed of phospholipid bilayers enclosing aqueous compartments [2]. The amphiphilic property of phospholipids, which display hydrophilic polar heads and lipophilic tails, allows the encapsulation of hydrophilic compounds in the aqueous space and lipophilic compounds in the lipid bilayer [3]. The biocompatibility, bioavailability, high loading capacity, ease of production, and sustained release of therapeutic agents are other properties that stand out [4]. Conventional liposomes composed of neutral lipids were the first generation of lipid vesicles to be used by the pharmaceutical industry. In turn, cationic liposomes represent the newest generation of liposomes and have been used in gene therapy [5].

Despite several advantages related to the use of liposomes as delivery systems, they have some drawbacks that restrict their therapeutic potential. While liposomes have been successfully used to reduce the toxicity of therapeutic agents, the vesicles themselves can induce toxicity. Dozens of in vivo studies have described the toxicity associated with the administration of one or just a few doses of cationic liposomes [6–8]. However, these reports lack information regarding the long-term toxicity, which is crucial considering the therapeutic regime of several pathologies, such as chronic diseases, that require the repeated administration of therapeutic agents to ensure sustained drug levels for extended periods [9].

Thereby, we conducted the first prolonged systemic toxicity study by intravenously administering 10 doses of neutral and cationic liposomes to wild-type mice over 3 weeks to better understand the effect of multi-doses administration of this lipid based nanocarriers in vivo. Bare NPs were tested without any targeting ligand to focus this study on evaluating the nanocarriers' toxicity upon repeated administration. Lipid vesicles were characterized physicochemically in terms of hydrodynamic diameter, polydispersity index (PDI), and zeta potential. The long-term stability at storage conditions was also evaluated for over 4 months. Mice mortality, variations in body weights, glucose levels, motor abilities, microscopic urinalyses, liposome–blood interaction, and organ weight and morphology were assessed to evaluate potential liposome-induced toxic effects. Histopathological examinations were also performed, and liver injury markers in blood were quantified.

2. Results and Discussion

2.1. Physicochemical Characterization of Liposomes

The physicochemical properties of the neutral and cationic LUVs were evaluated in terms of hydrodynamic diameter, PDI, and zeta potential values, as shown in Table 1. While neutral liposomes exhibited a hydrodynamic diameter of 139 ± 13 nm, the cationic liposomes showed a significantly smaller average of 112 ± 3 nm ($p < 0.05$) (Table 1). Such a difference may be related to the distinct composition of the liposomes [10].

Table 1. Physicochemical properties of neutral and cationic liposomes in terms of hydrodynamic diameter, polydispersity index (PDI), and zeta potential.

Liposomes	Composition	Hydrodynamic Diameter (nm)	PDI	Zeta Potential (mV)
Neutral	DSPC:CHOL:DSPE-PEG(2000) amine	139 ± 13	0.22 ± 0.02	−1 ± 1
Cationic	DOTAP:CHOL	112 ± 3	0.13 ± 0.01	33 ± 2

It has been reported that the efficacy of a delivery system is closely related to the size of NPs since this property can affect the in vivo stability, blood circulation time, agent release, cell uptake, clearance, and toxicity of NPs. NPs larger than 200 nm have revealed to be quickly cleared from the bloodstream by the lymphatic system [11]. However, nanocarriers too small have been connected to higher toxicity as the NP surface area increases. Thus, an optimal diameter of around 100 nm has been identified, as particles around that size have shown decreased toxicity [1]. Such evidence proved that the produced formulations have mean sizes valid for delivery applications.

The size distribution of NPs was evaluated by assessing the PDI of formulations. All formulations presented PDI values lower than 0.2 (Table 1), suggesting that the lipid suspensions have homogenous sizes, and therefore are valid for delivery purposes [12]. However, the neutral liposomes showed PDI values significantly higher than the cationic liposomes ($p < 0.05$), probably due to the different techniques used to reduce the size of the vesicles. This data goes in line with a report by Ong et al., demonstrating that extruded liposomes present smaller PDI values than sonicated liposomes [13].

The surface charge of NPs is another key property to consider when designing delivery systems since it affects nanocarriers' in vivo internalization rate and toxicity. As expected, neutral LUVs showed a zeta potential close to zero mV, while cationic LUVs exhibited a zeta potential of 33 ± 2 mV (Table 1).

Liposome stability remains a major limitation for their clinical application. For that reason, it is crucial to ensure their stability during the production process and the duration of the experiments, since NPs tend to aggregate to attain a thermodynamically favorable state. If a NP product is expected to be commercialized, its physicochemical properties should be preserved during the storage period. Hence, a long-term stability study of the produced liposomes was performed at storage conditions (4 °C) over 4 months (Figure 1). Variations in some of these characteristics suggest that the structure of NPs is altered over time, which may be linked with the loss of their stability and potential activities [14]. From Figure 1, it is possible to observe that the physicochemical properties of the neutral liposomes remained constant ($p > 0.05$) for at least 4 months when stored at 4 °C in the buffered medium. Moreover, while neutral LUVs exhibited a mean d/d_0 value of approximately 1.1 over the 4 months study period, cationic vesicles presented a value of 3.9 at the experimental endpoint, indicating NPs aggregation. The d/d_0 value represents the ratio between the mean diameter of the NPs at each time point and the initial mean diameter, being an indicator of size variation [15]. However, the physicochemical properties of DOTAP:CHOL vesicles were not significantly changed over the first month of storage. After this time, cationic liposomes exhibited a mean diameter above 200 nm and a PDI over 0.4.

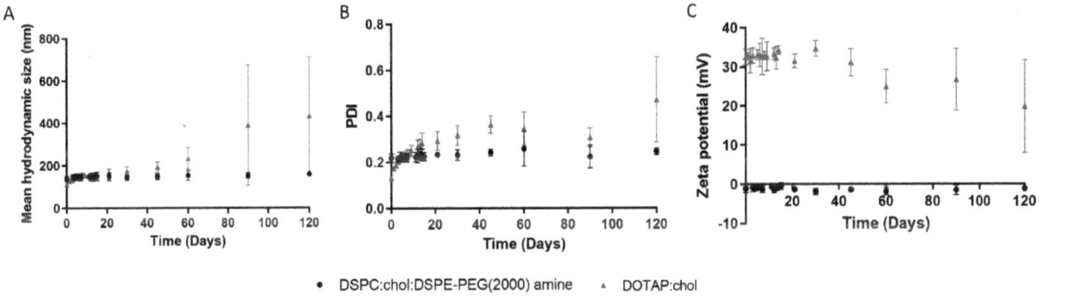

Figure 1. Physicochemical characterization of liposomes over 4 months in terms of (**A**) hydrodynamic diameter, (**B**) PDI, and (**C**) zeta potential values.

2.2. *Mice Survival and Clinical Observations*

The survival curves of mice repeatedly exposed to the different liposomes are shown in Figure 2. No mortality was registered among mice exposed to repeated doses of neutral liposomes, thus overlapping the survival curve of the control group (treated with PBS). However, a significant mortality rate was observed in mice treated with cationic liposomes, with an average of 27% mortality immediately after the first injection. Moreover, the mortality rate increased to 36% after the second injection. From the sixth to the tenth administration, mice treated with cationic liposomes displayed a survival rate of 55%. These results are in accordance with Chien et al. (2005) [16], which observed a 33% mortality rate after injecting three doses of cationic liposomes to male BALB/c mice. Despite the mortality observed in mice exposed to cationic liposomes, none exhibited alterations in fur appearance, eyes, sleep cycles, salivation, defecation, food and water intake, or other visible signs.

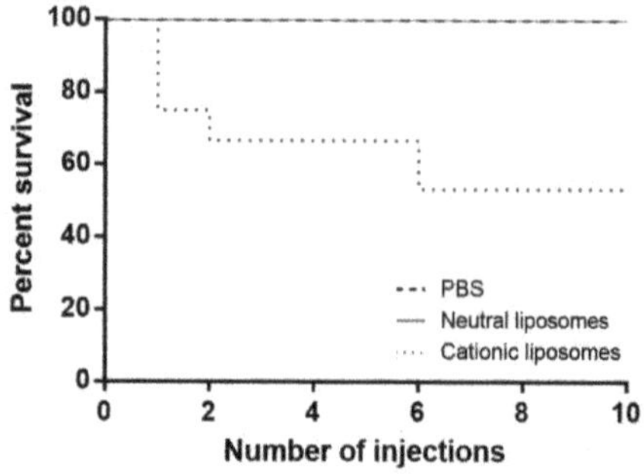

Figure 2. Effect of the repeated administration of PBS, neutral and cationic liposomes on mice survival.

2.3. Bodyweight

Bodyweight is frequently recorded in toxicology studies, since variations over 20% can be linked with toxic effects [17]. Thus, mice body weight was recorded before each administration and euthanasia (Supplemental Table S1). At the baseline, the PBS, neutral liposomes, and cationic liposomes groups showed an average body weight of 21.6 ± 1.3, 21.6 ± 1.4, and 21.2 ± 0.8, respectively, with no significant differences between the liposomes-treated and control mice ($p > 0.05$). Mice body weight remained stable until the end of the experiment ($p > 0.05$). Similar findings were obtained by Knudsen et al. (2015) [18] after administering a single dose of cationic liposomes to male Han Wistar rats.

2.4. Glucose Levels

Blood glucose represents another extensively used indicator in toxicological studies since variations in glucose levels are an established toxicity surrogate. Importantly, fluctuations in blood glucose concentrations can induce secondary toxic events, including glial toxicity, oxidative stress, and inflammatory processes [19]. Thus, the glucose levels of mice treated with repeated doses of PBS, neutral-, and cationic-lipid vesicles were monitored weekly and are shown in Supplemental Figure S1. Before starting the injection of LUVs, control, neutral, and cationic groups exhibited glucose levels of 135 ± 14, 126 ± 8, and 140 ± 10 mg/dL, respectively, with no significant differences between groups ($p > 0.05$). No significant variations were observed over the experiment in neutral and cationic liposomes-treated mice compared with the control group ($p > 0.05$), which is in concordance with a previous study [18].

2.5. Behavioral Tests

Behavioral monitoring is a sensitive way to assess the nervous system toxicosis induced by a tested drug or material [20]. In fact, variations in the behavioral responses of animals may be related to the impairment of sensory, motor, and cognitive aspects. The rotarod test is currently one of the most used behavior tests where the neurotoxicity or effect of a compound on animal behavior can be evaluated [21]. By monitoring the time rodents remain in the rotarod, motor coordination and balance defects can be detected [22]. Therefore, the rotarod test was performed before starting the NPs injection and 24 h-post-treatment. To complement the rotarod test, a forelimb grip strength test was performed 48 h post-treatment to evaluate the limb motor and neuromuscular function of experimental and control rodents [23]. The results of the rotarod and grip strength tests are shown in Figure 3A,B, respectively.

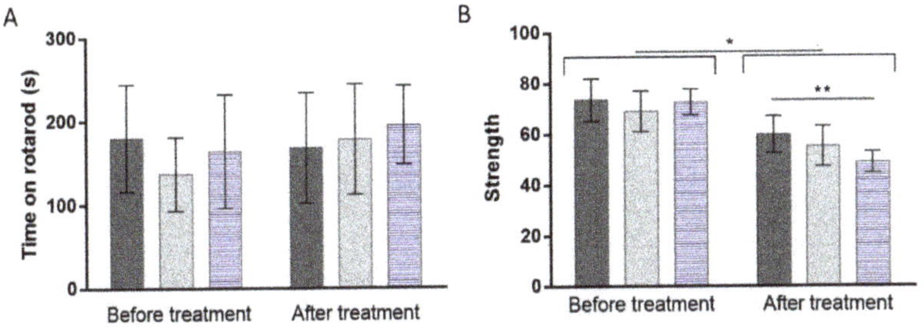

Figure 3. Effect of multi-dose administration of PBS (dark gray), neutral (light gray), and cationic liposomes (blue) on (**A**) rotarod and (**B**) grip strength performance. * $p < 0.05$, ** $p < 0.01$.

Concerning the rotarod test (Figure 3A), no significant variation in the latency to fall from the rotarod apparatus was detected after the repeated administration of both neutral and cationic vesicles compared to the control group ($p > 0.05$). These data suggest the absence of motor dysfunction due to liposome treatments. However, grip strength data (Figure 3B) revealed a significant reduction of the maximal muscle strength of mice after the repeated injection of PBS, neutral, and cationic liposomes ($p < 0.05$). Although variations on the maximal peak force may indicate motor neurotoxicity, the decreased grip strength of the control group suggests a lack of interest in the trial, potentially due to the excessive manipulation associated with repeated injections. Alternatively, rodents may get used to the manipulation, reducing their willingness to execute the task. Regardless, the repeated administration of cationic liposomes significantly declined the forelimb peak force values of mice by around 9.1% compared to the control group ($p < 0.01$), suggesting that these particular vesicles induce harmful effects on limb motor and neuromuscular function of mice.

2.6. Microscopic Urinalysis

The microscopic examination of urine is another common procedure to detect possible toxicity signals. Urinalysis identifies abnormal solutes, cells, casts, crystals, organisms, or particulate matter that may indicate some renal or systemic pathology. Supplemental Figure S2 shows the microscopic urinalysis of mice after the prolonged treatment of PBS, neutral, or positively charged liposomes. The urine of healthy animals or patients usually contains several chemicals that can be found in the form of crystals, and so, a small number of urine crystals become clinically irrelevant. However, the presence of abnormal crystals may indicate renal dysfunction. Some usually present crystals (triple phosphate) are pointed by black arrows in Supplemental Figure S2. In contrast, evidence of hippuric acid crystals was identified in the urine of mice treated with neutral liposomes.

In addition to crystals, some endothelial cells are also commonly present in the urine of healthy individuals. Red arrows in Supplemental Figure S2 depict some of these cells. However, other cell types are not expected to be found in urine, and thus, their presence is acknowledged as an indicator of health issues. An example of this are red blood cells (RBCs). When present in urine, RBCs are indicative of a disease condition known as hematuria. Supplemental Figure S2C (blue arrows) indicates some of the numerous RBCs present in the urine of mice treated with cationic LUVs, indicating damage at this level. Notably, hematuria was absent in the urine of the control and neutral liposome groups. Importantly, the RBCs identified in the cationic LUVs-treated mice's urine exhibited an unusual form with a spiked cell membrane, characteristic of acanthocytes [24]. This abnormal kind of RBCs possesses some spikes of varying lengths and widths irregularly located on the cell surface, as shown by the green arrows in Supplemental Figure S2D.

2.7. *Liposomes–Blood Interaction*

Before reaching target tissues or cells, liposomes injected intravenously first interact with blood components [25]. Thus, after observing a 27% mortality rate caused by the first injection of DOTAP:CHOL LUVs, an in vitro LUVs-blood interaction study was performed to identify the possible cause of such immediate deaths. Figure 4 shows blood samples from untreated mice mixed with PBS, neutral, or cationic liposomes. It is possible to observe that positively charged liposomes induced noticeable changes in blood, substantially increasing its turbidity and inducing coagulation (Figure 4C). In contrast, neither the increase of the turbidity nor the formation of clots was verified when PBS and neutral liposomes were mixed with blood (Figure 4A,B). Confirming the previous observations, a microscopic analysis of blood smears suggests that RBCs agglutinate in the presence of cationic liposomes (Supplemental Figure S3). These findings are in line with Senior's report [26], which also detected the increase in turbidity and the formation of clot-like mass upon the incubation of cationic liposomes with rat plasma. Furthermore, the authors revealed that the extent of plasma–liposomes interactions depend on the concentration of the phospholipid positive charge [26].

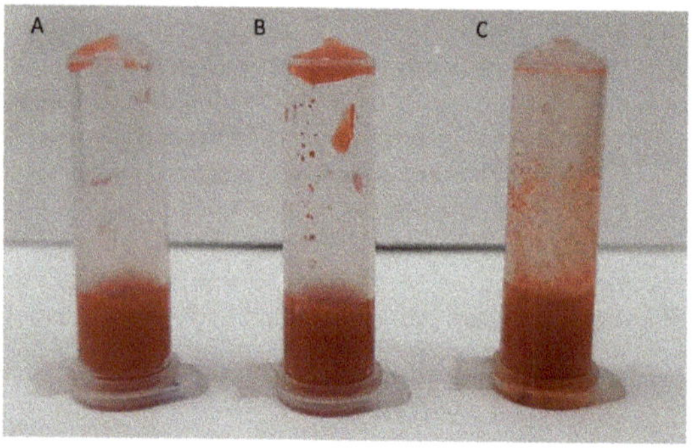

Figure 4. Ex vivo blood–liposome interaction. Blood from non-treated mice was mixed with either (**A**) PBS, (**B**) neutral, or (**C**) cationic liposomes.

The acute interaction between blood components and liposomes was also assessed in vivo by intravenously injecting one dose of DOTAP:CHOL LUVs into mice. Therefore, fresh blood was collected, and a blood smear was performed on a glass slides to analyze RBCs morphological alterations, several regions of the slide were observed, and the diameter or RBCs was measured in pixels using image software. The microscopic analysis of the blood smears of these mice shows that, after a single administration, positively charged liposomes induce morphological changes in RBCs (Supplemental Figure S4). Specifically, RBCs transitioned from a regular spherical shape (Supplemental Figure S4A) to irregular structures involving either fusiform (acuminocytes) (Supplemental Figure S4B, red arrows) or teardrop forms (dacrocytes) (Supplemental Figure S4B, blue arrows).

While numerous acuminocytes and dacrocytes were observed after a single dose of DOTAP:CHOL LUVs (Supplemental Figure S4B), such variations were less evident after repeated administration of cationic liposomes (Figure 5C). Instead, several fragmented RBCs (commonly called schistocytes) were identified in the blood smears of mice from the cationic liposomes group (Figure 5C, black arrows). Such structures are smaller than usual RBCs and typically irregularly shaped, and result from hemolysis (Figure 5C, red arrow). Hemolysis of erythrocytes caused by the interaction with cationic liposomes was previously observed in vitro [26]. No irregular structures were noticed in the groups treated with PBS (Figure 5A) and neutral liposomes (Figure 5B). Moreover, we observed high variability in the size of RBCs, a condition called anisocytosis (Supplemental Figure S5). Anisocytosis was quantified by assessing the RBC's mean width and the standard deviation of the gaussian distributions from the red cell distribution width (RDW) histograms using the

Measure Tool of the ImageJ software (National Institutes of Health, Bethesda, MD, USA). Details on these results are shown in Supplemental Figure S5 and Table 2. Overall, these findings suggest that neutral liposomes do not alter RDW compared to RBCs derived from control mice (Supplemental Figure S5, gray and black lines and bars). However, repeated injections of positively charged LUVs significantly affect RDW (Supplemental Figure S5, blue lines and bars). The data presented in Table 2 reveal a reduction in the average width of RBCs, likely due to the presence of several microcytic RBCs (erythrocytes smaller than usual). As expected, the cationic group displayed the largest standard deviation (Table 2), suggesting a more significant size variability of RBCs, i.e., anisocytosis [27]. This might be explained by the toxic effects exerted by cationic liposomes, which could modify RBCs membrane properties inducing cell adhesions and accelerated removal [28]. However, the alterations in RBCs size might be part of the normal physiological response to the loss of RBCs [29]. Consequently, two events should be occurring in these mice: (i) the faster production of RBCs to compensate low levels results in smaller RBCs due to the high demand for hemoglobin; and (ii) larger RBCs also appear to compensate the loss.

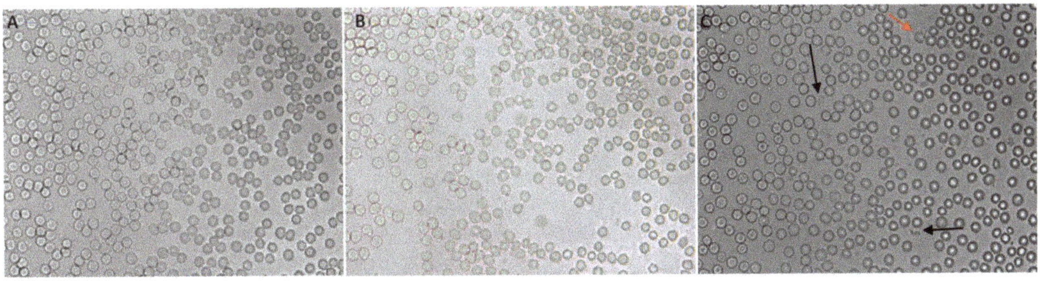

Figure 5. In vivo cationic liposomes–blood interaction. Microscopic images of blood smears from mice treated with (**A**) PBS, (**B**) neutral, and (**C**) cationic liposomes. Images obtained at a 40× magnification. Black and red identify schistocytes and hemolysis, respectively.

Table 2. Effect of the repeated administration of PBS, neutral, and cationic liposomes on the mean width of red blood cells (RBCs).

	PBS Group	Neutral Group	Cationic Group
Mean width of RBCs (pixel)	44.7 ± 2.6	44.6 ± 2.6	43.4 ± 3.1

The surface charge has been pointed out as a determining factor affecting the NPs hemocompatibility [30]. Han et al. (2012) [31] revealed that the electrostatic interactions between cationic NPs and the erythrocyte membrane cause erythrocyte agglutination. The functionalization of the NPs surface with negatively charged groups reduced the erythrocyte, aggregating effects of the NPs [31]. In turn, Zhao et al. (2011) revealed that modifying the liposomes surface with PEG molecules may shade the positive charge of the NPs, thus avoiding the toxic blood–liposomes interactions [32].

2.8. Organ Weight and Morphology

The comparison of the organ weight between substance-treated and control groups is extensively used to assess harmful effects [33]. In fact, organ weight is one of the most sensitive markers of toxicity since organ damage does not always translate into modifications in its morphology [34]. The absolute weight of the brain, lung, liver, kidney, and spleen was recorded at necropsy (Figure 6A). The brain, liver, and kidney weight and size of mice treated with neutral and cationic liposomes did not significantly change compared to the control group ($p > 0.05$). However, a significant reduction of the absolute lung weight was observed in mice treated with cationic LUVs-treated. Interestingly, the absolute weight of the spleen significantly increased in both liposome-treated groups. This variation was accompanied by an increase in the spleen dimensions in both liposomes-treated groups ($p < 0.05$) (Figure 6B). No major macroscopic changes were observed in the brain, lung, liver, kidney, or spleen after the repeated administration of liposomes.

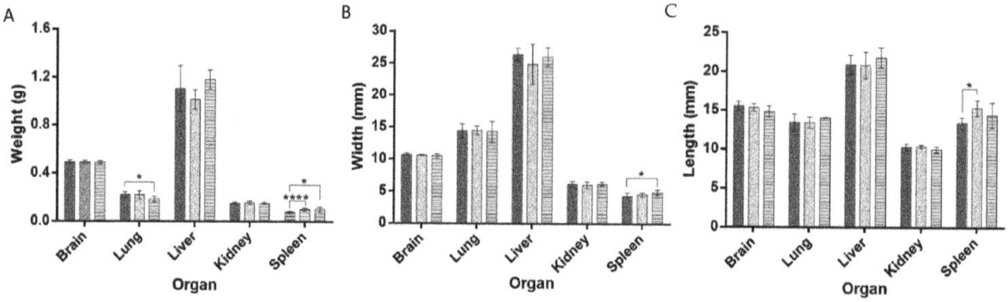

Figure 6. (**A**) Absolute organ weight, (**B**) organ width, and (**C**) organ length of mice treated with repeated doses of PBS (dark gray), neutral (light gray), and cationic (blue) liposomes. * $p < 0.05$, **** $p < 0.0001$.

2.9. Histopathological Examination

Histopathological studies of several tissues, including liver, lung, kidney, and spleen, were performed. While no alterations were noticed in the tissues of neutral LUVs-treated mice, the histopathological examination revealed that cationic liposomes induce alterations at the hematological level and inflammatory components. The spleen revealed extravascular hematopoiesis observed as diffuse hyperplasia of the red pulp (Supplemental Figure S6). In addition, an evident enrichment in megakaryocytes (Figure 7C, blue arrowhead) was observed in the spleen of mice treated with cationic liposomes compared with animals challenged with neutral liposomes or PBS. While some extra-medullar hematopoiesis is normal in rodents (especially in mice), an increase in this feature may result from induced hematotoxicity. The presence of hemosiderin (brown pigment) (Figure 7C, red arrowhead) in the spleens of cationic liposomes-treated mice may result from hemolytic anemia [35]. It is conceivable that since these are non-PEGylated liposomes, the NPs are recognized relatively fast by the spleen due to binding to proteins such as immunoglobulins, complement proteins and apolipoproteins [18]. Supporting these observations, the lungs of mice treated with cationic liposomes also showed a large population of brown pigmented alveolar macrophages (Figure 7). This could be explained by the high levels of damaged RBCs induced by cationic liposomes. These results agree with the modification of the morphology observed in both organs (Figure 6). Similar findings have been found after the acute administration of cationic nanoparticles [18,36]. Increased DNA damage in both lung and spleen after a single administration of cationic liposomes was observed in a previous study [18]. Moreover, cationic liposomes have been associated with dose-dependent toxicity and pulmonary inflammation. Dokka et al. (2000) demonstrated that cationic liposomes induce the generation of reactive oxygen species in lung cells, causing inflammation and toxicity [7].

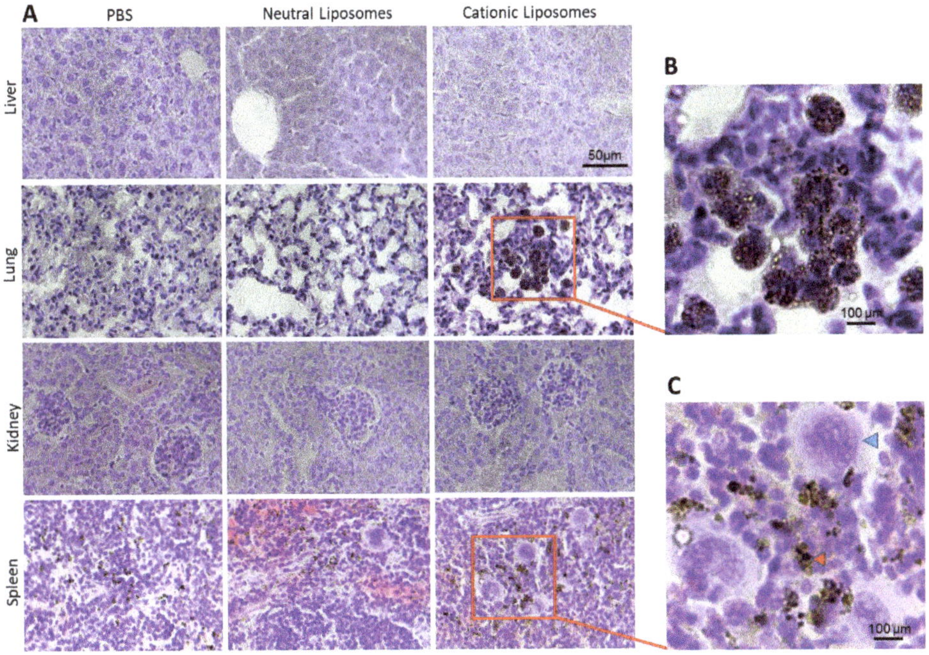

Figure 7. (**A**) Histopathological analysis of liver, lung, kidney, and spleen from mice treated with PBS, neutral, or cationic liposomes (bar depicts 50 µm) (10× magnification). (**B**) Magnification of a lung area from mice treated with cationic liposomes displaying brown pigment (hemosiderin) contained within alveolar macrophages. (**C**) Magnification of a spleen area from mice treated with cationic liposomes depicting brown pigmentation (hemosiderin, red arrowhead) and megakaryocytes (blue arrowhead). Bar in (**B**,**C**) represents 100 µm (40× magnification).

Importantly, the above-mentioned alterations are in line with the anisocytosis observed in blood smears (Supplemental Figure S3), the increased hematuria characterized by the presence of shape-altered RBCs in the urine of mice treated with cationic liposomes (Supplemental Figure S2), and the agglutination of fresh blood induced by cationic liposomes in vitro (Figure 4). No evident alterations were observed in the liver and kidneys (Supplemental Figure S6 and Figure 7).

2.10. Serum Biochemistry

The liver is the organ that processes most of the substances introduced into the organism. As such, toxic compounds or molecules may exert their toxicity at the liver level. To explore potential liver-induced toxicity, alterations in the levels of liver proteins such as aspartate aminotransferase (AST) and alanine aminotransferase (ALT) were assessed in the blood of experimental and control mice. In agreement with the data presented in Figure 7, no changes in AST and ALT levels were found between any of the groups included in this study (Figure 8). These data suggest that the liver is not critically damaged by liposomes and support the idea that the toxicity induced by cationic liposomes is mainly associated with RBCs.

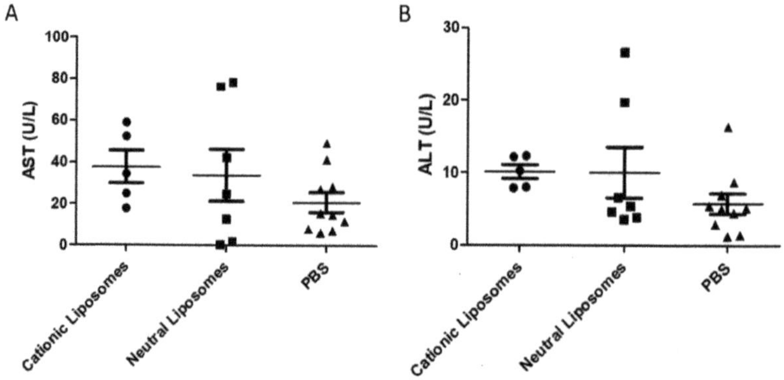

Figure 8. Plasma levels of (**A**) AST and (**B**) ALT in the blood of mice treated with either PBS (triangles), neutral (squares), or cationic liposomes (circles).

3. Materials and Methods

3.1. Chemicals

1,2-distearoyl-sn-glycero-3-phosphocholine (DSPC, MW 790, CN 850365P), cholesterol (CHOL, MW 387, CN 700000P), 2-distearoyl-sn-glycero-3-phosphoethanolamine-N-[amino(polyethylene glycol)-2000] (ammonium salt) (DSPE-PEG(2000) amine, MW 2791, CN 880128P) and 1,2-dioleoyl-3-trimethylammonium-propane (chloride salt) (DOTAP, MW 699, CN 890890P) were purchased from Avanti Polar Lipids, Inc. (Alabaster, AL, USA). Chloroform was obtained from Sigma-Aldrich (St. Louis, MO, EUA) (CN 25693). Phosphate buffered saline (PBS, 10×, pH 7.0–7.2, 0.067 M, CN SH30256.01) was acquired from GE Healthcare Life Sciences (HyClone™, Logan, UT, USA). Heparin (sodium salt, 1000 units/mL, CN 25021-400-30) was purchased from Sagent (Schaumburg, IL, USA).

3.2. Preparation of Liposomes

Neutral liposomes were produced by the thin-film hydration method by sonication [37]. Briefly, DSPC, CHOL, and DSPE-PEG(2000)amine were dissolved in chloroform at a molar ratio of 52:45:3. Then, the organic solvent was evaporated under a nitrogen stream. The produced film was hydrated with PBS at 37 °C (66 mM). To reduce the size, the suspension was sonicated for 40 min (1-min ON, 1-min OFF, 40% of amplitude) in an ice bath using an ultrasonic processor UP400S (Hielscher, Berlin, Germany).

Cationic liposomes were also produced by the thin-film hydration method followed by extrusion [38]. DOTAP and CHOL (molar ratio 85:15) were dissolved in chloroform, and a thin lipid film was obtained after the evaporation of the organic solvent under a nitrogen stream. The dried lipid film was hydrated with PBS at 37 °C (17 mM) and vortexed for 10 min. To reduce the vesicles' size, the suspension was extruded eleven times through Nuclepore™ (Maidstone, UK) track-etch polycarbonate membranes with a pore size of 100 nm.

3.3. Experimental Animals, Grouping, and Dosing Regime

Thirty-three adult female wild-type mice (C57Bl6) aged between 3–4 months were obtained from Jackson's laboratories (Bar Harbor, ME, USA). Only female mice were used in the present study to avoid possible variability of the results induced by sex differences. Five to six mice were housed per polypropylene ventilated cage in a room at 22 °C, humidity (40–60%), and a 12/12 h light/dark cycle. Animals were fed with standard mice pellet feed and water ad libitum in the animal facility of the Center for Laboratory Animal Medicine and Care (CLAMC) at UTHealth (Houston, TX, USA). Mice were housed for 48 h before starting the experiments. To promote animal welfare and reproducible experimental results, the rodents were allowed a period of 72 h to acclimate. The animal protocol was reviewed and approved by the Animal Welfare Committee (AWC) of the University of Texas Health Science Center at Houston (UTHealth) (approval number AWC-19-0061). All the experiments were performed according to the institutional guidelines.

The animals were randomly distributed into three groups receiving either vehicle (PBS), neutral or cationic liposomes (11/group). All groups received 10 doses of 200 µL over 3 weeks (administrations held on Mondays, Wednesdays, and Fridays). The doses and duration of treatment were selected according to previous studies [16,18].

3.4. Animal Survival, Clinical Observation, Body Weight, and Glucose Levels

Mice were examined daily for clinical signs of toxicity and mortality. The clinical observation included changes in fur, eyes, mucous membranes, lacrimation, and unusual breathing patterns. The body weight (BW) was recorded as an objective measurement before each administration and necropsy. Glucose levels were measured before the first injection and at euthanasia and monitored weekly.

3.5. Behavioral Tests

3.5.1. Rotarod Test

The rotarod test was performed before starting the injections and 24 h after the last administration to detect any defects in motor coordination. Following an accelerated speed test protocol, mice were placed into a rotating rod (Med Associates Inc., Fairfax, VA, USA), and the latency to fall was recorded. Succinctly, mice were placed on the rotarod apparatus, rotating at an increasing speed from 4 to 40 rpm, in a trial of 300 s. The latency to fall of 3 trials was recorded. A rest interval of 120 s between each trial was employed to avoid the animals' fatigue. Two successive animal rotations clinging to the rotarod were registered as latency to fall measurement. Before the first experiment, mice were helped to stay in the correct position for 30 s at a constant speed of 4 rpm to avoid false positives of animals turning, falling, or jumping.

3.5.2. Forelimb Grip Strength Test

Defects on rodents' limb motor and neuromuscular function were evaluated using a forelimb grip strength test. This test was performed before starting the injections and 48 h post-treatment, allowing an interval rest of 24 h from the rotarod test to avoid mice fatigue. A grip strength meter grid was manufactured to perform this experiment. Concisely, mice were held by the tail and placed horizontally over the grid until the animal forepaws clings. The animals were smoothly pulled back by the tail, and the maximal grip strength value displayed on the screen was recorded. A constant velocity was applied to ensure the repeatability of the test. This procedure was repeated 9 times, with a rest time of 120 s every 3 measurements. The forelimb grip strength values were recorded as the average of the 9 measurements.

3.6. Microscopic Urinalysis

In the morning following the last administration, three animals from each group were randomly chosen, and urine was collected for microscopic urinalysis. The microscopic examination was performed using a DMI6000B microscope (Leica, Buffalo Grove, IL, USA). Briefly, a 10 µL drop of urine was placed on a glass microscope slide and covered with a coverslip. The presence of microscopic elements, such as red and white blood cells, epithelial cells, casts, crystals, bacteria, yeast, and clumps, was analyzed.

3.7. In Vitro Interaction between Blood and Liposomes

The blood was collected by cardiac puncture after being euthanized by CO_2 inhalation. Blood samples (200 µL) were mixed with 200 µL of DSPC:CHOL:PEG(2000) amine and DOTAP:CHOL LUVs (1:1 *v*/*v*). A control sample was prepared containing an identical volume of PBS. Blood turbidity changes, clot formation, and hemolysis were examined macroscopically. Then, blood smears of the mixtures (30 μL) were performed and observed using a DMI6000B microscope (Leica, Buffalo Grove, IL, USA).

3.8. Acute In Vivo Interaction between Blood and Liposomes

A group of adult female wild-type mice were injected with a single dose of DOTAP:CHOL LUVs. Animals were euthanized by an overdose of anesthesia, and the blood was collected by cardiac puncture. Animals injected with PBS were subjected to the same procedure and used as controls. Blood smears from both animal groups (30 μL) were performed and observed using a DMI6000B microscope (Leica, Buffalo Grove, IL, USA). The effect of a single dose of positively charged liposomes on the morphology of RBCs was evaluated.

3.9. Prolonged In Vivo Study to Assess the Interaction between Blood and Liposomes

After administering 10 doses of PBS, DSPC:CHOL:PEG(2000) amine, and DOTAP:CHOL LUVs, the surviving animals were euthanized 120 h after the last injection via CO_2 inhalation followed by cardiac puncture to collect the blood. Three blood samples (30 μL) of each group were randomly selected to perform blood smears. The morphology of RBCs was analyzed using a DMI6000B microscope (Leica, Buffalo Grove, IL, USA).

3.10. Necropsy, Organ Weight, and Morphology

Necropsy was performed immediately after euthanasia. Here, each animal's brain, lungs, liver, kidneys, and spleen were excised and examined macroscopically to identify possible signs of toxicity. The organs were washed with PBS, placed on an absorbent paper for a few seconds, and the absolute organ weight was determined. The dimensions of the organs were also recorded using an automatic digital caliper (Neiko, Wenzhou, China). For further histopathological studies, the organs were placed in a 10% neutral buffered formalin solution. The blood samples from cardiac punctures were collected into Eppendorf tubes containing sodium heparin as an anticoagulant. Blood samples were centrifuged at 3000 rpm for 15 min to collect the serum. Plasma samples were frozen in liquid nitrogen and then stored at −80 °C until used for the liver injury assessment.

3.11. Histopathological Examinations

Major organs were stored in 3.7% formaldehyde, paraffin-embedded, and sliced at 10 μm for hematoxylin-eosin staining following routine protocols [39]. Briefly, after deparaffinization and rehydration, tissue slices were stained with hematoxylin solution for 5 min in a dark container and rinsed with distilled water. Next, sections were stained with eosin solution for 30 s, followed by dehydration with alcohol and clearing with xylene. The mounted sections were visualized under light microscopy, and histopathological evaluation was performed for spleen, lung, liver, and kidney tissues. Stained slices were observed at low- and high-power magnifications (10× and 40×, respectively) using a Leica DMI6000 B microscope (Leica Microsystems, Buffalo Grove, IL). Representative photomicrographs were taken with a digital camera (DFC310FX Leica™, Wetzlar, Germany). Low- and high-power magnifications were used to qualitatively analyze the cell type content in the red pulp of the spleen, the micromorphological integrity, the presence of granuloma formation, and the extent of cellular infiltration exhibited by lungs, livers, and kidneys.

3.12. Quantification of Liver Injury Markers in Blood

The levels of two established liver injury biomarkers, ALT and AST, were measured via diagnostic enzyme assay kits (ATL kit: catalog # A524-150, lot 86154; AST kit: catalog # A559-150, lot 84022, both Teco Diagnostics, Anaheim, CA, USA) in blood plasma, according to the manufacturer's protocol. ALT and AST activity was determined by measuring the rate of oxidation of NADH throughout an enzymatic reaction sequence at a specific wavelength (340 nm) using a SpectraMax® iD3 Multi-Mode Microplate Reader (Molecular Devices, San José, CA, USA).

3.13. Statistical Analysis

All the results are expressed as mean ± standard deviation. The statistical analysis of data was performed using student's t-tests, with a confidence interval of 95%. Results whose p-values ≤ 0.05 were considered significantly different. Statistical analysis and data presentation were completed using Prism 8 (GraphPad Software Inc. La Jolla, CA, USA).

4. Conclusions

This study thoroughly characterized the potential toxicity of neutral and cationic liposomes after repeated intravenous administrations in rodents. Our results show that cationic liposomes are toxic, evidenced by a 45% lethality. According to the results, the toxicity induced by the repeated administration of the cationic liposomes appears to be associated with the adverse interactions of the lipid vesicles with anionic serum macromolecules. Consequently, substantial changes in the spleen and liver of the mice were noticed. Therefore, caution should be exercised when using cationic liposomes in vivo. Importantly, our results highlight the safety of neutral liposomes and support their use as drug shuttles, even when repeated doses of a therapeutic agent are needed to be administered for optimal effects.

Supplementary Materials: The following supporting information can be downloaded at: https://www.mdpi.com/article/10.3390/ph15060761/s1, Figure S1: Effect of the repeated administration of PBS (dark gray), neutral (light gray), and cationic liposomes (blue) on blood glucose levels; Figure S2: Microscopic urinalysis of mice treated with cationic and neutral liposomes; Figure S3: Microscopic images of blood smears after mixing blood and liposomes ex vivo; Figure S4: Acute in vivo cationic liposomes-blood interaction; Figure S5: Effect of prolonged administration of PBS (black), neutral (gray), and cationic liposomes (blue) on the red blood cell distribution width (RDW); Figure S6: Histopathological analysis of liver, lung, kidney, and spleen at low power magnification; Table S1: Effect of the repeated administration of PBS, neutral and cationic liposomes on mice body weight.

Author Contributions: Conceptualization, J.A.L. and R.M.; methodology, R.M.; validation, M.C.P.; formal analysis, S.A., J.A.L., C.S.G.C. and S.R.; investigation, all authors; resources, C.S. and M.C.P.; data curation, S.A.; writing—original draft preparation, S.A. and J.A.L.; writing—review and editing, C.S., R.M. and M.C.P.; supervision, R.M. and M.C.P.; funding acquisition, R.M. All authors have read and agreed to the published version of the manuscript.

Funding: This work was financially supported by: Base Funding—LA/P/0045/2020 (ALiCE), and UIDP/00511/2020 (LEPABE), funded by national funds through the FCT/MCTES (PIDDAC); Project 2SMART—engineered Smart materials for Smart citizens, with reference NORTE-01-0145-FEDER-000054, supported by Norte Portugal Regional Operational Programme (NORTE 2020), under the PORTUGAL 2020 Partnership Agreement, through the European Regional Development Fund (ERDF); Project EXPL/NAN-MAT/0209/2021, supported by FCT—Fundação para a Ciência e a Tecnologia; FCT supported S.A. under two grants (SFRH/BD/129312/2017 and COVID/BD/151869/2021) and J.A.L under the Scientific Employment Stimulus—Institutional Call—[CEECINST/00049/2018]; and a grant from NIH (1RF1AG059321-01A1) to R.M and C.S.

Institutional Review Board Statement: The animal protocol was reviewed and approved by the Animal Welfare Committee (AWC) of the University of Texas Health Science Center at Houston (UTHealth)(approval number AWC-19-0061). All the experiments were performed according to the institutional guidelines.

Informed Consent Statement: Not applicable.

Data Availability Statement: Data is contained within the article and Supplementary Material.

Acknowledgments: The authors would like to thank the animal care personnel from the Center for Laboratory Animal Medicine and Care (CLAMC) at UTHealth (Houston, TX, USA), for their valuable assistance.

Conflicts of Interest: The authors declare no conflict of interest.

References

1. Ramalho, M.J.; Andrade, S.; Loureiro, J.A.; Pereira, M.C. Nanotechnology to improve the Alzheimer's disease therapy with natural compounds. *Drug Deliv. Transl. Res.* **2019**, *10*, 380–402. [CrossRef] [PubMed]
2. Andrade, S.; Ramalho, M.J.; Loureiro, J.A.; Pereira, M.C. Liposomes as biomembrane models: Biophysical techniques for drug-membrane interaction studies. *J. Mol. Liq.* **2021**, *334*, 116141. [CrossRef]
3. Guimarães, D.; Cavaco-Paulo, A.; Nogueira, E. Design of liposomes as drug delivery system for therapeutic applications. *Int. J. Pharm.* **2021**, *601*, 120571. [CrossRef] [PubMed]
4. Liu, P.; Chen, G.; Zhang, J. A Review of Liposomes as a Drug Delivery System: Current Status of Approved Products, Regulatory Environments, and Future Perspectives. *Molecules* **2022**, *27*, 1372. [CrossRef]
5. Ewert, K.K.; Scodeller, P.; Simón-Gracia, L.; Steffes, V.M.; Wonder, E.A.; Teesalu, T.; Safinya, C.R. Cationic Liposomes as Vectors for Nucleic Acid and Hydrophobic Drug Therapeutics. *Pharmaceutics* **2021**, *13*, 1365. [CrossRef]
6. Li, Y.; Cui, X.-L.; Chen, Q.-S.; Yu, J.; Zhang, H.; Gao, J.; Sun, D.-X.; Zhang, G.-Q. Cationic liposomes induce cytotoxicity in HepG2 via regulation of lipid metabolism based on whole-transcriptome sequencing analysis. *BMC Pharmacol. Toxicol.* **2018**, *19*, 43. [CrossRef]
7. Dokka, S.; Toledo, D.; Shi, X.; Castranova, V.; Rojanasakul, Y. Oxygen Radical-Mediated Pulmonary Toxicity Induced by Some Cationic Liposomes. *Pharm. Res.* **2000**, *17*, 521–525. [CrossRef]
8. Yu, J.; Zhang, H.; Li, Y.; Sun, S.; Gao, J.; Zhong, Y.; Sun, D.; Zhang, G. Metabolomics revealed the toxicity of cationic liposomes in HepG2 cells using UHPLC-Q-TOF/MS and multivariate data analysis. *Biomed. Chromatogr.* **2017**, *31*, e4036. [CrossRef]
9. Singh, A.P.; Biswas, A.; Shukla, A.W.; Maiti, P. Targeted therapy in chronic diseases using nanomaterial-based drug delivery vehicles. *Signal Transduct. Target. Ther.* **2019**, *4*, 33. [CrossRef]
10. Garbuzenko, O.; Barenholz, Y.; Priev, A. Effect of grafted PEG on liposome size and on compressibility and packing of lipid bilayer. *Chem. Phys. Lipids* **2005**, *135*, 117–129. [CrossRef]
11. Hoshyar, N.; Gray, S.; Han, H.; Bao, G. The effect of nanoparticle size on in vivo pharmacokinetics and cellular interaction. *Nanomedicine* **2016**, *11*, 673–692. [CrossRef] [PubMed]
12. Danaei, M.; Dehghankhold, M.; Ataei, S.; Hasanzadeh Davarani, F.; Javanmard, R.; Dokhani, A.; Khorasani, S.; Mozafari, M.R. Impact of Particle Size and Polydispersity Index on the Clinical Applications of Lipidic Nanocarrier Systems. *Pharmaceutics* **2018**, *10*, 57. [CrossRef] [PubMed]
13. Ong, S.G.M.; Chitneni, M.; Lee, K.S.; Ming, L.C.; Yuen, K.H. Evaluation of Extrusion Technique for Nanosizing Liposomes. *Pharmaceutics* **2016**, *8*, 36. [CrossRef] [PubMed]
14. Ramalho, M.J.; Loureiro, J.A.; Coelho, M.A.N.; Pereira, M.C. Factorial Design as a Tool for the Optimization of PLGA Nanoparticles for the Co-Delivery of Temozolomide and O6-Benzylguanine. *Pharmaceutics* **2019**, *11*, 401. [CrossRef]
15. Ramalho, M.J.; Loureiro, J.A.; Gomes, B.; Frasco, M.F.; Coelho, M.A.N.; Pereira, M.C. PLGA nanoparticles for calcitriol delivery. In Proceedings of the 2015 IEEE 4th Portuguese Meeting on Bioengineering (ENBENG), Porto, Portugal, 26–28 February 2015; IEEE: Porto, Portugal.
16. Chien, P.-Y.; Wang, J.; Carbonaro, D.; Lei, S.; Miller, B.; Sheikh, S.; Ali, S.M.; Ahmad, M.U.; Ahmad, I. Novel cationic cardiolipin analogue-based liposome for efficient DNA and small interfering RNA delivery in vitro and in vivo. *Cancer Gene Ther.* **2004**, *12*, 321–328. [CrossRef] [PubMed]
17. Lim, H.-S.; Seo, Y.S.; Ryu, S.M.; Moon, B.C.; Choi, G.; Kim, J.-S. Two-Week Repeated Oral Dose Toxicity Study of Mantidis Ootheca Water Extract in C57BL/6 Mice. *Evid.-Based Complement. Altern. Med.* **2019**, *2019*, 6180236. [CrossRef]
18. Knudsen, K.B.; Northeved, H.; Kumar, P.E.K.; Permin, A.; Gjetting, T.; Andresen, T.L.; Larsen, S.; Wegener, K.M.; Lykkesfeldt, J.; Jantzen, K.; et al. In vivo toxicity of cationic micelles and liposomes. *Nanomed. Nanotechnol. Biol. Med.* **2015**, *11*, 467–477. [CrossRef]
19. Quincozes-Santos, A.; Bobermin, L.D.; de Assis, A.M.; Gonçalves, C.-A.; Souza, D.O. Fluctuations in glucose levels induce glial toxicity with glutamatergic, oxidative and inflammatory implications. *Biochim. Biophys. Acta BBA Mol. Basis Dis.* **2017**, *1863*, 1–14. [CrossRef]
20. National Research Council. *Toxicity Testing: Strategies to Determine Needs and Priorities*; National Academies Press: Washington, DC, USA, 1984.
21. Dunham, W.N.; Miya, T.S. A Note on a Simple Apparatus for Detecting Neurological Deficit in Rats and Mice. *J. Am. Pharm. Assoc. (Sci. Ed.)* **1957**, *46*, 208–209. [CrossRef]
22. Sills, G.J.; Brodie, M.J. Antiepileptic Drugs | Preclinical Drug Development in Epilepsy. In *Encyclopedia of Basic Epilepsy Research*; Schwartzkroin, P.A., Ed.; Academic Press: Oxford, UK, 2009; pp. 97–103.
23. Nevins, M.E.; Nash, S.A.; Beardsley, P.M. Quantitative grip strength assessment as a means of evaluating muscle relaxation in mice. *Psychopharmacology* **1993**, *110*, 92–96. [CrossRef]
24. Heine, G.H.; Sester, U.; Girndt, M.; Köhler, H. Acanthocytes in the urine: Useful tool to differentiate diabetic nephropathy from glomerulonephritis? *Diabetes Care* **2004**, *27*, 190–194. [CrossRef] [PubMed]
25. Harashima, H.; Kiwada, H. Interactions of Liposomes with Cells In Vitro and In Vivo: Opsonins and Receptors. *Curr. Drug Metab.* **2001**, *2*, 397–409. [CrossRef]
26. Senior, J.H.; Trimble, K.R.; Maskiewicz, R. Interaction of positively-charged liposomes with blood: Implications for their application in vivo. *Biochim. Biophys. Acta (BBA)—Biomembr.* **1991**, *1070*, 173–179. [CrossRef]

27. Lippi, G.; Cervellin, G.; Sanchis-Gomar, F. Red blood cell distribution width: A marker of anisocytosis potentially associated with atrial fibrillation. *World J. Cardiol.* **2019**, *11*, 292–304. [CrossRef] [PubMed]
28. Nishiguchi, E.; Okubo, K.; Nakamura, S. Adhesion of Human Red Blood Cells and Surface Charge of the Membrane. *Cell Struct. Funct.* **1998**, *23*, 143–152. [CrossRef]
29. O'Connell, K.E.; Mikkola, A.M.; Stepanek, A.M.; Vernet, A.; Hall, C.D.; Sun, C.C.; Yildirim, E.; Staropoli, J.F.; Lee, J.T.; Brown, D.E. Practical murine hematopathology: A comparative review and implications for research. *Comp. Med.* **2015**, *65*, 96–113.
30. de la Harpe, K.M.; Kondiah, P.P.; Choonara, Y.E.; Marimuthu, T.; du Toit, L.C.; Pillay, V. The hemocompatibility of nanoparticles: A review of cell–nanoparticle interactions and hemostasis. *Cells* **2019**, *8*, 1209. [CrossRef]
31. Han, Y.; Wang, X.; Dai, H.; Li, S. Nanosize and Surface Charge Effects of Hydroxyapatite Nanoparticles on Red Blood Cell Suspensions. *ACS Appl. Mater. Interfaces* **2012**, *4*, 4616–4622. [CrossRef]
32. Qi, X.; Zhao, W.; Zhuang, S. Comparative study of the in vitro and in vivo characteristics of cationic and neutral liposomes. *Int. J. Nanomed.* **2011**, *6*, 3087–3098. [CrossRef]
33. Michael, B.; Yano, B.; Sellers, R.S.; Perry, R.; Morton, D.; Roome, N.; Johnson, J.K.; Schafer, K. Evaluation of Organ Weights for Rodent and Non-Rodent Toxicity Studies: A Review of Regulatory Guidelines and a Survey of Current Practices. *Toxicol. Pathol.* **2007**, *35*, 742–750. [CrossRef]
34. Piao, Y.; Liu, Y.; Xie, X. Change Trends of Organ Weight Background Data in Sprague Dawley Rats at Different Ages. *J. Toxicol. Pathol.* **2013**, *26*, 29–34. [CrossRef] [PubMed]
35. Suttie, A.W. Histopathology of the Spleen. *Toxicol. Pathol.* **2006**, *34*, 466–503. [CrossRef] [PubMed]
36. Mendonça, M.C.P.; Radaic, A.; Garcia-Fossa, F.; da Cruz-Höfling, M.A.; Vinolo, M.A.R.; de Jesus, M.B. The in vivo toxicological profile of cationic solid lipid nanoparticles. *Drug Deliv. Transl. Res.* **2019**, *10*, 34–42. [CrossRef] [PubMed]
37. Andrade, S.; Ramalho, M.J.; Loureiro, J.A.; Pereira, M.C. Interaction of natural compounds with biomembrane models: A biophysical approach for the Alzheimer's disease therapy. *Colloids Surf. B Biointerfaces* **2019**, *180*, 83–92. [CrossRef] [PubMed]
38. Andrade, S.; Loureiro, J.A.; Pereira, M.C. Vitamin B12 Inhibits Aβ Fibrillation and Disaggregates Preformed Fibrils in the Presence of Synthetic Neuronal Membranes. *ACS Chem. Neurosci.* **2021**, *12*, 2491–2502. [CrossRef] [PubMed]
39. Duran-Aniotz, C.; Moreno-Gonzalez, I.; Gamez, N.; Perez-Urrutia, N.; Vegas-Gomez, L.; Soto, C.; Morales, R. Amyloid pathology arrangements in Alzheimer's disease brains modulate in vivo seeding capability. *Acta Neuropathol. Commun.* **2021**, *9*, 56. [CrossRef]

pharmaceuticals

MDPI

Article

Phytosomes as a Plausible Nano-Delivery System for Enhanced Oral Bioavailability and Improved Hepatoprotective Activity of Silymarin

Ravi Gundadka Shriram [1], Afrasim Moin [2], Hadil Faris Alotaibi [3], El-Sayed Khafagy [4,5], Ahmed Al Saqr [4], Amr Selim Abu Lila [6,*] and Rompicherla Narayana Charyulu [1,*]

1 Department of Pharmaceutics, NGSM Institute of Pharmaceutical Sciences, Nitte (Deemed to be University), Mangalore 575018, Karnataka, India; ravigs1991@gmail.com
2 Department of Pharmaceutics, College of Pharmacy, University of Hail, Hail 81442, Saudi Arabia; a.moinuddin@uoh.edu.sa
3 Department of Pharmaceutical Sciences, College of Pharmacy, Princess Nourah bint Abdul Rahman University, Riyadh 11671, Saudi Arabia; hfalotaibi@pnu.edu.sa
4 Department of Pharmaceutics, College of Pharmacy, Prince Sattam bin Abdulaziz University, Al-Kharj 11942, Saudi Arabia; e.khafagy@psau.edu.sa (E.-S.K.); a.alsaqr@psau.edu.sa (A.A.S.)
5 Department of Pharmaceutics and Industrial Pharmacy, Faculty of Pharmacy, Suez Canal University, Ismailia 41522, Egypt
6 Department of Pharmaceutics and Industrial Pharmacy, Faculty of Pharmacy, Zagazig University, Zagazig 44519, Egypt
* Correspondence: a.abulila@uoh.edu.sa (A.S.A.L.); narayana@nitte.edu.in (R.N.C.)

Citation: Shriram, R.G.; Moin, A.; Alotaibi, H.F.; Khafagy, E.-S.; Al Saqr, A.; Abu Lila, A.S.; Charyulu, R.N. Phytosomes as a Plausible Nano-Delivery System for Enhanced Oral Bioavailability and Improved Hepatoprotective Activity of Silymarin. *Pharmaceuticals* **2022**, *15*, 790. https://doi.org/10.3390/ph15070790

Academic Editors: Ana Catarina Silva, João Nuno Moreira and José Manuel Sousa Lobo

Received: 7 June 2022
Accepted: 22 June 2022
Published: 24 June 2022

Abstract: Silymarin, a phyto-constituent derived from the plant *Silybum marianum*, has been widely acknowledged for its hepatoprotective activities. Nevertheless, its clinical utility is adversely hampered by its poor water-solubility and its limited oral bioavailability. The aim of this study was to investigate the efficacy of phospholipid-based phytosomes for enhancing the oral bioavailability of silymarin. The phytosomes were prepared using the solvent evaporation technique and were optimized using a full factorial design. The optimized silymarin phytosomal formulation was then characterized for particle size, surface morphology, aqueous solubility, and in vitro drug release. Furthermore, in vivo antioxidant activity, hepatoprotective activity and oral bioavailability of the optimized formula were investigated in a rat model. The prepared silymarin phytosomes were discrete particles with a porous, nearly smooth surface and were 218.4 ± 2.54 nm in diameter. In addition, the optimized silymarin phytosomal formulation showed a significant improvement in aqueous solubility (~360 μg/mL) compared to pure silymarin and manifested a higher rate and extent of silymarin release from the optimized formula in dissolution studies. The in vivo assessment studies revealed that the optimized silymarin phytosomal formulation efficiently exerted a hepatoprotective effect in a CCl_4-induced hepatotoxicity rat model via restoring the normal levels of antioxidant enzymes and ameliorating cellular abnormalities caused by CCl_4-intoxication. Most notably, as compared to pure silymarin, the optimized silymarin phytosomal formulation significantly improved silymarin oral bioavailability, as indicated by a 6-fold increase in the systemic bioavailability. Collectively, phytosomes might represent a plausible phospholipid-based nanocarrier for improving the oral bioavailability of phyto-constituents with poor aqueous solubility.

Keywords: anti-oxidant activity; hepatoprotective effect; phospholipid; phytosomes; Silymarin

1. Introduction

Traditionally, herbal medications, often known as phyto-pharmaceuticals, had been widely used in many countries for the management and treatment of many health disorders [1]. Globally, herbal medicine has gained cumulative popularity in modern medical practice because of their availability along with their diverse therapeutic applications [2].

Nevertheless, despite the fact that plant extracts and phyto-constituents may exert excellent in vitro bioactivity, they usually show poor in vivo effects due to their large molecular sizes and/or low lipid solubility, making them less absorbable and having poor bioavailability [3,4].

Silymarin is a natural polyphenolic flavonoid compound extracted from milk thistle (*Silybum marianum*) seeds [5]. Silymarin has been proved to exert supreme therapeutic activity in the treatment of a variety of liver disorders such as chronic liver disease, cirrhosis, and hepatocellular carcinoma [6]. In addition, a mounting body of literature has emphasized the therapeutic potential of silymarin as an anti-inflammatory, antioxidant, hypoglycemic, anticancer, and antiviral agent [7,8]. Furthermore, recent encouraging results have underscored the neuroprotective effect of silymarin in the management of neurodegenerative diseases such as traumatic brain injury and Alzheimer's disease [9,10]. Nevertheless, despite clinical trials demonstrating that silymarin is safe at large dosages, up to 1500 mg/day in humans, it has limitations such as limited water-solubility, poor bioavailability, and poor intestinal absorption [11], which collectively could constrain its widespread utilization in many clinical settings.

The application of nanotechnology appears to be a potential way to amplify the therapeutic activity of the active herbal extract via improving its bioavailability and promoting a prolonged drug release at the site of absorption. Many strategies have been adopted to enhance the aqueous solubility and the systemic bioavailability of active phyto-constituents following oral administration, including nanoemulsion, solid lipid nanoparticles, polymeric nanoparticles, liposomes, inclusion complexation, etc. [11–14]. Among these potential strategies, phytosomes, also known as phyto-phospholipid complexes, have emerged as an encouraging strategy to improve the bioavailability of active phyto-constituents. Phytosomes are vesicular drug delivery systems that could enhance the absorption and bioavailability of poorly water-soluble drugs [15]. They are prepared by complexing the naturally active phyto-constituent with phospholipids [3]. Unlike other lipid-based vesicular systems, the bioactive phyto-constituents represents an integral part of vesicular membrane by being anchored to the polar head of the phospholipid via a chemical (hydrogen) bond, rather than been entrapped within the aqueous core or phospholipid bilayers of vesicular membrane. Importantly, phytosomes offer several advantages, including increased drug encapsulation, improved stability (chemical bonds are formed between the polar head of the amphiphile molecule and the phytoconstituent), and improved bioavailability [16]. In addition, a faster absorption rate results in a smaller dose of active components required to exert the intended pharmacological effect. Telange et al. [17] reported that loading the polyphenolic flavonoid apigenin onto a phytosomal formulation significantly enhanced its aqueous solubility, and oral bioavailability and showed a superior hepatoprotective effect, compared to pure apigenin. Similarly, Rathee et al. [18] evaluated the antidiabetic potential of polyherbal extracts loaded onto phosphatidylcholine-based phytosomes. The authors demonstrated that polyherbal extract-loaded phytosomes efficiently induced remarkable antidiabetic activity in streptozotocin-nicotinamide-induced rat models, which was comparable to that of a standard hypoglycemic drug metformin.

The aim of the present work was to enhance the absorption and oral bioavailability of silymarin via its formulation within a phytosomal nanocarrier system. A two-factor, three-level full factorial design was adopted to formulate and optimize silymarin-loaded phytosomes. The optimized formulation showed porous, nearly smooth surface particles within the nano-size range. In addition, the optimized formula showed a remarkable improvement in aqueous solubility of loaded silymarin, compared to pure silymarin. Most importantly, the optimized silymarin phytosomal formulation efficiently improved silymarin oral bioavailability and exerted a superior hepatoprotective effect in a CCl_4-induced hepatotoxicity rat model, compared to plain silymarin.

2. Results and Discussion

2.1. Preparation of Silymarin Phytosomal Complex

The stable silymarin phytosomal complex with the phospholipid was formulated using the solvent evaporation method. A preliminary examination of the investigated process parameters indicated that the drug-to-phospholipid and reaction temperature had a significant impact on the particle size and drug content of the produced phytosomes. Accordingly, a three-level, two-factor full factorial design was adopted for the formulation and optimization of the silymarin phytosomal complex. In the current study, a total of 9 runs (Table 1) were formulated by altering two independent formulation variables; drug-to-phospholipid (X_1) and reaction temperature (X_2) and their impact on two dependent formulation parameters; particle size (Y_1) and drug content (Y_2) was assessed. The estimated values from the experimental trials revealed that the particle size fluctuated from 220.2 ± 1.27 to 494.2 ± 6.64 nm, while the drug content ranged from 67.3 ± 2.64 to 92.4 ± 3.51%. The fitted polynomial equations relating the responses (particle size and drug content) to the altered formulation variables are summarized in the following equations:

$$Y_1 = 222.14 + 29.47\,X_1 - 49.43\,X_2 + 2.02\,X_1X_2 + 58.43\,X_1^2 + 133.83\,X_2^2$$

$$Y_2 = 91.38 - 0.133\,X_1 + 3.62\,X_2 - 2.25\,X_1X_2 - 3.57\,X_1^2 - 11.32\,X_2^2$$

Table 1. Experimental design matrix of the full factorial design with experimental results.

X_1 (*w:w*)	X_2 (°C)	Y_1 (nm)	Y_2 (*w/w*%)
+1	−1	494.2 ± 6.64	67.3 ± 2.64
−1	+1	329.6 ± 4.21	81.7 ± 3.47
0	−1	402.8 ± 3.87	75.6 ± 2.92
+1	+1	395.8 ± 2.45	78.7 ± 2.43
0	+1	313.1 ± 4.69	83.5 ± 3.38
−1	−1	436.1 ± 5.92	70.3 ± 2.79
0	0	220.2 ± 1.27	92.4 ± 3.51
−1	0	255.3 ± 1.52	89.2 ± 3.68
+1	0	307.8 ± 3.95	85.4 ± 3.74

X_1: drug:phospholipid ratio; X_2: the reaction temperature; Y_1: particle size; and Y_2: drug content. Data represents mean ± SD of three independent experiments.

The obtained polynomial equations can be utilized to extract conclusions based on the magnitude of coefficient and the mathematical sign it carries. A negative sign signifies an antagonistic effect, whilst a positive sign signifies a synergistic effect of the factor on the selected response.

Response surface plots and contour plots were also used to determine the significance and amplitude of the tested dependent factors on the independent responses (Figure 1). The response surface and contour plots revealed that the studied parameters; drug-to-phospholipid (X_1) and reaction temperature (X_2), had a significant impact on both formulation responses; particle size (Y_1) and drug content (Y_2). It was evident that the particle size decreased as the drug:phospholipid ratio increased from 1:1 to 1:2. A further increase in the ratio to 1:3 was found to increase the particle size. Similarly, the drug content (%) was found to be increased upon increasing drug:phospholipid ratio from 1:1 to 1:2. A further increase in drug:phospholipid ratio to 1:3 significantly decreased the drug content. In addition, the reaction temperature exerted significant effects on both particle size and drug content. Phytosomes prepared at a reaction temperature of 70 °C showed the smallest particle size, and the highest drug content, compared to phytosomes prepared at a higher reaction temperature (75 °C). Similar findings were reported by Telange et al. who demonstrated that both drug:phospholipid ratio and reaction temperature could significantly affect the entrapment efficiency of the polyphenolic flavonoid, apigenin, within soybean phosphatidylcholine-based phytosomes [17].

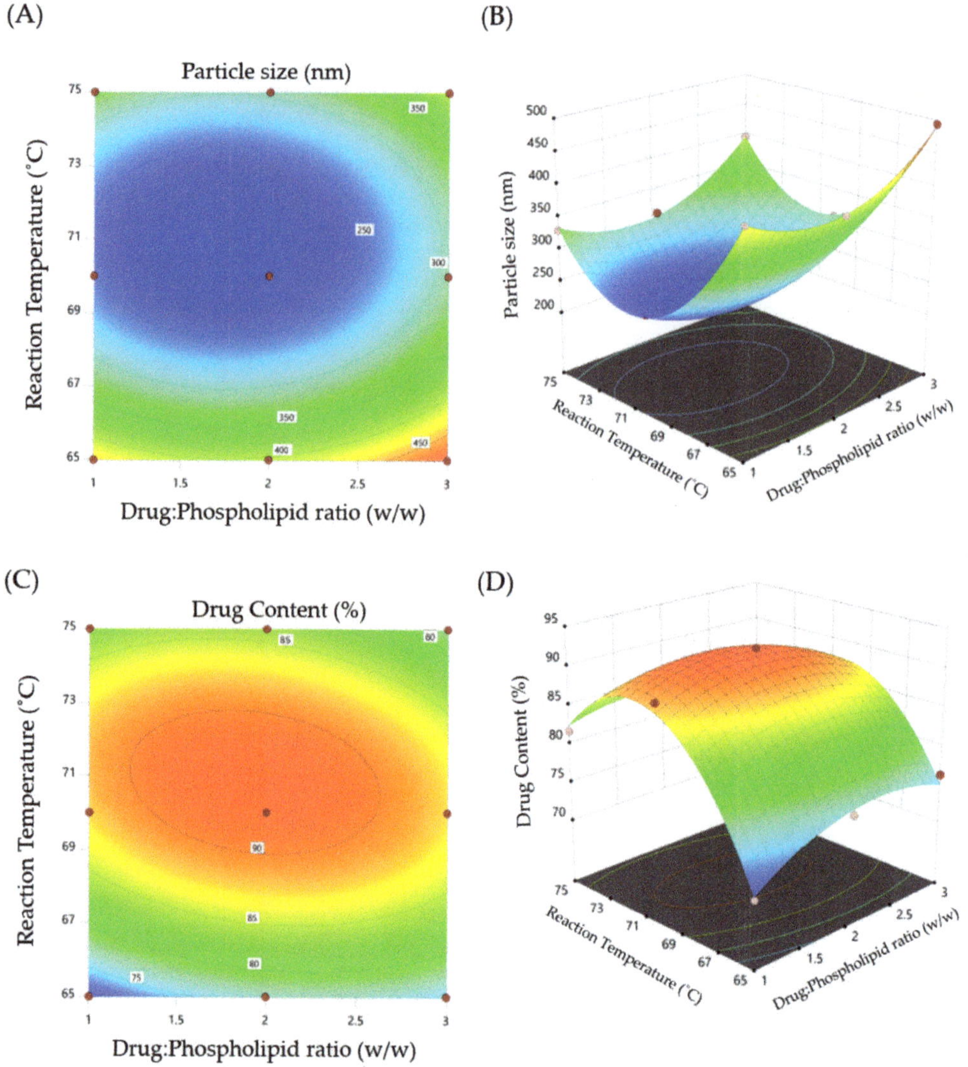

Figure 1. (**A**) Contour plot of particle size (Y_1); (**B**) 3D surface plot for Y_1; (**C**) contour plot of drug content (Y_2); and (**D**) 3D surface plot for Y_2.

2.2. Optimization of Silymarin Phytosomal Complex

A desirability approach was adopted to obtain an optimized phytosomal formulation with desired responses, such as minimum particle size and maximum drug content. Out of the generated solutions, the optimized formula was selected based on the desirability values (near to 1). The optimized phytosomal formula selected under the aforementioned constrains was obtained at a drug:phospholipid ratio of 1:1.93 and a reaction temperature of 70.8 °C. The particle size and drug content (%) of the formulated optimized silymarin phytosomal complex were 218.4 ± 2.54 nm and 90.21 ± 4.03%, respectively, which were close to predicted values (215.8 nm and 91.68%) of the phytosomal complex obtained at a desirability value of 0.984.

2.3. Evaluation of Silymarin Phytosomal Complex

2.3.1. Average Particle Size, Polydispersity Index and Zeta Potential

Particle size, PDI, and zeta potential are considered the main parameters that dictate the effective distribution and physical stability of the lipidic nanocarrier systems in a liquid medium [19]. In this study, the optimized silymarin phytosomes had a particle size of 218.4 ± 2.54 nm with PDI of 0.256 ± 0.02, indicating a narrow range of particle size distribution (Figure S1).

Zeta potential is a key determinant of stability of colloidal dispersions. It has been reported that a zeta potential value greater than ±30 mV is desired for an electrostatically stable formulation [20]. Zeta potential relies on the type and composition of the phospholipid used in the formulation. The optimized silymarin phytosomes had a zeta potential value of −30.8 mV (Figure S2), indicating good physical stability of the formulated phytosomes. Such relatively high zeta potential was attributed to the presence of a negatively charged phosphate group in the polar head of the phospholipid [21].

2.3.2. Surface Morphology

The surface morphology of the optimized silymarin phytosomal formulation was studied using SEM and TEM analysis. The SEM image of optimized silymarin phytosomes disclosed discrete particles with a porous and nearly smooth surface (Figure 2A), compared to the crystalline surface of pure silymarin (Figure 2B). This might account for the improved solubility of phytosomal vesicles compared to the pure drug. Further, when these optimized silymarin phytosomes were dispersed in distilled water, vesicular nanostructures were formed without any aggregation or decomposition, as evidenced by TEM images (Figure 2C), suggesting the formation of well-formed discrete vesicles.

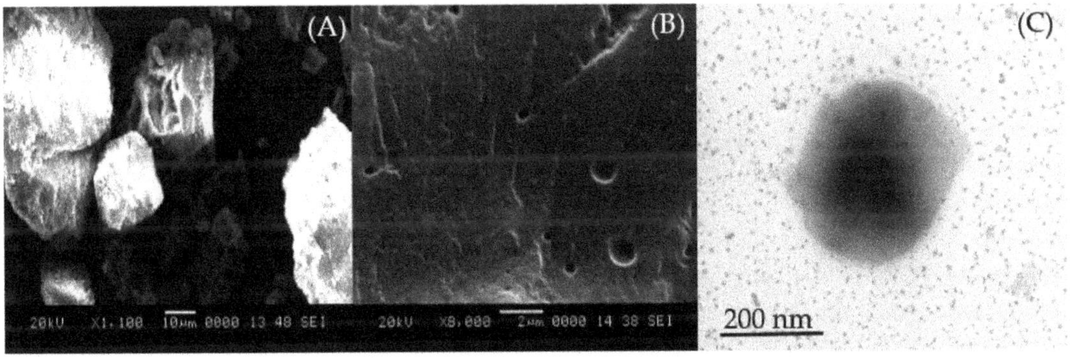

Figure 2. SEM image of (**A**) silymarin and (**B**) optimized silymarin phytosomes. (**C**) TEM image of optimized silymarin phytosomes.

2.4. Structural Characterization Silymarin Phytosomal Complex

2.4.1. Fourier Transform Infrared Spectroscopy (FTIR)

FTIR spectroscopy is a valuable tool for identifying the interaction between different components in the same formulation. Accordingly, the formation of the silymarin-phospholipid phytosomal complex was confirmed by the FTIR spectroscopy via matching the spectrum of the complex with the spectra of individual components used for the preparation of phytosomes. The FTIR spectra of silymarin, SPC, physical mixture of silymarin + SPC, and optimized silymarin phytosomal formulation are depicted in Figure 3. The FTIR spectrum of silymarin showed characteristic absorption peaks at 3647 cm^{-1} (O—H), 2876 cm^{-1} (C—H), 1643 cm^{-1} (C=O), and 1513 cm^{-1} (aromatic C=C). The FTIR spectrum of SPC unveiled characteristic absorption peaks at 2922 cm^{-1} and 2853 cm^{-1} (C—H, fatty acid chain), 1737 cm^{-1} (C=O, fatty acid ester), 1227 cm^{-1} (P=O), and 1048 cm^{-1}

(P—O—C). The spectrum of physical mixture of silymarin + SPC retained almost all the characteristic peaks of individual components. Of interest, remarkable changes were observed in the spectrum of the optimized silymarin phytosomal formulation. Broadening of the stretching absorption band of phenolic (O—H) of silymarin, along with the disappearance of characteristic absorption peaks at 1227 cm^{-1} and 1048 cm^{-1} for SPC in the phytosomal formulation suggests the occurrence of weak intermolecular interactions (H-bonding formation) between silymarin and SPC during the formation of the phytosomal complex. These results are in alignment with that of Hooresfand et al. [22], who demonstrated the formation of a weak bond between rutin and phospholipids during the formation of drug-phospholipid phytosomal complexes.

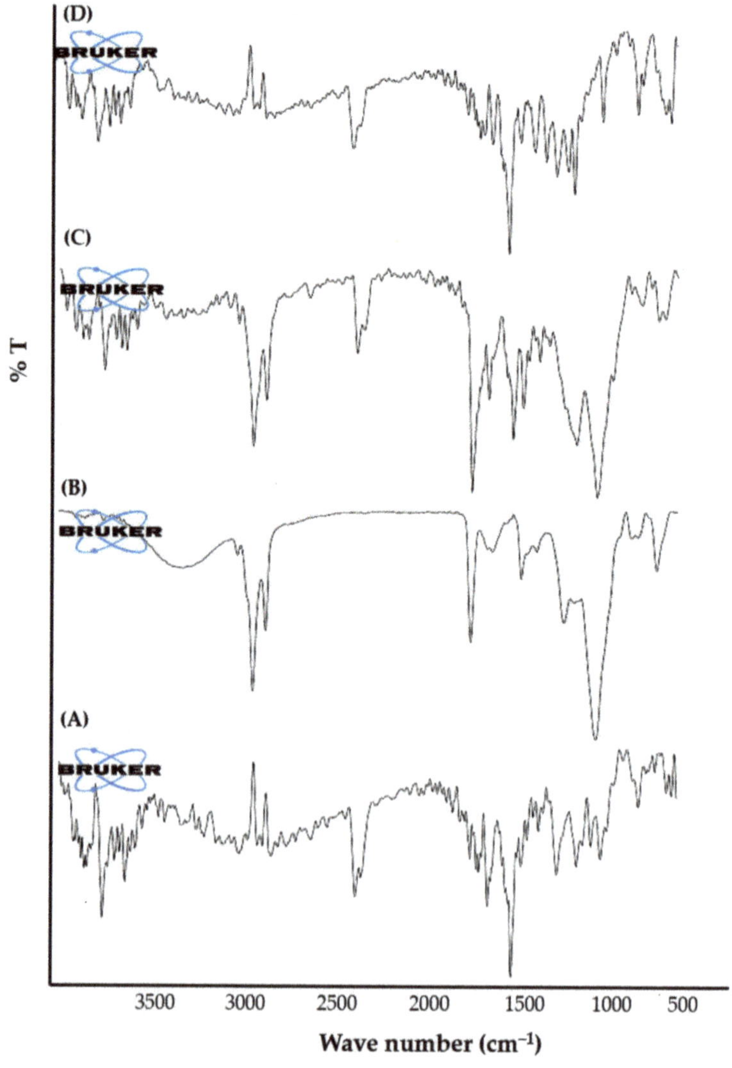

Figure 3. FTIR spectra of (**A**) silymarin; (**B**) SPC; (**C**) physical mixture of silymarin + SPC; and (**D**) optimized silymarin phytosomal formulation.

2.4.2. Differential Scanning Calorimetry (DSC)

Thermal analysis is a widely used approach to characterize the solid-state matter in the complex form. In differential scanning calorimetry (DSC), determination of changes in solid-state properties with respect to temperature change could provide useful information regarding the stability, degradation, and melting of tested materials [17]. Most importantly, DSC analysis could also afford information regarding drug-excipient interactions. DSC thermograms of silymarin, SPC, physical mixture of silymarin + SPC, and optimized silymarin phytosomal formulation are depicted in Figure 4. The thermogram of silymarin (Figure 4A) exhibited a sharp endothermal melting peak at 167.25 °C, indicating the crystalline nature of pure silymarin. The thermogram of SPC showed a sharp endothermal peak at 87.39 °C (Figure 4B) corresponding to the gel-to-liquid crystal state transition [23]. The thermogram of the physical mixture of silymarin + SPC (Figure 4C) showed a remarkable shift in the endothermic peaks of both silymarin and SPC towards lower temperatures (128.92 °C, and 79.51 °C, respectively). Of interest, the thermogram of the optimized silymarin phytosomal complex revealed the disappearance of the sharp endothermal peaks of both silymarin and SPC, and the appearance of a new peak broad endothermal peak at 74.23 °C. These results suggest that a stable silymarin-phospholipid phytosomal complex was formed via weak intermolecular interactions, van der Waals interactions, and/or hydrogen bonding, between silymarin and SPC. These interactions may allow the fatty acid chains of phospholipid to freely spin and enwrap silymarin molecules at a molecular level [24].

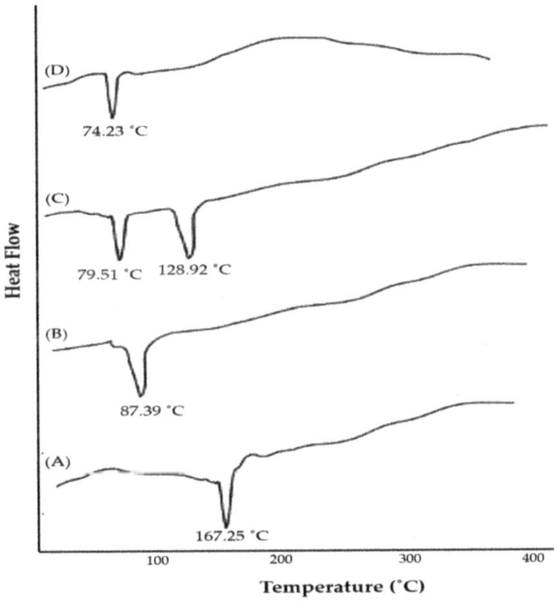

Figure 4. DSC thermograms of (**A**) silymarin; (**B**) SPC; (**C**) physical mixture of silymarin + SPC; and (**D**) optimized silymarin phytosomal formulation.

2.4.3. X-ray Powder Diffractometry (XRD)

The molecular crystallinity of the optimized silymarin phytosomes was determined using the X-ray powder diffractometry technique. The X-ray diffractograms of silymarin, SPC, and the optimized silymarin phytosomal formulation are depicted in Figure 5. The X-ray diffractogram of silymarin exhibited intense and sharp peaks at 2θ = 13.16°, 14.45°, 22.56°, and 26.74°, indicating the crystalline nature of silymarin (Figure 5A). On the other hand, the X-ray diffractogram of SPC manifests a single, relatively broad diffraction peak at 2θ = 20.05°, indicating the amorphous nature of SPC (Figure 5B). Of interest, the X-ray diffractogram of the optimized silymarin phytosomal formulation showed a single broad peak at 2θ = 21.13° (Figure 5C), which was similar to that of SPC, suggesting that silymarin in the optimized phytosomal formula is molecularly dispersed in a phospholipid matrix in the amorphous form. Similar results were reported by Cai et al., who demonstrated the change in the crystallinity of the cholinesterase inhibitor, huperzine A, from the crystalline state to the amorphous state upon complexing with phospholipids [25].

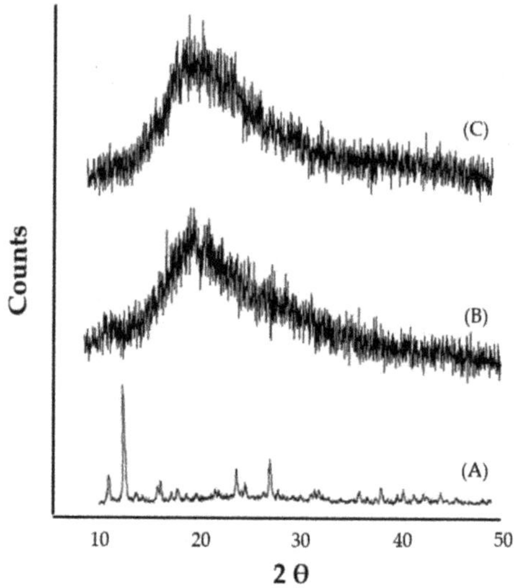

Figure 5. X-ray diffractograms of (**A**) silymarin; (**B**) SPC; and (**C**) optimized silymarin phytosomal formulation.

2.5. Solubility Study

Solubility and partition coefficients are two crucial factors that dictate the in vivo fate of orally administered drugs. Generally, orally administered drugs cannot be overly lipophilic as this will lead to poor absorption. Silymarin is a hydrophobic compound that shows very poor bioavailability due to its poor water solubility [26]. The results of aqueous solubility of pure silymarin and the silymarin-phospholipid phytosomal complex are summarized in Table 2. As depicted in Table 2, silymarin shows poor aqueous solubility in distilled water (45.7 μg/mL). On the other hand, a significant increase was observed in the aqueous solubility of the silymarin phytosomal complex (358.8 μg/mL) in comparison with pure silymarin ($p < 0.001$). This increased solubility of the silymarin phytosomal formulation might be attributed, on the one hand, to the change in drug crystallinity to the amorphous state upon complexing with phospholipid as confirmed by X-ray diffraction analysis, and on the other hand, to the amphiphilic nature of phytosomal formulation.

Table 2. Solubility of pure silymarin and optimized silymarin phytosomal formulation in water and phosphate buffer pH 7.4.

Medium	Solubility (μg/mL)	
	Pure Silymarin	**Optimized Silymarin Phytosome**
Water	45.73 ± 2.4	358.79 ± 9.4
n-octanol	129.29 ± 1.5	568.54 ± 8.5

Data represent mean ± SD of three independent experiments.

Generally, drugs with balanced water solubility and lipid solubility could efficiently penetrate the cell membrane lipid bilayer and thereby exert their pharmacological actions.

Besides its enhancing effect on the aqueous solubility of silymarin, the phytosomal formulation was found to enhance the lipid solubility of silymarin as well. The silymarin phytosomal formulation showed a ~4.5-fold increase in lipid (n-octanol) solubility, compared to the pure drug (Table 2). The enhanced lipid solubility of silymarin formulated within phytosomes might be ascribed to the engagement of polar heads of the drug and phospholipid in the complex (H-bond) formation, whilst the two long fatty chains of phospholipid molecules did not engage in the complex process and were freely rotatable, forming a lipophilic surface that bestowed the silymarin phytosomal formulation with lipid soluble characteristics [27]. Collectively, these results suggest the efficacy of silymarin-phospholipid phytosomal complexes in, not only enhancing the aqueous solubility of the lipophilic drug, silymarin, but in lipid solubility as well, promoting higher drug permeation through biological membranes with subsequent improvements in the oral bioavailability of the drug.

2.6. Dissolution Study

Figure 6 shows the dissolution profiles of pure silymarin and the optimized silymarin phytosomal formulation in a phosphate buffer pH 7.4. It was observed that the drug release pattern of pure silymarin and the optimized silymarin phytosomal formulation was similar up to 8 h. After 8 h, a plateau state was observed in the case of pure silymarin showing a maximum of 45% drug released at the end of 24 h. Unlike pure silymarin, the optimized silymarin phytosomal formulation exhibited sustained drug release; reaching 70.8% at the end of 24 h. The increased drug release from the optimized phytosomal formulation might be ascribed to the physicochemical changes that occurred upon complexing the drug with phospholipid, which increased the solubility of the complex compared to the pure silymarin, as evidenced by in vitro solubility studies.

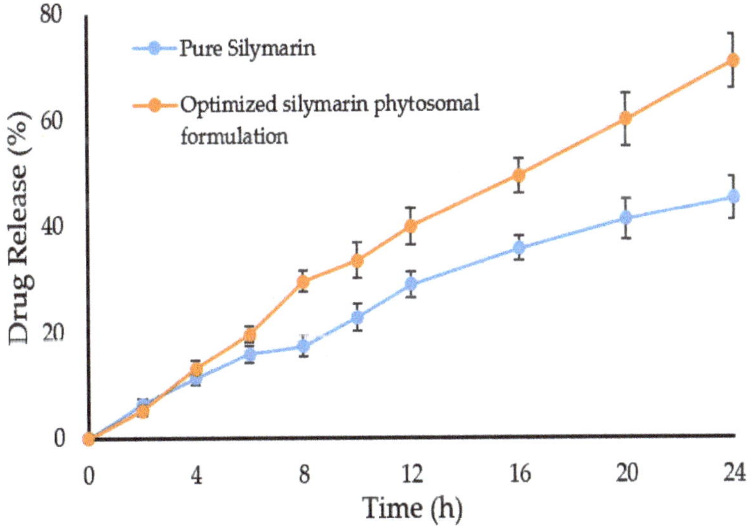

Figure 6. In vitro drug release profile of pure silymarin and optimized silymarin phytosomal formulation in phosphate buffer pH 7.4. Values are mean ± SD (n = 3).

To gain an insight into the release kinetics of silymarin from the silymarin phytosomal formulation, the release data were fitted into different kinetic models. In vitro release data revealed that drug release from the phytosomal formulation followed the Higuchi model; indicating that drug release is diffusion controlled.

2.7. *In Vivo Hepatoprotective Effect of Silymarin-Phospholipid Phytosomal Complex*

The liver is the major organ of metabolism and excretion that is involved in the detoxification process. Liver damage is one of the major health problems that is caused by various hepatotoxins. Carbon tetrachloride (CCl_4) is a hepatotoxin that has been commonly utilized in animal studies. In vivo, CCl_4 is converted by hepatic CYP450 enzymes producing reactive oxidant species that harm important organs such as the liver, kidney, heart, and brain [28], and reduce the activity of serum antioxidant enzymes via the generation of robust amounts of free radicals, which ultimately leads to the lipid peroxidation of cellular membranes. In the present study, hepatotoxicity was induced in the rats by using CCl_4, and the hepatoprotective effect of either pure silymarin or silymarin-phospholipid phytosomal complexes, in terms of normalizing serum levels of hepatic markers, was investigated. As summarized in Table 3, the serum levels of hepatic marker enzymes such as SGPT, SGOT, SALP, and total bilirubin were significantly elevated ($p < 0.01$), compared to non-CCL_4 intoxicated normal rats, confirming the hepatic damage caused by CCl_4. On the other hand, pre-treatment with pure silymarin for 7 days remarkably protected the animals from the hepatotoxic effect of CCl_4 as manifested by a considerable decrease in serum levels of marker enzymes, compared to CCl_4-intoxicated rats. Of interest, pre-treatment of animals with silymarin-phospholipid phytosomal complexes for 7 consecutive days nearly restored the serum levels of tested hepatic markers to the normal levels of negative control group (Table 3). These findings imply the superior hepatoprotective effect of silymarin phytosomes compared to that of pure silymarin.

Table 3. Hepatic marker enzymes levels following treatment with plain silymarin and optimized silymarin phytosomal formulation in CCl_4-intoxicated rat model.

Hepatic Antioxidant Enzyme	Group—I (Normal Control)	Group—II (CCl_4-Intoxicated Rats)	Group—III (Plain Silymarin)	Group—IV (Optimized Silymarin Phytosomes)
SGPT (U/L)	42.77 ± 1.82 **	134.37 ± 3.61	95.68 ± 3.56 **	57.35 ± 2.73 **
SGOT (U/L)	38.22 ± 2.71 **	97.76 ± 3.38	75.19 ± 3.22 *	46.88 ± 2.25 **
SALP (U/L)	141.53 ± 2.26 **	267.64 ± 3.29	221.77 ± 3.41 *	159.43 ± 3.55 **
Total bilirubin (mg/dL)	0.66 ± 0.03 **	1.41 ± 0.02	0.95 ± 0.02 **	0.72 ± 0.01 **

Data are mean ± SD ($n = 6$). * $p < 0.05$ and ** $p < 0.01$ vs. CCl_4-intoxicated rats. SGPT: serum glutamate pyruvate transaminase; SGOT: serum glutamate oxaloacetate transaminase; SALP: serum alkaline phosphatase.

2.8. *In Vivo Antioxidant Activity of Silymarin-Phospholipid Phytosomal Complex*

Globally, silymarin is considered one of the most commonly used natural compounds for the treatment of hepatic diseases owing to its antioxidant, antifibrotic, and anti-inflammatory activities [29]. Accordingly, in order to address the antioxidant potential effect of silymarin-phospholipid phytosomal complex, the levels of antioxidant enzymes, namely, glutathione reductase (GRD), reduced glutathione (GSH), glutathione S transferase (GST), glutathione peroxidase (GPx), catalase (CAT), and superoxide dismutase (SOD) were assayed in liver homogenates of CCl_4-treated and naïve rats. The effect of either pure silymarin or silymarin-phospholipid phytosomal complexes antioxidant biochemical paradigms is depicted in Table 4. It was evident that CCl_4 intoxication ensued a significant reduction ($p < 0.01$) in the levels all the tested antioxidant enzymes in liver homogenates compared to naïve control rats. In contrast, pre-treatment with pure silymarin for 7 consecutive days substantially ($p < 0.05$) reduced the CCl_4-induced drop in GSH, GPx, and CAT levels. Most importantly, pre-treatment with optimized silymarin phytosomes efficiently protected the animals from the CCl_4-induced drop in all tested antioxidant enzymes. The levels of all tested antioxidant enzymes (GSH, GPx, GST, GRD, SOD, and CAT) in liver homogenates were comparable to that of the naïve negative control group. These results suggest that optimized silymarin phytosomes could efficiently exert a hepatoprotective effect against CCl_4-induced intoxication via restoring the normal levels of antioxidant enzymes.

Table 4. Effect of plain silymarin and optimized silymarin phytosomes on antioxidant enzymes.

Hepatic Antioxidant Enzyme	Group—I (Normal Control)	Group—II (CCl_4-Intoxicated Rats)	Group—III (Plain Silymarin)	Group—IV (Optimized Silymarin Phytosomes)
GSH (nmol/mg protein)	49.16 ± 3.99 **	18.86 ± 1.28	29.37 ± 2.34 *	41.22 ± 2.15 **
GPx (nmol/mg protein)	332.23 ± 4.91 **	193.76 ± 3.71	244.35 ± 4.27 *	302.43 ± 3.33 **
GST (nmol/mg protein)	296.43 ± 4.73 **	165.28 ± 3.45	210.55 ± 4.28	264.88 ± 4.23 **
GRD (nmol/mg protein)	21.16 ± 1.54 **	7.89 ± 0.95	13.26 ± 1.54	18.47 ± 1.21 **
SOD (U/mg protein)	7.41 ± 0.11 **	4.21 ± 0.14	5.03 ± 0.22	6.21 ± 0.03 **
CAT (U/mg protein)	212.85 ± 2.87 **	95.46 ± 3.42	140.15 ± 3.76 *	187.29 ± 2.58 **

Data represent mean ± SD (n = 6). * $p < 0.05$ and ** $p < 0.01$ vs. CCl_4-intoxicated rats. GSH: glutathione; GPx: glutathione peroxidase; GST: glutathione S transferase; GRD: glutathione reductase; SOD: superoxide dismutase; and CAT: catalase.

To gain further insight into the antioxidant potential of silymarin-phospholipid phytosomal complexes, quantitative evaluation of malondialdehyde (MDA), a major lipid peroxidation product, was determined via thiobarbituric acid reactive substances (TBARS) assays [30]. As shown in Figure 7, CCl_4 intoxication triggered potent lipid peroxidation (LPO), as manifested by significantly ($p < 0.01$) elevated levels of MDA in CCL_4-intoxicated rats compared to naïve normal rats. In addition, pre-treatment with pure silymarin failed to protect the rats from CCL_4-triggred lipid peroxidation, as evidenced by comparable levels of MDA in both silymarin-pretreated CCL_4-intoxicated rats and positive control (CCL_4-intoxicated) rats. On the other hand, pre-treatment with silymarin-phospholipid phytosomal complexes significantly ($p < 0.01$) abrogated the CCl_4-induced increase of MDA levels. Cytochrome P 450-dependent monooxygenases is known to process the accumulated CCl_4 to trichloromethyl (CCl_3) radicals in the hepatic parenchymal cells [31]. Besides its role in the alkylation of cellular proteins, CCl_3 causes the polyunsaturated fatty acids to produce lipid peroxides, which could induce hepatotoxicity and alter hepatic marker enzyme levels [32,33]. In this study, the optimized silymarin phytosomal formulation showed the potential to ameliorate all cellular changes induced by CCl_4-intoxication. The optimized silymarin phytosomal efficiently restored all CCl_4-elevated rat liver function marker enzymes, resisted the CCl_4-induced reduction in antioxidant enzymes and significantly abrogated the CCl_4-induced increase in MDA levels. Collectively, these results underscore the reactive oxygen species (ROS) scavenging ability of silymarin phytosomal formulation, which efficiently helps in overcoming the oxidative damage/stress elicited by CCl_4-intoxication in rat models.

2.9. Histopathological Studies

Histological examination of rat liver tissues was adopted to assess the effect of pure silymarin or the optimized silymarin phytosomal formulation on CCl_4-induced liver damage. As shown in Figure 8, liver tissue of non CCl_4-intoxicated control rats showed well-preserved cellular structure with clear cytoplasm, indicating healthy functional liver cells. On the other hand, in CCl_4-intoxicated rats, obvious degeneration of parenchymal cells and fatty tissues with severe damage in the central lobular area was observed, underscoring the hepatotoxic effect of CCl_4. Pre-treatment with pure silymarin resulted in a moderate hepatoprotective effect as manifested by a remarkable decrease in fatty tissue degeneration and parenchymal cells damage. Of interest, the optimized silymarin phytosomal formulation efficiently protected liver tissue from the hepatotoxic effect of CCl_4. Normal hepatic cells with a well-restored cytoplasm and central vein were observed in the liver section of silymarin phytosomes-pre-treated rats. These findings suggest that the optimized silymarin phytosomal formulation could efficiently restore the normal anatomy of hepatic cells, presumably, via the augmented antioxidant potential of silymarin.

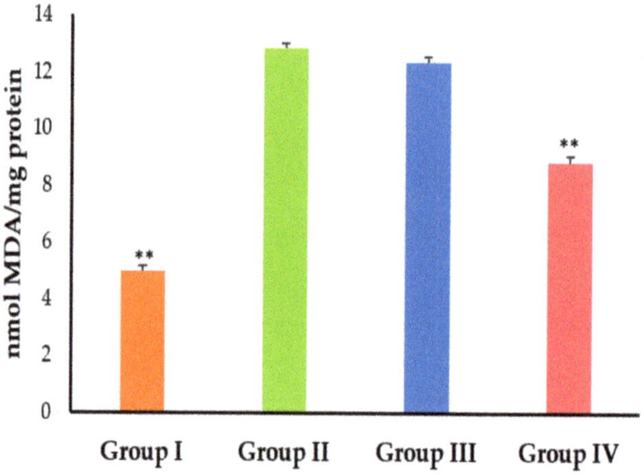

Figure 7. Effect of pure silymarin and optimized silymarin phytosomal formulation on lipid peroxidase (nmoles of MDA released/g tissue). Group I represents a negative control (treated with Tween 20 (1% *v*/*v*); Group II represents CCl_4-intoxicated rats (treated with CCl_4 + olive oil (1:1.5 mL/kg)); Group III represents CCl_4-intoxicated rats treated with plain silymarin; and Group 4 represents CCl_4-intoxicated rats treated with optimized silymarin phytosomal formulation. Data are mean ± SD ($n = 6$). ** $p < 0.01$ vs. CCl_4-intoxicated rats.

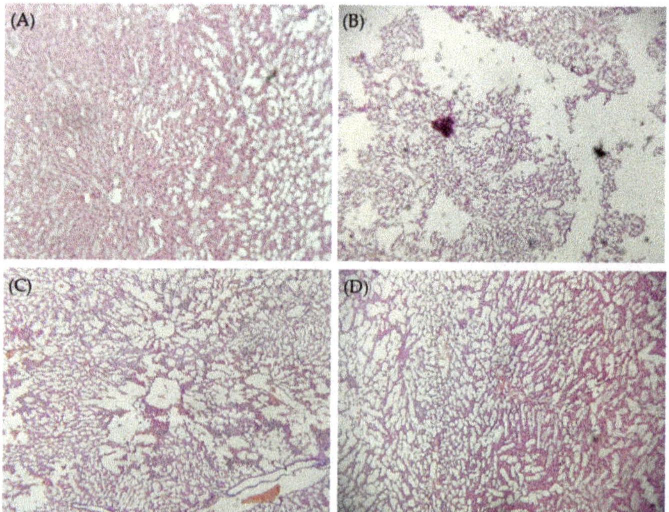

Figure 8. Histological micrographs of liver tissue of **(A)** negative control (treated with Tween 20 (1% *v*/*v*); **(B)** CCl_4-intoxicated rats (treated with CCl_4 + olive oil (1:1.5 mL/kg)); **(C)** CCl_4-intoxicated rats treated with plain silymarin and **(D)** CCl_4-intoxicated rats treated with optimized silymarin phytosomal formulation. 100× magnification.

2.10. Pharmacokinetics Study

To gain an insight into the underlying mechanism of the enhanced in vivo hepatoprotective effect of silymarin-phospholipid phytosomal complexes compared to pure silymarin, the in vivo pharmacokinetics of either plain silymarin (100 mg/Kg) or the optimized silymarin phytosomal formulation (100 mg/kg silymarin) were investigated in Wistar rats following oral administration. Figure 9 represents the mean plasma silymarin concentrations as a function of time. As depicted in Figure 9, plasma levels of plain silymarin were very low, presumably, due to its poor aqueous solubility, which might hinder its proper absorption. In contrast, a significant elevation in the plasma concentration of silymarin was observed in animals treated with the optimized silymarin phytosomal formulation. Such relatively higher plasma drug concentrations of silymarin from the phytosomal formulation following oral administration might be ascribed to the enhanced drug absorption from the phytosomal formulation owing to the amphiphilic nature of the formulation. Of note, phytosomes succeeded to maintain silymarin plasma concentrations at remarkably higher levels for a prolonged period of time (up to 24 h post administration).

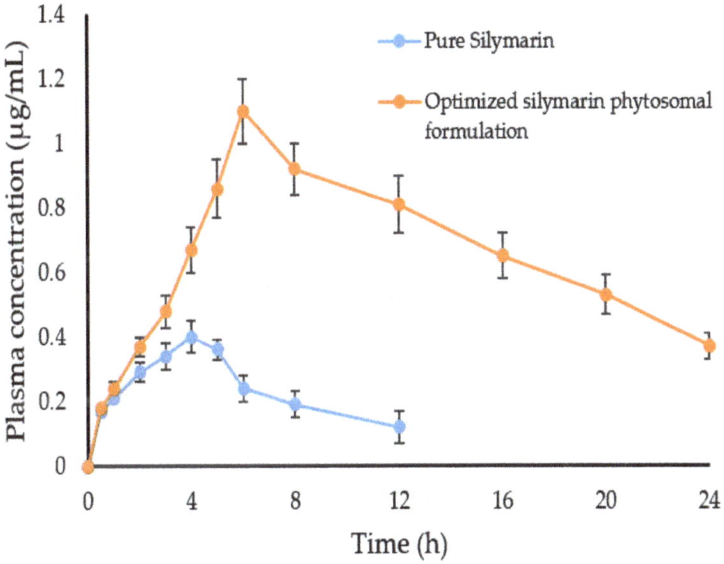

Figure 9. Mean plasma concentration-time profile of pure silymarin (100 mg/kg, p.o.) and optimized silymarin phytosomes (~100 mg/kg silymarin, p.o). Data are mean ± SD (n = 6).

The key pharmacokinetic parameters of silymarin are illustrated in Table 5. As depicted in Table 5, the optimized silymarin phytosomal formulation showed a significantly higher peak concentration (C_{max} = 1.1 ± 0.12 µg/mL) compared to the plain drug (C_{max} = 0.4 ± 0.10 µg/mL), indicating higher absorption of the drug from the optimized formulation. In addition, the optimized silymarin phytosomal formulation exhibited a longer half-life ($t_{1/2}$) and mean residence time (MRT) compared to the plain drug. The MRT of plain silymarin and the optimized silymarin phytosomal formulation were 9.44 ± 1.2 h and 20.43 ± 1.8 h, respectively. Such longer residence and/or prolonged duration of action of the optimized silymarin phytosomal formulation might be ascribed to the reduced systemic clearance of the optimized silymarin phytosomal formulation (Cl = 4.48 ± 0.77 mL·h^{-1}) compared to the plain drug (Cl = 26.03 ± 1.9 mL·h^{-1}). Most importantly, the mean relative bioavailability of the optimized silymarin phytosomal formulation was ~6-fold that of the plain drug. Such observed improvements in silymarin relative bioavailability following oral administration of the optimized silymarin phytosomal formulation can be accredited to the presence of phospholipid, which could efficiently enhance silymarin aqueous solubility, leading to increased intestinal absorption. In addition, complexation of the drug within the amphiphilic phospholipid-based vesicular carrier was reported to shield the drug from hepatic first-pass metabolism, and thereby, enhance its systemic bioavailability [17].

Table 5. Pharmacokinetic parameters of pure silymarin and (100 mg/kg, p.o.) and optimized silymarin phytosomes (~100 mg/kg silymarin, p.o).

Pharmacokinetic Parameters	Pure Silymarin	Optimized Silymarin Phytosomes
C_{max} (μg mL^{-1})	0.40 ± 0.10	1.10 ± 0.21 **
T_{max} (h)	4.0	6.0 **
$AUC_{0\text{-}t}$ (μg mL^{-1} h)	2.80 ± 0.71	45.76 ± 1.41 **
$AUC_{0\text{-}\infty}$ (mL^{-1} h)	3.84 ± 0.91	22.33 ± 2.13
Elimination half-life ($t_{1/2}$) (h)	6.01 ± 0.70	12.31 ± 0.96 **
Elimination rate constant (K_{el}) (h^{-1})	0.12 ± 0.02	0.06 ± 0.01 **
Mean residance time (MRT) (h)	9.44 ± 1.10	20.43 ± 1.76 **
Clearance (Cl) (mL·h^{-1})	26.03 ± 1.93	4.48 ± 0.77 **
Volume of distribution (V_d) (mL^{-1})	255.48 ± 12.33	79.53 ± 8.11 **

Data are mean ± SD (n = 6). ** $p < 0.01$.

3. Materials and Methods

3.1. Materials

Soybean phosphatidyl choline (Phospholipon® 90 G; 98% phopsphatidylcholine content) was received as a gift sample from Lipoid GmbH (Ludwigshafen, Germany). Silymarin was procured from Yucca Enterprises (Mumbai, India). Orthophosphoric acid, ethanol, methanol, chloroform, acetonitrile, carbon tetrachloride, and Tween 20 were obtained from Hi-Media Laboratory Ltd. (Mumbai, India). Liver function test kits and the TBARS assay kit were purchased from Aspen Laboratories (Delhi, India). All chemicals/reagents used in this study were of analytical or HPLC grade.

3.2. Preparation of Silymarin Phytosomal Complex

Silymarin-phospholipid complexes (silymarin phytosomes) were prepared by the solvent evaporation technique, as previously described [34]. In brief, accurately weighed quantities of silymarin and soybean phosphatidylcholine (SPC) were placed in a 200 mL flask and dissolved in 50 mL ethanol. Silymarin-phospholipid complexes were prepared in different weight/weight ratios (1:1. 1:2 and 1:3). The solution was then refluxed at 65 °C, 70 °C, or 75 °C with the help of a rotary evaporator for 2 h. The resultant solution was concentrated in order to attain a thin lipid film. The obtained silymarin-phospholipid phytosomal complex was dried under vacuum to remove any traces of the solvent. The dried silymarin-phospholipid phytosomal complex was then transferred into light-resistant glass vials, purged with nitrogen gas and stored at room temperature.

3.3. Design of Experiments

A full factorial design (Design Expert® software; Version 11.0.3.0) was utilized to investigate the impact of two independent formulation factors, namely, drug:phospholipid ratio (X_1, w:w) and reaction temperature (X_2, °C), on two dependent responses, namely, particle size (Y_1) and drug content (Y_2). The two independent variables (X_1 and X_2) were studied at three levels, denoted by the letters -1 (low), 0 (middle), and +1 (upper), resulting in a 3^2-factorial design with nine independent experimental runs (Table 1). The results of the experiments were analyzed implementing a mathematical model defined by the polynomial equation given below:

$$Y = b_0 + b_1X_1 + b_2X_2 + b_{12}X_1X_2 + b_{11}{X_1}^2 + b_{22}{X_2}^2$$

where, Y is the dependent response and b is the regression coefficient of the independent variable X. X_1 and X_2 are the main factors, while X_1X_2 represents the interaction between main factors. X_1^2 and X_2^2 are the polynomial terms.

3.4. Evaluation of Silymarin Phytosomes

3.4.1. Average Particle Size, Polydispersity Index and Zeta Potential

The average particle size, polydispersity index (PDI), and zeta potential of the prepared phytosomal formulations were determined by dynamic light scattering (DLS) and electrophoretic light scattering (ELS) techniques, respectively, using Malvern Zetasizer Nano-ZS (ZEN3600, Malvern Instrument Ltd., Malvern, UK) [35].

3.4.2. Surface Morphology

The surface morphology of the optimized silymarin phytosomal formulation was studied by scanning electron microscopy (SEM) and transmission electron microscopy (TEM). The SEM sample was prepared onto double-sided adhesive tape with phytosomal powder spread over it, placed on an aluminum stub, and observed using JEOL-JSM 6380LA SEM (JEOL Ltd., Tokyo, Japan) [36]. For TEM, the phytosomal powder sample was diluted in distilled water (1:20) and sonicated using a probe sonicator (Vibra-Cell™ Sonicator, Newtown, CT, USA) for 3 min. The sonicated sample was cast on a 300 mesh copper grid (carbon type-B) and allowed to adsorb as a thin liquid film by removing excess sample using filter paper, stained with uranyl acetate solution (2% *w*/*v*), and dried overnight under vacuum. This stained liquid film was observed under JEOL-JEM-100S TEM (JEOL Ltd., Tokyo, Japan) with an operating voltage 200 kV [37].

3.4.3. Estimation of Drug Content

The amount of silymarin incorporated within the formulated phytosomal complex was estimated by a spectrophotometric method. Briefly, an accurately weighed quantity of phytosomal complex (5 mg) was dispersed in 5 mL of chloroform; where the formulated phytosomes dissolve in chloroform, while non-complexed silymarin remains insoluble. Upon filtering the dispersion, non-complexed silymarin was separated as a solid residue, dried and re-dissolved in methanol [38]. The concentration of free non-complexed silymarin was determined spectrophotometrically at λ_{max} of 286 nm using UV-visible spectrophotometer (Shimazu, Tokyo, Japan). Drug content (%) was calculated using the following formula:

$$\text{Drug content } (\%) = \frac{\text{Total amount of Silymarin} - \text{amount of free Silymarin}}{\text{Total amount of Silymarin}} \times 100$$

3.4.4. Fourier Transform Infrared Spectroscopy (FTIR)

The chemical interaction between phytosomal components was studied using an infrared (IR) spectra matching approach using a FTIR spectrometer (Alpha Bruker, Berlin, Germany). The IR spectrum of the pure silymarin, soybean phosphatidyl choline (SPC), physical mixture of silymarin and SPC (1:1), and optimized silymarin phytosomal formulation was obtained by scanning within the wavelength range of 4000 to 500 cm^{-1} [39].

3.4.5. Differential Scanning Calorimetry (DSC)

Thermograms of silymarin, SPC, physical mixture of silymarin and SPC, and optimized silymarin phytosomal formulation were recorded on differential scanning colorimeter (TGA/DSC-SDT Q600, TA Instruments, New Castle, DE, USA). The thermal behavior was investigated by heating 2 mg of the individual samples at a heating rate of 10 °C/min from 25 °C to 400 °C in a covered sample pan under a nitrogen purge of 60 mL/min [40].

3.4.6. X-ray Powder Diffractometry (XRD)

X-ray diffractograms of silymarin, SPC, and optimized silymarin phytosomal formulation were recorded in X-ray diffractometer (Rigaku mini flex 600, Hokkaido, Japan) to study the molecular crystallinity. The instrument was adjusted at 40 kV tube voltage, 40 mA tube current, and 5–50° scanning angle of 2θ with a 1°/min step width [41].

3.5. *Solubility Study*

The apparent solubility of the samples was determined by adding excess amounts of silymarin, and optimized silymarin phytosomal formulation to 5 mL of distilled water or n-octanol into sealed glass containers at 25 ± 1 °C. The solution was then agitated for 24 h and further centrifuged for 30 min at 5000 rpm. Further, 1 mL of the filtrate was diluted up to 10 mL with respective solvents and then analyzed spectrophotometrically at λ_{max} of 286 nm [27].

3.6. *In Vitro Dissolution Study*

The in vitro dissolution profile of the silymarin phytosomal complex was carried out using the dialysis bag method to determine the drug release from the formulation. Briefly, 10 mg of pure silymarin and a definite weight of optimized silymarin phytosomal formulation, equivalent to 10 mg silymarin, were placed in the dialysis bags. The bags were placed in glass vials enclosing 100 mL of phosphate buffer pH 7.4. The glass vials were agitated at 50 rpm and 37 ± 1 °C. At predetermined time points, 2 mL samples were withdrawn from the glass vials and were interchanged with an equal volume of fresh buffer to retain the sink condition. The collected samples were filtered, suitably diluted, and analyzed using a UV spectrophotometer (Shimadzu, Tokyo, Japan) at 286 nm. To study the drug release mechanism from the formulation, the in vitro release data was fitted into different in vitro kinetic release models.

3.7. *In Vivo Studies*

3.7.1. Animals

Male Wistar rats (175–200 g) were used in this investigation. All animal experiments were reviewed and approved by the Animal Ethics Committee of N.G.S.M Institute of Pharmaceutical Sciences (NGSMIPS/IAEC/140). The rats were adapted to laboratory conditions by housing in groups of 7–8 in rat-breeding plastic tubs with stainless steel straight wired lid, at 22 ± 2 °C and 50 ± 10% relative humidity with a 12/12 h light-dark cycle for 10 days prior to experiments.

3.7.2. In Vivo Hepatoprotective and Antioxidant Activity Studies

Wistar rats were randomly categorized into 4 groups (n = 6). The first group (negative control group) was treated orally with an aqueous solution of Tween 20 (1% *v*/*v*) for 7 days. The second group received an aqueous solution of Tween 20 (1% *v*/*v*) orally for 7 days followed by a single i.p. dose of a mixture of carbon tetrachloride (CCl_4) and olive oil (1:1.5 mL/kg) on the 7th day, and served as a positive control group. The third group was treated orally with silymarin suspension (100 mg/kg/day) for 7 days, followed by a single i.p. dose of a mixture of CCl_4 and olive oil on the 7th day. The last group was treated orally with optimized silymarin phytosomal suspension (100 mg silymarin/kg/day) for 7 days, followed by a single i.p. dose of a mixture of CCl_4 and olive oil on the 7th day. At 24 h post CCL_4 intoxication, blood samples were collected, centrifuged and sera samples were separated. Liver function test (LFT) was assessed by quantitative determination of liver marker enzymes such as serum glutamate pyruvate transaminase (SGPT), serum glutamate oxaloacetate transaminase (SGOT), serum alkaline phosphatase (SALP), and total bilirubin.

For biochemical estimation of liver antioxidant enzymes, animals were euthanized post blood samples collection. The livers were dissected, rinsed with ice-cold saline, and were subjected to homogenization with 0.1M Tris HCl buffer (pH 7.4). The liver homogenate was centrifuged, and the supernatant was subjected to glutathione reductase (GRD), reduced glutathione (GSH), glutathione peroxidase (GPx), glutathione S transferase (GST), superoxide dismutase (SOD), and catalase (CAT). Lipid peroxidation was also estimated by quantifying the amount of malondialdehyde (MDA) in the liver homogenates using thiobarbituric acid reactive substance (TBARS) assay [30]. This assay involves the reaction of MDA with thiobarbituric acid (TBA) forming a pink chromogen (TBARS), which is measured at 530 nm. The concentration of MDA is expressed as nM of MDA/mg of protein.

3.7.3. Histopathological Studies

For histopathological observation, the dissected animal livers were stored in 10% *v*/*v* neutral buffered formalin. Later, the haematoxylin and eosin-stained liver sections were prepared and observed under Zeiss Primo Star microscope (Carl-Zeiss, Oberkochen, Germany).

3.7.4. In Vivo Pharmacokinetic Studies

For pharmacokinetic studies, Wistar rats were categorized into two groups ($n = 6$); control group receiving pure silymarin (100 mg/kg) and treatment group receiving optimized silymarin phytosomal formulation (100 mg silymarin/kg). At scheduled time points post-administration (0.5, 1, 2, 3, 4, 5, 6, 8, and 12 h), blood samples (500 μL) were collected from the retro-orbital plexus in heparinized tubes and centrifuged at 3000 rpm for 10 min to obtain plasma. Then, 200 μL of separated plasma samples was mixed with 1 mL methanol. The mixture was heated at 75 °C for 30 min and was further centrifuged at 4000 rpm for 30 min using a cooling centrifuge. The supernatant was filtered using a 0.22 μm membrane filter and drug concentration was quantified by HPLC analysis, as described previously [42]. Pharmacokinetic parameters of silymarin, including maximum plasma concentration (C_{max}), time required to reach a maximum concentration (t_{max}), elimination half-life ($t_{1/2}$), elimination rate constant (K_{el}), volume of distribution (V_d), clearance (Cl), and area under the plasma concentration-time curve ($AUC_{0–24h}$) were calculated using PK Solver 2.0 software. Furthermore, the bioavailability of optimized silymarin phytosomal formulation relative to that of pure silymarin was calculated.

3.8. Statistical Analysis

All data are presented as mean ± SD. Statistical analysis was performed using Student's *t*-test and one way analysis of variance (ANOVA). Statistical significance was defined at p values less than 0.05.

4. Conclusions

The present study manifested the potential of amphiphilic phospholipid-based phytosomes for enhancing the solubility, absorption, oral bioavailability, and in vivo hepatoprotective activity of the polyphenolic phyto-constituent, silymarin. Silymarin phytosomes were prepared using the solvent evaporation method and optimized using a full factorial design. The optimized silymarin phytosomal formulation efficiently enhanced the aqueous solubility of silymarin and sustained in vitro drug release for up to 24 h compared to the plain drug. In addition, in a CCl_4-induced hepatotoxicity rat model, compared to the plain drug, the optimized silymarin phytosomal formulation showed superior hepatoprotective effects as manifested by efficient restoration of normal levels of antioxidant enzymes and ameliorating all cellular changes induced by CCl_4-intoxication. Most importantly, the optimized silymarin phytosomal formulation significantly improved silymarin oral bioavailability as evidenced by a ~6-fold increase in systemic bioavailability compared to pure silymarin. Collectively, our results emphasize the utility of phospholipid-based phytosomes in improving the aqueous solubility, oral bioavailability, and thereby the pharmacological activities of poorly soluble phyto-constituents.

Supplementary Materials: The following supporting information can be downloaded at: https://www.mdpi.com/article/10.3390/ph15070790/s1, Figure S1: Particle size distribution of optimized silymarin phytosomal formulation; Figure S2: Zeta potential of optimized silymarin phytosomal formulation.

Author Contributions: Conceptualization, R.N.C. and A.S.A.L.; methodology, R.G.S. and A.M.; software, A.A.S., E.-S.K. and H.F.A.; formal analysis, A.A.S., E.-S.K., H.F.A. and A.M.; investigation, R.G.S., A.A.S., E.-S.K. and H.F.A.; resources, A.A.S. and H.F.A.; writing—original draft preparation, R.G.S., E.-S.K. and A.S.A.L.; writing—review and editing, A.S.A.L.; supervision, R.N.C.; funding acquisition, H.F.A. All authors have read and agreed to the published version of the manuscript.

Funding: This work was supported by Princess Nourah bint Abdulrahman University researchers supporting project number (PNURSP2022R205), Princess Nourah bint Abdulrahman University, Riyadh, Saudi Arabia.

Institutional Review Board Statement: The animal study protocol was approved by the Institutional Animal Ethics Committee of N.G.S.M Institute of Pharmaceutical Sciences (NGSMIPS/IAEC/140).

Informed Consent Statement: Not applicable.

Data Availability Statement: Data is contained within the article and supplementary material.

Acknowledgments: The authors extend their appreciation to Princess Nourah bint Abdulrahman University, Riyadh, Saudi Arabia for supporting this work under researcher supporting project number (PNURSP2022R205).

Conflicts of Interest: The authors declare no conflict of interest.

References

1. Bhatt, A. Phytopharmaceuticals: A new drug class regulated in India. *Perspect. Clin. Res.* **2016**, *7*, 59–61. [CrossRef] [PubMed]
2. Ekor, M. The growing use of herbal medicines: Issues relating to adverse reactions and challenges in monitoring safety. *Front. Pharmacol.* **2014**, *4*, 177. [CrossRef] [PubMed]
3. Lu, M.; Qiu, Q.; Luo, X.; Liu, X.; Sun, J.; Wang, C.; Lin, X.; Deng, Y.; Song, Y. Phyto-phospholipid complexes (phytosomes): A novel strategy to improve the bioavailability of active constituents. *Asian J. Pharm. Sci.* **2019**, *14*, 265–274. [CrossRef] [PubMed]
4. Aqil, F.; Munagala, R.; Jeyabalan, J.; Vadhanam, M.V. Bioavailability of phytochemicals and its enhancement by drug delivery systems. *Cancer Lett.* **2013**, *334*, 133–141. [CrossRef]
5. Abdallah, M.H.; Abu Lila, A.S.; Shawky, S.M.; Almansour, K.; Alshammari, F.; Khafagy, E.-S.; Makram, T.S. Experimental Design and Optimization of Nano-Transfersomal Gel to Enhance the Hypoglycemic Activity of Silymarin. *Polymers* **2022**, *14*, 508. [CrossRef]
6. Federico, A.; Dallio, M.; Loguercio, C. Silymarin/Silybin and Chronic Liver Disease: A Marriage of Many Years. *Molecules* **2017**, *22*, 191. [CrossRef]
7. Ramasamy, K.; Agarwal, R. Multitargeted therapy of cancer by silymarin. *Cancer Lett.* **2008**, *269*, 352–362. [CrossRef]
8. Liu, C.-H.; Jassey, A.; Hsu, H.-Y.; Lin, L.-T. Antiviral Activities of Silymarin and Derivatives. *Molecules* **2019**, *24*, 1552. [CrossRef]
9. Borah, A.; Paul, R.; Choudhury, S.; Choudhury, A.; Bhuyan, B.; Das Talukdar, A.; Dutta Choudhury, M.; Mohanakumar, K.P. Neuroprotective potential of silymarin against CNS disorders: Insight into the pathways and molecular mechanisms of action. *CNS Neurosci. Ther.* **2013**, *19*, 847–853. [CrossRef]
10. Pérez, H.J.; Carrillo, S.C.; García, E.; Ruiz-Mar, G.; Pérez-Tamayo, R.; Chavarría, A. Neuroprotective effect of silymarin in a MPTP mouse model of Parkinson's disease. *Toxicology* **2014**, *319*, 38–43. [CrossRef]
11. Di Costanzo, A.; Angelico, R. Formulation Strategies for Enhancing the Bioavailability of Silymarin: The State of the Art. *Molecules* **2019**, *24*, 2155. [CrossRef]
12. Martínez-Ballesta, M.; Gil-Izquierdo, Á.; García-Viguera, C.; Domínguez-Perles, R. Nanoparticles and Controlled Delivery for Bioactive Compounds: Outlining Challenges for New "Smart-Foods" for Health. *Foods* **2018**, *7*, 72. [CrossRef]
13. Yang, B.; Dong, Y.; Wang, F.; Zhang, Y. Nanoformulations to Enhance the Bioavailability and Physiological Functions of Polyphenols. *Molecules* **2020**, *25*, 4613. [CrossRef]
14. Kotta, S.; Khan, A.W.; Pramod, K.; Ansari, S.H.; Sharma, R.K.; Ali, J. Exploring oral nanoemulsions for bioavailability enhancement of poorly water-soluble drugs. *Expert Opin. Drug Deliv.* **2012**, *9*, 585–598. [CrossRef]
15. Alharbi, W.S.; Almughem, F.A.; Almehmady, A.M.; Jarallah, S.J.; Alsharif, W.K.; Alzahrani, N.M.; Alshehri, A.A. Phytosomes as an Emerging Nanotechnology Platform for the Topical Delivery of Bioactive Phytochemicals. *Pharmaceutics* **2021**, *13*, 1475. [CrossRef]
16. Barani, M.; Sangiovanni, E.; Angarano, M.; Rajizadeh, M.A.; Mehrabani, M.; Piazza, S.; Gangadharappa, H.V.; Pardakhty, A.; Mehrbani, M.; Dell'Agli, M.; et al. Phytosomes as Innovative Delivery Systems for Phytochemicals: A Comprehensive Review of Literature. *Int. J. Nanomed.* **2021**, *16*, 6983–7022. [CrossRef]

17. Telange, D.R.; Patil, A.T.; Pethe, A.M.; Fegade, H.; Anand, S.; Dave, V.S. Formulation and characterization of an apigenin-phospholipid phytosome (APLC) for improved solubility, in vivo bioavailability, and antioxidant potential. *Eur. J. Pharm. Sci.* **2017**, *108*, 36–49. [CrossRef]
18. Rathee, S.; Kamboj, A. Optimization and development of antidiabetic phytosomes by the Box-Behnken design. *J. Liposome Res.* **2018**, *28*, 161–172. [CrossRef]
19. Bannunah, A.M.; Vllasaliu, D.; Lord, J.; Stolnik, S. Mechanisms of Nanoparticle Internalization and Transport Across an Intestinal Epithelial Cell Model: Effect of Size and Surface Charge. *Mol. Pharm.* **2014**, *11*, 4363–4373. [CrossRef]
20. Al Saqr, A.; Khafagy, E.S.; Alalaiwe, A.; Aldawsari, M.F.; Alshahrani, S.M.; Anwer, M.K.; Khan, S.; Lila, A.S.A.; Arab, H.H.; Hegazy, W.A.H. Synthesis of Gold Nanoparticles by Using Green Machinery: Characterization and In Vitro Toxicity. *Nanomaterials* **2021**, *11*, 808. [CrossRef]
21. Hou, Z.; Li, Y.; Huang, Y.; Zhou, C.; Lin, J.; Wang, Y.; Cui, F.; Zhou, S.; Jia, M.; Ye, S.; et al. Phytosomes loaded with mitomycin C-soybean phosphatidylcholine complex developed for drug delivery. *Mol. Pharm.* **2013**, *10*, 90–101. [CrossRef]
22. Hooresfand, Z.; Ghanbarzadeh, S.; Hamishehkar, H. Preparation and Characterization of Rutin-loaded Nanophytosomes. *Pharm. Sci.* **2015**, *21*, 145–151. [CrossRef]
23. Ohtake, S.; Schebor, C.; Palecek, S.P.; de Pablo, J.J. Phase behavior of freeze-dried phospholipid–cholesterol mixtures stabilized with trehalose. *Biochim. Biophys. Acta-Biomembr.* **2005**, *1713*, 57–64. [CrossRef]
24. Yanyu, X.; Yunmei, S.; Zhipeng, C.; Qineng, P. The preparation of silybin-phospholipid complex and the study on its pharmacokinetics in rats. *Int. J. Pharm.* **2006**, *307*, 77–82. [CrossRef]
25. Cai, X.; Luan, Y.; Jiang, Y.; Song, A.; Shao, W.; Li, Z.; Zhao, Z. Huperzine A-phospholipid complex-loaded biodegradable thermosensitive polymer gel for controlled drug release. *Int. J. Pharm.* **2012**, *433*, 102–111. [CrossRef]
26. Sherikar, A.; Siddique, M.U.M.; More, M.; Goyal, S.N.; Milivojevic, M.; Alkahtani, S.; Alarifi, S.; Hasnain, M.S.; Nayak, A.K. Preparation and Evaluation of Silymarin-Loaded Solid Eutectic for Enhanced Anti-Inflammatory, Hepatoprotective Effect: *In Vitro-In Vivo* Prospect. *Oxidative Med. Cell. Longev.* **2021**, *2021*, 1818538. [CrossRef]
27. Zeng, Q.P.; Liu, Z.H.; Huang, A.W.; Zhang, J.; Song, H.T. Preparation and characterization of silymarin synchronized-release microporous osmotic pump tablets. *Drug Des. Devel. Ther.* **2016**, *10*, 519–531. [CrossRef] [PubMed]
28. Khan, R.A.; Khan, M.R.; Sahreen, S.; Shah, N.A. Hepatoprotective activity of Sonchus asper against carbon tetrachloride-induced injuries in male rats: A randomized controlled trial. *BMC Complement. Altern. Med.* **2012**, *12*, 90. [CrossRef] [PubMed]
29. Vargas-Mendoza, N.; Madrigal-Santillán, E.; Morales-González, A.; Esquivel-Soto, J.; Esquivel-Chirino, C.; García-Luna, Y.; González-Rubio, M.; Gayosso-de-Lucio, J.A.; Morales-González, J.A. Hepatoprotective effect of silymarin. *World J. Hepatol.* **2014**, *6*, 144–149. [CrossRef] [PubMed]
30. Ohkawa, H.; Ohishi, N.; Yagi, K. Assay for lipid peroxides in animal tissues by thiobarbituric acid reaction. *Anal. Biochem.* **1979**, *95*, 351–358. [CrossRef]
31. Li, X.-X.; Zheng, Q.-C.; Wang, Y.; Zhang, H.-X. Theoretical insights into the reductive metabolism of CCl4 by cytochrome P450 enzymes and the CCl4-dependent suicidal inactivation of P450. *Dalton Trans.* **2014**, *43*, 14833–14840. [CrossRef]
32. Kim, H.J.; Bruckner, J.V.; Dallas, C.E.; Gallo, J.M. Effect of dosing vehicles on the pharmacokinetics of orally administered carbon tetrachloride in rats. *Toxicol. Appl. Pharmacol.* **1990**, *102*, 50–60. [CrossRef]
33. Glende, E.A., Jr.; Hruszkewycz, A.M.; Recknagel, R.O. Critical role of lipid peroxidation in carbon tetrachloride-induced loss of aminopyrine demethylase, cytochrome P-450 and glucose 6-phosphatase. *Biochem. Pharmacol.* **1976**, *25*, 2163–2170. [CrossRef]
34. Gnananath, K.; Sri Nataraj, K.; Ganga Rao, B. Phospholipid Complex Technique for Superior Bioavailability of Phytoconstituents. *Adv. Pharm. Bull.* **2017**, *7*, 35–42. [CrossRef]
35. Soliman, W.E.; Khan, S.; Rizvi, S.M.D.; Moin, A.; Elsewedy, H.S.; Abulila, A.S.; Shehata, T.M. Therapeutic Applications of Biostable Silver Nanoparticles Synthesized Using Peel Extract of Benincasa hispida: Antibacterial and Anticancer Activities. *Nanomaterials* **2020**, *10*, 1954. [CrossRef]
36. Bhattacharyya, S.; Ahammed, S.M.; Saha, B.P.; Mukherjee, P.K. The gallic acid-phospholipid complex improved the antioxidant potential of gallic acid by enhancing its bioavailability. *AAPS PharmSciTech* **2013**, *14*, 1025–1033. [CrossRef]
37. Vasanth, S.; Dubey, A.; Ravi, G.S.; Lewis, S.A.; Ghate, V.M.; El-Zahaby, S.A.; Hebbar, S. Development and Investigation of Vitamin C-Enriched Adapalene-Loaded Transfersome Gel: A Collegial Approach for the Treatment of Acne Vulgaris. *AAPS PharmSciTech* **2020**, *21*, 61. [CrossRef]
38. Tan, Q.; Liu, S.; Chen, X.; Wu, M.; Wang, H.; Yin, H.; He, D.; Xiong, H.; Zhang, J. Design and evaluation of a novel evodiamine-phospholipid complex for improved oral bioavailability. *AAPS PharmSciTech* **2012**, *13*, 534–547. [CrossRef]
39. Singh, E.; Osmani, R.A.M.; Banerjee, R.; Abu Lila, A.S.; Moin, A.; Almansour, K.; Arab, H.H.; Alotaibi, H.F.; Khafagy, E.S. Poly ε-Caprolactone Nanoparticles for Sustained Intra-Articular Immune Modulation in Adjuvant-Induced Arthritis Rodent Model. *Pharmaceutics* **2022**, *14*, 519. [CrossRef]
40. Al Saqr, A.; Wani, S.U.D.; Gangadharappa, H.V.; Aldawsari, M.F.; Khafagy, E.S.; Lila, A.S.A. Enhanced Cytotoxic Activity of Docetaxel-Loaded Silk Fibroin Nanoparticles against Breast Cancer Cells. *Polymers* **2021**, *13*, 1416. [CrossRef]

41. Moin, A.; Wani, S.U.D.; Osmani, R.A.; Abu Lila, A.S.; Khafagy, E.S.; Arab, H.H.; Gangadharappa, H.V.; Allam, A.N. Formulation, characterization, and cellular toxicity assessment of tamoxifen-loaded silk fibroin nanoparticles in breast cancer. *Drug Deliv.* **2021**, *28*, 1626–1636. [CrossRef]
42. Wu, J.W.; Lin, L.C.; Hung, S.C.; Chi, C.W.; Tsai, T.H. Analysis of silibinin in rat plasma and bile for hepatobiliary excretion and oral bioavailability application. *J. Pharm. Biomed. Anal.* **2007**, *45*, 635–641. [CrossRef]

pharmaceuticals

MDPI

Article

Targeting Colorectal Cancer Cells with Niosomes Systems Loaded with Two Anticancer Drugs Models; Comparative In Vitro and Anticancer Studies

Shaymaa Wagdy El-Far [1,*], Hadel A. Abo El-Enin [2,*], Ebtsam M. Abdou [3,†], Ola Elsayed Nafea [4] and Rehab Abdelmonem [5,†]

1 Division of Pharmaceutical Microbiology, Department of Pharmaceutics and Industrial Pharmacy, College of Pharmacy, Taif University, P.O. Box 11099, Taif 21944, Saudi Arabia
2 Department of Pharmaceutics and Industrial Pharmacy, College of Pharmacy, Taif University, P.O. Box 11099, Taif 21944, Saudi Arabia
3 Department of Pharmaceutics, National Organization of Drug Control and Research (NODCAR), Giza P.O. Box 12511, Egypt; ebtsamabdou83@gmail.com
4 Department of Clinical Pharmacy, College of Pharmacy, Taif University, P.O. Box 11099, Taif 21944, Saudi Arabia; oenafea@tu.edu.sa
5 Department of Industrial Pharmacy, College of Pharmaceutical Sciences and Drug Manufacturing, Misr University for Science and Technology (MUST), 6th of October City P.O. Box 12566, Egypt; drrahoba@yahoo.com
* Correspondence: shfar@tu.edu.sa (S.W.E.-F.); hadel.a@tu.edu.sa (H.A.A.E.-E.)
† These authors contributed equally to this work.

Abstract: Colorectal cancer (CRC) is considered one of the most commonly diagnosed malignant diseases. Recently, there has been an increased focus on using nanotechnology to resolve most of the limitations in conventional chemotherapy. Niosomes have great advantages that overcome the drawbacks associated with other lipid drug delivery systems. They are simple, cheap, and highly stable nanocarriers. This study investigated the effectiveness of using niosomes with their amphiphilic characteristics in the incorporation of both hydrophilic and hydrophobic anticancer drugs for CRC treatment. Methods: Drug-free niosomes were formulated using a response surface D-optimal factorial design to study the cholesterol molar ratio, surfactant molar ratio and surfactant type effect on the particle size and Z-potential of the prepared niosomes. After numerical and statistical optimization, an optimized formulation having a particle size of 194.4 ± 15.5 nm and a Z-potential of 31.8 ± 1.9 mV was selected to be loaded with Oxaliplatin and Paclitaxel separately in different concentrations. The formulations with the highest entrapment efficiency (EE%) were evaluated for their drug release using the dialysis bag method, in vitro antitumor activity on HT-29 colon cancer cell line and apoptosis activity. Results: Niosomes prepared using d-α-tocopheryl polyethylene glycol 1000 succinate (TPGS) at a molar ratio 4, cholesterol (2 molar ratio) and loaded with 1 molar ratio of either Oxaliplatin or Paclitaxel provided nanosized vesicles (278.5 ± 19.7 and 251.6 ± 18.1 nm) with a Z-potential value (32.7 ± 1.01 and 31.69 ± 0.98 mV) with the highest EE% (90.57 ± 2.05 and 93.51 ± 2.97) for Oxaliplatin and Paclitaxel, respectively. These formulations demonstrated up to 48 h drug release and increased the in vitro cytotoxicity and apoptosis efficiency of both drugs up to twice as much as free drugs. Conclusion: These findings suggest that different formulation composition parameters can be adjusted to obtain nanosized niosomal vesicles with an accepted Z-potential. These niosomes could be loaded with either hydrophilic drugs such as Oxaliplatin or hydrophobic drugs such as Paclitaxel. Drug-loaded niosomes, as a unique nanomicellar system, could enhance the cellular uptake of both drugs, resulting in enhanced cytotoxic and apoptosis effects against HT-29 colon cancer cells. Oxaliplatin–niosomes and Paclitaxel–niosomes can be considered promising alternative drug delivery systems with enhanced bioavailability of these two anticancer drugs for colorectal cancer treatment.

Citation: El-Far, S.W.; Abo El-Enin, H.A.; Abdou, E.M.; Nafea, O.E.; Abdelmonem, R. Targeting Colorectal Cancer Cells with Niosomes Systems Loaded with Two Anticancer Drugs Models; Comparative In Vitro and Anticancer Studies. *Pharmaceuticals* **2022**, *15*, 816. https://doi.org/10.3390/ph15070816

Academic Editors: Ana Catarina Silva, João Nuno Moreira and José Manuel Sousa Lobo

Received: 6 June 2022
Accepted: 25 June 2022
Published: 30 June 2022

Keywords: Colorectal Cancer; Niosomes; Oxaliplatin; Paclitaxel; d-α-tocopheryl polyethylene glycol 1000 succinate (TPGS)

1. Introduction

Colorectal cancer (CRC) is a serious cancer type that is considered one of the most recently diagnosed malignant diseases. The incidence and mortality rates were higher in men than in women, especially in developed countries. In addition to its high mortality rate, it still ranks fifth in all tumor-related diseases and third in the United States among diagnosed male and female patients [1]. Colorectal cancer primary therapy management is surgery, but in non-metastatic disease (stages I–III), chemotherapy is used as adjuvant therapy in stage II disease and the majority of stage III and in the metastatic colorectal cancer progress patients [2,3].

Oxaliplatin is used for colorectal cancer treatment and could be used in the treatment of other tumors. It is the third-generation organo-platinum compound that could be used as a monotherapy or in combination with 5-fluorouracil (5-FU) for colorectal carcinoma treatment. Oxaliplatin is a monoclonal antibody that targets the epidermal growth factor receptor, triggers the immobilization of the mitotic cell cycle in colorectal tumor cells, and induces apoptosis [4,5]. Oxaliplatin monotherapy for colorectal cancer untreated patients produces response rates of about 12% to 24%, while for relapsed or refractory advanced colorectal cancer patients, it is from 10% to 11% [6].

Oxaliplatin is slightly soluble in water with a narrow therapeutic index drug; therefore, small changes in the dose can greatly affect the clinical efficacy and toxicity [7,8]. Oxaliplatin's toxicity is the peripheral sensory neuropathy, which is mainly two types. The first is acute sensory neuropathy and is exacerbated by cold temperatures (e.g., laryngopharyngeal dysesthesia), and it is completely reversible. After 24 weeks of Oxaliplatin administration, cumulative and frequent sensory neuropathy occurs. Chronic sensory neuropathy, the second type, slowly reverses after treatment is discontinued, and this side effect represents its dose-limiting toxicity [9]. These limitations of systemic toxicity and lower therapeutic index activity are mainly attributed to the high drug accumulation in erythrocytes compared to the lower drug accumulation in tumor tissues following intravenous administration [10].

Paclitaxel has been reported as an effective chemotherapy in the treatment of colorectal cancer [11]. At low doses, it regulates glutaminolysis, which inhibits tumor cell growth. It inhibits the tumor cells' proliferation and angiogenesis and enhances apoptosis. The mechanism of action is closely related to its ability to promote the polymerization of tubulin into microtubules by binding microtubules and stabilizing cell division [12–14].

The lower oral Paclitaxel bioavailability (<10%) is observed due to efflux of the drug by the multidrug transporter P-glycoprotein (Pgp) and excessive hepatic metabolism by the cytochrome P450 system [15]. In addition, Paclitaxel is highly lipophilic, insoluble in water, and lacks ionizable functional groups; therefore, changing pH does not enhance its solubility, and it cannot be used in a pharmaceutically different form [16].

Recently, there has been an increased focus on using nanotechnology to develop novel and targeted drug delivery systems. The unique properties of the nanosized drug delivery systems that arise from the small-sized particles and the large surface area of the vesicles may lead to improve the drugs' passive targeting properties. Additionally, the latter helps in maintaining more drug-loaded vesicles into tumor cells by enhancing the permeability and retention effect. They enhance the dose efficacy and reduce the side effects [17] and help in using the chemotherapy at low concentrations [18], which resolves most of the limitations in conventional chemotherapy [19].

Niosomes are a type of nanoparticle drug delivery systems known as non-ionic surfactant vehicles (NSVs). Niosomes act as self-assembly closed spheroidal structures of non-ionic amphiphiles in the aqueous medium [20]. They have the ability to entrap both hydrophilic and hydrophobic drugs in their core and between the bilayers, respectively [21].

Therefore, it is considered a good drug delivery system for many active agents as phytochemicals, extracts, drugs, and many anticancer drugs (e.g., methotrexate, doxorubicin, and cisplatin) [22,23]. Niosomes are considered simple, cheap, and highly stable nanocarriers compared to many other nanocarriers which could be used in treatment and diagnosis in cancer therapy [24]. They have great advantages that overcome the drawbacks associated with other lipid drug delivery systems as liposomes, as they have greater chemical stability, long shelf life, high purity, content uniformity, low cost, and convenient storage [25]. They have the ability to prolong the circulation of entrapped drugs, minimize drug degradation and inactivation after administration, which helps in preventing undesirable side effects and toxicity, increase drug bioavailability, and target the entrapped drug in the pathological area [26–28].

Therefore, we were interested in using niosomes to enhance Oxaliplatin and Paclitaxel anti-colorectal cancer activity and decrease their toxicity. Despite the significant progress in studying the efficiency of niosomes in improving the anticancer activity of the commonly used chemotherapy agents, there are some limitations to measure niosome efficiency in the treatment of colorectal cancer, especially for Oxaliplatin. In spite of the efficacy of niosomes in incorporating hydrophilic drugs, they are still not examined for Oxaliplatin. Previous studies prepared Paclitaxel in a variety of niosome formulations [24,29,30], but they did not consider the efficiency of niosomes in improving anti-colorectal cancer activity.

In this study, we aimed to investigate the effect of using different non-ionic surfactants (Span 60, Tween 80, and TPGS), which were reported for their ability to facilitate the anticancer drugs' activity [31–34], in different ratios to formulate nanosized vesicles with accepted Z-potential. These vesicles could be optimized to incorporate both hydrophilic (Oxaliplatin) and hydrophobic (Paclitaxel) colorectal anticancer drugs with high EE%, extended drug release, cytotoxic effect against HT-29 cells, and apoptosis efficiency. To our knowledge, this is considered the first report on comparing the efficacy of niosomes in the incorporation of both hydrophilic and hydrophobic colorectal anticancer drugs.

2. Results and Discussion

2.1. Drug-Free Niosomes Preparation and Optimization

Niosomes are a promising drug delivery system for cancer therapy as they help in targeting the drug to the cancer cells, increasing the treatment duration with reducing the severe side toxic effects and improving the drug stability [35]. Reducing the particle size and increasing the entrapped drug in the niosomes vesicles improves the drug cytotoxicity in cancer cells [36].

Niosomes were prepared using a thin film hydration method, as it is the most suitable, simple, and reproducible method for the preparation of multilamellar non-ionic niosomal vesicles. It is usually accompanied by sonication to acquire niosomes with a narrow size distribution [37].

Different non-ionic surfactants were used to optimize the drug-free niosomal formulations regarding the particle size and the Z-potential value. CHOL was used in a proper amount to achieve the most stable formulation due to its interaction with non-ionic surfactants, resulting in improvement of the niosomal vesicles' mechanical strength and permeability to water [38,39], in addition to stability under severe stress conditions [40].

Preparing vesicular carriers with a small particle size was one of the main concerns in this study, as the average size of lipid/nonionic surfactant vesicles is an important parameter with respect to the physical properties and biological fate of niosomes and their entrapped substances [41]. The prepared drug-free formulations had different particle sizes that ranged from 189.2 ± 13.4 nm to 293.3 ± 17.2 nm; see Table 1. The polydispersity index (PDI) of all the prepared niosomes formulations was <0.3, which is considered acceptable for lipid-based vesicles and indicates the formulation homogeneity [42].

Table 1. Experimental runs, independent and dependent variables of the factorial experimental design of drug-free niosomes.

Runs	Factors (Independent Variables)			Responses (Dependent Variables)		
	CHOL Ratio (*w*/*w*)	Surfactant Ratio (*w*/*w*)	Surfactant Type *	Particle Size (nm)	Z-Potential (mV)	PDI
F1	1.00	3.00	Span 60	242.5 ± 22.4	(−) 29.3 ± 1.8	0.158 ± 0.01
F2	1.00	4.00	Span 60	198.2 ± 18.6	(−) 31.4 ± 1.6	0.214 ± 0.04
F3	1.50	3.25	Span 60	232.1 ± 15.7	(−) 30.4 ± 2.1	0.256 ± 0.11
F4	2.00	3.00	Span 60	293.3 ± 17.2	(−) 30.2 ± 1.7	0.247 ± 0.21
F5	2.00	4.00	Span 60	251.2 ± 20.3	(−) 32.1 ± 1.9	0.165 ± 0.06
F6	1.00	3.00	TPGS	265.3 ± 18.4	(−) 29.1 ± 1.7	0.146 ± 0.04
F7	1.00	3.50	TPGS	241.2 ± 16.7	(−) 30.2 ± 2.2	0.132 ± 0.03
F8	1.50	3.00	TPGS	231.5 ± 18.2	(−) 29.8 ± 2.4	0.189 ± 0.14
F9	2.00	4.00	TPGS	194.4 ± 15.5	(−) 31.8 ± 1.9	0.175 ± 0.20
F10	2.00	3.00	TPGS	221.2 ± 21.3	(−) 30.2 ± 1.6	0.211 ± 0.07
F11	2.00	3.50	TPGS	198.1 ± 17.8	(−) 31.5 ± 1.8	0.241 ± 0.31
F12	1.00	4.00	Tween 80	241.7 ± 19.8	(−) 30.6 ± 2.4	0.257 ± 0.45
F13	1.00	3.00	Tween 80	261.4 ± 22.6	(−) 28.8 ± 2.1	0.237 ± 0.25
F14	1.50	3.00	Tween 80	228.3 ± 19.5	(−) 28.9 ± 1.5	0.198 ± 0.41
F15	1.50	3.50	Tween 80	203.1 ± 17.9	(−) 30.3 ± 1.8	0.269 ± 0.09
F16	2.00	4.00	Tween 80	189.2 ± 13.4	(−) 31.5 ± 2.2	0.222 ± 0.17
F17	2.00	3.00	Tween 80	228.4 ± 16.4	(−) 30.7 ± 2.1	0.243 ± 0.29

* Surfactant type; hydrophilic–lipophilic balance (HLB) value: Span 60 (HLB;4.7), TPGS (HLB; 13.2), Tween 80 (HLB; 15).

All the studied factors were found to have a significant effect on the particle size of the prepared drug-free niosomes with significant interaction between the CHOL ratio (X1) and surfactant type (X3), Table 2 and Figure 1; the final equation in terms of coded factors was:

$$\text{Particle size} = +208.82 - 6.05 \times A - 17.64 \times B + 11.24 \times C[1] - 6.42 \times C[2] - 1.87 \times AB + 32.00 \times AC[1] - 6.68 \times AC[2] - 3.83 \times BC[1] + 0.92 \times BC[2] + 16.40 \times A^2 + 9.57 \times B^2$$

Table 2. The design expert results of all response variables.

Source	Particle Size (nm)		Z-Potential (mV)	
	F	*p*-Value	F	*p*-Value
Model	68.78	<0.0001	12.67	0.0058
A: CHOL ratio	23.40	0.0047	33.52	0.0022
B: Surfactant ratio	236.62	<0.0001	92.89	0.0002
C: Surfactant type	31.81	0.0014	3.40	0.1168
AB	1.86	0.2313	1.17	0.3288
AC	178.48	<0.0001	0.78	0.5055
BC	3.05	0.1359	0.85	0.4817
A^2	49.58	0.0009	0.56	0.4872
B^2	12.94	0.0156	0.32	0.5939
Adequate precision	29.912		12.934	
R^2	0.9934		0.9654	
Adjusted R^2	0.9790		0.8892	
Predicted R^2	0.8413		0.5883	
SD	4.11		0.34	
%CV	1.78		1.12	

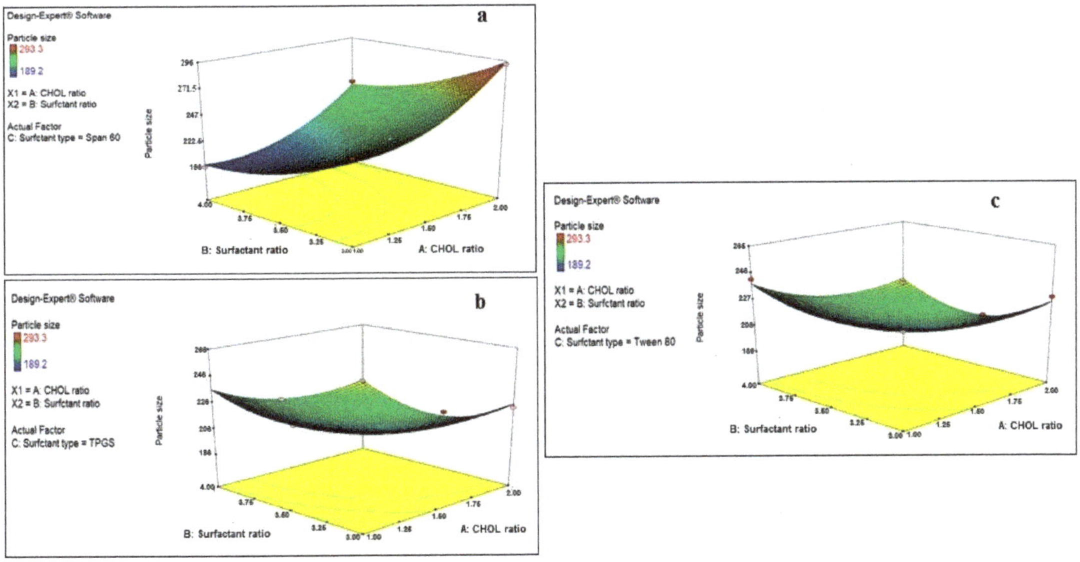

Figure 1. Effect of CHOL and surfactant ratio on the particle size of drug-free niosomes at different surfactant types ((**a**): Span 60, (**b**): TPGS, (**c**): Tween 80).

Regarding the effect of the CHOL ratio on the particle size of the prepared drug-free niosomes, a higher CHOL ratio resulted in a significant decrease in the particle size of niosomes formulated with TPGS and Tween 80 surfactants, while it resulted in an increase in the particle size of niosomes formulated with Span 60 surfactant. Cholesterol is an amphipathic rigid molecule with an inverted cone shape, which makes it able to be intercalated between the fluid hydrocarbon chains of the bilayer membrane with its hydrophilic head oriented toward the aqueous surface and aliphatic chain line up parallel to the hydrocarbon chains in the center of the bilayer of vesicles, resulting in increasing the chain order of the liquid-state bilayer and strengthening the nonpolar tail of the non-ionic surfactant [41,43]. For niosomes, the vesicle formation is governed by the hydrophobic interaction between the surfactant and the stabilizing agent, CHOL [44].

Span 60 is known to be more hydrophobic than TPGS and Tween 80, as it has an HLB value of 4.7, while the others have values of 13.2 and 15, respectively. This results in a reduction in the surface free energy associated with the increased lipophilicity [45], which makes Span 60 require less amounts of CHOL to form rigid vesicles. This is in accordance with what was reported previously: that Span 60 could form niosomes either without the addition of CHOL or with small quantities that only maintained the rigidity of niosomes membrane [21]. In addition, with Span 60, higher amounts of CHOL increase the niosomes' rigidity, which makes them more resistant to the effect of sonication on particle size reduction [46]. Unlike Span 60, TPGS and Tween 80 surfactants require larger amounts of CHOL, which would increase the hydrophobicity and decrease the surface energy, resulting in vesicles with smaller particle sizes. In addition, the hydrogen bonding between the carbonyl group of Tween 80 and the hydroxyl group of CHOL essentially governs the rigidity of the niosomes [47].

A higher surfactant ratio resulted usually in significant lower particle size. This may be related either to the formation of mixed micelles, at higher surfactant amounts, instead of niosomal vesicles, as mixed micelles have lower particle size [48], or to more strengthening of the steric resistance on the vesicle surface due to surfactant adsorption resulting in a lower particle size [49]. TPGS is known to increase the compressibility of the vesicular bilayer as a result of dehydration, when present in high concentrations, and decrease the bilayer defects in the niosomes, resulting in decreasing the particle size [50].

Regarding the effect of different factors on the Z-potential of the prepared drug-free niosomes, both CHOL and surfactant ratio have a positive effect on the Z-potential, while surfactant type has a non-significant effect with non-significant interaction between any two factors, Table 2 and Figure 2, with the final equation in terms of coded factors as:

$$ZP = +30.61 + 0.55 \times A + 0.94 \times B + 0.16 \times C\,[1] + 0.17 \times C\,[2] - 0.12 \times AB - 0.15 \times AC\,[1] - 7.407 \times 10^{-3} \times AC\,[2] + 0.040 \times BC\,[1] + 0.13 \times BC\,[2 + 0.14 \times A^2 - 0.12 \times B^2$$

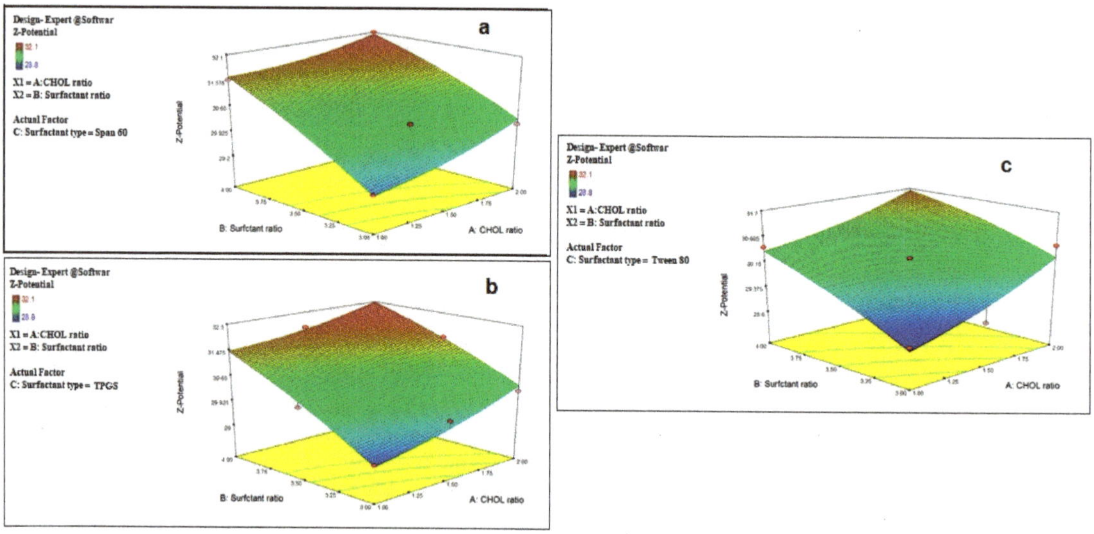

Figure 2. Effect of CHOL and surfactant ratio on the Z-potential of drug-free niosomes at different surfactant types ((**a**): Span 60, (**b**): TPGS, (**c**): Tween 80).

Z-potential is an important label for the identification of the prepared nanoparticle physical stability. The system with a Z-potential value around ±30 mV is considered stable [48] due to increasing the repulsion force between the particles, which can overcome the van der Waals attractive forces and hence prevent particles aggregation [51].

Although the prepared niosomes do not include the charge inducer additive, they were found to have accepted negative Z-potential values which ranged from -28.8 ± 2.1 to -32.1 ± 1.9 mV. This might be attributed to the preferential adsorption of hydroxyl ions of the used non-ionic surfactants at the vesicle surface, thus imparting a negative charge to the vesicles surface [41,52,53], and due to the effect of CHOL, as it was reported to impart a negative surface charge on the vesicles' surface [54]. This can also be related to the surface energy of the vesicles due to the HLB values of the surfactant, as it was reported that an increase in the surface energy of the vesicles leads to an increase in the values of Z-potential toward negative [45].

2.2. Optimization of the Prepared Drug-Free Niosomes

Responses constraints (particle size was minimized and Z-potential was maximized) were applied to determine the optimum levels of the variables through numerical optimization. The prepared optimized formulations were characterized, and no major residual error was found, indicating the validity of numerical optimization for this study. Different solutions were obtained with the first one having a desirability of 1, as shown in Figure 3, at which the formulation has a particle size of 186.9 nm and a Z-potential of -32.25 mV and consists of TPGS surfactant in a molar ratio of 3.99 with a CHOL molar ratio of 1.91.

These results can be represented by F9, which was selected for drug loading. The selected particle size could improve the phagocytosis by macrophages and prolong the plasma drug concentration [55].

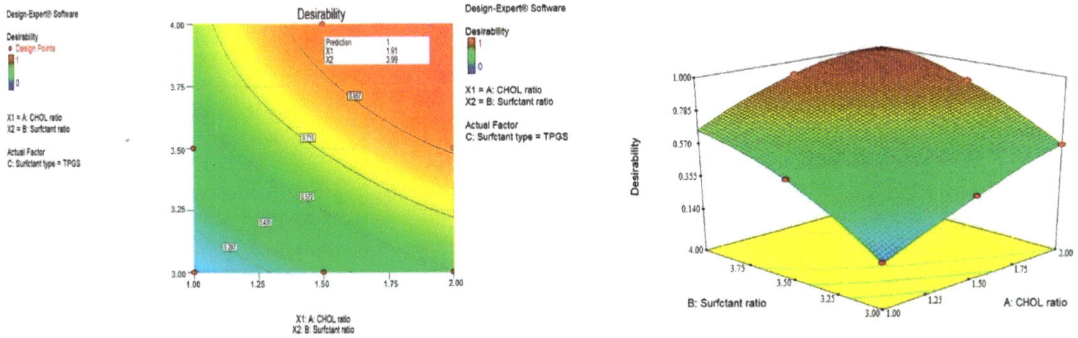

Figure 3. Optimization of the prepared drug-free niosomes.

2.3. *Preparation and Evaluation of Drug-Loaded Niosomes*

Both drugs, Oxaliplatin and Paclitaxel, could be successfully encapsulated separately into the optimized niosomes formulation with different drug concentrations. To ensure the encapsulation capacity of the prepared niosomes, EE% was determined. As represented in Table 3, increasing the drug ratio from 0.5 to 1 resulted in a significant increase in the EE% for both drugs, with p values = 0.0024 and 0.0175 for Oxaliplatin and Paclitaxel, respectively. This was in accordance with reported studies that higher drug concentrations enhance drug entrapment efficiency, as it imparts a driving force for the drug to be encapsulated into the vesicles [56]. There was no difference between the drug concentration in the supernatant before and after the addition of acetonitrile, indicating that there were no niosomes suspended in the supernatant, and all of them were resting in the dialysis bag.

Table 3. Effect of drug concentration on EE%, particle size, and Z-potential of the prepared drug-loaded niosomes.

Drug Loaded (Molar Ratio)	Oxaliplatin–TPGS Niosomes				Paclitaxel–TPGS Niosomes			
	EE%	Particle Size (nm)	Z-Potential (mV)	PDI	EE%	Particle Size (nm)	Z-Potential (mV)	PDI
0.5	77.19 ±2.68	236.4 ± 22.3	−31.7 ± 0.96	0.236 ± 0.07	83.82 ± 3.13	227.4 ± 16.3	−30.91 ± 0.45	0.283 ± 0.04
1	90.57 ±2.05	278.5 ± 19.7	−32.7 ± 1.01	0.264 ± 0.05	93.51 ± 2.97	251.6 ± 18. 1	−31.69 ± 0.98	0.273 ± 0.08
2	91.03 ±2.80	285.8 ± 23.5	−33.25 ± 1.41	0.295 ± 0.07	93.31 ± 3.31	258.6 ± 13.3	−32.99 ± 1.08	0.287 ± 0.09

Paclitaxel was significantly entrapped in a higher amount than Oxaliplatin at the same drug ratio, p value < 0.05. Theoretically, Paclitaxel, a water-insoluble drug, is placed into hydrophobic tail groups (more hydrophobic drug), while Oxaliplatin is placed in the aqueous core, since Oxaliplatin is more soluble in water. One of the possible reasons for the high entrapped amounts of both drugs might be correlated to the interaction between the drug and the surfactants, which could locate the drug into both hydrophobic tail groups and the aqueous interior part of niosomes.

Further increase in the drug concentration from 1 to 2% did not significantly increase the EE% for both drugs (p value = 0.09512 and 0.8297 for Oxaliplatin and Paclitaxel, respectively). This may be attributed to the saturation of the drug within the lipid bilayer of the niosomes, as the excess drug will be scattered between the niosomal pellets and the precipitate [57]. This was also affected by constant concentrations of CHOL and surfactant, which would yield a certain number of vesicles with limited drug loading. This finding indicates the suitability of the selected noisome formulae to encapsulate both hydrophilic and hydrophobic drugs.

The particle size and Z-potential of the prepared drug-loaded niosomes were measured, as shown in Table 3. It was found that increasing the drug concentration from 0.5 to 1 led to a significant increase in the vesicles size ($p < 0.05$), which is in direct correlation with the drug EE%. Drug encapsulation into the niosomal vesicles usually increases their particle size, which may be related to the interaction of the drug with the surfactant head groups, resulting in increasing the charge and mutual repulsion of the surfactant bilayers, thereby increasing the vesicle size [58]. Further increase in the drug concentration did not significantly affect the particle size ($p > 0.05$) of drug-loaded niosomes of either drug. The Z-potential was not significantly changed after loading the niosomes with either Oxaliplatin or Paclitaxel. Depending on these results, drug-loaded niosomes with each drug at a molar ratio of 1 for both drugs were selected for further evaluation. It is worthy here to mention that the PDI values of all the prepared drug-loaded niosomes were less than 0.3, indicating homogenous size distribution.

2.4. In Vitro Drug Release

The release pattern of Oxaliplatin–TPGS niosomes and Paclitaxel–TPGS niosomes in comparison with the free drugs is shown in Figure 4. Both drugs were released from the prepared niosomes at a higher rate than their free drugs. For Oxaliplatin–TPGS niosomes, 87.5 ± 1.99% was released after 24 h compared to 19.4 ± 1.76% from the free drug. For Paclitaxel–TPGS niosomes, 80.81 ± 2.98% was released after 24 h compared to 14.77 ± 0.98% from the free drug. The High EE% and small particle size of the prepared niosomes may be the reason for higher drug release from the prepared niosomes in addition to the hydrophilicity of the TPGS outer shell. The small vesicles size partitions the drug in nanosized particles (<300 nm). In addition, the presence of the surfactant as TPGS, which has a high HLB value and high concentration, facilitated the penetration of release medium to the niosomes surface and into the cores, thus improving the drug release pattern.

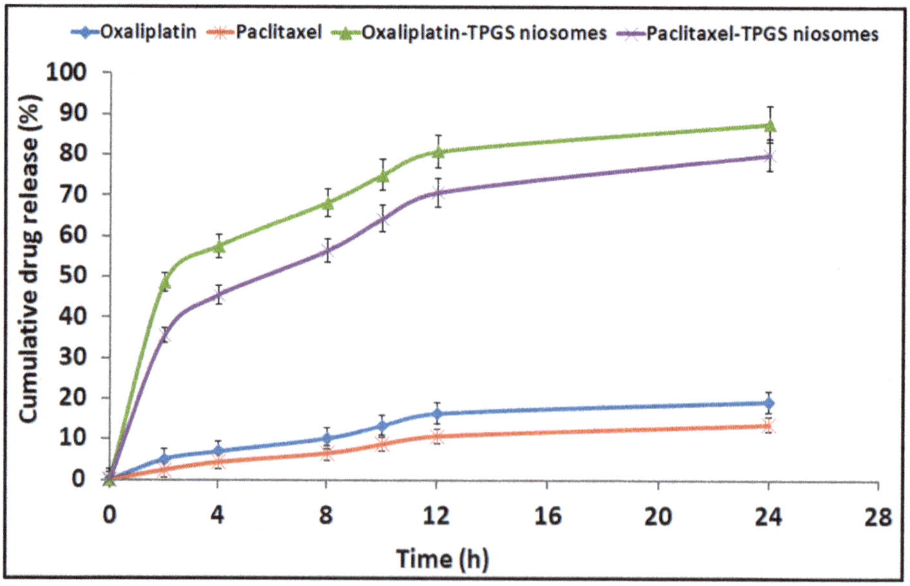

Figure 4. In vitro cumulative drug release profile from Oxaliplatin–TPGS niosomes, Paclitaxel–TPGS niosomes, Oxaliplatin free drug and Paclitaxel free drug.

The in vitro release pattern of both drugs from the prepared niosomes showed a bi-phasic pattern with an initial burst release followed by sustained release. The high first burst release pattern showed more than 40% at the first 4 h (57.53 ± 0.22% and 45.41 ± 0.43% for Oxaliplatin and Paclitaxel, respectively), which is attributed to the release of the unentrapped and adsorbed drug on the niosomes vesicles' surface [59]. The second release pattern shows a sustaining release rate for both drugs for 28 h. The significant difference in the second release pattern was due to the bilayered systems such as niosomes, as the drug release occurs by diffusion of the drug from the inner core and passage through the bilayer. In addition, the presence of CHOL, which stabilizes the niosomal bilayer membrane, thus enhances the extended drug release behavior [60]. This sustained behavior of drug release can provide prolonged in vivo drug action while decreasing the dosage frequency.

To determine the effective mechanisms assisting the drugs release from the prepared niosomes formulations, kinetic data were analyzed to express the best fitting mathematical model. Zero-order, first-order, Higuchi diffusion, and Korsmeyer–Peppas models were applied; the correlation coefficients (R^2) are summarized in Table 4. The best-fit model for both drugs' release from the prepared niosomes formulations was the Higuchi diffusion model. The latter indicated that the drugs release was a controlled diffusion process based on Fick's law; i.e., it depends on the time square root. The slow release was previously reported to have a beneficial in reducing the toxic side effects of the entrapped drugs [61,62].

Table 4. Different mathematical models of in vitro release data (means ± SD, n = 3).

Formulation	Correlation Coefficient (R^2)			
	Zero Order	1st Order	Higuchi Diffusion	Korsmeyer–Peppas
Oxaliplatin–TPGS–niosomes	0.6114 ± 0.034	0.8715 ± 0.027	0.8871 ± 0.021	0.8844 ± 0.011
Paclitaxel–TPGS–niosomes	0.7164 ± 0.021	0.9006 ± 0.014	0.9475 ± 0.011	0.942 ± 0.015

2.5. *Transmission Electron Microscopy (TEM)*

The morphology of the prepared niosomes is shown in Figure 5. All vesicles had a spherical uni-lamellar morphology with a smooth boundary and homogenous particle size. There was an absence of any aggregation between the nanoparticles, indicating their stability against Oswald ripening by globular collapsing [63].

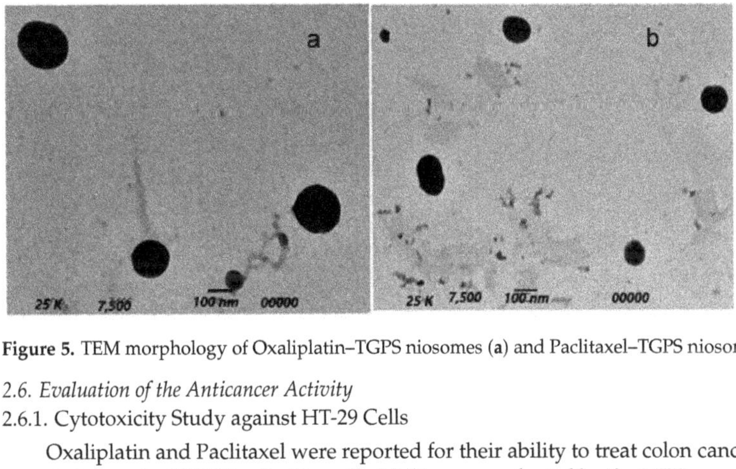

Figure 5. TEM morphology of Oxaliplatin–TGPS niosomes (**a**) and Paclitaxel–TGPS niosomes (**b**).

2.6. *Evaluation of the Anticancer Activity*

2.6.1. Cytotoxicity Study against HT-29 Cells

Oxaliplatin and Paclitaxel were reported for their ability to treat colon cancer. They were tested against HT-29 cells. The cell viability was evaluated by the MTT assay method and compared to the results of plain niosomes and free drugs. The tested formulations (Oxaliplatin–TPGS–niosomes and Paclitaxel–TPGS–niosomes) enhanced their cytotoxicity effect on the colorectal cancer cells. The cytotoxic effect of niosomes in HT-29 cells lines was approximately two-fold compared to that of their free drugs. All tested formulations showed a dose-dependent effect, as shown in Figure 6. The IC_{50} values of Oxaliplatin–TPGS–niosomes, Paclitaxel–TPGS–niosomes, drug-free niosomes (F9), Oxaliplatin solution, and Paclitaxel solution were calculated from the Figure 6 and were found to be 11.86 μg/mL, 7.18 μg/mL, 68.52 μg/mL, 23.56 μg/mL, 19.98 μg/mL, respectively. The significant decrease in the IC_{50} for the prepared niosomes relative to the free drug, about two folds for Oxaliplatin and about three folds for Paclitaxel, is remarkable and indicative of the ability of niosomal formulations to enhance the cellular uptake of both drugs. The significant efficacy of plain niosomes is suggested to be related to TPGS, which is a non-ionic surfactant that has an inhibitory efflux mechanism through ATPase inhibition and subsequent ATP depletion [64,65].

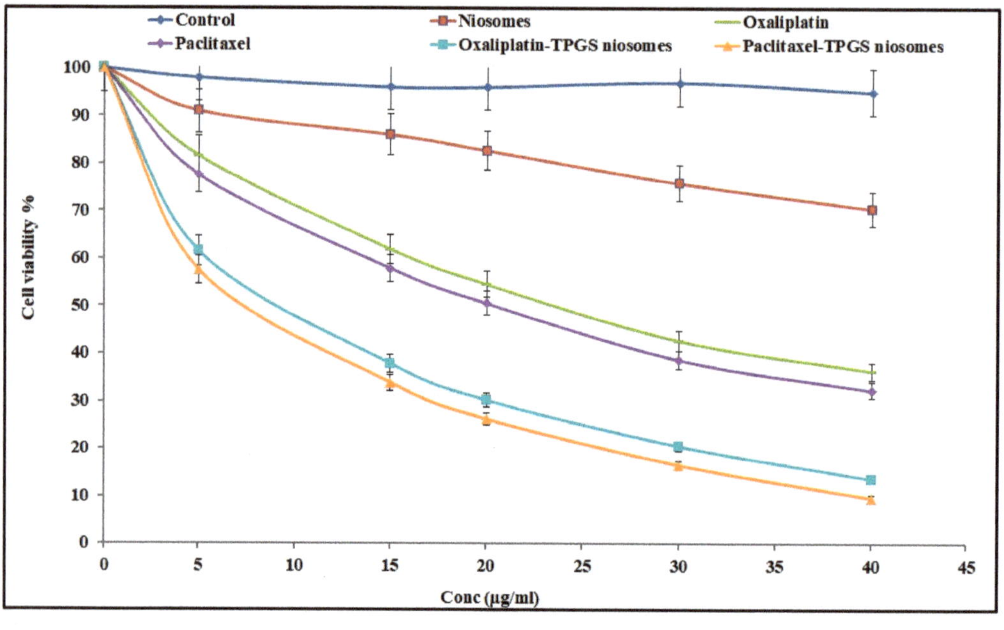

Figure 6. The cytotoxic effect of Oxaliplatin–TPGS–niosomes, Paclitaxel–TPGS–niosomes, drug-free niosomes (F9), Oxaliplatin solution and Paclitaxel solution at various concentrations against HT-29 cells for 24 h ($n = 3$, mean ± SD) ($p < 0.05$).

In general, niosomes formulations improved the cancer cell uptake and enhanced the cytotoxicity of both drugs. The high concentration of TPGS enhanced the drug uptake by cancer cells and extended its therapeutic effect. These results are in agreement with what was previously reported: that nanoparticles' cytotoxic effect is mediated by the internalization and subsequent release of the anticancer drug from nanoparticles intracellularly [64]. There were no significant differences between the cytotoxicity effect represented by IC_{50} value and the cytotoxicity percent of both Oxaliplatin–TPGS–niosomes and Paclitaxel–TPGS–niosomes at the same concentrations ($p < 0.5$). Therefore, niosomes are considered a good targeting carrier system for drug therapy in colorectal cancer for both drugs.

2.6.2. Apoptosis Analysis

The anticancer drugs' toxicity could be convoluted by apoptosis mechanism [66]. Figure 7 shows the apoptosis result related to the effect of different tested formulations. The apoptotic activity of niosome formulations (Oxaliplatin–TPGS–niosomes and Paclitaxel–TPGS–niosomes) was remarkably higher than that of their free drugs and plain noisome formulation. The noticed free niosomes apoptotic activity was due to the presence of TPGS. It was reported that TPGS can induce cancer cell apoptosis through different mechanisms, either by helping in the destruction and inhibition of the mitochondrial respiratory complex [67] or through induction of DNA damage or oxidation of lipid, protein, and enzyme, leading to cell destruction [68]. This is in agreement with previously reported findings that TPGS has been approved by the FDA as a P-glycoprotein (P-gp) inhibitor, which is an extracellular transporter that influences the pharmacokinetics (PK) of various compounds. Thus, TPGS could enhance the bioavailability and reverse MDR (modified drug release) [66,67,69]. The latter explains the higher niosomes-mediated delivery of the drugs to the cancer cells than the free drugs. It was reported previously that using non-ionic surfactants for niosomes preparation is promising due to their inhibitory effect of p-glycoprotein, which significantly increases the bioavailability of some anticancer drugs [70,71]. The niosomes' vesicles size also plays an important role in their cell penetration and, consequently, absorption and targeting, as particles with sizes less than 200 nm show higher cellular drug uptake for cancer therapy [72,73]. In addition, the presence of CHOL in the niosomes' structure could enhance cellular uptake due to the interaction between CHOL and the biological membranes [74]. There was no significant difference between the effect of Oxaliplatin–TPGS–niosomes and Paclitaxel–TPGS–niosomes ($p < 0.05$). These results demonstrate that niosomes represent a promising drug delivery system for anticancer drugs in colorectal cancer therapy. It could also be used to target tumor cells and prolong circulation in the body.

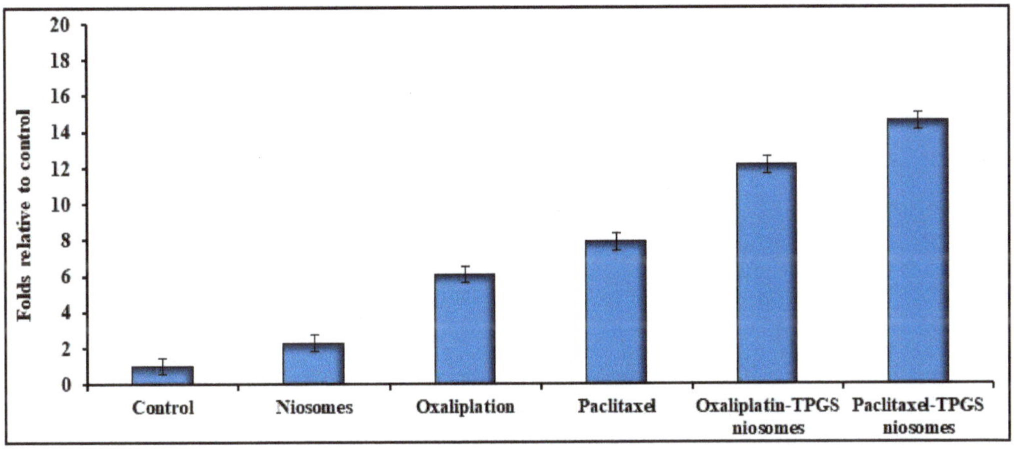

Figure 7. Effects of Oxaliplatin–TPGS–niosomes, Paclitaxel–TPGS–niosomes, drug-free niosomes (F9), Oxaliplatin solution and Paclitaxel solution therapy on apoptosis in HT-29 cancer cell line (IC_{50} values µg/mL) for 24 h treatment in HT-29 cells ($p < 0.05$ compared to control).

It is worthy here to mention that our results are comparable to the results of previous approaches that have been published about using nanotechnology formulations, other than niosomes, in enhancing the cytotoxic effect and decreasing the side effects of both Oxaliplatin and Paclitaxel. For example, Jabalera et al. formulated Oxaliplatin as biomimetic magnetic nanoparticles (BMNPs), and when they were tested against HT-29 cells, they induced about a two-fold decrease in the IC_{50} value compared to the Oxaliplatin solution [75]. Tummala et al. prepared Oxaliplatin immune-hybrid nanoparticles (OIHNPs) to deliver Oxaliplatin for colorectal cancer treatment, and these nanoparticles resulted in a significant increase in the cellular uptake compared to the free drug when they were tested on HT-29 cells [59]. On the other side, Zhen et al. found that the IC_{50} of Paclitaxel-loaded cationic liposomes synthesized by linoleoyl tails was at least two fold lower than that of cationic liposomes synthesized by oleoyl tails at every tested Paclitaxel content [76].

3. Materials and Methods

3.1. Materials

Oxaliplatin, Paclitaxel, Cholesterol, Span 60, Tween 80 and d-α-tocopheryl polyethylene glycol 1000 succinate (TPGS) were bought from Sigma-Aldrich Co. (St. Louis, MO, USA). All other chemicals were of analytical grade and were purchased from El-Gomhoria Co., Cairo, Egypt. The chemical structure of the used drugs and non-ionic surfactants is mentioned in Supplementary Material.

The colon cancer cell line HT-29 was cultured in Dulbecco's modified Eagle's medium, which contained 4.5 g of glucose per liter and 10% fetal bovine serum (FBS) (Thermofisher Scientific, Waltham, MA, USA). The culture media contained 100 units/mL of penicillin and 100 g/mL of streptomycin. The cells were kept at 37 °C with 5% CO_2. Prior to treatment with various agents, the cells were cultured in fresh media containing 10% FBS for cell growth and MTT studies.

3.2. Experimental Design

To define the optimally selected factors that produce niosomes with minimal particle size and the required Z-potential, response surface D-optimal factorial design was employed to statistically investigate the effect of different formulation variables on the properties of the prepared drug-free niosomes using Design-Expert® software (version 7; Stat-Ease, Inc., Minneapolis, MN, USA). Three independent factors were screened at three different levels as follows: cholesterol (CHOL) molar ratio (X1) at 3, 3.5, and 4, surfactant molar ratio (X2) at 1, 1.5, and 2, and surfactant type (X3) at Span 60, TPGS and Tween 80. Two independent variables were evaluated, which were particle size (Y1) and Zeta potential (Z-potential) (Y2). The design parameters and constraints are shown in Table 5, and their detailed composition is reported in Table 5.

Table 5. Factorial design of drug-free niosomes composition.

Factors		Levels	
		Low (−1)–High (1)	
A (X1): Cholesterol (molar ratio)	3	3.5	4
B (X2): Surfactant (molar ratio)	1	1.5	2
C (X3): Surfactant type	Span 60	TPGS	Tween 80
	Responses		
(Y1): Particle size (PS)		Minimize	
(Y2): Zeta potential (Z-potential)		Maximize	

3.3. Preparation of Drug-Free Niosomes

Drug-free niosomes were prepared by a thin film hydration method [20,77]. Nonionic surfactants (Span 60, TPGS and Tween 80) and CHOL were accurately weighed separately and dissolved in 10 mL chloroform then transferred to a round-bottom flask. The residual solvent was allowed to evaporate under reduced pressure using a rotary evaporator (Rotavap, Type R-110, Buchi, Switzerland) at 150 rpm and 65 °C for 2 h until the formation of a thin lipid film on the inner flask wall. After thin film formation, the dried film was then hydrated using 10 mL phosphate buffer saline pH 7.4 pre-heated to 65 °C with rotation for 1 h until dispersion was obtained. The dispersion was left to equilibrate at 25 °C overnight and then subjected to sonication using a probe sonicator (Sonifier® 250 Branson, MO, USA) in an ice-bath for three intermitted intervals, each one for 5 min. Dispersions were kept in a tightly closed container at 4 °C for evaluation.

3.4. Particle Size and Z-Potential Analysis

The particle size, estimated by dynamic light scattering (DLS), and Z-potential of the prepared drug-free niosomes were measured by a Zeta-sizer (Zeta-sizer Ver. 7.01, Malvern

Instruments, Worcestershire, UK) after appropriate dilution of the samples with de-ionized water (1:10) to avoid multi-scattering phenomena using standard operation methods. All measurements were conducted in triplicate at 25 ± 1 °C. Results were recorded as the mean ± SD.

3.5. Preparation of Drug-Loaded Niosomes

Based on statistical optimization of the prepared drug-free niosomes, one formulation having the minimal particle size and maximum Z-potential was selected to be loaded separately with the two drugs: Oxaliplatin and Paclitaxel. Drug-loaded niosomes were prepared in the same method as the drug-free niosomes (Section 3.3), while the drug was added in different amounts: 0.5, 1, and 2 molar ratios. Paclitaxel was dissolved in the organic phase (10 mL chloroform), while Oxaliplatin was dissolved in the pre-heated phosphate buffer saline pH 7.4 (65 °C).

3.6. Evaluation of the Prepared Drug-Loaded Niosomes

3.6.1. Drug Entrapment Efficiency (EE%)

The drug entrapment efficiency in the prepared drug-loaded niosomes was determined using the dialysis technique against phosphate-buffered saline (PBS, pH 7.4) for separation of the non-entrapped drug from the niosomes dispersion [78,79]. From each formulation, 3 mL of niosomal suspension was dropped into a dialysis bag (M.Wt. cut off: 12000. Medicell, London, UK). The bag was immersed into a beaker containing 100 mL phosphate-buffered saline (PBS, pH 7.4) with constant stirring at 4 °C. After every 30 min, samples were withdrawn, and the concentration of the free drugs was measured spectrophotometrically (Schimadzu spectrophotometer, Model UV-1601, Marsiling Industrial Estate, Singapore) at 260 nm and 227 nm for Oxaliplatin and Paclitaxel, respectively. Dialysis was complete when no more drugs were detectable in the recipient solution. The percentage of drug entrapment in the drug-loaded niosomes was calculated according to the following equation [80].

$$\text{Drug Entrapment \%} = [(\text{Total Drug} - \text{Drug in the supernatant})/\text{Total Drug}] \times 100$$

All the measurements were calculated three times, and results were represented as mean ± SD.

For confirmative studies, 1 mL of acetonitrile was added to 5 mL of supernatant with stirring to lyse any present niosomes into the supernatant. The solution was filtered, properly diluted with PBS (pH 7.4), and the drugs concentration was measured spectrophotometrically.

3.6.2. Measurement of the Particle Size and Z-Potential of Drug-Loaded Niosomes

The mean vesicles size and Z-potential value of the prepared drug-loaded niosomes formulations were calculated as previously described in Section 3.4. Results were recorded as the mean ± SD.

3.6.3. In Vitro Drug Release Study

To study the release pattern of both drugs from the prepared drug-loaded niosomes, an in vitro release study was performed using the dialysis bag method applying the sink conditions [22]. Two milliliters of either Oxaliplatin–TPGS niosomes or Paclitaxel–TPGS niosomes were placed in a dialysis bag of 50 mm flat width and 10 k Da, MWCO. The both-ended closed bag was placed in a conical flask containing 150 mL PBS pH 7.4 containing 1% sodium lauryl sulfate as a medium. The whole assembly was shaken using a thermostatically controlled shaker (PSU-20i Orbital Multi-Platform Shaker, Grant Instruments (Cambridge) Ltd., Thomas Scientific, Swedesboro, NJ, USA) at 37 °C and 50 rpm. Samples were withdrawn at 2 h intervals for 24 h and immediately replaced with pre-heated fresh medium to maintain the sink conditions. The cumulative amount released was determined spectrophotometrically at 260 nm and 227 nm for Oxaliplatin and Paclitaxel, respectively, and the cumulative amount released was calculated. The same method was repeated with the drug-free niosomes to be used as a blank. For comparative study, the release pattern of both pure drugs separately was studied in the same method. All measurements were calculated three times and results were represented as mean ± SD. Different models as zero-order, first-order, Higuchi diffusion, and Korsmeyer–Peppas were applied to evaluate the drug release pattern and determine the kinetics model that expresses the drug release mechanism from the prepared formulations [81].

3.6.4. Transmission Electron Microscopy (TEM)

Morphological examination of the optimized Paclitaxel–niosomes and Oxaliplatin–niosomes was conducted using Transmission Electron Microscope (TEM) (JEOL JEM1230, Tokyo, Japan). A drop of each formulation was placed on a carbon-coated copper grid to leave a thin film, which was negatively stained with 1% phosphotungstic acid (PTA). The grid was left to dry, and samples were scanned under the transmission electron microscope operating at an accelerating voltage of 80 kV.

3.7. Evaluation of the Anticancer Activity for the Selected Paclitaxel-Niosomes and Oxaliplatin-Niosomes

3.7.1. Cytotoxicity Study against HT-29 Cells

The cytotoxicity study on HT-29 (human colon adenocarcinoma) cells using an MTT (tetrazolium salt 3-[4,5-demethylthiazol-2-yl]-2-5-diphenlytetrazolium bromide) colorimetric method was completed for the following formulations: Oxaliplatin–TPGS niosomes, Paclitaxel–TPGS niosomes, drug-free niosomes (F9); Oxaliplatin and Paclitaxel solutions were used as positive controls. HT-29 cells were seeded in 96-well plates at a density of 5×10^3 cells and then incubated for 24 h at 37 °C. The tested cells were treated with series concentrations of the tested formulations (all containing an equivalent concentration) separately for 24 h at 37 °C. Cell viability was evaluated with MTT on a Synergy 2 Multi-Detection Microplate Reader by BioTek Instruments, Inc at 570 nm. Six independent experiments were conducted, and the inhibitory concentration (50%) (IC_{50}) was determined. Results were expressed as mean ± SD compared to the negative control of untreated cells (100% proliferation) [82].

3.7.2. Cell Apoptosis and Cell Cycle Assay of HT-29 Cells

The TUNEL method was used to analyze the ability of the selected niosomal formulations to induce apoptosis in HT-29 cells. The following formulations: Oxaliplatin–TPGS niosomes, Paclitaxel–TPGS niosomes, and drug-free niosomes (F9) were tested; Oxaliplatin and Paclitaxel solutions were used as positive controls. Sigma plot software was used to obtain the best-fit straight line, and the cellular apoptosis was expressed in folds relative to control cells (the untreated cells). The cells were seeded in 6-well plates and were treated with IC_{50} values of all the tested treatments and incubated for 24 h [83]. Six independent experiments were conducted, and results were expressed as mean ± SD.

3.8. Statistical Analysis

All data were expressed as the mean of triplicate ± standard deviation (SD). The formulation design and evaluation were performed using the Design-Expert 13® Software, Version 13.2.03, 2021, Stat-Ease, USA. One-way ANOVA was applied to assess the formulation factors' effect on the selected niosomes formulations characters considering $p \leq 0.05$ statistically significant.

4. Conclusions

Different formulation variables could be optimized to obtain niosomal vesicles having a low particle size and an accepted Z-potential. Optimized niosomes prepared by the thin-film hydration method using TPGS surfactant in a molar ratio of 4 along with cholesterol in a molar ratio of 2 were loaded with either Oxaliplatin or Paclitaxel in different molar ratios, and those with a molar ratio of 1 resulted in the highest EE% values, 90.57 ± 2.05

and 93.51 ± 2.97, respectively. Delivering both drugs as vesicular niosomes helped in modifying their release rate compared to their free drugs, as they showed extended drug release, which could lead to a decrease in their toxicity. The encapsulation of Oxaliplatin and Paclitaxel into the niosomes particles markedly enhanced their cytotoxicity effect along with apoptosis efficiency up to two to three fold compared to their free drugs. Therefore, niosomes preparation using non-ionic surfactant with certain anti-colorectal cancer activity as TPGS could be considered a unique nanomicellar system for high encapsulating and delivering hydrophilic drug such as Oxaliplatin and hydrophobic drug such as Paclitaxel with improving their therapy outcomes against colorectal cancer, taking into consideration cost effect.

Supplementary Materials: The following supporting information can be downloaded at: https://www.mdpi.com/article/10.3390/ph15070816/s1.

Author Contributions: H.A.A.E.-E. Designed the experiments, collected, analyzed the data and drafted the manuscript (written and reviewing). S.W.E.-F. Fund acquisition and final draft revision. O.E.N. Final draft revision. R.A. Final draft revision and E.M.A. Collected and analyzed the data and drafted the manuscript (written and reviewing). All authors are contributed in the final manuscript revision. All authors have read and agreed to the published version of the manuscript.

Funding: This work was supported by the Deanship of Scientific Research, Taif University, Taif, Saudi Arabia, grant number 20215.

Institutional Review Board Statement: Not applicable.

Informed Consent Statement: Not applicable.

Data Availability Statement: Data is contained within the article and supplementary material.

Acknowledgments: The authors would also like to acknowledge the financial support offered by Taif University Deanship of Scientific Research for Supporting this Project under project number (20215), Taif University, Taif, Saudi Arabia.

Conflicts of Interest: The authors declare no conflict of interest.

References

1. Pacal, I.; Karaboga, D.; Basturk, A.; Akay, B.; Nalbantoglu, U. A comprehensive review of deep learning in colon cancer. *Comput. Biol. Med.* **2020**, *126*, 104003. [CrossRef] [PubMed]
2. Caan, B.J.; Meyerhardt, J.A.; Brown, J.C.; Campbell, K.L.; Feliciano, E.M.C.; Lee, C.; Ross, M.C.; Quinney, S.; Quesenberry, C.; Sternfeld, B. Recruitment strategies and design considerations in a trial of resistance training to prevent dose-limiting toxicities in colon cancer patients undergoing chemotherapy. *Contemp. Clin. Trials* **2020**, *101*, 106242. [CrossRef] [PubMed]
3. Narvekar, M.; Xue, H.Y.; Eoh, J.Y.; Wong, H.L. Nanocarrier for poorly water-soluble anticancer drugs—Barriers of translation and solutions. *Aaps Pharmscitech* **2014**, *15*, 822–833. [CrossRef] [PubMed]
4. Nukatsuka, M.; Nakagawa, F.; Takechi, T. Efficacy of combination chemotherapy using a novel oral chemotherapeutic agent, TAS-102, with oxaliplatin on human colorectal and gastric cancer xenografts. *Anticancer Res.* **2015**, *35*, 4605–4615. [PubMed]
5. Zoetemelk, M.; Ramzy, G.M.; Rausch, M.; Nowak-Sliwinska, P. Drug-drug interactions of irinotecan, 5-fluorouracil, folinic acid and oxaliplatin and its activity in colorectal carcinoma treatment. *Molecules* **2020**, *25*, 2614. [CrossRef]
6. Petrelli, F.; Coinu, A.; Ghilardi, M.; Cabiddu, M.; Zaniboni, A.; Barni, S. Efficacy of oxaliplatin-based chemotherapy+ bevacizumab as first-line treatment for advanced colorectal cancer. *Am. J. Clin. Oncol.* **2015**, *38*, 227–233. [CrossRef]
7. Ibrahim, A.; Hirschfeld, S.; Cohen, M.H.; Griebel, D.J.; Williams, G.A.; Pazdur, R. FDA drug approval summaries: Oxaliplatin. *Oncologist* **2004**, *9*, 8–12. [CrossRef]
8. Zhu, L.; Chen, L. Progress in research on paclitaxel and tumor immunotherapy. *Cell. Mol. Biol. Lett.* **2019**, *24*, 40. [CrossRef]
9. Semrad, T.J.; Fahrni, A.R.; Gong, I.Y.; Khatri, V.P. Integrating chemotherapy into the management of oligometastatic colorectal cancer: Evidence-based approach using clinical trial findings. *Ann. Surg. Oncol.* **2015**, *22*, 855–862. [CrossRef]
10. Ahmed, F.; Kumari, S.; Kondapi, A.K. Evaluation of antiproliferative activity, safety and biodistribution of oxaliplatin and 5-fluorouracil loaded lactoferrin nanoparticles for the management of colon adenocarcinoma: An in vitro and an in vivo study. *Pharm. Res.* **2018**, *35*, 178. [CrossRef]
11. Zhou, J.; Chang, L.; Guan, Y.; Yang, L.; Xia, X.; Cui, L.; Yi, X.; Lin, G. Application of circulating tumor DNA as a non-invasive tool for monitoring the progression of colorectal cancer. *PLoS ONE* **2016**, *11*, e0159708. [CrossRef] [PubMed]
12. Lv, C.; Qu, H.; Zhu, W.; Xu, K.; Xu, A.; Jia, B.; Qing, Y.; Li, H.; Wei, H.-J.; Zhao, H.-Y. Low-dose paclitaxel inhibits tumor cell growth by regulating glutaminolysis in colorectal carcinoma cells. *Front. Pharmacol.* **2017**, *8*, 244. [CrossRef] [PubMed]

13. Einzig, A.I.; Neuberg, D.; Wiernik, P.H.; Grochow, L.B.; Ramirez, G.; O'Dwyer, P.J.; Petrelli, N.J. Phase II trial of paclitaxel in patients with advanced colon cancer previously untreated with cytotoxic chemotherapy: An eastern cooperative oncology group trial (PA286). *Am. J. Ther.* **1996**, *3*, 750–754. [CrossRef]
14. Ye, J.; Jiang, X.; Dong, Z.; Hu, S.; Xiao, M. Low-concentration PTX And RSL3 inhibits tumor cell growth synergistically by inducing ferroptosis in mutant p53 hypopharyngeal squamous carcinoma. *Cancer Manag. Res.* **2019**, *11*, 9783. [CrossRef] [PubMed]
15. Shanmugam, T.; Joshi, N.; Ahamad, N.; Deshmukh, A.; Banerjee, R. Enhanced absorption, and efficacy of oral self-assembled paclitaxel nanocochleates in multi-drug resistant colon cancer. *Int. J. Pharm.* **2020**, *586*, 119482. [CrossRef] [PubMed]
16. Singla, A.K.; Garg, A.; Aggarwal, D. Paclitaxel and its formulations. *Int. J. Pharm.* **2002**, *235*, 179–192. [CrossRef]
17. Kang, L.; Gao, Z.; Huang, W.; Jin, M.; Wang, Q. Nanocarrier-mediated co-delivery of chemotherapeutic drugs and gene agents for cancer treatment. *Acta Pharm. Sin. B* **2015**, *5*, 169–175. [CrossRef]
18. Laraib, U.; Sargazi, S.; Rahdar, A.; Khatami, M.; Pandey, S. Nanotechnology-based approaches for effective detection of tumor markers: A comprehensive state-of-the-art review. *Int. J. Biol. Macromol.* **2021**, *195*, 356–383. [CrossRef]
19. ud Din, F.; Aman, W.; Ullah, I.; Qureshi, O.S.; Mustapha, O.; Shafique, S.; Zeb, A. Effective use of nanocarriers as drug delivery systems for the treatment of selected tumors. *Int. J. Nanomed.* **2017**, *12*, 7291. [CrossRef]
20. Dehaghi, M.H.; Haeri, A.; Keshvari, H.; Abbasian, Z.; Dadashzadeh, S. Dorzolamide loaded niosomal vesicles: Comparison of passive and remote loading methods. *Iran. J. Pharm. Res.* **2017**, *16*, 413.
21. Kulkarni, P.; Rawtani, D.; Barot, T. Formulation and optimization of long acting dual niosomes using box-Behnken experimental design method for combinative delivery of ethionamide and D-cycloserine in tuberculosis treatment. *Colloids Surf. A Physicochem. Eng. Asp.* **2019**, *565*, 131–142. [CrossRef]
22. Muzzalupo, R.; Tavano, L.; La Mesa, C. Alkyl glucopyranoside-based niosomes containing methotrexate for pharmaceutical applications: Evaluation of physico-chemical and biological properties. *Int. J. Pharm.* **2013**, *458*, 224–229. [CrossRef] [PubMed]
23. Kanaani, L. Effects of cisplatin-loaded niosomal nanoparticleson BT-20 human breast carcinoma cells. *Asian Pac. J. Cancer Prev.* **2017**, *18*, 365.
24. Barani, M.; Hajinezhad, M.R.; Sargazi, S.; Rahdar, A.; Shahraki, S.; Lohrasbi-Nejad, A.; Baino, F. In vitro and in vivo anticancer effect of pH-responsive paclitaxel-loaded niosomes. *J. Mater. Sci. Mater. Med.* **2021**, *32*, 147. [CrossRef]
25. Hao, Y.-M. Entrapment and release difference resulting from hydrogen bonding interactions in niosome. *Int. J. Pharm.* **2011**, *403*, 245–253. [CrossRef] [PubMed]
26. Pachuau, L.; Roy, P.K.; Zothantluanga, J.H.; Ray, S.; Das, S. Encapsulation of bioactive compound and its therapeutic potential. In *Bioactive Natural Products for Pharmaceutical Applications*; Springer: Berlin/Heidelberg, Germany, 2021; pp. 687–714.
27. Verma, A.; Tiwari, A.; Saraf, S.; Panda, P.K.; Jain, A.; Jain, S.K. Emerging potential of niosomes in ocular delivery. *Expert Opin. Drug Deliv.* **2020**, *18*, 55–71. [CrossRef]
28. Heidari, F.; Akbarzadeh, I.; Nourouzian, D.; Mirzaie, A.; Bakhshandeh, H. Optimization and characterization of tannic acid loaded niosomes for enhanced antibacterial and anti-biofilm activities. *Adv. Powder Technol.* **2020**, *31*, 4768–4781. [CrossRef]
29. Pourmoghadasiyan, B.; Tavakkoli, F.; Beram, F.M.; Badmasti, F.; Mirzaie, A.; Kazempour, R.; Rahimi, S.; Larijani, S.F.; Hejabi, F.; Sedaghatnia, K. Nanosized paclitaxel-loaded niosomes: Formulation, in vitro cytotoxicity, and apoptosis gene expression in breast cancer cell lines. *Mol. Biol. Rep.* **2022**, *49*, 3597–3608. [CrossRef]
30. Malla, S.; Neupane, R.; Boddu, S.H.; Abou-Dahech, M.S.; Pasternak, M.; Hussein, N.; Ashby, C.R., Jr.; Tang, Y.; Babu, R.J.; Tiwari, A.K. Application of nanocarriers for paclitaxel delivery and chemotherapy of cancer. In *Paclitaxel*; Elsevier: Amsterdam, The Netherlands, 2022; pp. 73–127.
31. Li, H.; Yan, L.; Tang, E.K.; Zhang, Z.; Chen, W.; Liu, G.; Mo, J. Synthesis of TPGS/curcumin nanoparticles by thin-film hydration and evaluation of their anti-colon cancer efficacy in vitro and in vivo. *Front. Pharmacol.* **2019**, *10*, 769. [CrossRef]
32. Weiszhár, Z.; Czúcz, J.; Révész, C.; Rosivall, L.; Szebeni, J.; Rozsnyay, Z. Complement activation by polyethoxylated pharmaceutical surfactants: Cremophor-EL, Tween-80 and Tween-20. *Eur. J. Pharm. Sci.* **2012**, *45*, 492–498. [CrossRef]
33. El-Menshawe, S.F.; Sayed, O.M.; Abou Taleb, H.A.; Saweris, M.A.; Zaher, D.M.; Omar, H.A. The use of new quinazolinone derivative and doxorubicin loaded solid lipid nanoparticles in reversing drug resistance in experimental cancer cell lines: A systematic study. *J. Drug Deliv. Sci. Technol.* **2020**, *56*, 101569. [CrossRef]
34. Tu, Y.S.; Sun, D.M.; Zhang, J.J.; Jiang, Z.Q.; Chen, Y.X.; Zeng, X.H.; Huang, D.E.; Yao, N. Preparation and characterisation of andrographolide niosomes and its anti-hepatocellular carcinoma activity. *J. Microencapsul.* **2014**, *31*, 307–316. [CrossRef] [PubMed]
35. Haley, B.; Frenkel, E. Nanoparticles for drug delivery in cancer treatment. *Urol. Oncol.* **2008**, *26*, 57–64. [CrossRef]
36. Tavano, L.; Vivacqua, M.; Carito, V.; Muzzalupo, R.; Caroleo, M.C.; Nicoletta, F. Doxorubicin loaded magneto-niosomes for targeted drug delivery. *Colloids Surf. B Biointerfaces* **2013**, *102*, 803–807. [CrossRef] [PubMed]
37. Ge, X.; Wei, M.; He, S.; Yuan, W.-E. Advances of non-ionic surfactant vesicles (niosomes) and their application in drug delivery. *Pharmaceutics* **2019**, *11*, 55. [CrossRef]
38. Ritwiset, A.; Krongsuk, S.; Johns, J.R. Molecular structure and dynamical properties of niosome bilayers with and without cholesterol incorporation: A molecular dynamics simulation study. *Appl. Surf. Sci.* **2016**, *380*, 23–31. [CrossRef]
39. Hinz, H.; Kuttenreich, H.; Meyer, R.; Renner, M.; Fründ, R.; Koynova, R.; Boyanov, A.; Tenchov, B. Stereochemistry and size of sugar head groups determine structure and phase behavior of glycolipid membranes: Densitometric, calorimetric, and X-ray studies. *Biochemistry* **1991**, *30*, 5125–5138. [CrossRef]

40. Liu, T.; Guo, R.; Hua, W.; Qiu, J. Structure behaviors of hemoglobin in PEG 6000/Tween 80/Span 80/H_2O niosome system. *Colloids Surf. A Physicochem. Eng. Asp.* **2007**, *293*, 255–261. [CrossRef]
41. Essa, E.A. Effect of formulation and processing variables on the particle size of sorbitan monopalmitate niosomes. *Asian J. Pharm.* **2010**, *4*, 227. [CrossRef]
42. Danaei, M.; Dehghankhold, M.; Ataei, S.; Hasanzadeh Davarani, F.; Javanmard, R.; Dokhani, A.; Khorasani, S.; Mozafari, M. Impact of particle size and polydispersity index on the clinical applications of lipidic nanocarrier systems. *Pharmaceutics* **2018**, *10*, 57. [CrossRef]
43. Teaima, M.H.; El Mohamady, A.M.; El-Nabarawi, M.A.; Mohamed, A.I. Formulation and evaluation of niosomal vesicles containing ondansetron HCL for trans-mucosal nasal drug delivery. *Drug Dev. Ind. Pharm.* **2020**, *46*, 751–761. [CrossRef] [PubMed]
44. Sahu, A.K.; Mishra, J.; Mishra, A.K. Introducing Tween-curcumin niosomes: Preparation, characterization and microenvironment study. *Soft Matter* **2020**, *16*, 1779–1791. [CrossRef] [PubMed]
45. Kamboj, S.; Saini, V.; Bala, S. Formulation and characterization of drug loaded nonionic surfactant vesicles (niosomes) for oral bioavailability enhancement. *Sci. World J.* **2014**, *2014*, 959741. [CrossRef] [PubMed]
46. Shah, P.; Goodyear, B.; Haq, A.; Puri, V.; Michniak-Kohn, B. Evaluations of quality by design (QbD) elements impact for developing niosomes as a promising topical drug delivery platform. *Pharmaceutics* **2020**, *12*, 246. [CrossRef]
47. Roy, A.; Pyne, A.; Pal, P.; Dhara, S.; Sarkar, N. Effect of Vitamin E and a long-chain alcohol n-octanol on the carbohydrate-based nonionic amphiphile sucrose monolaurate formulation of newly developed niosomes and application in cell imaging. *ACS Omega* **2017**, *2*, 7637–7646. [CrossRef]
48. Aziz, D.E.; Abdelbary, A.A.; Elassasy, A.I. Implementing central composite design for developing transdermal diacerein-loaded niosomes: Ex vivo permeation and in vivo deposition. *Curr. Drug Deliv.* **2018**, *15*, 1330–1342. [CrossRef]
49. Wang, C.; Cui, B.; Guo, L.; Wang, A.; Zhao, X.; Wang, Y.; Sun, C.; Zeng, Z.; Zhi, H.; Chen, H. Fabrication and evaluation of lambda-cyhalothrin nanosuspension by one-step melt emulsification technique. *Nanomaterials* **2019**, *9*, 145. [CrossRef]
50. De Silva, L.; Fu, J.-Y.; Htar, T.T.; Muniyandy, S.; Kasbollah, A.; Kamal, W.H.B.W.; Chuah, L.-H. Characterization, optimization, and in vitro evaluation of Technetium-99m-labeled niosomes. *Int. J. Nanomed.* **2019**, *14*, 1101. [CrossRef]
51. Alzubaidi, A.F.; El-Helw, A.-R.M.; Ahmed, T.A.; Ahmed, O.A. The use of experimental design in the optimization of risperidone biodegradable nanoparticles: In vitro and in vivo study. *Artif. Cells Nanomed. Biotechnol.* **2017**, *45*, 313–320. [CrossRef]
52. Mohamed, M.I.; Kassem, M.A.; Khalil, R.M.; Younis, M.; Danvish, A.; Salama, A.; Wagdi, M. Enhancement of the anti-inflammatory efficacy of betamethasone valerate via niosomal encapsulation. *Biointerface Res. Appl. Chem.* **2021**, *11*, 14640–14660.
53. Junyaprasert, V.B.; Teeranachaideekul, V.; Supaperm, T. Effect of charged and non-ionic membrane additives on physicochemical properties and stability of niosomes. *Aaps Pharmscitech* **2008**, *9*, 851–859. [CrossRef] [PubMed]
54. Owodeha-Ashaka, K.; Ilomuanya, M.O.; Iyire, A. Evaluation of sonication on stability-indicating properties of optimized pilocarpine hydrochloride-loaded niosomes in ocular drug delivery. *Prog. Biomater.* **2021**, *10*, 207–220. [CrossRef] [PubMed]
55. Fang, S.; Pei, Y. Stealth PEG-PHDCA niosomes: Effects of chain length of PEG and particle size on niosome surface properties, in vitro drug release, phagocytic uptake, in vivo pharmacokinetics and antitumor activity. *J. Pharm. Sci.* **2006**, *95*, 1873–1887.
56. Aboul-Einien, M.H.; Kandil, S.M.; Abdou, E.M.; Diab, H.M.; Zaki, M.S. Ascorbic acid derivative-loaded modified aspasomes: Formulation, in vitro, ex vivo and clinical evaluation for melasma treatment. *J. Liposome Res.* **2020**, *30*, 54–67. [CrossRef] [PubMed]
57. Arzani, G.; Haeri, A.; Daeihamed, M.; Bakhtiari-Kaboutaraki, H.; Dadashzadeh, S. Niosomal carriers enhance oral bioavailability of carvedilol: Effects of bile salt-enriched vesicles and carrier surface charge. *Int. J. Nanomed.* **2015**, *10*, 4797.
58. Devi, S.G.; Udupa, N. Niosomal sumartriptan succinate for nasal administration. *Indian J. Pharm. Sci.* **2000**, *62*, 479.
59. Tummala, S.; Gowthamarajan, K.; Satish Kumar, M.; Wadhwani, A. Oxaliplatin immuno hybrid nanoparticles for active targeting: An approach for enhanced apoptotic activity and drug delivery to colorectal tumors. *Drug Deliv.* **2016**, *23*, 1773–1787. [CrossRef]
60. Jadon, P.S.; Gajbhiye, V.; Jadon, R.S.; Gajbhiye, K.R.; Ganesh, N. Enhanced oral bioavailability of griseofulvin via niosomes. *Aaps Pharmscitech* **2009**, *10*, 1186–1192. [CrossRef]
61. Bayindir, Z.S.; Yuksel, N. Characterization of niosomes prepared with various nonionic surfactants for paclitaxel oral delivery. *J. Pharm. Sci.* **2010**, *99*, 2049–2060. [CrossRef]
62. Choi, J.U.; Maharjan, R.; Pangeni, R.; Jha, S.K.; Lee, N.K.; Kweon, S.; Lee, H.K.; Chang, K.-Y.; Choi, Y.K.; Park, J.W. Modulating tumor immunity by metronomic dosing of oxaliplatin incorporated in multiple oral nanoemulsion. *J. Control. Release* **2020**, *322*, 13–30. [CrossRef]
63. Gokhale, J.P.; Mahajan, H.S.; Surana, S.J. Quercetin loaded nanoemulsion-based gel for rheumatoid arthritis: In vivo and in vitro studies. *Biomed. Pharmacother.* **2019**, *112*, 108622. [CrossRef] [PubMed]
64. Zaki, N.M. Augmented cytotoxicity of hydroxycamptothecin-loaded nanoparticles in lung and colon cancer cells by chemosensitizing pharmaceutical excipients. *Drug Deliv.* **2014**, *21*, 265–275. [CrossRef] [PubMed]
65. Batrakova, E.V.; Kabanov, A.V. Pluronic block copolymers: Evolution of drug delivery concept from inert nanocarriers to biological response modifiers. *J. Control. Release* **2008**, *130*, 98–106. [CrossRef] [PubMed]
66. Ahmadi, F.; Derakhshandeh, K.; Jalalizadeh, A.; Mostafaie, A.; Hosseinzadeh, L. Encapsulation in PLGA-PEG enhances 9-nitro-camptothecin cytotoxicity to human ovarian carcinoma cell line through apoptosis pathway. *Res. Pharm. Sci.* **2015**, *10*, 161.

67. Yang, C.; Wu, T.; Qi, Y.; Zhang, Z. Recent advances in the application of vitamin E TPGS for drug delivery. *Theranostics* **2018**, *8*, 464. [CrossRef]
68. Fan, Z.; Jiang, B.; Shi, D.; Yang, L.; Yin, W.; Zheng, K.; Zhang, X.; Xin, C.; Su, G.; Hou, Z. Selective antitumor activity of drug-free TPGS nanomicelles with ROS-induced mitochondrial cell death. *Int. J. Pharm.* **2021**, *594*, 120184. [CrossRef]
69. Dong, J.; Qin, Z.; Zhang, W.-D.; Cheng, G.; Yehuda, A.G.; Ashby, C.R., Jr.; Chen, Z.-S.; Cheng, X.-D.; Qin, J.-J. Medicinal chemistry strategies to discover P-glycoprotein inhibitors: An update. *Drug Resist. Updates* **2020**, *49*, 100681. [CrossRef]
70. Zografi, G.; Schott, H.; Swarbrick, J. Interfacial phenomena. In *Remington: The Science and Practice Pharmacy*; Mark Publishing: Easton, PA, USA, 1995.
71. Zhang, S.; Morris, M.E. Efflux transporters in drug excretion. In *Drug Delivery: Principles and Applications*; Wiley: Hoboken, NJ, USA, 2005; pp. 381–398.
72. Biswas, S.; Torchilin, V.P. Nanopreparations for organelle-specific delivery in cancer. *Adv. Drug Deliv. Rev.* **2014**, *66*, 26–41. [CrossRef]
73. Demirbolat, G.M.; Altintas, L.; Yilmaz, S.; Degim, I.T. Development of orally applicable, combinatorial drug–loaded nanoparticles for the treatment of fibrosarcoma. *J. Pharm. Sci.* **2018**, *107*, 1398–1407. [CrossRef]
74. Mahale, N.B.; Thakkar, P.D.; Mali, R.G.; Walunj, D.R.; Chaudhari, S.R. Niosomes: Novel sustained release nonionic stable vesicular systems—An overview. *Adv. Colloid Interface Sci.* **2012**, *183–184*, 46–54. [CrossRef]
75. Jabalera, Y.; Garcia-Pinel, B.; Ortiz, R.; Iglesias, G.; Cabeza, L.; Prados, J.; Jimenez-Lopez, C.; Melguizo, C. Oxaliplatin–biomimetic magnetic nanoparticle assemblies for colon cancer-targeted chemotherapy: An in vitro study. *Pharmaceutics* **2019**, *11*, 395. [CrossRef] [PubMed]
76. Zhen, Y.; Ewert, K.K.; Fisher, W.S.; Steffes, V.M.; Li, Y.; Safinya, C.R. Paclitaxel loading in cationic liposome vectors is enhanced by replacement of oleoyl with linoleoyl tails with distinct lipid shapes. *Sci. Rep.* **2021**, *11*, 7311. [CrossRef] [PubMed]
77. Durak, S.; Esmaeili Rad, M.; Alp Yetisgin, A.; Eda Sutova, H.; Kutlu, O.; Cetinel, S.; Zarrabi, A. Niosomal drug delivery systems for ocular disease—Recent advances and future prospects. *Nanomaterials* **2020**, *10*, 1191. [CrossRef] [PubMed]
78. Tavano, L.; Muzzalupo, R.; Mauro, L.; Pellegrino, M.; Andò, S.; Picci, N. Transferrin-conjugated pluronic niosomes as a new drug delivery system for anticancer therapy. *Langmuir* **2013**, *29*, 12638–12646. [CrossRef]
79. Tavano, L.; Muzzalupo, R.; Trombino, S.; Cassano, R.; Pingitore, A.; Picci, N. Effect of formulations variables on the in vitro percutaneous permeation of Sodium Diclofenac from new vesicular systems obtained from Pluronic triblock copolymers. *Colloids Surf. B Biointerfaces* **2010**, *79*, 227–234. [CrossRef]
80. Waddad, A.Y.; Abbad, S.; Yu, F.; Munyendo, W.L.L.; Wang, J.; Lv, H.; Zhou, J. Formulation, characterization and pharmacokinetics of Morin hydrate niosomes prepared from various non-ionic surfactants. *Int. J. Pharm.* **2013**, *456*, 446–458. [CrossRef]
81. Mircioiu, C.; Voicu, V.; Anuta, V.; Tudose, A.; Celia, C.; Paolino, D.; Fresta, M.; Sandulovici, R.; Mircioiu, I. Mathematical modeling of release kinetics from supramolecular drug delivery systems. *Pharmaceutics* **2019**, *11*, 140. [CrossRef]
82. Galaup, A.; Opolon, P.; Bouquet, C.; Li, H.; Opolon, D.; Bissery, M.-C.; Tursz, T.; Perricaudet, M.; Griscelli, F. Combined effects of docetaxel and angiostatin gene therapy in prostate tumor model. *Mol. Ther.* **2003**, *7*, 731–740. [CrossRef]
83. Ren, Y.; Li, X.; Han, B.; Zhao, N.; Mu, M.; Wang, C.; Du, Y.; Wang, Y.; Tong, A.; Liu, Y. Improved anti-colorectal carcinomatosis effect of tannic acid co-loaded with oxaliplatin in nanoparticles encapsulated in thermosensitive hydrogel. *Eur. J. Pharm. Sci.* **2019**, *128*, 279–289. [CrossRef]

pharmaceuticals

MDPI

Article

Central Composite Optimization of Glycerosomes for the Enhanced Oral Bioavailability and Brain Delivery of Quetiapine Fumarate

Randa Mohammed Zaki [1,2,*], Munerah M. Alfadhel [1], Manal A. Alossaimi [3], Lara Ayman Elsawaf [3], Vidya Devanathadesikan Seshadri [4], Alanood S. Almurshedi [5], Rehab Mohammad Yusif [6,7] and Mayada Said [8]

1 Department of Pharmaceutics, College of Pharmacy, Prince Sattam Bin Abdulaziz University, P.O. Box 173, Al-Kharj 11942, Saudi Arabia; m.alfadhel@psau.edu.sa
2 Department of Pharmaceutics and Industrial Pharmacy, Faculty of Pharmacy, Beni-Suef University, Beni-Suef P.O. Box 62514, Egypt
3 Department of Pharmaceutical Chemistry, College of Pharmacy, Prince Sattam Bin Abdulaziz University, P.O. Box 173, Al-Kharj 11942, Saudi Arabia; m.alossaimi@psau.edu.sa (M.A.A.); lolahappy71@yahoo.com (L.A.E.)
4 Department of Pharmacology and Toxicology, College of Pharmacy, Prince Sattam Bin Abdulaziz University, P.O. Box 173, Al-Kharj 11942, Saudi Arabia; v.adri@psau.edu.sa
5 Department of Pharmaceutics, College of Pharmacy, King Saud University, P.O. Box 2457, Riyadh 11451, Saudi Arabia; marshady@ksu.edu.sa
6 Department of Pharmaceutics, Faculty of Pharmacy, Mansoura University, Mansoura P.O. Box 35516, Egypt; rehabyusif@yahoo.com
7 Department of Pharmaceutics and Pharmaceutical Technology, College of Pharmacy, Taibah University, P.O. Box 30039, Al-Madinah Al-Munawarah 41477, Saudi Arabia
8 Department of Pharmaceutics and Industrial Pharmacy, Faculty of Pharmacy, Cairo University, Cairo P.O. Box 11562, Egypt; mayada.mohamed@pharma.cu.edu.sa
* Correspondence: r.abdelrahman@psau.edu.sa; Tel.: +20-11-51093936

Citation: Zaki, R.M.; Alfadhel, M.M.; Alossaimi, M.A.; Elsawaf, L.A.; Devanathadesikan Seshadri, V.; Almurshedi, A.S.; Yusif, R.M.; Said, M. Central Composite Optimization of Glycerosomes for the Enhanced Oral Bioavailability and Brain Delivery of Quetiapine Fumarate. *Pharmaceuticals* **2022**, *15*, 940. https://doi.org/10.3390/ph15080940

Academic Editors: Ana Catarina Silva, João Nuno Moreira and José Manuel Sousa Lobo

Received: 7 June 2022
Accepted: 19 July 2022
Published: 29 July 2022

Abstract: This study aimed to formulate and statistically optimize glycerosomal formulations of Quetiapine fumarate (QTF) to increase its oral bioavailability and enhance its brain delivery. The study was designed using a Central composite rotatable design using Design-Expert® software. The independent variables in the study were glycerol % w/v and cholesterol % w/v, while the dependent variables were vesicle size (VS), zeta potential (ZP), and entrapment efficiency percent (EE%). The numerical optimization process resulted in an optimum formula composed of 29.645 (w/v%) glycerol, 0.8 (w/v%) cholesterol, and 5 (w/v%) lecithin. It showed a vesicle size of 290.4 nm, zeta potential of −34.58, and entrapment efficiency of 80.85%. The optimum formula was further characterized for DSC, XRD, TEM, in-vitro release, the effect of aging, and pharmacokinetic study. DSC thermogram confirmed the compatibility of the drug with the ingredients. XRD revealed the encapsulation of the drug in the glycerosomal nanovesicles. TEM image revealed spherical vesicles with no aggregates. Additionally, it showed enhanced drug release when compared to a drug suspension and also exhibited good stability for one month. Moreover, it showed higher brain C_{max}, AUC_{0-24}, and $AUC_{0-\infty}$ and plasma AUC_{0-24} and $AUC_{0-\infty}$ in comparison to drug suspension. It showed brain and plasma bioavailability enhancement of 153.15 and 179.85%, respectively, compared to the drug suspension. So, the optimum glycerosomal formula may be regarded as a promising carrier to enhance the oral bioavailability and brain delivery of Quetiapine fumarate.

Keywords: schizophrenia; quetiapine fumarate; glycerosomes; central composite rotatable design; bioavailability; pharmacokinetic

1. Introduction

Schizophrenia is a chronic and severe mental disorder, defined by positive (hallucinations and delusions), negative (disruption of normal behavior and emotion), and cognitive (difficulties in memory and attention) symptoms [1]. Symptoms of schizophrenia start in adulthood and continue throughout life [2]. These symptoms can be managed by an antipsychotic drug, especially atypical antipsychotic drugs [2]. Among atypical antipsychotic drugs Quetiapine fumarate (QTF), QTF, is a second-generation atypical antipsychotic drug that has broader efficiency than traditional antipsychotics and many other atypical antipsychotic drugs [3]. It is a dibenzothiazepine derivative [2]. It is effective against positive and negative symptoms of schizophrenia with good neurocognition properties [4,5]. The exact mechanism of action of QTF is unknown, but it is thought to block nerve receptors for many neurotransmitters, restricting communications between nerves. This action could be done by combining dopamine type 2 and serotonin type 2 (5HT2) receptor antagonism. QTF also has an antidepressant activity which could be due to the effect of its metabolite N-desalkyl quetiapine fumarate on selective norepinephrine reuptake inhibition and 5-HT1A and 5-HT7 receptor activity [6]. Many clinical trials showed that QTF has an acceptable safety profile [7]. It was approved for first-line treatment of schizophrenia [8]. It also showed effectiveness in bipolar mania [9].

The oral route is the most common route for drug delivery, but many factors may affect drug absorption and bioavailability, like pH of the GIT, drug solubility, residence time, and hepatic first-pass metabolism [10]. QTF has an oral bioavailability of 9%, which is related to its high hepatic metabolism resulting in reduced brain concentration [11]. QTF suffers from low water solubility, especially at higher pH, and as a result, reduced absorption is anticipated at higher pH [12]. QTF has a plasma half-life of 6 h, and as a result, it needs frequent dosing to maintain effective therapeutic concentration [12]. Schizophrenia treatment via the oral route is very challenging due to the presence of a protective blood-brain barrier (BBB), complex tight junctions that make sealing for the paracellular pathway, and P-glycoprotein, which reduces the amount delivered of many drugs into the brain. QTF is a P-glycoprotein substrate that suffers from reduced brain concentration following oral administration [13]. Therefore, the incorporation of QTF in lipid-based nanoformulations like glycerosomes may overcome the overmentioned limitations. GLSMs could protect the encapsulated drug from degradation in the GIT [14]. They also can target the lymphatic system owing to their lipid nature [15,16]. Many drugs could be orally delivered through the lymphatic system, which avoids hepatic first-pass metabolism [17,18]. It was reported that lipid-containing nanoparticles could enhance the uptake of drugs into the lymphatic circulation, which could be related to their small size and lipid nature [14].

Nanoformulations have many advantages for brain delivery like their flexibility [19], increased solubility of drugs [20], the release of the drug in a controlled manner [21], crossing and overcoming the BBB, and targeting the drugs into the brain [19], which is desired for drugs treating mental illness like schizophrenia [22]. This results in increasing the concentrations of drugs in the brain tissues and cells with the consequence of increasing their bioavailability [22].

Glycerosomes (GLSMs) are a new generation of liposomes containing phospholipids, water, and varying concentrations of glycerol (10–30 *w*/*v*%) [23]. Glycerol is non-toxic, harmless, and non-irritating and so is safely used. GLSMs can encapsulate both hydrophilic and hydrophobic drugs [24]. They differ from liposomes by being more stable and having greater fluidity than liposomes [23]. The increased fluidity of GLSMs is related to the presence of glycerol in high percent, which makes modifications to the bilayer membrane [25]. This increased fluidity can aid in better penetration into the brain tissue. GLSMs may contain cholesterol which increases the stability of the bilayer [25]. GLSMs are prepared by the same common techniques used for liposome preparations [23,26].

Our work aimed to develop QTF glycerosomes to enhance the oral bioavailability and brain delivery of QTF.

2. Results and Discussion

2.1. Evaluation of QTF Glycerosomal Formulations

2.1.1. Measurement of Vesicle Size VS, PDI, and ZP

The VS of various glycerosomal formulations varied between 110.23 to 321.51 nm, as evident in Table 1. The smaller the particle, the larger the surface area available for drug absorption and penetration into the brain [27]. The effects of Glycerol concentration (X1) and cholesterol concentration (X2) on VS are shown in Figures 1A and 2A.

The linear model was the most suitable one to be fitted to VS data (p-value = 0.0041) with a small difference between the adjusted and predicted R^2 (less than 0.2), which ensures the validity of the model [28] and high adequate precision of 9.66 (greater than 4); this indicated that the model was able to navigate the design space as shown in Table 2 [29].

Table 1. Composition of Different Coded formulations with their responses in Central Composite Design for optimization of QTF loaded GLSMs.

Formula Code	Independent Variables		Dependent Variables			
	Glycerol conc (*w*/*v*%) (X1)	Cholesterol conc (*w*/*v*%) (X2)	VS (nm) (Y1)	PDI	ZP (mV) (Y2)	EE% (Y3)
G1	5.86	0.5	110.23 ± 6.48	0.248 ± 0.067	−20.3 ± 0.92	28.31 ± 1.74
G2	10	0.2	130.25 ± 7.47	0.268 ± 0.142	−21.8 ± 1.73	43.21 ± 3.62
G3	10	0.8	161.55 ± 10.72	0.174 ± 0.054	−27.35 ± 2.61	54.42 ± 2.18
G4	20	0.08	115.42 ± 5.43	0.125 ± 0.021	−19.1 ± 1.23	32.3 ± 1.26
G5	20	0.5	238.02 ± 4.73	0.402 ± 0.023	−30.4 ± 2.42	66.2 ± 2.81
G6	20	0.92	283.56 ± 11.23	0.281 ± 0.126	−34.4 ± 1.89	73.2 ± 1.34
G7	30	0.2	232.30 ± 7.82	0.265 ± 0.134	−31.4 ± 2.26	65.79 ± 2.64
G8	30	0.8	321.51 ± 4.73	0.345 ± 0.084	−37.7 ± 1.82	78.08 ± 3.21
G9	34.14	0.5	228.42 ± 6.29	0.352 ± 0.078	−29.1 ± 2.35	64.3 ± 4.32

VS: vesicle size, ZP: zeta potential, PDI: polydispersity index, EE%: entrapment efficiency percent, Data represented as mean ± SD (n = 3).

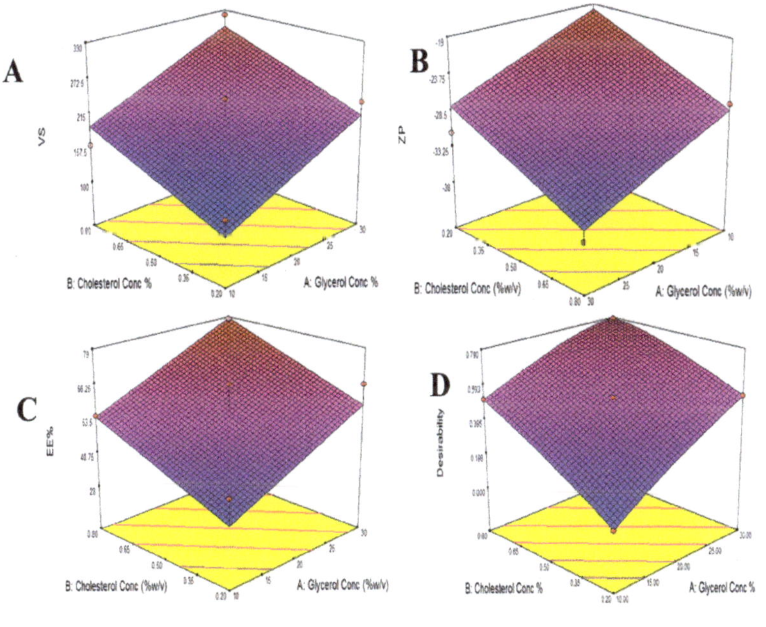

Figure 1. Response surface plot for the effect of Glycerol concentration and Cholesterol concentration on VS (**A**), ZP (**B**), EE% (**C**), and Desirability (**D**).

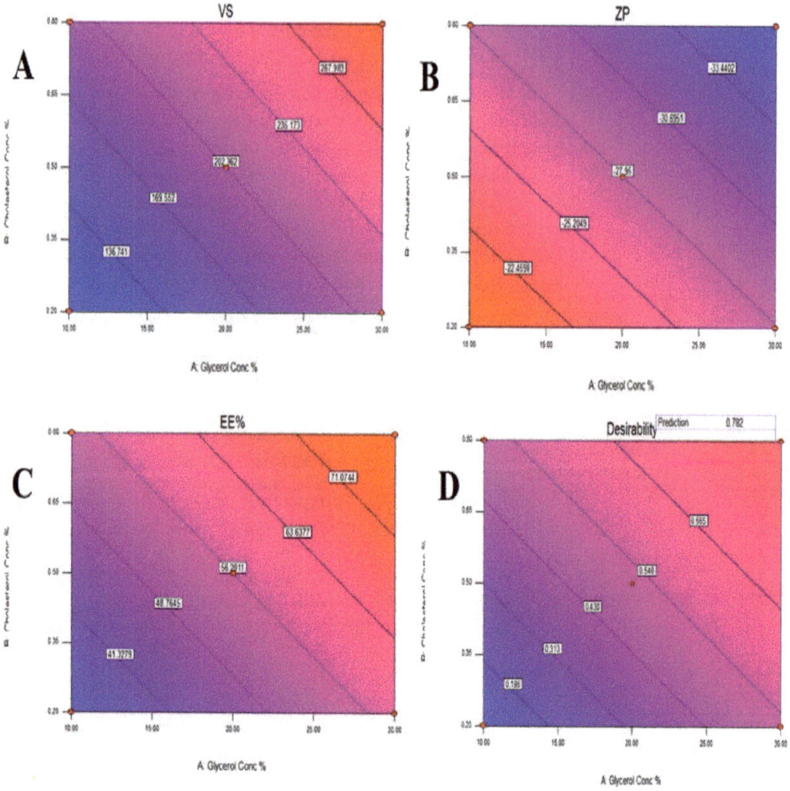

Figure 2. Contour plot for the effect of Glycerol concentration and Cholesterol concentration on Vesicles size (**A**), Zeta potential (**B**), Entrapment efficiency% (**C**), and Desirability (**D**).

Table 2. Output data of Central Composite Design of QTF loaded GLSMs.

Dependent Variables	R^2	Adjusted R^2	Predicted R^2	Adequate Precision
Y1: VS (nm)	0.8393	0.7858	0.6387	9.6576
Y2: ZP (mV)	0.8245	0.7660	0.5859	9.1957
Y3: EE %	0.7880	0.7174	0.5272	8.1482

VS: vesicle size, ZP: zeta potential, EE%: entrapment efficiency percent.

The effect of the studied factors on VS could be studied using the following equation:

$$VS = 202.36 + 53.64\ X1 + 44.79\ X2 \quad (1)$$

It was evident from ANOVA analysis, as represented in Table 3, that both Glycerol concentration (X1) and cholesterol concentration (X2) significantly affected VS values with (p-values = 0.0051 and 0.0115, respectively), where the increase in both glycerol and cholesterol concentrations led to a significant increase in VS as revealed by the positive sign of their coefficients in the correlation equation. However, as per Equation (1), the high regression coefficient of Glycerol concentration (X1) indicated a higher impact than cholesterol concentration (X2) on VS.

Table 3. ANOVA for Central Composite Design of QTF loaded GLSMs.

Dependent Variable	Source	SS	Df	Mean Square	F Value	*p*-Value
Y1	Model	39,069.40	2	19,534.70	15.67	0.0041
	X1	23,020.78	1	23,020.78	18.47	0.0051
	X2	16,048.63	1	16,048.63	12.87	0.0115
Y2	Model	271.36	2	135.68	14.10	0.0054
	X1	131.18	1	131.18	13.63	0.0102
	X2	140.18	1	140.18	14.56	0.0088
Y3	Model	2006.51	2	1003.26	11.15	0.0095
	X1	1179.46	1	1179.46	13.11	0.0111
	X2	827.05	1	827.05	9.19	0.0230

Y1: VS (nm), Y2: ZP (mV), Y3: EE%, X1: Glycerol concentration (*w*/*v*%), X2: Cholesterol concentration (*w*/*v*%), SS: sum of squares, df: degree of freedom.

The increase in VS with the increase in glycerol concentration could be explained by the sticky nature of glycerol. It increased the viscosity of the dispersion, which made it difficult for size reduction during sonication. Moreover, it loosens the packing of the glycerosomal lipid bilayer membrane, which results in decreased curvature of the bilayer, and as a result, bigger vesicles are formed [23,26].

Moreover, it was noted that at lower concentrations of cholesterol, the order of the lipid bilayer chain is increased, which resulted in close packing and, as a result, the size decreased. However, due to its hydrophobic nature, increasing its concentration led to increased hydrophobicity of the bilayer and disturbance of the lipid membrane of GLSMs and, as a result, increased vesicle size in an attempt to reach thermodynamic stability. In addition, cholesterol increased the rigidity of the GLSMs membrane, which resulted in resistance to size reduction during the sonication step [30]. This explained the positive impact of cholesterol on vesicle size.

PDI points out the magnitude of the size diversity and is expressed by values between 0 and 1 [29]. As shown in Table 1, the PDI values of the prepared glycerosomal formulations lay between 0.13 and 0.40; this could indicate that the size distribution was within the acceptable limits for the prepared glycerosomal dispersions [29].

ZP indicates the physical stability of the glycerosomal formulations. The larger the value of the ZP, The larger the repulsion forces between vesicles, which resulted in reduced aggregation and increased stability of the system [31].

As shown in Table 1, The ZP of different glycerosomal formulations ranged from −19.1 to −37.7 mV. This could point out that the prepared glycerosomal formulations were physically stable [29]. The effects of Glycerol concentration (X1) and cholesterol concentration (X2) on ZP are illustrated in Figures 1B and 2B.

The data of ZP were fitted to a linear model (p-values < 0.0058) with an adequate high precision (9.1957) and a difference between the adjusted and predicted R^2 of less than 0.2. The following equation could relate the effect of the studied factors on ZP:

$$ZP = 27.95 + 4.05\ X1 + 4.19\ X2 \quad (2)$$

It was shown from the ANOVA analysis in Table 3 that both glycerol (X1) and cholesterol (X2) concentrations significantly affected ZP (p-values = 0.0109 and 0.0094, respectively). Both X1 and X2 significantly increased the ZP absolute values and this was confirmed by their positive regression coefficients as per Equation (2). However, cholesterol concentration (X2) showed a higher impact on ZP values than glycerol concentration (X1) due to its higher regression coefficient value as in Equation (2).

Increasing ZP absolute values with increasing glycerol concentration could be related to its interaction with polar heads of the phospholipids in the lipid bilayer which resulted in a change in the orientation of molecules and affected the total surface charge of the vesicles [32]. Furthermore, The rise in the ZP absolute values with the increase in cholesterol concentration could be due to its ability to modify the surface charge of the vesicles preventing vesicle aggregation and increasing their stability [24,33].

2.1.2. Measurement of EE%

The EE% of various glycerosomal formulations varied between 28.3 to 78.1%, as shown in Table 1, confirming successful encapsulation for the drug in the GLSMs so that glycerol-containing nanovesicles can be utilized as a successful delivery system for QTF. The effects of glycerol concentration (X1) and cholesterol concentration (X2) on EE% are represented in Figures 1C and 2C.

The EE% data were best analyzed using a linear model (p-values < 0.0095) where the adequate precision is high (8.1482). In addition, a less than 0.2 difference between the adjusted and predicted R^2 was found. The following equation could make a relationship between the studied factors on EE%:

$$EE\% = 56.2 + 12.14\ X1 + 10.17\ X2 \quad (3)$$

It was evident from the ANOVA analysis that both glycerol and cholesterol concentrations significantly affected the EE% (p-values = 0.0111 and 0.0230, respectively), where both had positive impacts on the EE% values. However, Glycerol concentration (X1) showed a higher impact than cholesterol concentration (X2) on EE% due to its higher regression coefficient as per Equation (3).

The increase in EE% with the increase in Cholesterol concentration could be referred to as the lipophilic nature of the drug, which increased its integration in the lipid phase containing lipophilic cholesterol [26]. Additionally, Cholesterol increases the rigidity of the lipid bilayer membrane, controls permeability, and enhances vesicle stability [26]. So, increasing cholesterol concentrations reduced the leakage of the entrapped drug, consequently enhancing the EE%.

Output data of Central Composite Design of QTF loaded GLSMs is shown in Table 2. ANOVA for Central Composite Design of QTF loaded GLSMs is shown in Table 3.

2.2. Statistical Analysis, Optimization, and Validation

Design Expert® software was used to perform A numeric analysis to make a selection of an optimum glycerosomal formulation, where VS was minimized while ZP and EE% were maximized. This optimization process showed an optimum glycerosomal formulation with a desirability of 0.781 (Figures 1D and 2D). It was composed of 29.645 (w/v%) glycerol, 0.799 (w/v%) cholesterol and 5 (w/v%) lecithin. The predicted values of VS, ZP, and EE% were 298.882 nm, −35.997 mV, and 78.079%, respectively, as shown in Figure 3. The optimum formula was then prepared, followed by its validation as demonstrated in Table 4 with a % relative error of less than 5% from the predicted values shown by the design expert software, indicating the fitness of the model [34].

Table 4. Validation of the optimum formula.

	VS (nm)	ZP (mV)	EE%
Predicted value	298.88	−35.997	78.08
Experimental value	290.4	−34.58	80.85
% Relative error	2.84	3.94	3.55

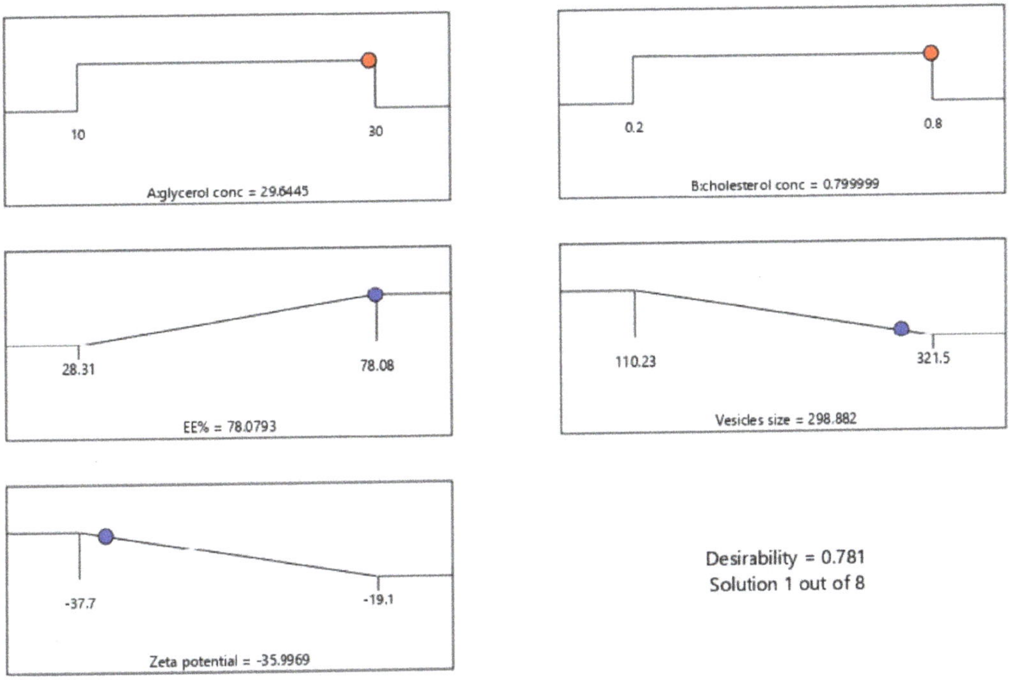

Figure 3. The composition of the optimized formula and its predicted responses according to Central Composite Design.

2.3. *Evaluation of the Optimum QTP Formula*

2.3.1. Differential Scanning Calorimetry (DSC)

DSC thermograms of pure QTF, a physical mixture of lecithin, cholesterol, and QTF, and the optimum glycerosomal formula are shown in Figure 4. Pure QTP showed a sharp endothermic peak at 182.95 °C, indicating its melting point in crystal form (Figure 4A) [35]. The drug's endothermic peak was well preserved in its physical mixture with lecithin and cholesterol (Figure 4B) with changes in the form of shifting of the temperature of the melt or broadening. It is familiar that the quantity of materials used, particularly in drug excipient mixtures, may affect the peak shape and enthalpy. So, these small changes in the melting endotherm of the drug may be resulted from mixing the drug with the excipients, which reduced the purity of each component in the mixture and this may not necessarily refer to potential incompatibility [10,36,37]. Therefore, it could be concluded that QTF is compatible with excipients used in the formulation. In addition, the optimum glycerosomal formula (Figure 4C) showed a broad endothermic peak with a decrease in the intensity, indicating encapsulation for the drug and its conversion into an amorphous form. Besides, changes in the drug crystallinity may lead to shifts in the melting point [38].

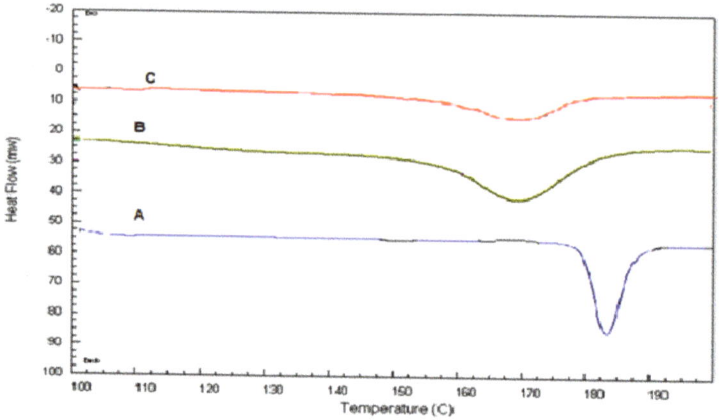

Figure 4. DSC thermograms of A: Pure QTF, B: lecithin, cholesterol, and QTF physical mixture, C: the optimized formula.

2.3.2. X-ray Diffraction Study (XRD)

XRD spectra of pure QTF and the optimum formula were illustrated in (Figure 5). The XRD of pure QTF showed sharp peaks at 2θ scattered angles of 16°, 20°, 21°, 22°, and 23° indicating its crystalline nature (Figure 5A). However, a decrease in the intensity of some drug peaks and disappearance of others was noted in the XRD spectrum of the optimized formula (Figure 5B), probably due to the encapsulation of the drug within GLSMs nanovesicles. These results support the prediscussed DSC results [39].

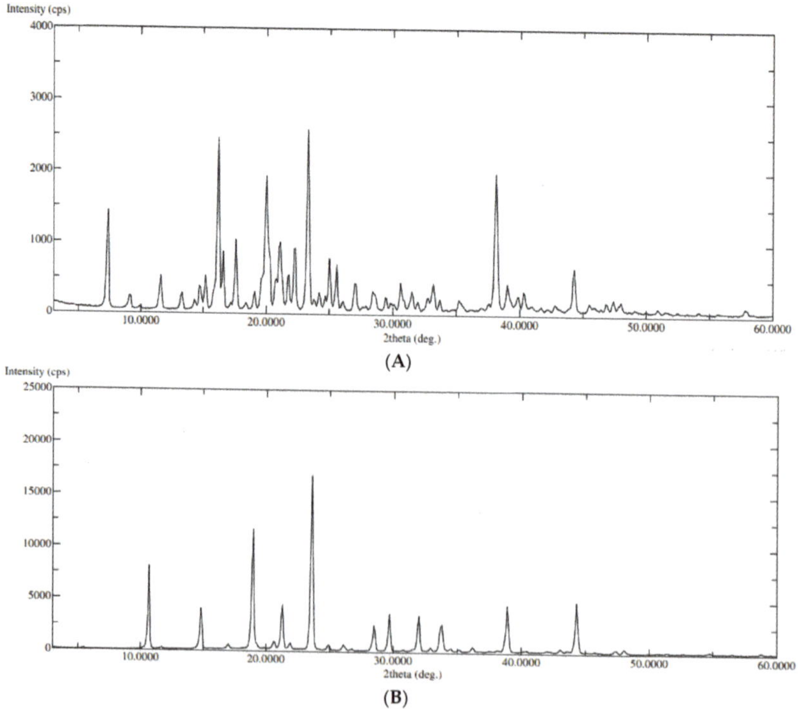

Figure 5. XRD of (**A**): pure QTF, (**B**): the optimized formula.

2.3.3. Transmission Electron Microscopy (TEM)

TEM image showed small spherical vesicles, as shown in Figure 6. There were no aggregates that indicated good physical stability of the dispersion and could be related to the high ZP on the surfaces of the vesicles, which induces repulsion between the adjacent GLSMs [29,40–42]. Moreover, GLSMs showed an average dimension of 272.83 ± 36.21 nm.

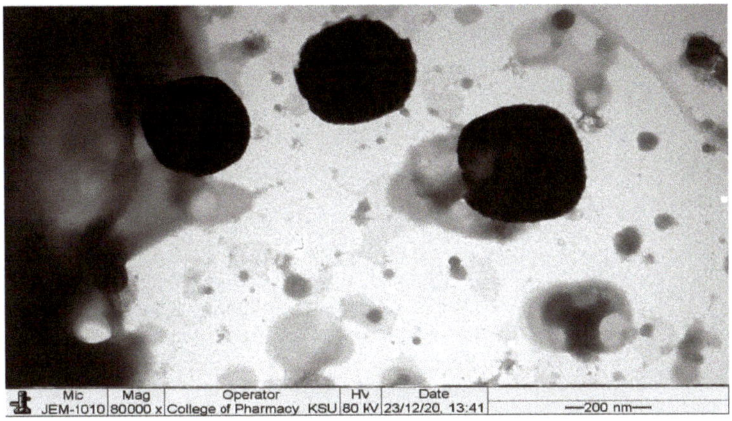

Figure 6. TEM image of the optimized formula.

2.3.4. In-Vitro Release

Figure 7 shows the release profile of the optimum GLSM formula in comparison to QTF suspension. The optimum formula showed enhanced QTF release in comparison to the drug suspension. This could be related to the amphiphilic properties of phosphatidylcholine used in glycersomes formation [26,43]. Moreover, the reduction in vesicle size of the glycerosomal formulation may increase the drug release. Vesicle size affects drug release from GLSMs, where a higher release rate was obtained by smaller vesicles than larger sized ones [26,44]. Our results comply with the results obtained by Salem et al., who showed a significant enhancement of the release of drugs from GLSMs in comparison to drug suspension [26].

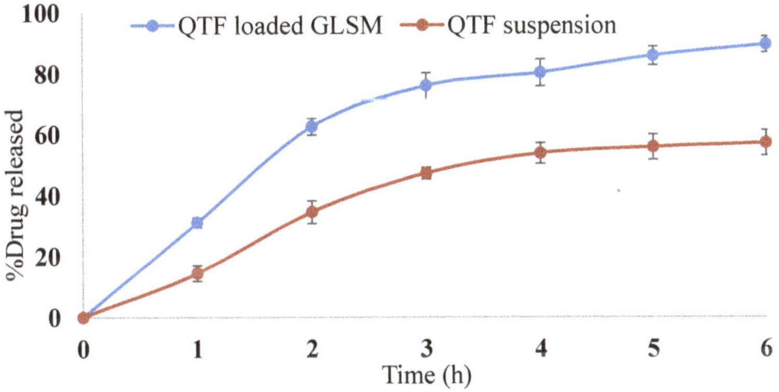

Figure 7. In vitro release profile of QTF from QTF loaded GLSMs and QTF suspension.

2.3.5. Effect of Aging

Table 5 demonstrates the effect of storage for one month on the stability of the optimum glycerosomal formula. There were no significant changes in VS, ZP, and EE% at all-time points (7 and 30 days), which indicates good stability of the optimum GLSM formula during storage for one month at 4 °C. The slight decrease in EE% may be due to the presence of glycerol which enhances the flexibility and loosen the packing of the glycerosomal lipid bilayer, which results in leakage of drug from GLSMs. However, there was a slight increase in vesicle size, which may be attributed to the hydrophilic nature of glycerol, so an increase in the water uptake of the vesicle bilayers thus increases vesicle size.

Table 5. The effect of storage at 4 °C for one month on VS, ZP, and EE% of the optimized formula.

Responses	Fresh	After 7 Days	After 30 Days
VS (nm)	290.41 ± 10.43	292.93 ± 13.43	300.34 ± 12.38
ZP (mV)	−34.58 ± 2.13	−34.24 ± 1.88	−33.67 ± 1.65
EE%	81.23 ± 2.43	80.85 ± 3.98	79.46 ± 3.01

2.4. *In-Vivo Bioavailability of the Optimized QTP Glycerosomal Formula*

The mean QTF concentrations in rat brains and plasma upon administration of the optimum GLSM formula and aqueous drug suspension are shown in Figure 8. The optimum GLSM formula showed a significantly higher brain C_{max}, $AUC_{0–24}$, and $AUC_{0–\infty}$ in comparison to QTF suspension with p-values of 0.0477, 0.003, and 0.003, respectively, as pointed out in Table 6. It also showed a significantly higher plasma $AUC_{0–24}$ and $AUC_{0–\infty}$ in comparison to QTF suspension with p-values of 0.004 and 0.049, respectively, as shown in Table 6. The optimum GLSM formula showed brain and plasma bioavailability enhancement of 153.15 and 179.85%, respectively, compared to the drug suspension [29]. These obtained findings could indicate the ability of the optimum GLSM formula to enhance the oral bioavailability and brain delivery of QTF in comparison to a drug suspension, which could be related to the lipophilic nature of the formula, which reduced first-pass metabolism [45,46]. In addition to the enhanced solubility of QTF within the formula, the small vesicle size of the optimum GLSM formula and increased fluidity of the GLSM lipid bilayer membrane due to the presence of glycerol which led to better penetration into the brain tissue. It was also reported that polar lipids such as phospholipids are associated with proteins in the structural membranes due to the structural similarity with biomembranes, which resulted in facilitating drug transport across BBB [11,47].

Table 6. Pharmacokinetic Parameters of QTF in the brain after oral administration of QTF suspension and QTF Loaded GLSMs.

Pharmacokinetic Parameters	Brain Data		Plasma Data	
	QTF Suspension	QTF Loaded GLSMs	QTF Suspension	QTF Loaded GLSMs
$t_{1/2}$ (h)	13.009 ± 2.59	12.835 ± 5.88	31.291 ± 3.783	47.859 ± 17.880
T_{max} (h)	4.000 ± 0.00	4.666 ± 1.15	2.666 ± 0.577	3.333 ± 0.577
C_{max} (μg/mL)	33.393 ± 4.33	49.806 ± 11.69	8.933 ± 2.656	14.953 ± 8.304
$AUC_{0–24}$ (μg.h/mL)	318.126 ± 13.82	489.753 ± 41.78	131.998 ± 12.020	178.406 ± 6.108
$AUC_{0–\infty}$ (μg.h/mL)	496.187 ± 39.28	759.934 ±167.91	341.538 ± 19.888	614.155 ± 169.148
MRT (h)	21.983 ± 4.19	21.949 ± 8.70	46.772 ± 6.694	69.418 ± 25.772
% Bioavailability Enhancement	153.15		179.82	

C_{max}: maximum plasma concentration, T_{max}: time to reach maximum plasma concentration, AUC: the area under the curve; MRT: mean residence time. Data represented as mean ± SD (n = 3).

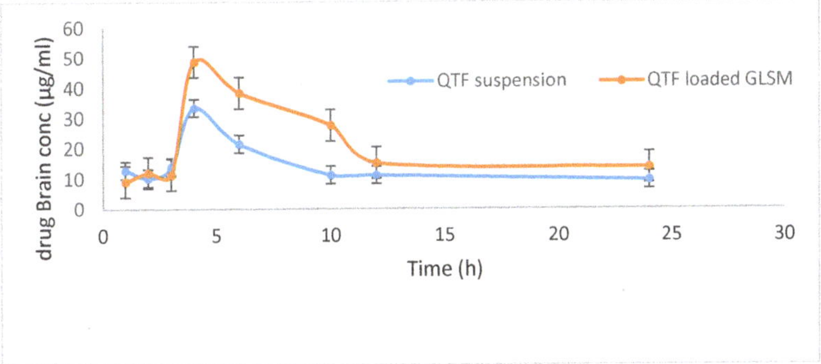

(A)

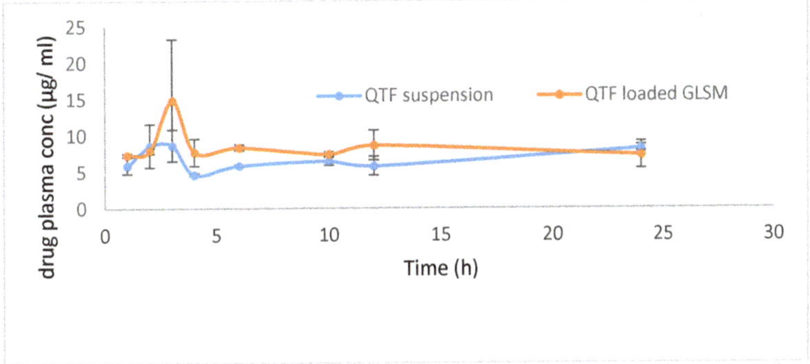

(B)

Figure 8. QTF mean brain concentration (**A**) and mean plasma concentration (**B**) after oral administration of QTF suspension, and QTF Loaded GLSMs.

3. Materials and Methods

3.1. Materials

Quetiapine fumarate (QTF) was gifted by the Al jazeera pharmaceuticals Co. Lecithin, cholesterol, and glycerol were purchased from Sigma-Aldrich (Saint Louis, MO, USA). Acetonitrile for HPLC $\geq$ 99.9% (Sigma-Aldrich®, Saint Louis, MO, USA). Methanol HPLC grade, Diethyl ether HPLC grade, and Chloroform HPLC grade were purchased from (Sigma-Aldrich®, Saint Louis, MO, USA). HPLC grade water was obtained from a Milli-Q ultrapure Water system. Orthophosphoric acid for HPLC 85–90% (Fluka®, Buchs, Switzerland). Sodium hydroxide pellets (Sigma-Aldrich®, Saint-Quentin-Fallavier, France). Nylon membrane filter type 0.45 µm HNWP was purchased from (Merck, Darmstadt, Germany).

3.2. Statistical Design of QTF Loaded GLSMs

This study was designed using a central composite rotatable design to address the effect of different variables of formulation on QTF-loaded GLSMs characteristics using Design Expert® software (Ver. 7, Stat-Ease, Minneapolis, MN, USA). The independent variables were glycerol concentration (X1) which ranged from 10 to 30 w/v% and cholesterol concentration (X2), which lay between 0.2 to 0.8 w/v%. This resulted in 9 experimental runs. QTF was kept constant in all formulations at a concentration of 1 w/v%. The dependent variables were vesicle size (VS) (Y1), ZP (Y2), and EE% (Y3). Table 7 shows the independent (low and high level) and dependent variables. Table 1 shows the composition of QTF-loaded GLSMs.

Table 7. Central Composite Design for optimization of QTF loaded GLSMs.

Independent Variables	Levels	
	Low	High
Glycerol concentration $w/v\%$ (X1)	10	30
Cholesterol concentration $w/v\%$ (X2)	0.2	0.8
Dependent values (Responses)	Desirability	
Vesicle size (Y1)	Minimize	
Zeta potential (Y2)	Maximize	
Entrapment efficiency (Y3)	Maximize	

3.3. Preparation of QTF Glycerosomal Formulations

GLSMs were prepared by thin film hydration technique [23] using lecithin as a lipid in a concentration of 5 ($\%w/v$) based on a pre-screening study. Lecithin, cholesterol, and 100 mg QTF were dissolved in 10 mL ethanol in a flask with a round bottom. A rotary evaporator (Buchi Rotavapor R-200, Allschwil, Switzerland) was used to evaporate the organic solvent under reduced pressure at a temperature of 40 °C and 90 rpm. Then, 10 mL phosphate buffer pH (7.4) containing different concentrations of glycerol was used to hydrate the film, followed by sonication for 10 min using an ultrasonicator (Model 3510; Branson Ultrasonics, Danbury, CT, USA).

3.4. Evaluation of QTF Glycerosomal Formulations

3.4.1. Measurement of Vesicles Size (VS), Polydispersity Index (PDI), and Zeta Potential (ZP)

Zetasizer Nano ZS instrument (Malvern Instruments, Worcestershire, UK)was used to measure the VS, PDI, and ZP of the prepared QTP-loaded GLSMs at 25 °C after appropriate dilution with distilled water [39,42,48]. The measurements were done in triplicate.

3.4.2. Measurement of Entrapment Efficiency (EE%)

The prepared glycerosomal formulations were centrifuged at 17,000 rpm for 1 h at 4 °C [48] by a cooling centrifuge (SIGMA 3–30 K, Sigma, Steinheim, Germany) to separate glycerosomal vesicles from the un-entrapped QTF. The concentration of QTF in the supernatant was determined after suitable dilutions using a UV spectrophotometer (Shimadzu UV-1800, Kyoto 604-8511, Japan) at the predetermined λ_{max} (254 nm). Validation of the method was done by calculating linearity within a range of concentration of 2.5 to 20 µg/mL (R^2 of 0.9994).

The EE% was calculated applying the equation [29,41,42].

$$\text{EE\%} = \frac{TD - FD}{TD} \times 100 \tag{4}$$

where EE% is the entrapment efficiency, *FD* and *TD* are the amounts of the free and total drugs, respectively.

The obtained nanoparticles in the bottom of the centrifuge tube were washed with phosphate buffer pH 7.4 and recentrifuged to remove the unentrapped drug. The washing of nanoparticles was repeated in triplicate to ensure the complete removal of the unentrapped drug. The purified nanoparticles were kept for further characterization.

3.5. Statistical Analysis, Optimization, and Validation

Factorial analysis of variance (ANOVA) was used to analyze the studied responses using Design Expert® software. A desirability function was used to select the optimum formula with the smallest VS and the highest ZP and EE%. For checking the validity of the used statistical models, The optimum formula was prepared and evaluated for VS, ZP, and

EE% and percentage relative errors were calculated between the obtained results and the predicted values using the following equation [34].

$$\% \text{ Relative error} = \frac{\text{predicted value} - \text{experimental value})}{\text{predicted value}} \times 100 \quad (5)$$

3.6. *Evaluation of the Optimum QTF Formula*

3.6.1. Differential Scanning Calorimetry (DSC)

DSC analysis was accomplished for pure QTF, a physical mixture of lecithin, cholesterol, and QTF, and the optimum formula using a differential scanning calorimeter (DSC N-650; Scinco, Liguria, Italy). Samples of about 5 mg were placed in the aluminum pan of the apparatus and subjected to heat at a rate of 10 °C/minute until 200 °C underflow of inert nitrogen.

3.6.2. X-ray Diffraction Study (XRD)

X-ray diffraction measurements of pure QTF and the optimum formula were performed using an Ultima IV Diffractometer (Rigaku Inc. Tokyo, Japan at College of Pharmacy, King Saud University, Riyadh, KSA). The XRD spectra were scanned in the range of 0–60° (2θ) at a rate of 10°/min speed.

3.6.3. Transmission Electron Microscopy (TEM)

A transmission electron microscope (TEM; JEOL JEM-1010, Tokyo, Japan) was used to visualize the morphology of the optimum formula as well as the dimensions of GLSMs. After diluting the samples suitably, they were put on a carbon-coated copper grid. Then, 2% *w/v* phosphotungstic acid was used to coat the samples. They were then kept in the air for 5 min to be dried. Then, a TEM operated under an acceleration voltage of 80 kV [49] and ×80,000 power of magnification was used to image the samples at room temperature. The measurement was repeated six times to calculate the average of GLSMs dimensions.

3.6.4. In-Vitro Release

The release of QTF from the optimum glycerosomal formula compared to drug suspension was studied by placing an amount of each formula equivalent to 5 mg QTF in the dialysis bags. Then it was suspended in a 250 mL dissolution medium (phosphate buffer pH (7.4)) [50] in the dissolution apparatus (Pharm Test, Hainburg, Germany) at a temperature of 37 °C with stirring at 100 rpm. The amount of QTF was quantified at different time points by withdrawing 5 mL from the dissolution media at 1, 2, 3, 4, 5, and 6 h and instantly replaced with an equal amount of fresh media. Then, the concentration of QTF in the collected samples was quantified using a UV spectrophotometer at 254 nm. The measurements were done three times, and the percent of QTP released at different time points was determined as follows [51]:

$$\text{Qn} = \frac{Cn \times Vr + \sum_{i=1}^{n-1} Ci \times Vs}{initial\ drug\ content} \quad (6)$$

where Qn: Percent of QTF released cumulatively

Cn: Concentration of QTP in the dissolution medium at the *n*th sample

Vr: Volume of dissolution medium

Vs: Volume of sample

$\sum_{i=1}^{n-1} Ci$: The summation of the concentrations measured previously

The release profile of the optimum QTF-loaded GLSMs in comparison to drug suspension was made by making a plot between the percentage of QTF released (Q_n) at different time points vs. corresponding time.

3.6.5. Effect of Aging

The stability of the optimum QTF-loaded GLSMs was assessed as a function of time regarding VS, ZP, and EE% after keeping the formulation in an air-tight vial, kept away from light at 4 °C for one month [52].

3.7. In-Vivo Bioavailability of the Optimized QTF Loaded GLSMs

3.7.1. Study Design

The study was done on male Wistar albino rats weighing 140 ± 20 g. They were kept in a temperature-controlled room (22 ± 2 °C) in cages of polypropylene. Standardized pellet feed and clean drinking water were supplied to them. The study was approved by the Institutional Animal Ethical Committee (IAEC) number 202010001 of CPCSEA (Committee for Control and Supervision of Experiments on Animals), Prince Sattam Bin Abdulaziz University. A total of 96 rats were used in the study. They were divided into two groups. The first group was for QTF aqueous suspension and the second group was for the optimum QTF-loaded GLSMs. All animals were fasted for 18 h before receiving any doses. Dosing animals orally is done by the method described by Kuentz [53]. For each group, six animals were kept as control and the rest of the animals received an oral dose equivalent to 20 mg/kg body weight of QTF suspension and optimum QTF-loaded GLSMs, respectively [54,55]. At different time intervals 1, 2, 3, 4, 6, 12, and 24 h following administration of both QTF suspension and optimum QTF loaded GLSMs, six animals were sacrificed from each group by being cervically decapitated, followed by the collection of blood in commercially available anti-coagulant treated tubes for plasma separation. The tubes containing spray-dried Heparin/EDTA anticoagulants are used to separate plasma from the blood. The tube was centrifuged at 2000× *g* for 10 min. Ref. [56] a refrigerated centrifuge was used to separate cells from the plasma by centrifugation for 10 min at 1000–2000× *g*. After that, plasma was immediately conveyed using a Pasteur pipette into polypropylene. While handling the samples, they should be kept at 2–8 °C. Plasma was divided into 0.5 mL aliquots and stored at −20 °C or lower for further use [56]. While the brain was instantly dissected out and washed with cold saline and known amounts of tissues were homogenized at 5000 rpm with appropriate ice-cold buffer in a Teflon homogenizer for 10 min. The plasma and homogenized brain samples were subjected to HPLC evaluation for absorbed quetiapine.

3.7.2. HPLC Assay of QTF in Plasma and Brain

To prepare the serum samples for HPLC analysis, 10 µg/mL of lamotrigine (internal standard) and 0.1 mL of NaOH (0.1 M) were added to 100 µL of serum, and the Valcon tubes were shaken for 1 min as the first step. For the second step, 5 mL of diethyl ether was added and vortexed for 5 min and mixed for 5 min, and the mixtures were then centrifuged at 3000 rpm for 6 min at room temperature. For the third step, 4 mL was carefully suctioned from the upper layer of ether; then, the remaining mixture was extracted once again using 5 mL of diethyl ether. For the fourth step, 4 mL was carefully suctioned from the upper layer of ether and then added together with the previous extract; the evaporation step was done at room temperature. Finally, the reconstitution of the residue with 100 µL of methanol was done then reconstituted samples were injected into the HPLC system [10].

For brain samples, about 1 mL of phosphate buffer (pH 3) was added to the brain homogenate, followed by vortexing. After that, 1 mL of 60% chloroform and 40% of methanol mixture was added to homogenate and mixed for 1 min, then centrifugation at 5000 rpm for 10 min at 4 °C. After that, the organic layer was separated into a tube, then the drug was extracted once again, and the extract was added to the previous one, followed by evaporation under vacuum. Finally, the residue was resuspended in 2 mL HPLC grade of 80% acetonitrile and 20% methanol mixture and then reconstituted samples were injected into the HPLC system [57].

For quantitative estimation of Quetiapine Fumarate in serum and brain samples, a Shimadzu HPLC system (SHIMADZU 1200 series HPLC system (Kyoto, Japan) equipped with a quaternary pump, online degasser, an autosampler (SHIMADZU1200, Kyoto, Japan) (model 20A), and separation in the final method was achieved on a Thermosil® C-18 column (250 mm × 4.6 mm i.d., 5 μm particle size) column (Thermo, USA). The operating temperature of the oven column was fixed at 30 °C. The system was equipped with SPD-20A/20AV UV-Vis detectors set at 254 nm. Isocratic elution was utilized with a mobile phase of 0.02 M of phosphate buffer (pH 5.5) mixed with acetonitrile in a ratio of 35:65. Finally, the 0.45 μm membrane filters were used to filter the mobile phase, then degassed by sonication for 15 min, prior to its use. The injection volume was 20 μL, and the flow rate was 1 mL/min with a total run time of 15 min. The liquid chromatography instrument was interfaced with a computer running LabSolutions software using Microsoft Windows 7. The concentrations of QTF in rat serum and brain samples were compared against a standard of QTF in the mobile phase [58].

3.7.3. Pharmacokinetic Analysis

A plot of the mean QTF plasma concentrations and brain concentrations was made against time. Both plasma and brain Pharmacokinetic parameters were calculated using WinNonlin software (version 1.5, Scientific Consulting, Inc., Rockville, MD, USA). Pharmacokinetic parameters include the peak plasma and brain concentrations (C_{max}) in addition to the time to reach these peaks (T_{max}). Additionally, the area under the curve till the last time (AUC_{0-24}) and till infinity ($AUC_{0-\infty}$) were determined using the trapezoidal rule. Moreover, the mean residence time (MRT) and the elimination half-life ($T_{1/2}$) were calculated. Results were expressed as mean values ± standard deviations. Then, ANOVA was used to analyze the obtained pharmacokinetic parameters to test the significant differences between both QTF suspension and optimum QTF-loaded GLSMs.

4. Conclusions

Glycerosomes (GLSMs) are a new generation of liposomes containing a high concentration of glycerol (10–30 *w*/*v*%). GLSMs have advantages over liposomes in being more stable and having greater fluidity than liposomes due to the presence of glycerol in high percent. This increased fluidity makes GLSMs more penetrable into the brain tissue than liposomes. GLSMs were prepared and subjected to an optimization process using a Face centered rotatable design on selecting the formula having the smallest vesicle size, the largest zeta potential, and entrapment efficiency. The optimum formula, which was composed of 29.645 *w*/*v*% glycerol, 0.8% cholesterol, and 5% lecithin, showed a vesicle size of 290.4 nm, a zeta potential of −34.58, and entrapment efficiency of 80.85%. It was also revealed that spherical vesicles by TEM with no aggregates indicated high stable systems that are confirmed by the stability study. Additionally, the optimum formula showed enhanced drug release when compared to a drug suspension. Moreover, it was subjected to a pharmacokinetic study where it showed enhanced brain and plasma bioavailability of QTF when compared to the drug suspension. Therefore, it could be concluded that QTF-loaded GLSMs are a promising new nanocarrier for the oral delivery of QTF.

Author Contributions: Conceptualization, R.M.Z., A.S.A. and R.M.Y.; data curation, R.M.Z., L.A.E., A.S.A., R.M.Y. and M.S.; formal analysis, R.M.Z., M.A.A., L.A.E. and M.S.; funding acquisition, M.M.A. and R.M.Y.; investigation, M.M.A., V.D.S. and M.S.; methodology, R.M.Z., M.A.A., L.A.E. and V.D.S.; project administration, M.M.A., M.A.A., L.A.E., R.M.Y. and M.S.; resources, M.M.A., M.A.A., V.D.S., R.M.Y. and M.S.; software, R.M.Z.; supervision, R.M.Z., M.M.A. and V.D.S.; validation, M.A.A.; visualization, M.A.A. and A.S.A.; writing—original draft, M.S.; writing—review and editing, R.M.Z., V.D.S., A.S.A. and R.M.Y. All authors have read and agreed to the published version of the manuscript.

Funding: This research received no external funding.

Institutional Review Board Statement: The study was conducted according to the guidelines of the Declaration of Helsinki and approved by the Institutional Animal Ethical Committee (IAEC) number 202010001 of CPCSEA (Committee for Control and Supervision of Experiments on Animals), Prince Sattam Bin Abdulaziz University, approved on 20 January 2022.

Informed Consent Statement: Not applicable.

Data Availability Statement: The data is contained in the manuscript.

Acknowledgments: The authors extend their appreciation to the Deanship of Scientific Research, Prince Sattam Bin Abdulaziz University, Al-Kharj, Saudi Arabia.

Conflicts of Interest: The authors declare no conflict of interest.

References

1. Bülbül, E.Ö.; Mesut, B.; Cevher, E.; Öztaş, E.; Özsoy, Y. Product transfer from lab-scale to pilot-scale of quetiapine fumarate orodispersible films using quality by design approach. *J. Drug Deliv. Sci. Technol.* **2019**, *54*, 101358. [CrossRef]
2. Boche, M.; Pokharkar, V. Quetiapine nanoemulsion for intranasal drug delivery: Evaluation of brain-targeting efficiency. *AAPS PharmSciTech* **2017**, *18*, 686–696. [CrossRef]
3. Thompson, W.; Quay, T.A.; Rojas-Fernandez, C.; Farrell, B.; Bjerre, L.M. Atypical antipsychotics for insomnia: A systematic review. *Sleep Med.* **2016**, *22*, 13–17. [CrossRef]
4. Patel, N.; Baldaniya, M.; Raval, M.; Sheth, N. Formulation and development of in situ nasal gelling systems for quetiapine fumarate-loaded mucoadhesive microemulsion. *J. Pharm. Innov.* **2015**, *10*, 357–373. [CrossRef]
5. Karki, S.; Kim, H.; Na, S.-J.; Shin, D.; Jo, K.; Lee, J. Thin films as an emerging platform for drug delivery. *Asian J. Pharm. Sci.* **2016**, *11*, 559–574. [CrossRef]
6. Estevez-Carrizo, F.E.; Parrillo, S.; Ercoli, M.C.; Estevez-Parrillo, F.T. Single-dose relative bioavailability of a new quetiapine fumarate extended-release formulation: A postprandial, randomized, open-label, two-period crossover study in healthy Uruguayan volunteers. *Clin. Ther.* **2011**, *33*, 738–745. [CrossRef] [PubMed]
7. Hsiao, C.-C.; Chen, K.-P.; Tsai, C.-J.; Wang, L.-J.; Chen, C.-K.; Lin, S.-K. Rapid initiation of quetiapine well tolerated as compared with the conventional initiation regimen in patients with schizophrenia or schizoaffective disorders. *Kaohsiung J. Med. Sci.* **2011**, *27*, 508–513. [CrossRef] [PubMed]
8. Baig, M.R.; Wilson, J.L.; Lemmer, J.A.; Beck, R.D.; Peterson, A.L.; Roache, J.D. Enhancing completion of cognitive processing therapy for posttraumatic stress disorder with quetiapine in veterans with mild traumatic brain injury: A case series. *Psychiatr. Q.* **2019**, *90*, 431–445. [CrossRef] [PubMed]
9. Maan, J.S.; Ershadi, M.; Khan, I.; Saadabadi, A. *Quetiapine*; StatPearls Publishing: Tampa, FL, USA, 2021.
10. Narala, A.; Veerabrahma, K. Preparation, characterization and evaluation of quetiapine fumarate solid lipid nanoparticles to improve the oral bioavailability. *J. Pharm.* **2013**, *2013*, 265741. [CrossRef]
11. Khunt, D.; Shah, B.; Misra, M. Role of butter oil in brain targeted delivery of Quetiapine fumarate microemulsion via intranasal route. *J. Drug Deliv. Sci. Technol.* **2017**, *40*, 11–20. [CrossRef]
12. Shah, B.; Khunt, D.; Misra, M.; Padh, H. Application of Box-Behnken design for optimization and development of quetiapine fumarate loaded chitosan nanoparticles for brain delivery via intranasal route*. *Int. J. Biol. Macromol.* **2016**, *89*, 206–218. [CrossRef] [PubMed]
13. Shah, B.; Khunt, D.; Misra, M. Comparative evaluation of intranasally delivered quetiapine loaded mucoadhesive microemulsion and polymeric nanoparticles for brain targeting: Pharmacokinetic and gamma scintigraphy studies. *Future J. Pharm. Sci.* **2021**, *7*, 1–12. [CrossRef]
14. Ben Hadj Ayed, O.; Lassoued, M.A.; Sfar, S. Quality-by-Design Approach Development, Characterization, and In Vitro Release Mechanism Elucidation of Nanostructured Lipid Carriers for Quetiapine Fumarate Oral Delivery. *J. Pharm. Innov.* **2021**, 1–16. [CrossRef]
15. Lawless, E.; Griffin, B.T.; O'Mahony, A.; O'Driscoll, C.M. Exploring the impact of drug properties on the extent of intestinal lymphatic transport-in vitro and in vivo studies. *Pharm. Res.* **2015**, *32*, 1817–1829. [CrossRef]
16. Chaturvedi, S.; Garg, A.; Verma, A. Nano lipid based carriers for lymphatic voyage of anti-cancer drugs: An insight into the in-vitro, ex-vivo, in-situ and in-vivo study models. *J. Drug Deliv. Sci. Technol.* **2020**, *59*, 101899. [CrossRef]
17. Poonia, N.; Kharb, R.; Lather, V.; Pandita, D. Nanostructured lipid carriers: Versatile oral delivery vehicle. *Future Sci. OA* **2016**, *2*, FSO135. [CrossRef]
18. Pandya, P.; Giram, P.; Bhole, R.P.; Chang, H.-I.; Raut, S.Y. Nanocarriers based oral lymphatic drug targeting: Strategic bioavailability enhancement approaches. *J. Drug Deliv. Sci. Technol.* **2021**, *64*, 102585. [CrossRef]
19. Agrahari, V. The exciting potential of nanotherapy in brain-tumor targeted drug delivery approaches. *Neural Regen. Res.* **2017**, *12*, 197. [CrossRef]
20. Chopra, H.; Dey, P.S.; Das, D.; Bhattacharya, T.; Shah, M.; Mubin, S.; Maishu, S.P.; Akter, R.; Rahman, M.H.; Karthika, C. Curcumin nanoparticles as promising therapeutic agents for drug targets. *Molecules* **2021**, *26*, 4998. [CrossRef]

21. Herdiana, Y.; Wathoni, N.; Shamsuddin, S.; Muchtaridi, M. Drug release study of the chitosan-based nanoparticles. *Heliyon* **2021**, *8*, e08674. [CrossRef]
22. Zorkina, Y.; Abramova, O.; Ushakova, V.; Morozova, A.; Zubkov, E.; Valikhov, M.; Melnikov, P.; Majouga, A.; Chekhonin, V. Nano carrier drug delivery systems for the treatment of neuropsychiatric disorders: Advantages and limitations. *Molecules* **2020**, *25*, 5294. [CrossRef] [PubMed]
23. Manca, M.L.; Zaru, M.; Manconi, M.; Lai, F.; Valenti, D.; Sinico, C.; Fadda, A.M. Glycerosomes: A new tool for effective dermal and transdermal drug delivery. *Int. J. Pharm.* **2013**, *455*, 66–74. [CrossRef] [PubMed]
24. Zaru, M.; Manca, M.L.; Fadda, A.M.; Orsini, G. Glycerosomes and Use Thereof in Pharmaceutical and Cosmetic Preparations for Topical Applications. U.S. Patent No. 8,778,367, 15 July 2014.
25. Gupta, P.; Mazumder, R.; Padhi, S. Glycerosomes: Advanced liposomal drug delivery system. *Indian J. Pharm. Sci.* **2020**, *82*, 385–397. [CrossRef]
26. Salem, H.F.; Kharshoum, R.M.; Sayed, O.M.; Abdel Hakim, L.F. Formulation design and optimization of novel soft glycerosomes for enhanced topical delivery of celecoxib and cupferron by Box–Behnken statistical design. *Drug Dev. Ind. Pharm.* **2018**, *44*, 1871–1884. [CrossRef]
27. Bshara, H.; Osman, R.; Mansour, S.; El-Shamy, A.E.-H.A. Chitosan and cyclodextrin in intranasal microemulsion for improved brain buspirone hydrochloride pharmacokinetics in rats. *Carbohydr. Polym.* **2014**, *99*, 297–305. [CrossRef]
28. Abourehab, M.A.; Khames, A.; Genedy, S.; Mostafa, S.; Khaleel, M.A.; Omar, M.M.; El Sisi, A.M. Sesame oil-based nanostructured lipid carriers of nicergoline, intranasal delivery system for brain targeting of synergistic cerebrovascular protection. *Pharmaceutics* **2021**, *13*, 581. [CrossRef]
29. Said, M.; Aboelwafa, A.A.; Elshafeey, A.H.; Elsayed, I. Central composite optimization of ocular mucoadhesive cubosomes for enhanced bioavailability and controlled delivery of voriconazole. *J. Drug Deliv. Sci. Technol.* **2021**, *61*, 102075. [CrossRef]
30. Essa, E.A. Effect of formulation and processing variables on the particle size of sorbitan monopalmitate niosomes. *Asian J. Pharm. AJP* **2014**, *4*, 227–233. [CrossRef]
31. Salem, H.F.; Nafady, M.M.; Ali, A.A.; Khalil, N.M.; Elsisi, A.A. Evaluation of Metformin Hydrochloride Tailoring Bilosomes as an Effective Transdermal Nanocarrier. *Int. J. Nanomed.* **2022**, *17*, 1185. [CrossRef]
32. Vitonyte, J.; Manca, M.L.; Caddeo, C.; Valenti, D.; Peris, J.E.; Usach, I.; Nacher, A.; Matos, M.; Gutiérrez, G.; Orrù, G. Bifunctional viscous nanovesicles co-loaded with resveratrol and gallic acid for skin protection against microbial and oxidative injuries. *Eur. J. Pharm. Biopharm.* **2017**, *114*, 278–287. [CrossRef]
33. Md, S.; Alhakamy, N.A.; Aldawsari, H.M.; Husain, M.; Khan, N.; Alfaleh, M.A.; Asfour, H.Z.; Riadi, Y.; Bilgrami, A.L.; Akhter, M.H. Plumbagin-Loaded Glycerosome Gel as Topical Delivery System for Skin Cancer Therapy. *Polymers* **2021**, *13*, 923. [CrossRef] [PubMed]
34. Mazyed, E.A.; Abdelaziz, A.E. Fabrication of transgelosomes for enhancing the ocular delivery of acetazolamide: Statistical optimization, in vitro characterization, and in vivo study. *Pharmaceutics* **2020**, *12*, 465. [CrossRef] [PubMed]
35. Vadlamudi, H.C.; Yalavarthi, P.R.; Nagaswaram, T.; Rasheed, A.; Peesa, J.P. In-vitro and pharmacodynamic characterization of solidified self microemulsified system of quetiapine fumarate. *J. Pharm. Investig.* **2019**, *49*, 161–172. [CrossRef]
36. Westesen, K.; Bunjes, H.; Koch, M. Physicochemical characterization of lipid nanoparticles and evaluation of their drug loading capacity and sustained release potential. *J. Control. Release* **1997**, *48*, 223–236. [CrossRef]
37. Narendar, D.; Arjun, N.; Someshwar, K.; Rao, Y.M. Quality by design approach for development and optimization of Quetiapine Fumarate effervescent floating matrix tablets for improved oral bioavailability. *J. Pharm. Investig.* **2016**, *46*, 253–263. [CrossRef]
38. Sun, X.; Yu, Z.; Cai, Z.; Yu, L.; Lv, Y. Voriconazole composited polyvinyl alcohol/hydroxypropyl-β-cyclodextrin nanofibers for ophthalmic delivery. *PLoS ONE* **2016**, *11*, e0167961. [CrossRef]
39. Zaki, R.M.; Alfadhel, M.M.; Alshahrani, S.M.; Alsaqr, A.; Al-Kharashi, L.A.; Anwer, M.K. Formulation of Chitosan-Coated Brigatinib Nanospanlastics: Optimization, Characterization, Stability Assessment and In-Vitro Cytotoxicity Activity against H-1975 Cell Lines. *Pharmaceuticals* **2022**, *15*, 348. [CrossRef]
40. Dehghani, F.; Farhadian, N.; Golmohammadzadeh, S.; Biriaee, A.; Ebrahimi, M.; Karimi, M. Preparation, characterization and in-vivo evaluation of microemulsions containing tamoxifen citrate anti-cancer drug. *Eur. J. Pharm. Sci.* **2017**, *96*, 479–489. [CrossRef]
41. Said, M.; Elsayed, I.; Aboelwafa, A.A.; Elshafeey, A.H. Transdermal agomelatine microemulsion gel: Pyramidal screening, statistical optimization and in vivo bioavailability. *Drug Deliv.* **2017**, *24*, 1159–1169. [CrossRef]
42. Said, M.; Elsayed, I.; Aboelwafa, A.A.; Elshafeey, A.H. A novel concept of overcoming the skin barrier using augmented liquid nanocrystals: Box-Behnken optimization, ex vivo and in vivo evaluation. *Colloids Surf. B Biointerfaces* **2018**, *170*, 258–265. [CrossRef]
43. Li, J.; Wang, X.; Zhang, T.; Wang, C.; Huang, Z.; Luo, X.; Deng, Y. A review on phospholipids and their main applications in drug delivery systems. *Asian J. Pharm. Sci.* **2015**, *10*, 81–98. [CrossRef]
44. Salem, H.F.; Kharshoum, R.M.; Abdel Hakim, L.F.; Abdelrahim, M.E. Edge activators and a polycationic polymer enhance the formulation of porous voriconazole nanoagglomerate for the use as a dry powder inhaler. *J. Liposome Res.* **2016**, *26*, 324–335. [CrossRef]
45. Ahn, H.; Park, J.-H. Liposomal delivery systems for intestinal lymphatic drug transport. *Biomater. Res.* **2016**, *20*, 1–6. [CrossRef]

46. Vishwakarma, N.; Jain, A.; Sharma, R.; Mody, N.; Vyas, S.; Vyas, S.P. Lipid-based nanocarriers for lymphatic transportation. *AAPS PharmSciTech* **2019**, *20*, 1–13. [CrossRef]
47. Goel, S.; Ojha, N.K. Ashtang Ghrita: A noble Ayurveda drug for central nervous system. *J. Ayurveda Holist. Med. (JAHM)* **2015**, *3*, 18–24.
48. Zaki, R.M.; Ibrahim, M.A.; Alshora, D.H.; El Ela, A.E.S.A. Formulation and Evaluation of Transdermal Gel Containing Tacrolimus-Loaded Spanlastics: In Vitro, Ex Vivo and In Vivo Studies. *Polymers* **2022**, *14*, 1528. [CrossRef] [PubMed]
49. Salem, H.F.; Kharshoum, R.M.; Abou-Taleb, H.A.; Farouk, H.O.; Zaki, R.M. Fabrication and appraisal of simvastatin via tailored niosomal nanovesicles for transdermal delivery enhancement: In vitro and in vivo assessment. *Pharmaceutics* **2021**, *13*, 138. [CrossRef]
50. Hosseinzadeh, H.; Atyabi, F.; Dinarvand, R.; Ostad, S.N. Chitosan–Pluronic nanoparticles as oral delivery of anticancer gemcitabine: Preparation and in vitro study. *Int. J. Nanomed.* **2012**, *7*, 1851.
51. Habib, B.A.; Sayed, S.; Elsayed, G.M. Enhanced transdermal delivery of ondansetron using nanovesicular systems: Fabrication, characterization, optimization and ex-vivo permeation study-Box-Cox transformation practical example. *Eur. J. Pharm. Sci.* **2018**, *115*, 352–361. [CrossRef]
52. De Sá, F.A.P.; Taveira, S.F.; Gelfuso, G.M.; Lima, E.M.; Gratieri, T. Liposomal voriconazole (VOR) formulation for improved ocular delivery. *Colloids Surf. B Biointerfaces* **2015**, *133*, 331–338. [CrossRef]
53. Kuentz, M. Lipid-based formulations for oral delivery of lipophilic drugs. *Drug Discov. Today Technol.* **2012**, *9*, e97–e104. [CrossRef]
54. Ezzeldin, E.; Asiri, Y.A.; Iqbal, M. Effects of green tea extracts on the pharmacokinetics of quetiapine in rats. *Evid.-Based Complementary Altern. Med.* **2015**, *2015*, 615285. [CrossRef]
55. Gao, J.; Feng, M.; Swalve, N.; Davis, C.; Sui, N.; Li, M. Effects of repeated quetiapine treatment on conditioned avoidance responding in rats. *Eur. J. Pharmacol.* **2015**, *769*, 154–161. [CrossRef] [PubMed]
56. Thavasu, P.; Longhurst, S.; Joel, S.; Slevin, M.; Balkwill, F. Measuring cytokine levels in blood. Importance of anticoagulants, processing, and storage conditions. *J. Immunol. Methods* **1992**, *153*, 115–124. [CrossRef]
57. Upadhyay, P.; Trivedi, J.; Pundarikakshudu, K.; Sheth, N. Direct and enhanced delivery of nanoliposomes of anti schizophrenic agent to the brain through nasal route. *Saudi Pharm. J.* **2017**, *25*, 346–358. [CrossRef] [PubMed]
58. Belal, F.; Elbrashy, A.; Eid, M.; Nasr, J.J. Stability—Indicating HPLC method for the determination of quetiapine: Application to tablets and human plasma. *J. Liq. Chromatogr. Relat. Technol.* **2008**, *31*, 1283–1298. [CrossRef]